SECTION OUTLINE

The following is a list of the four major sections of the *Handbook of Biochemistry and Molecular Biology;* each consisting of one or more volumes.

SECTION A: PROTEINS

Volume I: Nomenclature, Amino Acids, Peptides and Polypeptides
Volume II: Nomenclature, Proteins
Volume III: Proteins

SECTION B: NUCLEIC ACIDS

Volume I: Nomenclature, Purines, Pyrimidines, Nucleotides, and Oligonucleotides, Nucleic Acids and Polynucleotides
Volume II: Nomenclature, Nucleic Acids, Enzymes Involved with Nucleic Acid Function, Genetics and Biology

SECTION C: LIPIDS, CARBOHYDRATES, STEROIDS

Volume I: Nomenclature, Lipids, Carbohydrates, Steroids

SECTION D: PHYSICAL AND CHEMICAL DATA

Volume I: Nomenclature, Physical and Chemical Data
Volume II: Nomenclature, Chromatography and Gel Filtration, Absorption Data, Fluorescence Bond Angles and Distances

All CRC Handbook volumes listed above are currently in print and available from CRC Press, Inc. 18901 Cranwood Parkway, Cleveland, Ohio 44128.

Cumulative Series Index for CRC Handbook of Biochemistry and Molecular Biology

3rd Edition

EDITOR

Gerald D. Fasman, Ph. D.

Rosenfield Professor of Biochemistry
Graduate Department of Biochemistry
Brandeis University
Waltham, Massachusetts

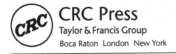

CRC Press
Taylor & Francis Group
Boca Raton London New York

CRC Press is an imprint of the
Taylor & Francis Group, an **informa** business

CRC Press
Taylor & Francis Group
6000 Broken Sound Parkway NW, Suite 300
Boca Raton, FL 33487-2742

Reissued 2019 by CRC Press

A Library of Congress record exists under LC control number:

Publisher's Note
The publisher has gone to great lengths to ensure the quality of this reprint but points out that some imperfections in the original copies may be apparent.

Disclaimer
The publisher has made every effort to trace copyright holders and welcomes correspondence from those they have been unable to contact.

ISBN 13: 978-0-367-26090-3 (hbk)
ISBN 13: 978-0-429-29142-5 (ebk)
ISBN 13: 978-0-367-26091-0 (pbk)

Visit the Taylor & Francis Web site at http://www.taylorandfrancis.com and the
CRC Press Web site at http://www.crcpress.com

PUBLISHER'S PREFACE

This volume which carries the designation "Cumulative Series Index," is the master key to the first eight volumes of the *CRC Handbook of Biochemistry and Molecular Biology*. It represents a reasonably effective solution of an inherent problem in the reference information field.

The problem itself is so deceptively simple that its statement seems almost a truism: a specific bit of objective data — commonly termed a "fact" — is useful information **only** when and if it is accessible. The greater the number of facts, the greater the difficulty of accessibility. Today, the total sum of human knowledge includes an almost infinite number of facts, and the number continues to expand with each moment of human experience.

The only feasible method of coping with a quantitative problem of this magnitude is to create an organizational structure which identifies and then classifies the individual facts according to logical or meaningful divisions, subdivisions, and sub-subdivisions, etc. In utilizing this method, we collect a large number of facts which are, in some manner, related to each other or related to some common subject, and make these facts available in book format. To further enhance the convenience of the process, the book is divided into sections usually called chapters; the chapters into paragraphs; and the paragraphs into sentences. Finally, for the rapid location of a specific fact within this structure, we provide an index which is a list of facts organized by alphabetical sequence.

In the reference information field, which may be appropriately defined as the collection, storage, and distribution of facts, the volume index has proven to be a practical and effective device to provide convenient accessibility to the fact content within the volume.

However, the publication of multivolume series, particularly in science and medicine, has created a new dimension to the problem of accessibility. Each volume within the series may contain facts which are relevant to a subject which appears in more than one volume. This, in turn, necessitates checking the index of each volume; but the larger the series, the greater the inconvenience of checking the index of each volume.

The obvious solution is to alphabetically merge all individual volume indexes into a single series index. As is often the case, a good idea is simple in concept but the implementation is difficult and complicated. In the production of this Series Index volume, it was necessary to establish viable principles for the merging of "three-tier" indexes; develop a coding system and computer program which would perform the actual task of merging; and finally to invest an enormous amount of dedicated and diligent man-hours to review and proofread the computer output to assure an acceptable level of quality and accuracy.

We are fully aware that this volume, which is the first Cumulative Series Index for the *CRC Handbook of Biochemistry and Molecular Biology*, will not meet our objectives in all respects. Hopefully, as we continue to acquire know-how in this specialized and rather sophisticated endeavor, assisted by comments and recommendations from users, future cumulative indexes will improve in quality and content. We are confident, however, that this volume is of great significance not only because it is a first effort, but even more, because it provides the world scientific community with convenient access to a large data base in the field of biochemistry and molecular biology.

B. J. Starkoff
President

INSTRUCTIONS FOR USE

PART I: SUBJECT ENTRIES

Part I is a straightforward merging of the indexes of all eight volumes of the Series. In the sample tiered entry that follows, the volume number is in bold-face type; it is followed by a colon and the page number in regular type:

Azurin
    amino acid composition, complete data, **07**: 505
    amino acid sequence, **07**: 498
    average hydrophobicity value, **01**: 215
    circular dichroism in near-UV region, at room tempera-
      ture, **07**: 144
    cyanogen bromide cleavage, **02**: 199
    luminescence of, table, **01**: 205
    molar absorptivity and-or absorbance values, **02**: 399
    molecular weights, stoichiometry and sources, **02**: 282

With the exception of certain eccentricities that occur in the merging of "three-tier" entries, this section contains no particular difficulties for the user.

PART II: CHEMICAL SUBSTANCES ENTRIES

Part II of this cumulative index does require some special "getting-used-to" by the user in order that he may take advantage of the vast amount of information provided by the computer. New sections have been created that were not in the previous indexes. In the sample tiered entry that follows, the center dot (•) indicates where the primary word *originally occurred* in the subject index entry:

Receptor
    acetylcholine •
      average hydrophobicity value, **01**: 210
    acetylcholine • protein
      circular dichroism in the UV region, **07**: 82
    lipopolysaccharides •
      circular dichroism in the UV region, **07**: 109

In other words, a new *section* of information ("Receptors") has been created by computer analyses of the original subject entries of the eight volumes. The word "receptor" did *not* occur as a primary entry in any of the previous books. Similarly, existing sections of the subject index have been expanded by this computer search of the data base.

It is clear that some problems will have arisen in the creation of this new information bank.

1. **Singular and Plural Entries**: Because the original indexes often included a term in both the singular and the plural forms, the Cumulative Series Index may have *two* separate blocks of entries about that term (for example, "Amino acid" and "Amino acids"). Please check both singular and plural forms of any chemical substance.
2. *See* **and** *See also* **Cross-references**: It is obvious that a merged index of many books may need extra cross-references that were not required in the separate volumes themselves. For this reason, *See* and *See also* cross-references have been added, but the user is encouraged to exercise his ingenuity in searching for all possible cross-references.

3. **Alphabetical Order of Entries:** The use of the computer to create this section has caused certain peculiarities in the interfiling of merged entries from the eight volumes. Specifically, two problems must be understood by the user of this index.

  a. **Compound Word Entries:** The computer has delineated three discreet sections for each compound entry — terms with a compound as a double word having a *hyphen* between the words, terms with a compound as a double word having a *space* between the words, and terms with a compound as a *merged* double word. An example of this follows:

N-Acetyl-DL-β-phenylalanine
  methyl ester
    UV spectra of, **01:** 193
N-Acetyl-DL-tryptophan
  methyl ester UV spectra, **01:** 192
  tryptophan; • methyl ester, UV spectra of, **01:** 192
N-Acetyl-L-tyrosine
  ethyl ester, UV spectra, **01:** 194
  ethyl ester anion, UV spectra, **01:** 195
} double word with hypen

Acetyl CoA synthetase
  Neurospora crassa mutant, **04:** 744
Acetyl hexosamine
  content of, in glyco-proteins, **02:** 258-274
  molar extinctions; • of aromatic amino acids,
    cystine and N-acetylcysteine, **01:** 186
N-acetyl methyl esters
  amino acids; UV absorption characteristics, • of
    aromatic types, cystine and N-acetylcysteine,
    01: 186
Acetyl ornithine transferase
  Neurospora crassa mutant, **04:** 745
} double word with space

N-Acetylalanine
  physical and chemical properties, **01:** 148
β-2-Acetylamino-2-deoxy-D-glucoside acetylamino-
    deoxyglucohydrolase
  enzymatic reactions, velocity and parameters, table, **05:**
    430-433
N-Acetylarginine
  physical and chemical properties, **01:** 132
} merged double word

Because of this computer "peculiarity" the user will have to check compound terms in all three sections, especially when looking for compounds in such major groups as "Acetyl," "Keto," "Methyl," and "Poly."

  b. **Chemical Prefixes:** Because the computer is programmed to ignore chemical prefixes in italics, it does not always ignore other prefixes and so may alphabetize terms under such prefixes as "30S" while ignoring such descriptive prefixes as "*c*" in a term like "*c*-reactive." The sample below shows this problem:

Protein *(continued)*
    quaternary structure of a molecule, definition, **02:** 77
    quaternary structure of molecule, definition, **01:** 73

incorrect filing under "R" ⟶ R17 coat-
    amino acid composition, complete data, **07:** 510

correct filing under "reactive" ⟶ c-reactive •
    molar absorptivity and-or absorbance values, **02:** 409
    subunit, constitution of, **02:** 337
    red-
    amino acid composition, complete data, **07:** 510

relaxing •
  molar absorptivity and-or absorbance values, **02:** 505
retinol-binding •
  average hydrophobicity value, **01:** 230
  circular dichroism
    UV and near UV region, **07:** 121, 160
  human, amino acid composition, **02:** 303
  molar absorptivity and-or absorbance values, **02:** 505
  optical rotatory dispersion in the UV region, **07:** 121
  properties of, **02:** 304
riboflavin-binding •
  average hydrophobicity value, **01:** 231
RNA, *see* Nucleic acids, Transfer RNA, TRNA
  (TRNA); • (wt %) in ribosomes from various
  sources, **04:** 472
RNA, *see* Nucleic acids, Transfer RNA, TRNA
  (TRNA); viral; code word table for the coat • gene,
  04: 340
30S ribosomal •
  amino acid composition, incomplete data, **07:** 514
  spectrophotometric determination, • concentration,
    short-wavelength UV, **08:** 197
sulfate-binding •
  amino acid composition, complete data, **07:** 510

incorrect filing under "S" ⟶ 30S ribosomal •

One major section in this index, "TRNA" (filed under "T"), was caused by such a computer eccentricity. The user will have to check compounds both *with* and *without* prefixes to find out if the term he is looking for is present in a "peculiar" place.

These are the only major problems associated with this index. Certain minor problems exist; however, they *are* minor and should pose no real difficulty for the user. The publisher welcomes any suggestions or corrections.

TABLE OF CONTENTS

Subject Entries 1

Chemical Substances Entries 120

Errata and Addenda 293

CRC Handbook Titles and Assigned Code Numbers

CODE NUMBER	TITLE
01	CRC Handbook of Biochemistry and Molecular Biology, 3rd Ed., Sect. A: Proteins, Vol. I
02	CRC Handbook of Biochemistry and Molecular Biology, 3rd Ed., Sect. A: Proteins, Vol. II
03	CRC Handbook of Biochemistry and Molecular Biology, 3rd Ed., Sect. B: Nucleic Acids, Vol. I
04	CRC Handbook of Biochemistry and Molecular Biology, 3rd Ed., Sect. B: Nucleic Acids, Vol. II
05	CRC Handbook of Biochemistry and Molecular Biology, 3rd Ed., Sect. C; Lipids, Carbohydrates, Steroids
06	CRC Handbook of Biochemistry and Molecular Biology, 3rd Ed., Sect. D: Physical and Chemical Data, Vol. I
07	CRC Handbook of Biochemistry and Molecular Biology, 3rd Ed., Sect. A: Proteins, Vol. III
08	CRC Handbook of Biochemistry and Molecular Biology, 3rd Ed., Sect. D: Physical and Chemical Data, Vol. II

Part I: Subject Entries

A

Abbreviations
  amino acid derivatives, journal reference to rules, 02: 87
  amino acids, table of, 01: 78, 02: 62
  chemical names, journal reference to rules, 02: 87
  corrinoid derivatives and vitamin B_{12}, 08: 16-17
  distinguished from symbols, 01: 6, 02: 6, 04: 6, 05: 6-9, 06: 6, 08: 6
  immunoglobulin, 02: 179
  journal titles, recommendations for use, 03: 62, 05: 17
  nucleic acids, journal reference to, 02: 87
  peptide hormones, list, 02: 177-178
  peptides, journal reference to rules, 02: 87
  polynucleotides, journal references to, 02: 87
  polypeptide chains, conformation, journal reference, 02: 87
  polypeptide chains, nomenclature rules, 01: 59-73, 02: 63-77
  polypeptides, sequential, 01: 333
  polypeptides, synthetic, journal reference, 02: 87
  pyrimidine photoproducts, proposals, 04: 51-57
  pyrimidine photoproducts, proposals for, 03: 51-57
  use of, in biochemical nomenclature, 01: 6-7, 03: 6, 7, 04: 6, 7, 05: 6, 7, 06: 6, 08: 6-7
  use of in biochemical nomenclature, 02: 6-7
Abrin; origin, structure, and characteristics as protein biosynthesis inhibitor, 04: 555
Abrine
  physical and chemical properties, 01: 148
Absidia
  G + C composition of DNA of, table arranged by specie, 04: 185
Absolute entropy, *see* Entropy, absolute
Absorbance
  transmission limits of common ions, 08: 196
Absorbance, UV and visible region, table of values, 02: 383-514
Absorbance bands
  compounds used in biochemical studies, 06: 123-129
Absorbances, molecular, *see* Molecular absorbances
Absorption, polyribonucleotides, use of tables in calculation of, 03: 596
Absorption coefficient, molar, *see* Molar absorptivity
Absorption data
  amides in water and in cyclohexane, 08: 141-143
  fluorescent polyene probes, 08: 211-212
  hemin and hematin spectra in ether, 08: 279
  metalloporphyrin methyl esters, 08: 278
  metalloporphyrins, 08: 279
  porphyrin dications in aqueous HCl, 08: 269-271
  porphyrin spectra in organic solvents, 08: 273-274
  porphyrins in various solutions, 08: 272
  pyridine hemochrome spectra, 08: 280
  UV, pyridoxine, pyridoxal and pyridoxamine derivatives, 08: 252-266
Absorptivity, mean residue, *see* Mean residue absorptivity
Acanthamoeba
  amino acid requirements for growth, table, 04: 641
  G + C composition of DNA of, table arranged by specie, 04: 228
Acetals, nomenclature rules, 05: 126-130, 132
β-Acetamido-L-alanine, *see* β-N-Acetyl-α-, β-diaminopropionic acid
3'-Acetamido-3'-deoxyadenosine, physicochemical constants, spectral, chemotherapeutic and biological properties, 03: 274
2-Acetamidoacrylic acid
  structure and symbols for those incorporated into synthetic polypeptides, 01: 97
Acetate buffer
  preparation of, 06: 372
  protonic activity tables, 06: 529-539
Acetic acid derivatives
  heat of proton ionization, pK, and related thermodynamic quantities, 06: 153-157
α Aceto-acid reductoisomerase
  Neurospora crassa mutant, 04: 751
Acetoacetate decarboxylase
  amino acid composition, complete data, 07: 505
  circular dichroism
    in near UV region, 07: 143
    in the UV region, 07: 82
  molar absorptivity and-or absorbance values, 02: 383
  optical rotatory dispersion
    in UV region, 07: 44
    in visible and near UV region, 07: 15
Acetoacetic acid decarboxylase
  average hydrophobicity value, 01: 210
Acetobacter
  amino acid requirements for growth, table, 04: 630
  G + C composition of DNA of, table arranged by specie, 04: 152-153
Acetonic acid
  heat of proton ionization, pK, and related thermodynamic quantities, 06: 157
Acetophenone
  heat of proton ionization, pK, and related thermodynamic quantities, 06: 157
Acetoxy-cycloheximide, origin, structure, and characteristic as protein biosynthesis inhibitor, 04: 555
β-N-Acetyl-α,β-diaminopropionic acid
  physical and chemical properties, 01: 119
N^{α}-Acetyl-2-fluorophenylalanine
  structure and symbols for those incorporated into synthetic polypeptides, 01: 97
N-Acetyl-β-D-glucosaminidase
  average hydrophobicity value, 01: 210
N-Acetyl-β-D-glucosaminidase-A, average hydrophobicity value, 01: 210
N-Acetyl-β-D-glucosaminidase-B, average hydrophobicity value, 01: 210
N-Acetyl-DL-β-phenylalanine methyl ester
  UV spectra of, 01: 193
N-Acetyl-DL-tryptophan methyl ester UV spectra, 01: 192
N-Acetyl-L-tyrosine ethyl ester, UV spectra, 01: 194
N-Acetyl-L-tyrosine ethyl ester anion, UV spectra, 01: 195
Acetyl CoA synthetase
  Neurospora crassa mutant, 04: 744

Acetyl hexosamine, content of, in glyco-proteins, **02:** 258-274

Acetyl ornithine transferase
Neurospora crassa mutant, **04:** 745

N-Acetylalanine
physical and chemical properties, **01:** 148

β-2-Acetylamino-2-deoxy-D-glucoside acetylamino-deoxyglucohydrolase
enzymatic reactions, velocity and parameters, table, **05:** 430-433

N-Acetylarginine
physical and chemical properties, **01:** 132

N-Acetylaspartic acid
physical and chemical properties, **01:** 148

Acetylcholine receptor
average hydrophobicity value, **01:** 210

Acetylcholine receptor protein
circular dichroism in the UV region, **07:** 82

Acetylcholinesterase
amino acid composition, incomplete data, **07:** 512
average hydrophobicity value, **01:** 210
molar absorptivity and-or absorbance values, **02:** 383
optical rotatory dispersion
in the UV region, **07:** 44
in the visible and near UV regions, **07:** 15
subunit, constitution of, **02:** 344

N-Acetylcysteine
UV absorption characteristics, **01:** 186

N⁴-Acetylcytidine
composition in various tRNA's, **04:** 428-441
isolation and detection of, in RNA, general remarks, **03:** 237
RNA, various, natural occurrence in, **03:** 222

N-Acetyldjenkolic acid
physical and chemical properties, **01:** 151

Acetylenic dicarboxylic acid diamide
physical and chemical properties, **01:** 121

N-Acetylglutamic acid
physical and chemical properties, **01:** 148

β-D-N-Acetylhexose amidase
placenta, human
subunit, constitution of, **02:** 333

O-Acetylhomoserine
physical and chemical properties, **01:** 122

Nα-Acetyllysine-N-methylamide
structure and symbols for those incorporated into synthetic polypeptides, **01:** 97

N-Acetylornithine
physical and chemical properties, **01:** 119

Acetylornithine γ-transaminase
average hydrophobicity value, **01:** 210

Acetylsalicylic acid
heat of proton ionization, pK, and related thermodynamic quantities, **06:** 179

O-Acetylserine sulfhydrase A
molar absorptivity and-or absorbance values, **02:** 383

O-Acetylserine sulfhydrylase A
amino acid composition, complete data, **07:** 505
average hydrophobicity value, **01:** 210

Achiral molecule, nomenclature for, **02:** 36-58, **03:** 28-33, **04:** 28-33, **05:** 33-38, **06:** 35, **08:** 35-40

Achiral molecule nomenclature for, **01:** 36-58

Achlya
G + C composition of DNA of, table arranged by specie, **04:** 185

Achromobacter
G + C composition of DNA of, table arranged by specie, **04:** 69-71

Achromobacteriaceae
G + C composition of DNA of, table arranged by genera and specie, **04:** 69-74

Achromycin, *see* Tetracycline

Achromycin 260, *see* Puromycin

Acid, *see also* Acids

Acid DNase, *see* Deoxyribonuclease I

α,-Acid glycoprotein
amino acid composition, incomplete data, **07:** 512
optical rotatory dispersion
UV region, **07:** 44
visible and near UV regions, **07:** 15

α₁-Acid glycoprotein
average hydrophobicity value, **01:** 210

Acid phosphatase
wheat bran
luminescence of, table, **01:** 206

Acid phosphomonoesterase I
prostate, human
subunit, constitution of, **02:** 333

Acid proteinase, *Aspergillus*, *see* Aspergillus acid, proteinase
optical rotatory dispersion
UV region, **07:** 48
visible and near UV regions, **07:** 18

Rhizopus acid proteinase
circular dichroism in the UV region, **07:** 121
optical rotatory dispersion in the UV region, **07:** 73

Acid value
polyol esters table, **05:** 515

Aciddminococcus
amino acid requirements for growth, table, **04:** 630
G + C composition of DNA of, table arranged by specie, **04:** 147

Acidemia
organic acid metabolism errors, characteristics, **01:** 326-327

Acidic brain protein
amino acid composition, incomplete data, **07:** 512

Acidic glycoprotein
circular dichroism in the UV region, **07:** 82

Acids, *see also* Acid
commercial strength, table of concentration data, **06:** 384
pK'ₐ values, table, **06:** 307-348

Acids, natural, derived from carbohydrates
chemical formula, **05:** 153-176
chromatography, **05:** 153-176
melting point, **05:** 153-176
specific rotation, **05:** 153-176

Aciduria
amino acid metabolism errors, characteristics, **01:** 317-324
organic acid metabolism errors, characteristics, **01:** 326-327

Adenosine *(continued)*
  pK'_a values, **06**: 330
  raman frequencies, table of values, **03**: 534-535
Adenosine and derivatives
  molal osmotic coefficients, **03**: 528
  UV spectra, **03**: 432-435
  UV spectral characteristics and acid dissociation constants, **03**: 413-414
Adenosine and nucleoside derivatives
  physical constants and spectral properties, index to, **03**: 69
Adenosine deaminase
  amino acid composition, complete data, **07**: 505
  optical rotatory dispersion
    UV region, **07**: 45
    visible and near UV regions, **07**: 16
Adenosine deaminase, average hydrophobicity value, **01**: 211
Adenosine monophosphate deaminase
  average hydrophobicity value, **01**: 211
Adenosine monophosphate nucleosidase
  average hydrophobicity value, **01**: 211
Adenosine nucleotide derivatives
  physical constants and spectral properties, index to , **03**: 72-73
Adenosine triphosphate, average hydrophobicity values, **01**: 211
Adenosine triphosphate sulfurylase
  molar absorptivity and-or absorbance values, **02**: 385
Adenosinetriphosphatase, *see also* ATPase
  optical rotatory dispersion
    UV region, **07**: 45
    visible and near UV regions, **07**: 16
Adenovirus
  molar absorptivity and-or absorbance values, **02**: 385
Adenovirus 2--VA RNA, nucleotide sequence model, **04**: 349
Adenylate cyclase
  average hydrophobicity value, **01**: 211
Adenylate kinase
  amino acid composition, complete data, **07**: 505
  optical rotatory dispersion
    UV region, **07**: 45
    visible and near UV regions, **07**: 16
Adenylic acid
  derivatives, UV spectral characteristics and acid dissociation constants, **03**: 416
Adenylosuccinase
  amino acid composition, complete data, **07**: 505
  Neurospora crassa mutant, **04**: 746
Adenylosuccinate-AMP-lyase
  average hydrophobicity value, **01**: 212
Adipic acid
  heat of proton ionization, pK, and related thermodynamic quantities, **06**: 160
ADP, *see* Adenylic acid
  pK'_a values, **06**: 330
Adrenal iron-sulfur protein
  amino acid composition, complete data, **07**: 505
Adrenochrome; origin, structure, and characteristic as protein biosynthesis inhibitor, **04**: 557

Adrenocorticotropic hormone
  circular dichroism in the UV region, **07**: 82
α_s-Adrenocorticotropic hormone
  optical rotatory dispersion in the visible and near UV regions, **07**: 16
Adrenocorticotropins, natural
  amino acid sequence, **07**: 375
Adrenodoxin
  amino acid sequence, **07**: 428
  average hydrophobicity value, **01**: 212
  circular dichroism in the UV region, **07**: 82
  molar absorptivity and-or absorbance values, **02**: 385
  optical rotatory dispersion in the UV region, **07**: 45
  table of cofactors, molecular weights, stoichiometry and sources, **02**: 279
Adrenodoxin reductase
  average hydrophobicity value, **01**: 212
Adsorption indicators, applications for several, **06**: 383
Aequorin
  amino acid composition, complete data, **07**: 505
  average hydrophobicity value, **01**: 212
  molar absorptivity and-or absorbance values, **02**: 385
Aerobacter
  amino acid requirements for growth, table, **04**: 630
Aerobacter (Enterobacter)
  G + C composition of DNA of, table arranged by specie, **04**: 104-105
Aerococcus
  G + C composition of DNA of, table arranged by specie, **04**: 127
Aeromonas
  G + C composition of DNA of, table arranged by specie, **04**: 153
Agaricus
  G + C composition of DNA of, table arranged by specie, **04**: 186
Agglutinin
  average hydrophobicity value, **01**: 212
  carbohydrate content, **02**: 270
  molar absorptivity and-or absorbance values, **02**: 385
  subunit, constitution of, **02**: 327, 335
Agnatha, DNA content per cell, **04**: 293
Agrobacterium
  amino acid requirements for growth, table, **04**: 630
  G + C composition of DNA of, table arranged by specie, **04**: 162-164
Alanine
  far ultraviolet absorption spectra
    aqueous solution at pH 5, **01**: 184
    neutral water, table, **01**: 185
    0.1 *M* sodium dodecyl sulfate, table, **01**: 185
  free acid in amniotic fluid in early pregnancy and at term, **01**: 327
  free acid in blood plasma of newborn infants and adults, **01**: 328
  nucleoside composition, table of values, **04**: 428
  nucleotide sequences of, **04**: 442-443
  pK'_a values, **06**: 318
  physical and chemical properties, **01**: 112
  requirements of, for growth of various microorganisms, table, **04**: 630-643

Alanine *(continued)*
specific rotatory dispersion constants, 0.1 M solution, **01:** 244
spectra, far UV, **01:** 184
symbols for atoms and bonds in side chains, **01:** 69, **02:** 73
α-Alanine
antagonists of, **01:** 177
heat of proton ionization, pK, and related thermodynamic quantities, **06:** 161
D-Alanine
antagonists of, **01:** 177
β-Alanine
antagonists of, **01:** 177
free acid in blood plasma of newborn infants and adults, **01:** 328
heat of proton ionization, pK, and related thermodynamic quantities, **06:** 161
hyperbetaalaninemia, effect of, **01:** 317
physical and chemical properties, **01:** 112
structure and symbols for those incorporated into synthetic polypeptides, **01:** 97
Alanine amino transferase
amino acid composition, complete data, **07:** 505
average hydrophobicity value, **01:** 212
Alanosine
physical and chemical properties, **01:** 134
2-Alanyl-3-isoxazolin-5-one
physical and chemical properties, **01:** 135
DL-Alanylglycine
heat capacity and entropy values, **06:** 110
Albizzine
physical and chemical properties, **01:** 132
Albumin
average hydrophobicity value, **01:** 212
bovine serum
luminescence of, table, **01:** 205
circular dichroism
in UV and near UV region, **07:** 83, 143
human serum
luminescence of, table, **01:** 205
molar absorptivity and-or absorbance values, **02:** 386-387
molecular parameters, **02:** 242
optical rotatory dispersion in the UV region, **07:** 45
refractive index increments, **02:** 372-373
Albumin, bovine
heat of proton ionization, pK, and related thermodynamic quantities, **06:** 183
Albumin, bovine serum
heat of proton ionization, pK, and related thermodynamic quantities, **06:** 161
Albumin, horse serum
calorimetric Δ H values accompanying conformational changes, **06:** 270
Albumin, plasma, *see also* Human plasma albumin; Plasma albumin
ligand binding
drugs, list of references, **02:** 568-574
endogenous ligands, list of references, **02:** 556-557
fatty acids, list of references, **02:** 558-562
inorganic anions, list of references, **02:** 563

measurement of, list of techniques, **02:** 555
metal ions, list of references, **02:** 563
steroids, list of references, **02:** 563-564
visible dyes, list of references, **02:** 564-568
Alcaligenes
G + C composition of DNA of, table arranged by specie, **04:** 71-73
Alcohol, retinol, *see* Retinol alcohol, Vitamin A
thumbprint, content in, **08:** 121
Alcohol dehydrogenase
amino acid sequence, **07:** 314-315
average hydrophobicity value, **01:** 212
molar absorptivity and-or absorbance values, **02:** 388
optical rotatory dispersion
UV region, **07:** 45
visible and near UV regions, **07:** 16
subunit, constitution of, **02:** 328, 330, 337, 338
table of cofactors, molecular weights, stoichiometry and sources, **02:** 284
Alcohols and other oxygen acids, pK'_a values, **06:** 315-317
Aldaric acids
chemical formula, **05:** 168-170
chromatography, **05:** 168-170
melting point, **05:** 168-170
nomenclature rules, **05:** 125-126
specific rotation, **05:** 168-170
Aldehyde dehydrogenase
amino acid composition, complete data, **07:** 505
molar absorptivity and-or absorbance values, **02:** 388
subunit, constitution of, **02:** 343
Aldehyde dehydrogenase, protein A
average hydrophobicity value, **01:** 212
Aldehyde oxidase
molar absorptivity and-or absorbance values, **02:** 389
table of cofactors, molecular weights, stoichiometry and sources, **02:** 278
Alditols, amino
chemical formula, **05:** 148-149
chromatography, **05:** 148-149
melting point, **05:** 148-149
specific rotation, **05:** 148-149
Alditols, natural
chemical formula, **05:** 139-142
chromatography, **05:** 139-142
melting point, **05:** 139-142
specific rotation, **05:** 139-142
Alditols, nomenclature rules, **05:** 119-120
Aldoketoses, nomenclature rules, **05:** 108-109
Aldolase, *see* Fructose-bisphosphate aldolase
average hydrophobicity value, **01:** 212
cofactors, molecular weights, stoichiometry, sources, **02:** 284
cyanogen bromide cleavage, **02:** 199
enzymatic activity, subcellular fractions, **02:** 698, 715
luminescence of, table, **01:** 205
molar absorptivity and-or absorbance values, **02:** 389
subunit, constitution of, **02:** 331, 335, 338, 377
viscosity, intrinsic, **02:** 721
Aldolase, 3-deoxy-2-keto-6-phosphogluconate
molar absorptivity and-or absorbance values, **02:** 390
Aldolase, fructose-1,6-diphosphate, average hydrophobicity values, **01:** 212

Aldolase, fructose diphosphate, average hydrophobicity
value, **01:** 212

Aldolase, L-Rhamnulose l-phosphate
molar absorptivity and-or absorbance values, **02:** 390

Aldolase C
subunit, constitution of, **02:** 338

Aldolase C, average hydrophobicity value, **01:** 212

Aldonic acids
chemical formula, **05:** 153-176
chromatography, **05:** 153-164
melting point, **05:** 153-164
nomenclature rules, **05:** 121-122
specific rotation, **05:** 153-164

Aldose l-epimerase
molar absorptivity and-or absorbance values, **02:** 390

Aldoses, natural
chemical formula, **05:** 181-217
chromatography, **05:** 181-217
melting point, **05:** 181-217
specific rotation, **05:** 181-217

Algae
amino acid requirements for growth, table, **04:** 630
DNA base compositions for, **04:** 236-237
DNA content per cell for various, table, **04:** 286
G + C composition of DNA of, table arranged by gen-
era and specie, **04:** 224-227

Algae, thallophyta, *see* Thallophyta; algae

Aliphatic acids, long-chain, and related compounds,
molecular dimensions, **05:** 498

Alkaline phosphatase
amino acid composition, complete data, **07:** 505
average hydrophobicity value, **01:** 213
carbohydrate content, **02:** 274
circular dichroism in the UV region, **07:** 83
molecular weights, stoichiometry and sources, **02:** 284
optical rotatory dispersion
UV region, **07:** 45
visible and near UV regions, **07:** 16
subunit, constitution of, **02:** 331, 335, 337

Aspergillus alkaline proteinase
optical rotatory dispersion
UV region, **07:** 48
visible and near UV regions, **07:** 18

Alkaline proteinase A and B, thermophilic, *Streptomyces,*
see *Trypsin, thermophilic Streptomyces*

Alkaline proteinase B
average hydrophobicity value, **01:** 213

Alkaloids and derivatives, pK'_a, **06:** 326-327

Alkyl derivatives of unmodified bases and nucleosides,
UV spectra of some, **03:** 420-447

Allantoicase
circular dichroism
in UV and near UV region, **07:** 83, 143
optical rotatory dispersion
UV region, **07:** 46
visible and near UV regions, **07:** 16

Alleles
Streptomyces coelicolor, **04:** 724-727

Allelic mutants, *Aspergillus nidulans,* **04:** 732-737

Allergen 1-B
amino acid composition, complete data, **07:** 505

Allergen (antigen K)
amino acid composition, complete data, **07:** 505

Alliin
physical and chemical properties, **01:** 151

Alliin lyase
molar absorptivity and-or absorbance values, **02:** 391

D-Alloenduracididine
physical and chemical properties, **01:** 164

Allograft, definition of, **04:** 884

D-Allohydroxyproline betaine, *see* Turcine

Alloisoleucine
structure and symbols for those incorporated into synthetic polypeptides, **01:** 97

Allomycin, physicochemical constants, spectral, chemotherapeutic and biological properties, **03:** 276

Allomycin; origin, structure, and characteristic as protein
biosynthesis inhibitor, **04:** 557

D-Allothreonine
physical and chemical properties, **01:** 164

Allyglycine
antagonism to cysteine, **01:** 177

S-Allylcysteine
physical and chemical properties, **01:** 151

S-Allylmercaptocysteine
physical and chemical properties, **01:** 151

Althiomycin; origin, structure, and characteristic as
protein biosynthesis inhibitor, **04:** 557

Aluminichrome
proton NMR and suggested conformations, **07:** 567

Aluminichrysin
proton NMR and suggested conformations, **07:** 568

Aluminicrocin
proton NMR and suggested conformations, **07:** 568

Aluminum, chemical resistance as used in ultracentrifuge
centerpieces, **08:** 429-430

Amandin
molar absorptivity and-or absorbance values, **02:** 392
refractive index increments, **02:** 373

Amanita
G + C composition of DNA of, table arranged by specie, **04:** 186

Amauroascus
G + C composition of DNA of, table arranged by specie, **04:** 186

Amicetin, *see also* Sacromycin

Amicetin, physicochemical constants, spectral, chemotherapeutic and biological properties, **03:** 277

Amicetin B, *see* Plicacetin

Amicetin B, physicochemical constants, spectral, chemotherapeutic and biological properties, **03:** 278

Amicetin; origin, structure, and characteristic as protein
biosynthesis inhibitor, **04:** 558

ω-Amidase
average hydrophobicity value, **01:** 213

Amide I and amide II components,[a] cm^{-1} (solid state)
prominent, table, **07:** 597

Amides
absorption data in water and in cyclohexane, **08:**
141-143
far ultraviolet absorption spectra
aqueous solution at pH 5, **01:** 184
neutral water, table, **01:** 185

Amides *(continued)*

0.1 *M* sodium dodecyl sulfate, table, **01:** 185

N-Amidinoglycyl, *see* Guanidinoacetyl

Amine buffers, structures and pK_a values, **06:** 368-369

Amine derivatives

heat of proton ionization, pK, and related thermodynamics quantities, **06:** 162-164

Amine oxidase

molar absorptivity and-or absorbance values, **02:** 392

table of cofactors, molecular weights, stoichiometry and sources, **02:** 282

Amines, pK'_a values, **06:** 322-326

α-Amino-γ-*N*-acetylaminobutyric acid

physical and chemical properties, **01:** 119

D-Amino-acid oxidase

molar absorptivity and-or absorbance values, **02:** 392

subunit, constitution of, **02:** 333

L-Amino-acid oxidase

molar absorptivity and, **02:** or absorbance values, **02:** 392

subunit, constitution of, **02:** 336

α-Amino-actanoic acid

physical and chemical properties, **01:** 115

α-Amino-ε-amidino caproic acid, *see* Indospicine

α-Amino-β-(2-amino-2-carboxyethylmercaptobutyric acid)

physical and chemical properties, **01:** 151

2-Amino-4-(2-amino-3-hydroxypropoxy)-but-3-enoic acid, *see* Rhizobitoxine

3-Amino-2-benzylpropionic acid

structure and symbols for those incorporated into synthetic polypeptides, **01:** 97

3-Amino-3-benzylpropionic acid

structure and symbols for those incorporated into synthetic polypeptides, **01:** 97

α-Amino-*n*-butyric acid

thumbprint, content in, **08:** 121

N-(3-Amino-3-carboxy-propyl)-β-carboxypyridinium betaine, *see also* Nicotianine

physical and chemical properties, **01:** 161

3-Amino-(3-carboxy-propyldimethylsulfonium)

physical and chemical properties, **01:** 151

3-Amino-3-carboxy-pyrrolidine, *see* Cucurbitine

α-Amino-γ-[2-(4-carboxy)-thiazolyl butyric acid]

physical and chemical properties, **01:** 152

2-Amino-2-carboxyethane-sulfonamide

antagonism to asparagine, **01:** 177

2-Amino-2-carboxyethyl-2-guanidineethyl hydrogen phosphate, *see* Lombricine

N-ε-(2-Amino-2-carboxyethyl)-lysine

physical and chemical properties, **01:** 119

N-δ-(2-Amino-2-carboxyethyl)-ornithine

physical and chemical properties, **01:** 119

3-Amino-3-carboxypropane-sulfonamide

antagonism to glutamine, **01:** 177

3-(3-Amino-3-carboxypropyl)uridine

composition in various tRNA's, **04:** 428-441

isolation and detection of, in RNA, general remarks, **03:** 241

RNA, various, natural occurrence in, **03:** 229

α-Amino-β-chlorobutyric acid

antagonism to leucine, **01:** 178

3'-Amino-3'-deoxyadenosine, physicochemical constants, spectral, chemotherapeutic and biological properties, **03:** 280

1-(3'-(γ-Amino-α-γ-dicarboxypropyl-amino)-propylazetidine-2-carboxylic acid, *see* Nicotianamine

2-Amino-4,4-dichlorobutyric acid

physical and chemical properties, **01:** 159

α-Amino-(2,5-dihydro-5-methyl) furan-2-acetic acid, *see* Furanomycin

2-Amino-4,5-dihydroxy pentanoic acid

physical and chemical properties, **01:** 122

α-Amino-β,β-dimethyl-γ-hydroxybutyric acid, *see* Pantonine

2-Amino-6-dimethylamino-4-hexynoic acid

structure and symbols for those incorporated into synthetic polypeptides, **01:** 98

2-Amino-3-dimethylaminopropionic acid

physical and chemical properties, **01:** 119

α-Amino-d-*N*-ethylglutaramic acid, *see* Theanine

2-Amino-3-ethylvaleric acid

structure and symbols for those incorporated into synthetic polypeptides, **01:** 98

2-Amino-3-formyl-3-pentenoic acid

physical and chemical properties, **01:** 112, 122

α-Amino-ε-guanidino-γ-hydroxy-hexenoic acid, *see* γ-Hydroxyhomoarginine

Amino-δ-guanidinovaleric acid, *see* Arginine

α-Amino-(*O*-guanidyl)-γ-hydroxybutyric acid, *see* Canavanine

α-Amino-δ-(guanylureido)-valeric acid, *see* Gigartinine

2-Amino-5-heptenoic acid

antagonism to methionine, **01:** 178

2-Amino-4,5-hexadienoic acid

physical and chemical properties, **01:** 113

2-Amino-4-hexenoic acid

antagonism to methionine, **01:** 178

physical and chemical properties, **01:** 113

2-Amino-4-hydroxy-hept-6-ynoic acid

physical and chemical properties, **01:** 113

2-Amino-6-hydroxy-4-methyl-4-hexenoic acid

physical and chemical properties, **01:** 113, 123

2-Amino-4-hydroxy-5-*N*-methylformamido-6-ribosylaminopyrimidine

physical constants and spectral properties, **03:** 116

2-Amino-4-hydroxy-5-*N*-methylformamido-6-ribosylaminopyrimidine 3' (2')-phosphate

physical constants and spectral properties, **03:** 195

4-Amino-3-hydroxy-6-methylheptanoic acid

structure and symbols for those incorporated into synthetic polypeptides, **01:** 98

2-Amino-4-hydroxy-methylhex-5-ynoic acid

physical and chemical properties, **01:** 113

α-Amino-γ-hydroxyadipic acid

physical and chemical properties, **01:** 122

α-Amino-ε-hydroxyaminohexanoic acid, *see* ε-Hydroxylaminonorleucine

2-Amino-6-hydroxyaminohexanoic acid

physical and chemical properties, **01:** 122

α-Amino-γ-hydroxybutyric acid, *see* Homoserine

α-Amino-β-hydroxybutyric acid, *see* Threonine

γ-Amino-β-hydroxybutyric acid
physical and chemical properties, **01:** 123
γ-Amino-β-hydroxybutyric acid betaine, *see* Carnitine
α-Amino-ε-hydroxycaproic acid
antagonism to lysine, **01:** 178
2-Amino-3-hydroxymethyl-3-pentenoic acid
physical and chemical properties, **01:** 113, 123
α-Amino-γ-hydroxypimelic acid
physical and chemical properties, **01:** 123
α-Amino-β-hydroxypropionic acid, *see* Serine
O-(2-Amino-3-hydroxypropyl)-homoserine, *see* Dihydrorhizobitoxine
α-Amino-δ-hydroxyvaleric acid
antagonism to ornithine, **01:** 178
physical and chemical properties, **01:** 123
2-Amino-3-(2-imidazolyl)propionic acid
structure and symbols for those incorporated into synthetic polypeptides, **01:** 98
α-Amino-β-(2-iminoimidazolidinyl)-propionic acid, *see*
D-Alloenduracididine, Enduracididine
α-Amino-β-3(indazole)-propionic acid
antagonism to Tryptophan, **01:** 179
α-Amino-β-3-indolepropionic acid, *see* Tryptophan
α-Amino-3-keto-5-isoxazolidine acetic acid, *see* Tricholomic acid
α-Amino-3-keto-4-isoxazoline-5-acetic acid, *see* Ibotenic
acid
α-Amino-β-ketobutyric acid
physical and chemical properties, **01:** 123
2-Amino-4-ketohexenoic acid, *see* 4-Ketonorleucine
α-Amino-β-mercaptopropionic acid, *see* Cysteine
2-Amino-4-methoxy-*trans*-3-butenoic acid
physical and chemical properties, **01:** 114
α-Amino-β-methyl-γ,δ-dihydroxyisocaproic acid
physical and chemical properties, **01:** 123
2-Amino-4-methyl-hexenoic acid
physical and chemical properties, **01:** 114
structure and symbols for those incorporated into synthetic polypeptides, **01:** 98
2-Amino-4-methyl-4-hexenoic acid
antagonism to phenylalanine, **01:** 179
physical and chemical properties, **01:** 114
structure and symbols for those incorporated into synthetic polypeptides, **01:** 98
2-Amino-4-methyl-5-hexenoic acid
physical and chemical properties, **01:** 114, 115
2-Amino-5-methyl-4-hexenoic acid
physical and chemical properties, **01:** 114
2-Amino-5-methyl-5-hexenoic acid
structure and symbols for those incorporated into synthetic polypeptides, **01:** 98
2-Amino-5-methyl-6-hydroxyhex-4-enoic acid
physical and chemical properties, **01:** 124
2-Amino-2-methyl-1,3-propanediol(ammediol) buffer,
preparation of, **06:** 376
α-Amino-β-methylaminopropionic acid
physical and chemical properties, **01:** 120
γ-Amino-α-methylene butyric acid
physical and chemical properties, **01:** 114
α-Amino-β-(2-methylene cyclopropyl)-propionic acid, *see*
Hypoglycin A

2-Amino-4-methylhexenoic acid
antagonism to leucine, **01:** 178
α-Amino-γ-methylthiobutyric acid, *see* Methionine
α-Amino-β-methylvaleric acid, *see* Isoleucine
1-Amino-2-nitrocyclopentane carboxylic acid
physical and chemical properties, **01:** 136
2-Amino-3-(*N*-nitrosohydroxyamino) propionic acid, *see*
Alanosine
α-Amino-β-oxalylaminopropionic acid
physical and chemical properties, **01:** 120
α-Amino-β-phenylbutyric acid
physical and chemical properties, **01:** 129
3-Amino-4-phenylbutyric acid
structure and symbols for those incorporated into synthetic polypeptides, **01:** 99
α-Amino-β-phenylethanesulfonic acid
antagonism to phenylalanine, **01:** 179
β-Amino-β-phenylpropionic acid
physical and chemical properties, **01:** 129
α-Amino-β-phosphonopropionic acid
physical and chemical properties, **01:** 161
2-Amino-4-pontynoic acid
physical and chemical properties, **01:** 115
1-Amino-D-proline
physical and chemical properties, **01:** 165
α-Amino-β-propionic acid, *see* Tyrosine hydroxyphenyl
2-Amino-3-(2-pyridyl)propionic acid
structure and symbols for those incorporated into synthetic polypeptides, **01:** 99
2-Amino-3-(2-pyrimidyl)propionic acid
structure and symbols for those incorporated into synthetic polypeptides, **01:** 99
α-Amino-ε-Trimethylamino adipic acid, *see* Laminine
2-Amino-6-(trimethylammonio)hexanoic acid
structure and symbols for those incorporated into synthetic polypeptides, **01:** 99
2-Amino-3-ureidopropionic acid, *see* Albizzine
Amino acid
Escherichia coli ribosomal proteins: 30 S, composition,
04: 476
Escherichia coli ribosomal proteins: 50 S, composition,
04: 477-478
sequence data, ribosomal proteins from *Escherichia coli*,
04: 479-481
Amino acid-carbohydrate linkages found in mammalian
glycoproteins, **05:** 281
Amino acid composition
proteinase inhibitors
animal sources, table, **02:** 649-653
microbial sources, **02:** 664
plant sources, table, **02:** 605-610
retinol-binding protein human, **02:** 303
Tamm-Horsfall glycoprotein, **02:** 303
urokinase, **02:** 302
amino acid composition, complete data, **07:** 509
circular dichroism in the UV region, **07:** 118
optical rotatory dispersion in the UV region, **07:** 70
Amino acid compositions
discussion, complete data, **07:** 504
references, complete data, **07:** 515-519
selected proteins, complete data, **07:** 504
tables, complete data, **07:** 505-514

Amino acid decarboxylase, aromatic
  average hydrophobicity value, **01:** 213
Amino acid group
  dimensions of, **02:** 742-758
D-Amino acid oxidase
  amino acid composition, complete data, **07:** 505
  average hydrophobicity value, **01:** 213
  circular dichroism in the UV region, **07:** 84
  optical rotatory dispersion
    UV region, **07:** 46
    visible and near UV regions, **07:** 17
L-Amino acid oxidase
  amino acid composition, complete data, **07:** 505
  optical rotatory dispersion in the UV region, **07:** 46
Amino acid replacements in naturally occurring (NM)
      and chemically induced (CM) mutants of TMV, lo-
      cation of some, **07:** 266-267
Amino acid sequence for selected proteins, **07:** 192-339
Amino acid sequences
  β_2 microglobulin, **02:** 305
  proteinase inhibitors
    animal sources, table, **02:** 656-659
    microbial source, **02:** 665
    plant sources, **02:** 611-617
  rules for one-letter notation, **02:** 59-62
Amino acid sequences, Tables, **07:** 341-349
Amino acid side chains
  dimensions of, **02:** 742-758
Amino acids, *see also* Aromatic amino acids, *also* specific
      acids
  abbreviations, table of, **01:** 78, **02:** 62
  aminoacidurias, characteristics of, table, **01:** 317-324
  antagonists, table of, **01:** 177-180
  aromatic
    luminescence of, table, **01:** 200
    luminescence of derivatives of, table, **01:** 201-203
  average hydrophobicity values for side chains, **01:** 209
  bond angles and distances for the grouping, **08:** 222
  chromatography, gas-liquid, data tables, **08:** 93-110
  chromatography, ion exchange
    ninhydrin positive compounds, elution behavior, **08:**
      122
    thumbprint, constituents of, **08:** 121
    urine, resolution of ninhydrin positive constituents, **08:**
      114-119
    variables, mathematical relationships, **08:** 112-113
  circular dichroism spectra of metal complexes of, **01:**
      245-315
  enthalpy of formation, table, **06:** 111-112
  entropies, absolute, table of values, **06:** 109
  entropies of formation, table of values, **06:** 109
  enzymatic activities, susceptibility of poly(α-amino
      acids), **01:** 393-396
  free acid in blood plasma of newborn infants and
      adults, table, **01:** 328
  free energy of formation, table of values, **06:** 111-112
  free energy of formation in aqueous solution at 25°C,
      06: 118
  free energy of solution in aqueous solution at 25°C, **06:**
      118
  heat capacities, table of values, **06:** 109
  heat of combustion, table of values, **06:** 111-112

  heats of solution in aqueous solution at 25°C, **06:**
      116-117
  α-Keto acids analogs of, properties, **01:** 181-182
  metabolic disease related, rapid short column
      chromatography, **08:** 128-129
  metabolism, errors of, table, **01:** 317-324
  molal activity coefficients, table of values, **06:** 119-120
  molecular absorbances of aromatic types, data, **01:**
      187-189
  naturally occurring
    physical and chemical properties, table, **01:** 111-166
    synonyms for, **01:** 111-166
  ninhydrin reaction, absorption ratios and product color
      constants, **08:** 123-124
  ninhydrin reactive, chromatographic positions, **08:** 126
  pK'_a values, **06:** 318-320
  peptic hydrolysis in human α- and β-chains, **02:** 216
  L-phosphorus-containing, physical and chemical proper-
      ties, **01:** 161-164
  pK values for several, in proteins, tables, **02:** 689-696
  plasma, normal or low, renal aminoacidurias, **01:**
      323-324
  poly(α-amino acids)
    enzymatic activities, susceptibility to, **01:** 393-396
    solubility, table, **01:** 393-396
  polymerized
    abbreviated nomenclature for, **01:** 91-95
    symbols for, use of, **01:** 13
  polymerized, use of symbols for, **02:** 13-14
  residue, notation, **02:** 63-64
  residue notation, **01:** 59-60
  sequences, rules for one-letter notation, **01:** 75-78, **02:**
      59-62
  solubilities in water at various temperatures, table of
      values, **06:** 115
  solubility in water, equation coefficient values for se-
      veral, **06:** 107-108
  solubility of poly(α-amino acids), table, **01:** 393-396
  spectra, far UV absorption, data, **01:** 184-185
  L-N-substituted, physical and chemical properties, **01:**
      148-151
  L-sulfur and selenium-containing, physical and chemical
      properties, **01:** 151-158
  symbols for, use of, **01:** 8-9, **02:** 8-9
  symbols for derivatives and peptides, **01:** 79-90
  synthetic
    structures and symbols for those incorporated into
      synthetic polypeptides, **01:** 96
  α,β-unsaturated, structure and properties, table, **01:** 175
  L-ureido, physical and chemical properties, **01:** 132-134
  UV absorption characteristics, N-acetyl methyl esters of
      aromatic types, cystine and N-acetylcysteine, **01:** 186
  UV spectra of derivatives of cysteine, cystine, histidine,
      phenylalanine, tyrosine, and tryptophan, **01:** 192-199
D-Amino acids
  physical and chemical properties, **01:** 164-166
Amino acids among 60 species, frequency of occurrence,
      at different positions along chain
  table, **07:** 288-291
L-Amino acids containing other nitrogenous groups, *see
      also* L-Aromatic amino acids
  physical and chemical properties, **01:** 134-135

Amino alditols, *see* Alditols, amino

α-Amino groups
   pK values in proteins, table, **02:** 693

ε-Amino groups
   pK values in proteins, table, **02:** 694

Amino protein group, chemical modification of
   reagents used, table of specificities, **02:** 203-204

Amino sugar, naturally occurring
   electrophoretic mobility, data for several systems, **05:** 359-370
   melting point, **05:** 359-370
   sources, **05:** 359-370
   specific rotation, **05:** 359-370
   structural formula, **05:** 359-370

Amino sugar acids
   chemical formula, **05:** 170-176
   chromatography, **05:** 170-176
   melting point, **05:** 170-176
   specific rotation, **05:** 170-176

α-Aminoacetic acid, *see* Glycine

Aminoacidurias
   primary overflow types, characteristics of, **01:** 317-322
   renal (transport) types, characteristics of, **01:** 323-324

α-Aminoadipic acid
   physical and chemical properties, **01:** 117

2-Aminoadipic acid
   structure and symbols for those incorporated into synthetic polypeptides, **01:** 97

3-Aminoadipic acid, **01:** 97
   structure and symbols for those incorporated into synthetic polypeptides, **01:** 97

β-Aminoalanine, *see* α,β-Diaminopropionic acid

Aminoalkyl adenylate; origin, structure, and characteristic as protein biosynthesis inhibitor, **04:** 558

p-Aminobenzoic acid
   biological characteristics, **08:** 302
   properties of, **08:** 293

γ-Aminobutryic acid betaine; *see* γ-Butyrobetaine

N-(4-Aminobutyl)-3-aminopropionic acid, *see* β-Putreanine

DL-3-Aminobutyramide; characteristics as protein biosynthesis inhibitor, **04:** 559

α-Aminobutyric acid
   antagonism to valine, **01:** 180
   free acid in amniotic fluid in early pregnancy and at term, **01:** 327
   physical and chemical properties, **01:** 112

γ-Aminobutyric acid
   physical and chemical properties, **01:** 112

D-α-Aminobutyric acid
   antagonism to D-Alanine, **01:** 177

β-Aminobutyric acid
   antagonism to β-Alanine, **01:** 177

2-Aminobutyric acid
   structure and symbols for those incorporated into synthetic polypeptides, **01:** 97

3-Aminobutyric acid
   structure and symbols for those incorporated into synthetic polypeptides, **01:** 97

4-Aminobutyric acid
   structure and symbols for those incorporated into synthetic polypeptides, **01:** 97

γ-Aminobutyrine, *see* α,γ-Diaminobutyric acid

6-Aminocaproic acid, *see* 6-Aminohexenoic acid

Aminochromes; origin, structure, and characteristics as protein biosynthesis inhibitor, **04:** 559

2-Aminocrotonic acid
   structure and symbols for those incorporated into synthetic polypeptides, **01:** 97

1-Aminocyclohexane-1-carboxylic acid
   structure and symbols for those incorporated into synthetic polypeptides, **01:** 97

3-Aminocyclohexane alanine
   antagonism to lysine, **01:** 178

1-Aminocyclopentane-1-carboxylic acid
   structure and symbols for those incorporated into synthetic polypeptides, **01:** 97

1-Aminocyclopropane-1-carboxylic acid
   physical and chemical properties, **01:** 112

α-Aminodimethyl-γ-butyrothetin, *see* S-Methylmethionine

α-Aminoethanesulfonic acid
   antagonism to α-Alanine, **01:** 177

2-Aminoethanesulfonic acid, *see* Taurine

S-(β-Aminoethyl)-cysteine
   antagonism to lysine, **01:** 178

2-Aminoethyl phosphonic acid, *see* Ciliatine

α-Aminoglutaramic acid, *see* Glutamine

α-Aminoglutaric acid, *see* Glutamic acid

3-Aminoglutaric acid
   physical and chemical properties, **01:** 117

α-Aminoheptenoic acid
   physical and chemical properties, **01:** 112

6-Aminohexanoic acid
   structure and symbols for those incorporated into synthetic polypeptides, **01:** 98

α-Aminoisoamylsulfonic acid
   antagonism to Leucine, **01:** 178

α-Aminoisobutanesulfonic acid
   antagonism to valine, **01:** 180

α-Aminoisobutyric acid
   antagonism to α-Alanine, **01:** 177
   physical and chemical properties, **01:** 113

β-Aminoisobutyric acid
   physical and chemical properties, **01:** 113

2-Aminoisobutyric acid
   structure and symbols for those incorporated into synthetic polypeptides, **01:** 98

α-Aminoisocaproic acid, *see* Leucine

α-Aminoisovaleric acid, *see* Valine

α-Aminolevulinic acid
   antagonism to aspartic acid, **01:** 177

Aminomethanesulfonic acid
   structure and symbols for those incorporated into synthetic polypeptides, **01:** 98

α-Aminomethanesulfonic acid
   antagonism to glycine, **01:** 177

4-Aminomethylbenzoic acid
   structure and symbols for those incorporated into synthetic polypeptides, **01:** 98

3-Aminomethylcyclohexane glycine
   antagonism to lysine, **01:** 178

8-Aminooctanoic acid
   structure and symbols for those incorporated into synthetic polypeptides, **01:** 98

Aminopeptidase
  average hydrophobicity value, **01:** 213
  enzymatic hydrolysis, conjugated proteins, **02:** 211
  molar absorptivity and-or absorbance values, **02:** 393
  molecular weights, stoichiometry and sources, **02:** 285
  subunit, constitution of, **02:** 346, 347
Aminopeptidase (cytosol)
  amino acid composition, complete data, **07:** 508
  circular dichroism in the UV region, **07:** 84
  optical rotatory dispersion
    UV region, **07:** 46
    visible and near UV regions, **07:** 17
Aminopeptidase (microsomal)
  molar absorptivity and-or absorbance values, **02:** 393
Aminopeptidase P
  molar absorptivity and-or absorbance values, **02:** 393
o-Aminophenylalanine
  antagonism to phenylalanine, **01:** 179
p-Aminophenylalanine
  antagonism to phenylalanine, **01:** 179
  antagonism to tyrosine, **01:** 180
(4-Amino)phenylalanine
  structure and symbols for those incorporated into synthetic polypeptides, **01:** 98
α-Aminopimelic acid
  physical and chemical properties, **01:** 117
2-Aminopimelic acid
  structure and symbols for those incorporated into synthetic polypeptides, **01:** 99
4-Aminopipecolic acid
  physical and chemical properties, **01:** 136
cis-3-Aminoproline
  physical and chemical properties, **01:** 136
α-Aminopropionic acid, *see* Alanine
β-Aminopropionic acid, *see* β-Alanine
α-Aminosuccinamic acid, *see* Asparagine
α-Aminosuccinic acid, *see* Aspartic acid
Aminotripeptidase, TP-2
  average hydrophobicity value, **01:** 213
3-Aminotyrosine
  structure and symbols for those incorporated into synthetic polypeptides, **01:** 99
Ammonia
  heat of proton ionization, pK, and related thermodynamic quantities, **06:** 167
  thumbprint, content in, **08:** 121
Amoeba
  amino acid requirements for growth, table, **04:** 641
  G + C composition of DNA of, table arranged by specie, **04:** 228
Amorphosporangium
  G + C composition of DNA of, table arranged by specie, **04:** 77
AMP
  heat of proton ionization, pK, and related thermodynamic quantities, **06:** 160
  pK'_a values, **06:** 330
D-AMP-3, *see* Thiamphenicol
AMP Deaminase
  subunit, constitution of, **02:** 344
Amphibia, satellite DNA's; buoyant density and G + C content of, table, **04:** 389-390

Amphibians
  DNA content per cell for various, table, **04:** 298-299
Amphotericin B
  UV spectra, formula, molecular weight, **08:** 184
Ampullariella
  G + C composition of DNA of, table arranged by specie, **04:** 77
Amylase
  average hydrophobicity values, **01:** 213
  enzymatic activity, subcellular fractions, **02:** 698, 714
  molar absorptivity, and-or absorbance values, **02:** 393
  table of cofactors, molecular weights, stoichiometry and sources, **02:** 278
α-Amylase
  amino acid composition, complete data, **07:** 505
  carbohydrate content, **02:** 274
  circular dichroism
    in UV and near UV region, **07:** 84, 143
  molar absorptivity and-or absorbance values, **02:** 393
  optical rotatory dispersion
    UV region, **07:** 46
    visible and near UV regions, **07:** 17
  refractive index increments, **02:** 374
  subunit, constitution of, **02:** 332
β-Amylase
  circular dichroism in the UV region, **07:** 84
  luminescence of, table, **01:** 205
  molar absorptivity and-or absorbance values, **02:** 394
  optical rotatory dispersion
    UV region, **07:** 47
    visible and near UV regions, **07:** 17
  subunit, constitution of, **02:** 340
α-Amylase, average hydrophobicity values, **01:** 213
α-Amylase-I, II, average hydrophobicity values, **01:** 213
Amylase PI, PII, PIII, average hydrophobicity values, **01:** 213
Analgesics, ligands binding to plasma albumin, **02:** 570
Anaplasma
  G + C composition of DNA of, table arranged by specie, **04:** 78
Anaplasmataceae
  G + C composition of DNA of, table arranged by genera and specie, **04:** 78
Androgens, structures and properties, **05:** 531-533
Angiosperms; buoyant density and G + C content of satellite DNAs for several species, table, **04:** 400-401
Angiotensin amide
  luminescence of, **01:** 204
Angiotensin I
  amino acid sequence, **07:** 375
Angiotensin II
  amino acid sequence, **07:** 375
Angiotensinogen
  amino acid sequence, **07:** 375
Angolamycin; origin, structure, and characteristic as protein biosynthesis inhibitor, **04:** 559
Angusticeps-type toxins, *see* Toxins, angusticeps-type
Angustmycin A, physicochemical constants, spectral, chemotherapeutic and biological properties, **03:** 282
Angustmycin C, physicochemical constants, spectral, chemotherapeutic and biological properties, **03:** 284

Arachidonic acid *(continued)*
  liberation phosphatidyl inositol, **08:** 320
  occurrence, **08:** 325
  precursor in prostaglandin biosynthesis, **08:** 334-338
Arachin
  molar absorptivity and-or absorbance values, **02:** 395
  refractive index increments, **02:** 374
  subunit, constitution of, **02:** 346
Arachniotus
  G + C composition of DNA of, table arranged by specie, **04:** 186
Archangiaceae
  G + C composition of DNA of, table arranged by genera and specie, **04:** 78
Archangium
  G + C composition of DNA of, table arranged by specie, **04:** 78
Arginase
  amino acid composition, incomplete data, **07:** 512
  bovine liver
    luminescence of, table, **01:** 205
  enzymatic activity, subcellular fractions, **02:** 698
  molar absorptivity and-or absorbance values, **02:** 395
  optical rotatory dispersion
    UV region, **07:** 47
    visible and near UV regions, **07:** 17
  subunit, constitution of, **02:** 335
Arginine
  antagonism to lysine, **01:** 178
  antagonists of, **01:** 177
  bond distances and angles for side chain, **08:** 222
  far ultraviolet absorption spectra
    aqueous solution at pH5, **01:** 184
    neutral water, table, **01:** 185
    0.1 *M* sodium dodecyl sulfate, table, **01:** 185
  free acid in amniotic fluid in early pregnancy and at term, **01:** 327
  free acid in blood plasma of newborn infants and adults, **01:** 328
  heat of proton ionization, pK, and related thermodynamic quantities, **06:** 169
  molar extinctions, **01:** 185
  nucleoside composition, table of values, **04:** 428
  nucleotide sequences of, **04:** 442-443
  pK'_a values, **06:** 318
  physical and chemical properties, **01:** 132
  requirements of, for growth of various microorganisms, table, **04:** 630-643
  spectra, far UV, **01:** 184
  symbols for atoms and bonds in side chains, **01:** 70, **02:** 74
  thumbprint, content in, **08:** 121
Arginine-specific carbamyl phosphate synthetase
  Neurospora crassa mutant, **04:** 740
Arginine-specific CPS-linked glutaminase
  Neurospora crassa mutant, **04:** 748
Arginine decarboxylase
  amino acid composition, complete data, **07:** 505
  average hydrophobicity value, **01:** 214
  molar absorptivity and-or absorbance values, **02:** 395
  subunit, constitution of, **02:** 345, 350

Arginine kinase
  amino acid composition, complete data, **07:** 505
  circular dichroism
    in UV and near UV region, **07:** 85, 143
  molar absorptivity and-or absorbance values, **02:** 395
  optical rotatory dispersion
    UV region, **07:** 47
    visible and near UV regions, **07:** 17
Arginine kinase, average hydrophobicity values, **01:** 214
Arginine vasopressin
  amino acid sequence, physical and biological properties, **07:** 197-198
Arginine vasotocin
  amino acid sequence, biological properties, **07:** 195-196
Argininosuccinase
  molar absorptivity and-or absorbance values, **02:** 396
  Neurospora crassa mutant, **04:** 755
  subunit, constitution of, **02:** 340
  synthetase
    Neurospora crassa mutant, **04:** 740
Argininosuccinic acid
  argininosuccinic aciduria, effect of, **01:** 317
Argininosuccinic aciduria
  characteristics of, **01:** 317
Aristeromycin, physicochemical constants, spectral, chemotherapeutic and biological properties, **03:** 295
Aromatic amino acids, *see also* Amino acids
L-Aromatic amino acids, *see also* L-Amino acid listing
  physical and chemical properties, **01:** 129-132
Arsenic acid
  heat of proton ionization, pK, and related thermodynamic quantities, **06:** 170
β-Arthraniloyl-α-aminopropionic acid, *see* Kynurenine
Arthrobacter
  G + C composition of DNA of, table arranged by specie, **04:** 97-99
Arthrobotrys
  G + C composition of DNA of, table arranged by specie, **04:** 186
Arthropoda
  deoxyribonucleic acids from, purine and pyrimidine distribution in, **04:** 266
  DNA content per cell for various, table, **04:** 291-293
Aryl sulfatase, *Neurospora crassa* mutant, **04:** 744
Aschelminthes
  deoxyribonucleic acids from, purine and pyrimidine distribution in, **04:** 264
Ascomycetes, DNA content per cell for various, table, **04:** 284
Ascorbate-2-sulfate, structure and properties, **08:** 281
Ascorbate oxidase
  circular dichroism in the UV region, **07:** 85
Ascorbic acid, *see also* Vitamin C
  biological characteristics, **08:** 283, 302
  structure and properties, **08:** 281, 293
L-Ascorbic acid, *see also* Vitamin C
  properties, **08:** 293
  UV spectra, formula, molecular weight, **08:** 149-150
Ascorbic acid oxidase
  amino acid composition, incomplete data, **07:** 512
Ascorbigen
  physical and chemical properties, **01:** 136

B

Bacillus subtilis (continued)
    genetic markers, designation of, **04:** 686-698
    morphogenetic markers, **04:** 699-701
    restriction and modification enzymes in several strains, recognition sequences for, **04:** 532-534
    revised linkage map, **04:** 686
    ribosomal RNA from, nucleotide composition, **04:** 409
    standard media for growth of, **04:** 649
Backusia
    G + C composition of DNA of, table arranged by specie, **04:** 189
Bacteria
    amino acid requirements for growth, table, **04:** 630
    G + C composition of DNA of, table, arranged by family, genera, specie, **04:** 69-183
    nearest neighbor frequencies, in DNA from various, **04:** 314-315
Bacteria, glycolipids of, structures and organisms, **05:** 373-393
Bacteria, gram-negative, lipopolysaccharides of
    sugar composition, **05:** 396-402
    sugar sequences, general structure, **05:** 403-412
Bacterial phages
    deoxyribonucleic acids from, purine and pyrimidine distribution in, **04:** 276-278
Bacterial protease, *see* Microbial metalloenzyme
Bacteriochlorophyll
    UV spectra, formula, molecular weight, **08:** 159
Bacteriochlorophyll-protein complex
    amino acid composition, complete data, **07:** 505
Bacteriocin DF_{13}, origin, structure, and characteristic as protein biosynthesis inhibitor, **04:** 561
Bacteriophage lambda (λ)
    Escherichia coli, genetic and molecular map, **04:** 678
Bacteriophage protein
    amino acid sequence of coat proteins, **07:** 261-262
    circular dichroism in the UV region, **07:** 86
    optical rotatory dispersion
        UV region, **07:** 48
        visible and near UV regions, **07:** 18
Bacteriophage T4
    genes
        gene product, **04:** 665-673
        molecular weight, **04:** 665-673
        mutant defect or function, **04:** 665-673
        restrictive host, **04:** 665-673
    linkage map, **04:** 664
Bacteriophage types
    viral DNA
        nucleotide sequences, **04:** 350-351
    viral RNA
        nucleotide sequences and models, **04:** 337-344
    virus-induced RNA
        nucleotide sequences and models, **04:** 346-348
Bacteriophages
    DNA content per cell for various, table, **04:** 307-308
Bacterium
    amino acid requirements for growth, table, **04:** 632
    G + C composition of DNA of, table arranged by specie, **04:** 105

Bacteroidaceae
    G + C composition of DNA of, table arranged by genera and specie, **04:** 86-87
Bacteroides
    amino acid requirements for growth, table, **04:** 632
    G + C composition of DNA of, table arranged by specie, **04:** 86-87
Baikiain
    physical and chemical properties, **01:** 137
Bamicetin, physicochemical constants, spectral, chemotherapeutic and biological properties, **03:** 301
Bamicetin; origin, structure, and characteristic as protein biosynthesis inhibitor, **04:** 561
Barbitol buffer, preparation of, **06:** 375
Barbiturates, ligands binding to plasma albumin, **02:** 569
Barbituric acid
    chemical structures and approved numbering schemes, **08:** 224
    pK'_a values, **06:** 330
Barbituric acid derivatives
    heat of proton ionization, pK, and related thermodynamic quantities, **06:** 171-172
Bases
    alkyl, UV spectral characteristics and pK_a values, **03:** 409-416
    commercial strength, table of concentration data, **06:** 384
    osmometry coefficients, vapor phase, **03:** 528-529
    pK'_a values, **06:** 307-348
    symbols for, use of, **03:** 8, **04:** 8
    UV spectra of unmodified, **03:** 420-447
Basic amino acid permease
    Neurospora crassa mutant, **04:** 755
Basic brain protein
    amino acid composition, incomplete data, **07:** 512
Basic plasma protein
    amino acid composition, complete data, **07:** 505
Basidiobolus
    amino acid requirements for growth, table, **04:** 640
    G + C composition of DNA of, table arranged by specie, **04:** 189
Bdellovibrio
    G + C composition of DNA of, table arranged by specie, **04:** 166
Beauveria
    G + C composition of DNA of, table arranged by specie, **04:** 189
Beckman rotors, construction data for isokinetic sucrose and glycerol gradients, **06:** 432-464
Bee venom protein
    amino acid sequences, **07:** 498
Beeswax fractions, composition of acids of, **05:** 504
Beijerinckia
    G + C composition of DNA of, table arranged by specie, **04:** 81
Bence-Jones protein
    circular dichroism in the UV region, **07:** 86
    optical rotatory dispersion
        UV region, **07:** 49
        visible and near UV regions, **07:** 18
Benzaldehyde derivatives, heat of proton ionization, pK, and related thermodynamic quantities, **06:** 172

Benzene derivatives, heat of proton ionization, pK, and related thermodynamic quantities, **06:** 172

Benzoic acid
pK'_a values, **06:** 313

Benzoic acid derivatives
heat of proton ionization, pK, and related thermodynamic quantities, **06:** 176-181

β-(2-Benzothienyl)alanine
antagonism to tryptophan, **01:** 179

S-Benzyl-β-mercaptopyruvic acid, properties of, **01:** 182

N-Benzylglutamine
antagonism to glutamine, **01:** 177

(α-Benzyl)phenylalanine
structure and symbols for those incorporated into synthetic polypeptides, **01:** 100

3-Benzyltyrosine
structure and symbols for those incorporated into synthetic polypeptides, **01:** 100

Berninamycin; origin, structure, and characteristic as protein biosynthesis inhibitor, **04:** 562

Betaine of thiol histidine, *see* Ergothionine

Betonicine
physical and chemical properties, **01:** 161

Bibliographic references in biochemical journals to CEBJ recommendations, **06:** 58

Bibliographic references in biochemical journals, CEBJ recommendations, **01:** 17-20, **02:** 17-20, **03:** 59-62, **04:** 59-62, **05:** 14-17, **08:** 58-61

Bifidobacterium
G + C composition of DNA of, table arranged by specie, **04:** 75, 115

Bile acids, structures and properties, **05:** 534-535

Bile pigments
pK'_a values, **06:** 348

Bile pigments, UV spectra and formulas, **08:** 169

Bilirubin
UV spectra, formula, molecular weight, **08:** 179

Binding sites, number of, for purified lectins, **02:** 547-551

Bio-Gel A® filtration media, table of properties, **08:** 130

Bio-Gel P® filtration media, table of properties, **08:** 131-132

Biochemical nomenclature, *see* Nomenclature, biochemical

Biochemical pathways, chart of, **04:** insert

Biosynthesis
prostaglandins, pathways diagram, **08:** 317
prostaglandins, properties of intermediates, thromboxanes and by-products, **08:** 332-341

Biotin
biological characteristics, **08:** 302
properties of, **08:** 293

Biotin carboxyl carrier protein
average hydrophobicity value, **01:** 215

Bird egg whites
proteinase inhibitors from, specificities and properties, **02:** 624-629

Birds
DNA content per cell for various, table, **04:** 300-301

satellite DNAs
buoyant density and G + C content of, table, **04:** 390-391

2,2'-Bis(3-hydroxymethylbut-2-enyl)ϵ-carotene
UV spectra, formula, molecular weight, **08:** 188

Bispora
G + C composition of DNA of, table arranged by specie, **04:** 189

Bispyridine ferroprotoporphyrin IX, *see* Pyridine hemochromogen
UV spectra, formula, molecular weight, **08:** 173

β,β-bis(Trifluoromethyl)alanine, *see* γ_6-Hexafluorovaline

Bjerkandera
G + C composition of DNA of, table arranged by specie, **04:** 189

Blakesleea
G + C composition of DNA of, table arranged by specie, **04:** 189

Blasticidin S, physicochemical constants, spectral, chemotherapeutic and biological properties, **03:** 303

Blasticidin S; origin, structure, and characteristic as protein biosynthesis inhibitor, **04:** 562

Blastocladiales
amino acid requirements for growth, table, **04:** 640

Blastocladiella
G + C composition of DNA of, table arranged by specie, **04:** 189

Blastocrithidia
G + C composition of DNA of, table arranged by specie, **04:** 228

Blastokinin
average hydrophobicity value, **01:** 215

Blood, mammalian and chicken
proteinase inhibitors from, specificity and properties, **02:** 636-641

Blood clotting factors
amino acid sequences, **07:** 350-354

Blood coagulation factors, nomenclature, **02:** 195

Blood coagulation protein
table of data and characteristics, **02:** 254-255

Blood plasma, *see also* Human plasma; Plasma
fibrin stabilizing factor system of, **02:** 670
free amino acid content, newborn infants and adults, table, **01:** 328

Blood proteins, human, demonstrating quantitative abnormality, **04:** 881

Blue copper proteins
resonance raman spectra, **07:** 589

Bluensomycin; origin, structure, and characteristic as protein biosynthesis inhibitor, **04:** 563

Boat conformation in stereochemistry, **01:** 42-43, **02:** 42-43, **04:** 34-35, **06:** 41, **08:** 41-42

Boiling point, fatty acids, **05:** 484-490

Bond angle
RNA molecules, values for two fragments, **04:** 465-468
standard polynucleotide double helices, **04:** 411-415

Bond angles
amino acid side chains, amino acid group, peptide linkage, **02:** 742-758

Bond angles, sugar unit, **05:** 472

Bond angles and distances
amino acid group, **08:** 222

Bond angles and distances *(continued)*
    amino acid side chains values for several, **08:** 222-223
    elements having biochemical importance, values for, **08:** 221
    peptide linkage, **08:** 222
    purines and pyrimidines, **08:** 224-227
Bond lengths
    amino acid side chains, amino acid group, peptide linkage, **02:** 742-758
    RNA molecules, values for two fragments, **04:** 465-468
    standard polynucleotide double helices, **04:** 411-415
Bond lengths, sugar unit, **05:** 472
Borax-NaOH buffer, preparation of, **06:** 376
Bordetella
    amino acid requirements for growth, table, **04:** 632
    G + C composition of DNA of, table arranged by specie, **04:** 91
Boric acid-borax buffer, preparation of, **06:** 376
Boric acid, heat of proton ionization, pK, related thermodynamic quantities, **06:** 182
Borrelia
    G + C composition of DNA of, table arranged by specie, **04:** 180
Borrelidin; origin, structure, and characteristic as protein biosynthesis inhibitor, **04:** 563
Botrytis
    G + C composition of DNA of, table arranged by specie, **04:** 190
Bottromycin A$_2$; origin, structure, and characteristic as protein biosynthesis inhibitor, **04:** 563
Bovine α thrombin A chain
    alignment of amino acid sequences homologous to, **07:** 342-343
Bovista
    G + C composition of DNA of, table arranged by specie, **04:** 190
Bowman-Birk inhibitor
    legume sources, specificity and properties, **02:** 588-589
    plant sources, amino acid composition, **02:** 606
Bradykinin group
    amino acid sequence, physical and biological properties, **07:** 222-235
Bradykininogen
    amino acid composition, incomplete data, **07:** 512
    average hydrophobicity value, **01:** 215
Brain
    molar absorptivity and-or absorbance values, **02:** 399
Brain acidic protein (S-100--)
    optical rotatory dispersion in the UV region, **07:** 49
Brain proteolipid protein
    optical rotatory dispersion
        UV region, **07:** 49
        visible and near UV regions, **07:** 19
Bredinin, physicochemical constants, spectral, chemotherapeutic and biological properties, **03:** 305
Brettanomyces
    G + C composition of DNA of, table arranged by specie, **04:** 190
Brevibacteriaceae
    G + C composition of DNA of, table arranged by genera and specie, **04:** 87-89

Brevibacterium
    G + C composition of DNA of, table arranged by specie, **04:** 87-89
Bromelain
    amino acid sequence, **07:** 356-357
    carbohydrate content, **02:** 274
    circular dichroism
        UV and near-UV region, **07:** 86, 144
    molar absorptivity and-or absorbance values, **02:** 399
    optical rotatory dispersion
        UV region, **07:** 49
        visible and near UV regions, **07:** 19
Bromophenylalanines
    antagonism to phenylalanine, **01:** 179
5-Bromouridine
    molal activity coefficients, **03:** 529
    molal osmotic coefficients, **03:** 528
Brucella
    amino acid requirements for growth, table, **04:** 632
    G + C composition of DNA of, table arranged by specie, **04:** 91
Brucellaceae
    G + C composition of DNA of, table arranged by genera and specie, **04:** 89-93
Bryamycin; origin, structure, and characteristic as protein biosynthesis inhibitor, **04:** 564
Bufanolide
    steroid nomenclature, use of term in, **05:** 65-66
Buffer solutions
    amine types, table of structures and pK_a values, **06:** 368-369
    enzyme studies, preparation of buffers for, **06:** 370-377
    equilibrium data measurement, recommendations, **06:** 95
    histochemical studies, preparation of buffers for, **06:** 370-377
    pH values at varying temperatures for several, **06:** 360-361
    preparation data for several, **06:** 358-359
    preparation instructions for several, **06:** 362-363
    protonic activity for several, **06:** 529-539
    standard primary, pH values and preparation, **06:** 354-355
α-Bungarotoxin
    average hydrophobicity value, **01:** 215
    circular dichroism in near-UV region, at room temperature, **07:** 145
β-Bungarotoxin
    circular dichroism in near-UV region, at room temperature, **07:** 145
Buoyant density
    calculation of GC composition from, **04:** 356
    DNA
        chloroplast, table of values, **04:** 356-358
        nuclear, table of values, **04:** 356-358
    DNA, cellular, values for several, **03:** 565-566
    DNA, T-even coliphage, **03:** 568
    DNA, viral, **03:** 560-562, 566-567
    nucleic acids, **03:** 565-566
    polynucleotides, **03:** 565-566
    polynucleotides, synthetic, **03:** 571-573
    ribosomes, from various sources, **04:** 472

Buoyant density *(continued)*
  RNA, viral, in the Cs_2SO_4 gradient, **03**: 569
  satellite DNAs
    amphibia, **04**: 389-390
    birds, **04**: 390-391
    crustaceae, **04**: 384-387
    insects, **04**: 380-384
    mammals, **04**: 391-399
    molluscs, **04**: 387
    plants, **04**: 399-402
    tunicates, **04**: 388
Butane derivatives
  heat of proton ionization, pK, and related thermodynamic quantities, **06**: 183
Butanoic acid derivatives
  heat of proton ionization, pK, and related thermodynamic quantities, **06**: 184-185
O-Butylhomoserine
  physical and chemical properties, **01**: 124
Butyric acid
  amino acid requirements for growth, table, **04**: 632
γ-Butyrobetaine
  physical and chemical properties, **01**: 161
Byssochlamys
  G + C composition of DNA of, table arranged by specie, **04**: 190

C

C3a Anaphylatoxin
  circular dichroism in the UV region, **07**: 84
C5a Anaphylatoxin
  circular dichroism in the UV region, **07**: 84
Cacodylate buffer
  preparation of, **06**: 373
  protonic activity tables, **06**: 529-539
Caffeine
  pK'_a values, **06**: 333
Caffeine, ligands binding to plasma albumin, **02**: 573
Calciferol, *see also* Vitamin D
  properties, **08**: 286
  UV spectra, formula, molecular weight, **08**: 152
Calcitonin
  average hydrophobicity value, **01**: 215
  molar absorptivity and-or absorbance values, **02**: 399
Calcitonins
  amino acid sequence, **07**: 383
Calcium-binding protein
  average hydrophobicity value, **01**: 215
  circular dichroism
    in UV and near-UV regions, **07**: 86, 145
Calcium-binding protein (high affinity)
  amino acid composition, incomplete data, **07**: 512
  circular dichroism in the UV region, **07**: 87
Calcium precipitable protein
  circular dichroism in the UV region, **07**: 87
Calibration techniques for optical instruments, **06**: 390-392
Calorimetry
  macromolecules, conformational changes of, ΔH values, **06**: 270-293

Calsequestrin
  circular dichroism in the UV region, **07**: 87
Canaline
  antagonism to ornithine, **01**: 178
  physical and chemical properties, **01**: 120
Canavanine
  antagonism to arginine, **01**: 177
  physical and chemical properties, **01**: 132
Canavanosuccinic acid
  physical and chemical properties, **01**: 132
Candida
  G + C composition of DNA of, table arranged by specie, **04**: 190-191
Canthaxanthin
  UV spectra, formula, molecular weight, **08**: 190
Carbamate kinase
  amino acid composition, complete data, **07**: 505
N-Carbamoyl-2-(*p*-hydroxyphenyl) glycine
  physical and chemical properties, **01**: 137
Carbamoylglycine, *see* Hydantoic acid
Carbamoylphosphate synthase
  molar absorptivity and-or absorbance values, **02**: 400
  subunit, constitution of, **02**: 345
O-Carbamyl-D-serine
  antagonism to *D*-Alanine, **01**: 177
  physical and chemical properties, **01**: 165
Carbamyl phosphate synthetase
  average hydrophobicity value, **01**: 215
S-Carbamylcysteine
  antagonism to glutamine, **01**: 177
O-Carbamylserine
  antagonism to glutamine, **01**: 177
Carbamyltaurine
  physical and chemical properties, **01**: 152
O-Carbazylserine
  antagonism to glutamine, **01**: 177
Carbocycles, fundamental, IUPAC rules for nomenclature, **05**: 60-64
Carbohydrate-amino acid linkages found in mammalian glycoproteins, **05**: 281
Carbohydrate-protein linkages, types, **02**: 257
Carbohydrate composition
  proteinase inhibitors, table of selected, **02**: 666-667
  Tamm-Horsfall glycoprotein, **02**: 303
Carbohydrate content
  glycoproteins
    blood group substances, table, **02**: 262-263
    body fluids, **02**: 267
    cell membrane, **02**: 266
    eggs, table of values, **02**: 268-269
    enzymes, table of values, **02**: 273-274
    hormones, table of values, **02**: 271-272
    milk, table of values, **02**: 268-269
    mucins, table, **02**: 262-263
    plants, table of values, **02**: 270
    plasma, human, table of values, **02**: 258
    plasma, nonhuman, table of values, **02**: 259-260
    tissues, table of values, **02**: 264-265
    viruses, enveloped, **02**: 267
  lectins, purified, table of values, **02**: 546-551
  proteinase inhibitors
    animal sources, **02**: 618-641

5-Carboxymethyluridine
  isolation and detection of, in RNA, general remarks, **03**: 241-242
  RNA, various, natural occurrence in, **03**: 230
Carboxypeptidase
  molar absorptivity and-or absorbance values, **02**: 402
  molecular weights, stoichiometry and sources, **02**: 284
Carboxypeptidase A
  amino acid composition, complete data, **07**: 505
  amino acid sequence, **07**: 338-339
  average hydrophobicity values, **01**: 216
  circular dichroism
    in UV and near-UV region, **07**: 87, 146
  cyanogen bromide cleavage, **02**: 199
  enzymatic hydrolysis of proteins, **02**: 209
  luminescence of, table, **01**: 205
  molar absorptivity and-or absorbance values, **02**: 402
  molecular weights, stoichiometry and sources, **02**: 283
  optical rotatory dispersion
    UV region, **07**: 50
    visible and near UV regions, **07**: 19
  structure, drawing of, **02**: 763
Carboxypeptidase B
  amino acid sequence, **07**: 338-339
  circular dichroism
    UV and near-UV region, **07**: 88, 146
Carboxypeptidase B, average hydrophobicity values, **01**: 216
Carboxypeptidase Y, average hydrophobicity value, **01**: 216
m-Carboxyphenyl-glycine
  physical and chemical properties, **01**: 165
m-Carboxyphenylalanine
  physical and chemical properties, **01**: 129
S-(2-Carboxypropyl)-cysteine
  physical and chemical properties, **01**: 152
β-(6-Carboxypyran-5-yl) alanine, *see* Stizolobic acid
Carboxytransphosphorylase
  average hydrophobicity value, **01**: 216
m-Carboxytyrosine, *see* 3-Carboxy-4-hydroxy-phenylalanine
Carcinogen-binding protein
  amino acid composition, incomplete data, **07**: 512
Cardanolide
  steroid nomenclature, use of term, **05**: 64-65
Cardiac glycosides, ligands binding to plasma albumin, **02**: 572
Carnitine
  physical and chemical properties, **01**: 161
Carnitine acetyltransferase
  optical rotatory dispersion
    UV region, **07**: 50
    visible and near UV regions, **07**: 19
Carnosine
  carnosinemia, effect of, **01**: 317
  imidazole aminoaciduria, effect of, **01**: 317
Carnosinemia
  characteristics of, **01**: 317
β-Carotene, *see also* Carotenoids
  properties, **08**: 286
  UV spectra, formula, molecular weight, **08**: 192

Carotenoids
  definition, **06**: 63, **08**: 63
  naturally-occurring, trivial names and structures, **06**: 74-90
  naturally occurring, trivial names and structures, **08**: 74-90
  nomenclature rules, **06**: 63-90, **08**: 63-90
Casein
  carbohydrate content, **02**: 268, 269
  molar absorptivity and-or absorbance values, **02**: 403
  optical rotatory dispersion
    UV region, **07**: 50
    visible and near UV regions, **07**: 19
α$_s$-Casein
  circular dichroism in the UV region; extrema between 185 and 250 NM^3, **07**: 88
β-Casein
  refractive index increments, **02**: 374
K-Casein component A
  amino acid composition, complete data, **07**: 505
α$_{S1,2}$-Caseins
  refractive index increments, **02**: 374
Cat
  deoxynucleotide polymerizing enzymes from, properties of, **04**: 539-544
Catalase
  amino acid composition, complete data, **07**: 506
  amino acid sequences of proteins, **07**: 308
  average hydrophobicity value, **01**: 216
  circular dichroism
    UV and near-UV region, **07**: 88, 146
  enzymatic activity, subcellular fractions, **02**: 699, 710
  molar absorptivity and-or absorbance values, **02**: 403
  optical rotatory dispersion
    UV region, **07**: 50
    visible and near UV regions, **07**: 20
  subunit, constitution of, **02**: 343
Catechol 2,3-dioxygenase
  amino acid composition, complete data, **07**: 508
  circular dichroism in the UV region, **07**: 88
  optical rotatory dispersion
    UV region, **07**: 50
    visible and near UV regions, **07**: 20
Catechol 2,3-dioxygenase (*meta*-pyrocatechase)
  circular dichroism in near-UV region, at room temperature, **07**: 146
Catechol 1,2-dioxygenase (pyrocatechase)
  amino acid composition, complete data, **07**: 509
  circular dichroism
    UV and near-UV region, **07**: 88, 146
  optical rotatory dispersion in the UV region, **07**: 50
Catenabacterium
  G + C composition of DNA of, table arranged by specie, **04**: 115
Catenulin, *see* Paromomycin
Caulobacter
  G + C composition of DNA of, table arranged by specie, **04**: 95
Caulobacteriaceae
  G + C composition of DNA of, table arranged by genera and specie, **04**: 95
CD, *see* Circular dichroism

CDP, *see* Cytidylic acid

Celesticetin; origin, structure, and characteristic as protein biosynthesis inhibitor, **04**: 564

Cell and cell constituents, range of weights, **08**: 424

K-cells
immunological response, **07**: 537

Cells for optical measurements, determination of path length, **06**: 391

Cellulase
amino acid composition, complete data, **07**: 506
circular dichroism in the UV region, **07**: 88
molar absorptivity and-or absorbance values, **02**: 404

Cellulomonas
G + C composition of DNA of, table arranged by specie, **04**: 99

Cellulosic ion exchanges, properties, **08**: 136-138

Centrifugation
density gradient, centrifugal force chart for rotors, **08**: 433
ultracentrifuge centerpiece materials, chemical resistence, **08**: 428-430
ultracentrifuge tubes, chemical resistence of, **08**: 434

Centrifugation, density gradient
isokinetic gradients, calculations and techniques for construction, **06**: 426-431
isokinetic gradients, sucrose and glycerol, data for construction
Beckman rotors, **06**: 432-464
Christ rotors, **06**: 465-479
geometrical parameters used in calculations, **06**: 428
International rotors, **06**: 480-488
MSE rotors, **06**: 489-518

Cenuloplasmin
molecular parameters, **02**: 245

Cephalosporin Pl; origin, structure, and characteristic as protein biosynthesis inhibitor, **04**: 565

Cephalosporinase
circular dichroism, **07**: 88
UV and near-UV region, **07**: 88, 155

Ceramide, generic term usage, **05**: 9

Ceratocystis
G + C composition of DNA of, table arranged by specie, **04**: 192

Cercospora
amino acid requirements for growth, table, **04**: 640
G + C composition of DNA of, table arranged by specie. **04**: 192

Cereal grains, proteinase inhibitors from, specificities and properties, **02**: 598-599

Cerebrocuprein
molar absorptivity and-or absorbance values, **02**: 404

Cerebroside, generic term usage, **05**: 10

Ceriporiopsis
G + C composition of DNA of, table arranged by specie, **04**: 192

Ceruloplasmin
amino acid composition, complete data, **07**: 506
circular dichroism in the UV region, **07**: 88
human
molar absorptivity and-or absorbance values, **02**: 404
molecular weight, stoichiometry and sources, **02**: 281

optical rotatory dispersion
UV region, **07**: 50
visible and near UV regions, **07**: 20

pig
molar absorptivity and-or absorbance values, **02**: 405

plasma, human
carbohydrate content, molecular weights, sedimentation coefficients, **02**: 258

rabbit
molar absorptivity and-or absorbance values, **02**: 405

rat
molar absorptivity and-or absorbance values, **02**: 405

serum, human
subunit, constitution of, **02**: 336

Cesium chloride solution, density values as a function of refractive index, **06**: 419-423

Chaetoceras
G + C composition of DNA of, table arranged by specie, **04**: 224

Chaetocladium
G + C composition of DNA of, table arranged by specie, **04**: 192

Chaetomella

Chaetomium
G + C composition of DNA of, table arranged by specie, **04**: 192-193

Chain conformation angles in polynucleotide double helices, **04**: 416

Chain length composition, herring oils and pilchard oil, **05**: 525

Chain weight
contractile proteins, table of values, **02**: 306

Chains, *see also* Side chains

Chair conformation in stereochemistry, **01**: 42, **02**: 42, **04**: 34, **06**: 41, **08**: 41

Chalcomycin; origin, structure, and characteristic as protein biosynthesis inhibitor, **04**: 565

Chara
G + C composition of DNA of, table arranged by specie, **04**: 224

Chartreusin; origin, structure, and characteristic as protein biosynthesis inhibitor, **04**: 566

Chemical formula, *see* Formula, chemical

Chemical shifts
dinucleoside monophosphates, **03**: 531-532
dinucleotides and oligonucleotides, **03**: 531-532
mononucleotides, data, **03**: 530
nucleosides, **03**: 530-533
polynucleotides, **03**: 533

Chemotherapeutic properties
antibiotics, nucleoside, **03**: 271-393

Chicken
deoxynucleotide polymerizing enzymes from, properties of, **04**: 539-544

Chimpanzee, MHC designation, **04**: 885

Chiral compounds, cyclitol nomenclature, **05**: 98

Chirality
carotenoid nomenclature, **06**: 72
definition and nomenclature rules, **01**: 34-58, **02**: 34-58, **06**: 33
sequence rule, use of, **01**: 61, **02**: 65

Chirality, definition and nomenclature rules, **03:** 26-50, **04:** 26-50, **08:** 33-41, 50-56

Chirality, definitions and nomenclature rules, **05:** 31-55

Chlamydia
  G + C composition of DNA of, table arranged by specie, **04:** 95

Chlamydiaceae
  G + C composition of DNA of, table arranged by genera and specie, **04:** 95

Chlamydobacteriaceae
  G + C composition of DNA of, table arranged by genera and specie, **04:** 95

Chlamydomonas
  G + C composition of DNA of, table arranged by specie, **04:** 224-225

Chloramphenicol
  UV spectra, formula, molecular weight, **08:** 181

Chloramphenicol; origin, structure, and characteristic as protein biosynthesis inhibitor, **04:** 566

Chlorella
  amino acid requirements for growth, table, **04:** 630
  G + C composition of DNA of, table arranged by specie, **04:** 225

Chloridium
  G + C composition of DNA of, table arranged by specie, **04:** 193

Chloroacetate buffer
  protonic activity tables, **06:** 529-539

Chlorobacteriaceae
  G + C composition of DNA of, table arranged by genera and specie, **04:** 96-97

Chlorobium
  G + C composition of DNA of, table arranged by specie, **04:** 96

Chlorobium, C_{555}
  amino acid sequence, **07:** 303

Chlorocruorin
  refractive index increments, **02:** 374

Chlorogonium
  G + C composition of DNA of, table arranged by specie, **04:** 225

δ-Chloroleucine
  antagonism to leucine, **01:** 178

Chloroperoxidase
  amino acid composition, incomplete data, **07:** 512
  carbohydrate content, **02:** 273

(4-Chloro)phenylalanine
  structure and symbols for those incorporated into synthetic polypeptides, **01:** 100

Chlorophenylalanines
  antagonism to phenylalanine, **01:** 179

Chlorophyll
  UV spectra, formula, molecular weight, **08:** 170-171

5-Chloropiperidazine-3-carboxylic acid
  physical and chemical properties, **01:** 159

Chloroplast chromosome, circular
  length and molecular weight, table of values, **04:** 359-360

Chloroplast nucleic acids, *see* Nucleic acid, chloroplast

Chloroplast ribosomal RNA, base composition, table, **04:** 361-362

Chloropseudomonas
  G + C composition of DNA of, table arranged by specie, **04:** 97

Chlortetracycline; origin, structure, and characteristic as protein biosynthesis inhibitor, **04:** 567

Choanephora
  G + C composition of DNA of, table arranged by specie, **04:** 193

Cholchisine-binding protein
  average hydrophobicity value, **01:** 216

Cholecalciferol, properties of, **08:** 287

Cholecystokinin-pancreozymin
  cyanogen bromide cleavage, **02:** 199

Cholesteryl esters, content in various animal tissues, **05:** 519-520

Choline
  biological characteristics, **08:** 302
  properties of, **08:** 294

Choline esterase, *see* Cholinesterase

Choline sulfatase
  Neurospora crassa mutant, **04:** 744

Cholinesterase
  carbohydrate content, **02:** 273
  circular dichroism in the UV region, **07:** 88
  molar absorptivity and-or absorbance values, **02:** 405
  molecular parameters, **02:** 245
  optical rotatory dispersion in the visible and near UV regions, **07:** 20
  subunit, constitution of, **02:** 345

Chondrine
  physical and chemical properties, **01:** 153

Chondrococcus
  G + C composition of DNA of, table arranged by specie, **04:** 145

Chondroitin sulfate
  table of data and characteristics, **02:** 686

Chondromyces
  G + C composition of DNA of, table arranged by specie, **04:** 150-151

Chondrostei, DNA content per cell, **04:** 293

Chordata
  deoxyribonucleic acids from, purine and pyrimidine distribution in, **04:** 268-273
  DNA content per cell for various, table, **04:** 293-305

Chorionic gonadotropin
  amino acid composition, complete data, **07:** 506
  amino acid sequence
    α subunit, **07:** 393-394, 402
    β subunit, **07:** 402
  circular dichroism in the UV region, **07:** 89
  molar absorptivity and-or absorbance values, **02:** 406
  subunit, constitution of, **02:** 327

Chorionic gonadotropin-α
  average hydrophobicity value, **01:** 216

Chorionic gonadotropin-β
  average hydrophobicity value, **01:** 216

Chorionic somatomammotropin
  circular dichroism
    UV and near-UV region, **07:** 89, 147

Chorismate mutase
  molar absorptivity and-or absorbance values, **02:** 406

Chorismate mutase-prephenate dehydratase
average hydrophobicity value, **01:** 216
Chorismic acid synthetase
Neurospora crassa mutant, **04:** 745
Chorismic mutase
Neurospora crassa mutant, **04:** 748
Christ rotors, construction data for isokinetic sucrose and
glycerol gradients, **06:** 465-479
Christmas factor
physical data and characteristics, **02:** 254-255
Chromatium
G + C composition of DNA of, table arranged by specie, **04:** 178-179
Chromatography
aldaric acids, **05:** 168-170
alditols, amino, **05:** 148-149
alditols, natural, **05:** 139-142
aldonic acids, **05:** 153-164
aldoses, natural, **05:** 181-217
amino acids, data tables, **08:** 93-110
peptides, references, **08:** 111
amino sugar acids, **05:** 170-176
antibiotics, nucleoside, **03:** 271-393
Brij 35 detergent, properties of, **08:** 216
gas-liquid
inosamines, **05:** 148-149
inositols, **05:** 142-147
inososes, **05:** 147
ion exchange, amino acids
ninhydrin positive compounds, elution behavior, **08:**
122
thumbprint, constituents of, **08:** 121
urine, resolution of ninhydrin positive constituents, **08:**
114-119
variables, mathematical relationship, **08:** 112-113
ketoses, natural, **05:** 226-239
ninhydrin reactive substances, positions, **08:** 126
porphyrins R_F values in 2,6-lutidine-water systems, **08:**
276
prostaglandin isolation applications, **08:** 344
prostaglandin precursors, isolation and detection, **08:**
327
rapid short column
amino acids related to metabolic diseases, elution
time, **08:** 128-129
uronic acids, **05:** 165-168
Chromobacterium
G + C composition of DNA of, table arranged by specie, **04:** 164
Chromosome, *see also* Haploid chromosome
Chromosome, circular chloroplast; length and molecular
weight, **04:** 359-360
Chromosome numbers, haploid, in fungi, table of values,
04: 874-877
Chymoelastase, guanidine stable
average hydrophobicity value, **01:** 217
Chymoelastase, lysine free
average hydrophobicity value, **01:** 216
Chymopapain-B[5]
amino acid sequence, **07:** 356-357

Chymosin
optical rotatory dispersion
UV region, **07:** 51
visible and near UV regions, **07:** 20
Chymotrypsin
calorimetric ΔH values accompanying conformational
changes, **06:** 274, 275
cyanogen bromide cleavage, **02:** 199
enzymatic hydrolysis, conjugated proteins, **02:** 211
enzymatic hydrolysis of proteins, **02:** 209
molar absorptivity and-or absorbance values, **02:** 406
specificity for hydrolysis of peptide bonds, **02:** 212
α-Chymotrypsin
circular dichroism, **07:** 89
UV and near-UV region, **07:** 89, 147
conformation, schematic drawing of, **02:** 762
luminescence of, table, **01:** 205
molar absorptivity and-or absorbance values, **02:** 406
optical rotatory dispersion
UV region, **07:** 51
visible and near UV regions, **07:** 20
refractive index increments, **02:** 374
Chymotrypsin, anionic
average hydrophobicity value, **01:** 217
Chymotrypsin A
molar absorptivity and-or absorbance values, **02:** 406
Chymotrypsin C
molar absorptivity and-or absorbance values, **02:** 406
Chymotrypsin II
average hydrophobicity value, **01:** 217
Chymotrypsin II, human
molar absorptivity and-or absorbance values, **02:** 406
Chymotrypsin inhibitor
lower animal sources, specificity and properties, **02:**
620-621
Chymotrypsin inhibitor I
subunit, constitution of, **02:** 327
Chymotrypsinogen
calorimetric ΔH values accompanying conformational
changes, **06:** 274-275
circular dichroism in the UV region, **07:** 89
molar absorptivity and-or absorbance values, **02:** 407
optical rotatory dispersion
UV region, **07:** 51
visible and near UV regions, **07:** 20
refractive index increments, **02:** 374
viscosity, intrinsic, **02:** 721
α-Chymotrypsinogen
heat capacity and entropy values, **06:** 110
molar absorptivity and-or absorbance values, **02:** 407
Chymotrypsinogen A
circular dichroism
UV and in near-UV region, **07:** 89, 147
luminescence of, table, **01:** 205
optical rotatory dispersion
UV region, **07:** 51
visible and near UV regions, **07:** 21
Chymotrypsinogen A, B, C
average hydrophobicity value, **01:** 217
molar absorptivity and-or absorbance values, **02:** 407

Chymotrypsinogen B
  optical rotatory dispersion
    UV region, 07: 51
    visible and near UV regions, 07: 21
Chymotryptic hydrolysis
  human globin, α-chains of, 02: 213
  proteins, condition for, 02: 214
Cilia protein, outer fibers
  amino acid composition, complete data, 07: 506
  optical rotatory dispersion in the visible and near UV
    regions, 07: 21
Ciliatine
  physical and chemical properties, 01: 161
Circinella
  G + C composition of DNA of, table arranged by spe-
    cie, 04: 193
Circular dichroic spectra
  nucleoproteins, graph, 06: 393
Circular dichroism
  characteristics of a single aromatic side chain of
    proteins in near-ultraviolet region, Table 1, 07: 142
  definition and formulae, 07: 4
  dinucleotides, graphs, 03: 472-527
  extrema and crossovers for 15 double-helical
    oligoribonucleotides, 03: 595
  extrema and crossovers for synthetic polynucleotides,
    03: 592-595
  intensities for native proteins at maxima in the near-
    ultraviolet region at room temperature, Table 2, 07:
    143-163
  mono- and oligosaccharides, table, 05: 465-468
  of various proteins, spectra, 07: 8-13
  polyribonucleotides, use of table in calculation of, 03:
    591
  polysaccharides, table, 05: 468-470
  reference values, tables, 07: 135-136, 138-139
  spectra
    amino acids, metal complexes of, 01: 245-315
    peptides, metal complexes of, 01: 245-315
    spectra of representative naturally occurring nucleic
      acids, 03: 591
    UV region: extrema between 185 and 250 NM, table,
      07: 82-129
Circular dichroism bands of aromatic amino acids and
    peptides
  in near-ultraviolet regions, discussion, 07: 167
  circular dichroism intensities at maxima in near-UV re-
    gion, at room temperature, table, 07: 163
Circular dichroism parameters
  dinucleoside monophosphates, 2'-O-methylated, 03: 471
  oligonucleotides of DNA, 03: 465-468
  oligonucleotides of RNA, 03: 461-465
Circular dichroism spectrophotometers, modern design of,
    08: 201-202
Circular dichrometers, calibration techniques for, 06: 391
cis,cis-Muconate lactonizing enzyme
  average hydrophobicity value, 01: 227
Citation of bibliographic references in biochemical jour-
    nals, CEBJ recommendations, 01: 17-20, 02: 17-20,
    03: 59-62, 04: 59-62, 05: 14-17, 06: 58, 08: 58-61

Citeromyces
  G + C composition of DNA of, table arranged by spe-
    cie, 04: 193
Citrate-phosphate buffer, preparation of, 06: 372
Citrate (si)-synthase
  circular dichroism in the UV region, 07: 89
  optical rotatory dispersion in the UV region, 07: 51
Citrate buffer, preparation of, 06: 371
Citrate condensing enzyme, see Citrate (si)-synthase
Citrate cycle; pathways chart, 04: insert
Citrate oxaloacetate lyase
  amino acid composition, incomplete data, 07: 512
Citrate synthase, see Citrate (si)-synthase
  molar absorptivity and-or absorbance values, 02: 407
  subunit, constitution of, 02: 333, 343
Citric acid
  heat of proton ionization, pK, and related thermody-
    namic quantities, 06: 188-189
  pK'_a values, 06: 309
Citrinin
  UV spectra, formula, molecular weight, 08: 164
Citrobacter
  G + C composition of DNA of, table arranged by spe-
    cie, 04: 105
Citrulline
  citrullinemia, effect of, 01: 318
  free acid in amniotic fluid in early pregnancy and at
    term, 01: 327
  free acid in blood plasma of newborn infants and
    adults, 01: 328
  physical and chemical properties, 01: 133
  structure and symbols for those incorporated into syn-
    thetic polypeptides, 01: 100
  thumbprint, content in, 08: 121
Citrullinemia
  characteristics of, 01: 318
Cladosporium
  amino acid requirements for growth, table, 04: 640
  G + C composition of DNA of, table arranged by spe-
    cie, 04: 193
Classification, glycolipids, 05: 416-423
Claviceps
  G + C composition of DNA of, table arranged by spe-
    cie, 04: 193
Clavicipitic acid
  physical and chemical properties, 01: 137
Clindamycin; origin, structure, and characteristic as
    protein biosynthesis inhibitor, 04: 567
Clostridiopeptidase B, see Clostridium histolyticum protei-
    nase B
Clostridium
  amino acid requirements for growth, table, 04: 633
  G + C composition of DNA of, table arranged by spe-
    cie, 04: 85-86
Clostripain, see Clostridium histolyticum proteinase B
Clupeine, Pacific herring
  amino acid sequences, 07: 498
CMP
  pK'_a values, 06: 330

Coagulation factors
  plasma, human
    carbohydrate content, molecular weight, sedimentation coefficients, **02:** 258
  plasma, nonhuman
    carbohydrate content, **02:** 260
Coagulation vitamins, properties of, **08:** 290
Coat proteins
  amino acid sequences, **07:** 261
Cobramine B
  amino acid composition, complete data, **07:** 506
Cobrotoxin
  circular dichroism
    UV and near-UV region, **07:** 89, 147
  optical rotatory dispersion in the UV region, **07:** 52
Cocaine
  pK'_a values, **06:** 326
Coccolithus
  G + C composition of DNA of, table arranged by specie, **04:** 225
Cocoonase
  average hydrophobicity value, **01:** 217
  molar absorptivity and-or absorbance values, **02:** 408
Code, genetic, table of codons, **04:** 896
Codeine
  pK'_a values, **06:** 326
Coding, effect of point mutations on, **04:** 894
Codons, genetic code, table, **04:** 896
Codons found in the MS_2 coat protein gene, **04:** 340
Coelenterata
  deoxyribonucleic acids from, purine and pyrimidine distribution in, **04:** 264
  DNA content per cell for various, table, **04:** 290
Coemansia
  G + C composition of DNA of, table arranged by specie, **04:** 194
Coenzyme Q
  nomenclature recommendations, **08:** 9-11
Coenzymes
  abbreviations, use of, **08:** 6
  abbreviations for, use of, **01:** 6, **02:** 6, **03:** 6, **06:** 6
  nomenclature, journal references for, **02:** 87
Coenzymes, use of abbreviations, **05:** 6
Coenzymes, use of abbreviations for, **04:** 6
Coffearin, *see* Trigonelline
Coformycin, physicochemical constants, spectral, chemotherapeutic and biological properties, **03:** 306
Cokeromyces
  G + C composition of DNA of, table arranged by specie, **04:** 194
Colchicine
  pK'_a values, **06:** 326
Colicin E₁
  circular dichroism in the UV region, **07:** 89
Colicin E₂
  circular dichroism in the UV region, **07:** 89
Colicin E₃
  circular dichroism in the UV region, **07:** 89
Colicin E3; origin, structure, and characteristic as protein biosynthesis inhibitor, **04:** 567
Colicin Iₐ-CA53
  average hydrophobicity value, **01:** 217

Colicin I_b-P9
  average hydrophobicity value, **01:** 217
Collagen
  amino acid composition, complete data, **07:** 506
  average hydrophobicity values, **01:** 217
  circular dichroism
    UV and spectra, **07:** 9, 89
  cross-linkage, **07:** 523
  cyanogen bromide cleavage, **02:** 199, 202
  heat capacity and entropy values, **06:** 110
  optical rotatory dispersion
    spectra, **07:** 9
    UV region, **07:** 52
  post-translational enzymes in, **07:** 524
  refractive index increments, **02:** 374
  selected amino acid analysis, **07:** 520-521
  subunit, constitution of, **02:** 342
Collagen chains
  amino acid sequences, **07:** 474-488
Collagenase
  circular dichroism in the UV region, **07:** 90
  enzymatic hydrolysis of proteins, **02:** 209
  molar absorptivity and-or absorbance values, **02:** 408
  optical rotatory dispersion
    UV region, **07:** 52
    visible and near UV regions, **07:** 21
Collagenase, average hydrophobicity values, **01:** 217
Collectotrichum
  amino acid requirements for growth, table, **04:** 640
Colletotrichum
  G + C composition of DNA of, table arranged by specie, **04:** 194
Colpidium
  G + C composition of DNA of, table arranged by specie, **04:** 228
Comamonas
  G + C composition of DNA of, table arranged by specie, **04:** 166
Conalbumin, *see* Ovotransferrin
  average hydrophobicity value, **01:** 217
  carbohydrate content, **02:** 268
  molar absorptivity and-or absorbance values, **02:** 408
  molecular weight, stoichiometry, source, function, **02:** 276
  refractive index increments, **02:** 374
α-Conarachin
  optical rotatory dispersion in the visible and near UV regions, **07:** 21
Concanavalin A
  amino acid composition, complete data, **07:** 506
  circular dichroism
    UV and near-UV region, **07:** 90, 147
  optical rotatory dispersion
    UV region, **07:** 52
    visible and near UV regions, **07:** 21
Concentration dependence
  Lorentz correction factors, values for several compounds, **06:** 396-403
  refractive index, values for several compounds, **06:** 395
  Sellmeier constants, values for several compounds, **06:** 395

Condensing enzyme
  Neurospora crassa mutant, **04**: 749
Configuration
  absolute, for cyclitols, **05**: 97-98
  polypeptide chemistry, use of term, **01**: 73, **02**: 77
  relative, for cyclitols, **05**: 93-94
Conformation
  polypeptide chemistry, use of term, **01**: 73, **02**: 77
  proteins, drawings illustrating, **02**: 760-766
Conformational map, typical, **01**: 67, **02**: 71
Conformer molecule in stereochemistry, **01**: 42-46, **02**: 42-46, **04**: 34-38, **06**: 41, **08**: 41-49
Congenic strains, definition of, **04**: 884
γ-Conglycinin
  circular dichroism in the UV region, **07**: 90
  optical rotatory dispersion
    UV region, **07**: 52
    visible and near UV regions, **07**: 21
Conjugated proteins, *see also* Proteins, conjugated
Conjugates, covalent protein, table of data, **01**: 208
Contractile protein
  molecular parameters, table, **02**: 306
Copolymers of repeating sequence, melting temperatures, **03**: 583-585
Copper phathalocyanine
  UV spectra, formula, molecular weight, **08**: 178
Coprinus
  amino acid requirements for growth, table, **04**: 640
  G + C composition of DNA of, table arranged by specie, **04**: 194
Coprinus radiatus
  mutants, biochemical, map of, **04**: 762
Cordycepin, physicochemical constants, spectral, chemotherapeutic and biological properties, **03**: 308
Corn (Zea mays), *see also* Maize
  deoxyribonucleic acids from, purine and pyrimidine distribution in, **04**: 259
Corrinoid protein
  average hydrophobicity value, **01**: 217
Corrinoids, *see also* Cyanocobalamin, Vitamin B₁₂
  nomenclature, journal references for, **02**: 87
  nomenclature and structures, **08**: 12-17
Corticoids, structures and properties, **05**: 536-538
Corticosteroid-binding globulin
  amino acid composition, complete data, **07**: 506
Corticosteroid-transporting protein
  plasma, nonhuman, carbohydrate content, **02**: 259
Corticotropin
  amino acid sequence, **07**: 385
  luminescence of, table, **01**: 205
Cortisol metabolites binding large protein
  amino acid composition, incomplete data, **07**: 512
Corynebacteriaceae
  G + C composition of DNA of, table arranged by genera and specie, **04**: 97-103
Corynebacterium
  amino acid requirements for growth, table, **04**: 633
  G + C composition of DNA of, table arranged by specie, **04**: 99-103
Cotton effect
  circular dichroism of helix, β and unordered form, spectra, **07**: 5

  definition, **07**: 5
  in UV region, protein conformation, spectra, **07**: 9
  optical rotatory dispersion of helix, β and unordered form, spectra, **07**: 5
Cotton effect, circular dichroism calculations, **03**: 461-465, 470
Coupling constants
  dinucleoside monophosphates, of the H1′ and H2′ protons, **03**: 531-532
  dinucleotides, of the H1′ and H2′ protons, **03**: 531-532
  mononucleotides, of the H1′ and H2′ protons, **03**: 530
  oligonucleotides, of the H1′ and H2′ protons, **03**: 531-532
  polynucleotides, of the H1′ and H2′ protons, **03**: 533
Covalent protein conjugates, *see also* Conjugated proteins; Proteins, covalent conjugates
Covalent radii of common elements, **08**: 221
Cow
  deoxynucleotide polymerizing enzymes from, properties of, **04**: 539-544
Crabs; buoyant density and G + C content of satellite DNAs for several varieties, **04**: 384-387
Creatine
  enthalpy and free energy of formation, **06**: 112
  heat capacity and entropy values, **06**: 110
  heat of combustion, **06**: 112
  pK'_a values, **06**: 318
Creatine kinase
  average hydrophobicity value, **01**: 217
  circular dichroism
    UV and near-UV region, **07**: 90, 148
  molar absorptivity and-or absorbance values, **02**: 409
  optical rotatory dispersion
    UV region, **07**: 52
    visible and near UV regions, **07**: 21
  subunit, constitution of, **02**: 330
Creatine phosphokinase, *see* Creatine, kinase
Creatinine
  enthalpy and free energy of formation, **06**: 112
  heat capacity and entropy values, **06**: 110
  heat of combustion, **06**: 112
Cricosphaera
  G + C composition of DNA of, table arranged by specie, **04**: 225
Crithidia
  amino acid requirements for growth, table, **04**: 641
  G + C composition of DNA of, table arranged by specie, **04**: 228
all-trans-Crocetin dimethyl ester
  UV spectra, formula, molecular weight, **08**: 194
Crotocin (Antibiotic T); origin, structure, and characteristic as protein biosynthesis inhibitor, **04**: 568
Crotocol; origin, structure, and characteristic as protein biosynthesis inhibitor, **04**: 568
Crotonase
  amino acid composition, complete data, **07**: 506
  average hydrophobicity value, **01**: 217
  molar absorptivity and-or absorbance values, **02**: 409
  subunit, constitution of, **02**: 338, 339
Crotonoside
  physical constants and spectral properties, **03**: 99

Crotoxin
average hydrophobicity value, **01:** 217
molar absorptivity and-or absorbance values, **02:** 409
Crotylalanine, *see* 2-Amino-5-heptenoic acid
Crotylglycine, *see* 2-Amino-4-hexenoic acid
Crustaceae, satellite DNAs; buoyant density and G + C
content of,table, **04:** 384-387
β-Crustacyanin
amino acid composition, complete data, **07:** 506
Cryoglobulin
molar absorptivity and-or absorbance values, **02:** 409
refractive index increments, **02:** 374
Cryptococcus
G + C composition of DNA of, table arranged by specie, **04:** 194-195
Cryptopleurine; origin, structure, and characteristic as
protein biosynthesis inhibitor, **04:** 569
Crystallin
molar absorptivity and-or absorbance values, **02:** 410,
411
α-Crystallin
circular dichroism in the UV region, **07:** 90
composite sequence, α chains, **07:** 503
optical rotatory dispersion
UV region, **07:** 52
visible and near UV regions, **07:** 21
variable positions, α chains, **07:** 502
γ-Crystallin
circular dichroism in the UV region, **07:** 90
optical rotatory dispersion in the UV region, **07:** 52
β-Crystallin
amino acid composition, complete data, **07:** 506
Ctenomyces
G + C composition of DNA of, table arranged by specie, **04:** 195
Cucurbitine
physical and chemical properties, **01:** 138
Cunninghamella
G + C composition of DNA of, table arranged by specie, **04:** 195
Cuproproteins
nomenclature rules, **02:** 121
Curvularia
amino acid requirements for growth, table, **04:** 640
G + C composition of DNA of, table arranged by specie, **04:** 196
γ-Cyano-α-aminobutyric acid
physical and chemical properties, **01:** 135
β-Cyanoalanine
physical and chemical properties, **01:** 134
structure and symbols for those incorporated into synthetic polypeptides, **01:** 100
Cyanocobalamin, *see also* Vitamin B$_{12}$
biological characteristics, **08:** 302
nomenclature and structure, **08:** 12-17
properties of, **08:** 294
UV spectra, formula, molecular weight, **08:** 144
N-(2-Cyanoethyl)glycine
structure and symbols for those incorporated into synthetic polypeptides, **01:** 100
Cyanogen bromide cleavage, peptides and proteins, table,
02: 199-202

Cyanomethemoglobin
UV and visible absorption spectra, **07:** 181
Cyanomethemoglobin, ferrihemoglobin cyanide, HiCN
UV spectra, molecular weight, **08:** 172
Cyclic polypeptides, *see* Polypeptides, cyclic, Polypeptides, cyclic
Cyclitol nomenclature
evolution of, **05:** 89-90
IUPAC recommendations, **05:** 91-98
Cyclitols
nomenclature, journal references for, **02:** 87
Cyclo fatty acids, physical and chemical characteristics,
05: 488-489
Cycloallin
physical and chemical properties, **01:** 153
Cyclobutane derivatives, proposals for abbreviations, **03:**
51-53, **04:** 51-53
1,4-Cyclohexadiene-1-alanine, *see*
2,5-Dihydrophenylalanine
β-(1,4-Cyclohexadienyl)alanine
structure and symbols for those incorporated into synthetic polypeptides, **01:** 100
Cyclohexane derivatives
heat of proton ionization, pK, and related thermodynamic quantities, **06:** 190
1-Cyclohexene-1-alanine
antagonism to phenylalanine, **01:** 179
Cycloheximide; origin, structure, and characteristic as
protein biosynthesis inhibitor, **04:** 569
Cyclohexylalanine
antagonism to phenylalanine, **01:** 179
β-(Cyclohexyl)alanine
structure and symbols for those incorporated into synthetic polypeptides, **01:** 100
α-(Cyclohexyl)glycine
structure and symbols for those incorporated into synthetic polypeptides, **01:** 100
β-Cyclohexylpyruvic acid
properties of, **01:** 181
Cycloleucine, *see* 1-Aminocyclopentane-1-carboxylic acid
Cyclonorleucine, *see* 1-Aminocyclohexane-1-carboxylic
acid
1-Cyclopentene-1-alanine
antagonism to phenylalanine, **01:** 179
3-Cyclopentene-1-alanine
antagonism to leucine, **01:** 178
2-Cyclopentene-1-glycine
antagonism to isoleucine, **01:** 178
3-Cyclopentene-1-glycine
antagonism to isoleucine, **01:** 178
Cyclopentene alanine
antagonism to leucine, **01:** 178
Cyclopentene glycine
antagonism to leucine, **01:** 178
β-(Cyclopentyl)alanine
structure and symbols for those incorporated into synthetic polypeptides, **01:** 101
α-(Cyclopentyl)glycine
structure and symbols for those incorporated into synthetic polypeptides, **01:** 101
D-Cycloserine
antagonism to *D*-Alanine, **01:** 177

D-Cycloserine *(continued)*
physical and chemical properties, **01**: 165
Cyclotella
G + C composition of DNA of, table arranged by specie, **04**: 225
Cylindrocephalum
G + C composition of DNA of, table arranged by specie, **04**: 196
Cylindrotheca
G + C composition of DNA of, table arranged by specie, **04**: 225
Cystathionase
amino acid composition, complete data, **07**: 506
average hydrophobicity value, **01**: 217
Cystathionase II
Neurospora crassa mutant, **04**: 749
Cystathionine
cystathioninuria, effect of, **01**: 318
Cystathionine S-(2-amino-2-carboxyethylhomocysteine)
physical and chemical properties, **01**: 151
Cystathionine γ-synthetase
amino acid composition, complete data, **07**: 506
Cystathioninuria
characteristics of, **01**: 318
Cysteamine to hypotaurine enzyme
amino acid composition, complete data, **07**: 506
Cysteic acid
antagonism to aspartic acid, **01**: 177
free acid in amniotic fluid in early pregnancy and at term, **01**: 327
physical and chemical properties, **01**: 153
Cysteine
active site peptides, **07**: 187
antagonists of, **01**: 177
far ultraviolet absorption spectra
aqueous solution at pH 5, **01**: 184
neutral water, table, **01**: 185
0.1 M sodium dodecyl sulfate, table, **01**: 185
heat of proton ionization, pK, and related thermodynamic quantities, **06**: 191
molar extinctions, **01**: 185
nucleoside composition, tables of values, **04**: 429
nucleotide sequences of, **04**: 442-443
pK'_a values, **06**: 318, 346
physical and chemical properties, **01**: 153
requirements of, for growth of various microorganisms, table, **04**: 630-643
symbols for atoms and bonds in side chains, **01**: 69, **02**: 73
UV spectra of, **01**: 197
Cysteine β 93 SH
pK values in human hemoglobin, **02**: 696
Cysteine desulfyhydrase
molar absorptivity and-or absorbance values, **02**: 412
subunit, constitution of, **02**: 342
Cysteine sulfinic acid
physical and chemical properties, **01**: 153
Cysteine synthase
molar absorptivity and-or absorbance values, **02**: 412
Cysteine synthetase
subunit, constitution of, **02**: 345

Cystine
antagonism to α,ε-Diaminopimelic acid, **01**: 177
cystinosis, nephropathic, effect of, **01**: 318
destruction of, during acid hydrolysis, **02**: 206
N,N'-diacetyl-L-cystine dimethyl ester, UV spectra of, **01**: 199
free acid in amniotic fluid in early pregnancy and at term, **01**: 327
free acid in blood plasma of newborn infants and adults, **01**: 328
pK'_a values, **06**: 318
physical and chemical properties, **01**: 153
requirements of, for growth of various microorganisms, table, **04**: 630-643
spectra, far UV, **01**: 184
symbols for atoms and bonds in side chains, **01**: 69, **02**: 73
thumbprint, content in, **08**: 121
UV absorption characteristics, **01**: 186
UV spectra of, **01**: 198
½Cystine
far ultraviolet absorption spectra
aqueous solution at pH 5, **01**: 184
neutral water, table, **01**: 185
0.1 M sodium dodecyl sulfate, table, **01**: 185
molar extinctions, **01**: 185
Cystine derivatives
heat of proton ionization, pK, and related thermodynamic quantities, **06**: 191
Cystine disulfoxide
physical and chemical properties, **01**: 153
Cystinosis, nephropathic
characteristics of, **01**: 318
Cystinuria, isolated
characteristics of, **01**: 323
Cystinuria type I
characteristics of, **01**: 323
Cystinuria type II
characteristics of, **01**: 323
Cystinuria type III
characteristics of, **01**: 323
Cystinyl compounds
longest wavelength disulfide circular dichroism band, **07**: 173
Cystoseira
G + C composition of DNA of, table arranged by specie, **04**: 225
Cytidine
bond angles and distances, **08**: 224
chemical structures and approved numbering schemes, **08**: 224
composition in various tRNA's, **04**: 428-441
molal activity coefficients, **03**: 529
molal osmotic coefficients, **03**: 528
pK'_a values, **06**: 330, 339
raman frequencies, table of values, **03**: 540-541
Cytidine and derivatives
UV spectra, **03**: 440-443
UV spectral characteristics and acid dissociation constants, **03**: 414-415

Cytidine and nucleoside derivatives
physical constants and spectral properties, index to, **03:** 70
Cytidine derivatives
heat of proton ionization, pK, and related thermodynamic quantities, **06:** 191
Cytidine nucleotide derivatives
physical constants and spectral properties, index to, **03:** 73
Cytidylic acid
derivatives, UV spectral characteristics and acid dissociation constants, **03:** 416
Cytisine
pK'_a values, **06:** 326
Cytochrome
average hydrophobicity values, **01:** 217-218
Cytochrome b
amino acid composition, complete data, **07:** 506
molar absorptivity and-or absorbance values, **02:** 412
Cytochrome b_2, *see* Lactate dehydrogenase (cytochrome b_2)
enzymatic activity, subcellular fractions, **02:** 707
subunit, constitution of, **02:** 343
Cytochrome b_5
circular dichroism
UV and near-UV region, **07:** 91, 148
optical rotatory dispersion
UV region, **07:** 53
visible and near UV regions, **07:** 22
Cytochrome b_{563}
circular dichroism
UV and near-UV region, **07:** 91, 148
Cytochrome c, *see also* Eukaryotic cytochromes c
amino acid composition, complete data, **07:** 506
amino acid sequence, **07:** 304-306
circular dichroism
UV and near-UV region, **07:** 91, 148
cyanogen bromide cleavage, **02:** 199
enzymatic activity, subcellular fractions, **02:** 702
molar absorptivity and-or absorbance values, **02:** 413
optical rotatory dispersion in the UV region, **07:** 53
Cytochrome c_A
circular dichroism in the UV region, **07:** 92
optical rotatory dispersion in the UV region, **07:** 53
Cytochrome c_1
circular dichroism
UV and near-UV region, **07:** 93, 150
molar absorptivity and-or absorbance values, **02:** 414
Cytochrome c_2
amino acid sequence, **07:** 294-298
cyanogen bromide cleavage, **02:** 199
molar absorptivity and-or absorbance values, **02:** 414
Cytochrome c_3
amino acid sequence, **07:** 299-301
optical rotatory dispersion in the UV region, **07:** 53
Cytochrome c_4
amino acid sequence, **07:** 301
Cytochrome c_5
amino acid sequence, **07:** 302
Cytochrome c_{550}
molar absorptivity and-or absorbance values, **02:** 414

Cytochrome c_{551}
cyanogen bromide cleavage, **02:** 199
molar absorptivity and-or absorbance values, **02:** 415
Cytochrome c_{552}
molar absorptivity and-or absorbance values, **02:** 415
Cytochrome c_7
amino acid sequence, **07:** 299-301
Cytochrome f
amino acid sequence, **07:** 304
Cytochrome p_{450}
optical rotatory dispersion in the UV region, **07:** 53
Cytochrome c, Fe^{+++}
circular dichroism in the UV region, **07:** 92
Cytochrome c oxidase
circular dichroism in the UV region, **07:** 93
optical rotatory dispersion in the UV region, **07:** 54
Cytochrome c peroxidase
molar absorptivity and-or absorbance values, **02:** 417
Cytochrome c
calorimetric ΔH values accompanying conformational changes, **06:** 275
Cytochrome oxidase, *see* Cytochrome c, oxidase
molar absorptivity and-or absorbance values, **02:** 417
subunit, constitution of, **02:** 340
table of cofactors, molecular weights, stoichiometry and sources, **02:** 283
Cytochromes
definition and nomenclature, **02:** 116-120
list of, **02:** 119
oxidation-reduction potentials, **06:** 132-137
Cytochromes in animals
molecular turnover, table, **07:** 559
Cytocuprein
apocytocuprein, human
molar absorptivity and-or absorbance values, **02:** 417
molar absorptivity and-or absorbance values, **02:** 417
Cytomycin, physicochemical constants, spectral, chemotherapeutic and biological properties, **03:** 310
Cytophaga
G + C composition of DNA of, table arranged by specie, **04:** 103-104
Cytophagaceae
G + C composition of DNA of, table arranged by genera and specie, **04:** 103-104
Cytoplasmic ribosomal RNA, base composition, table, **04:** 361-362
Cytosine
heat of proton ionization, pK, and related thermodynamic quantities, **06:** 191
pK'_a values, **06:** 330, 339
Cytosine and derivatives
physical constants and spectral properties, index to, **03:** 67
UV spectra, **03:** 427-428
UV spectral characteristics and acid dissociation constants, **03:** 412
Cytotoxins
amino acid sequences, **07:** 370-373
from venom of various snakes, **07:** 370-373
Cytovirin, physicochemical constants, spectral, chemotherapeutic and biological properties, **03:** 311

D

Dactylium
   G + C composition of DNA of, table arranged by specie, **04:** 196

Dactylosporangium
   G + C composition of DNA of, table arranged by specie, **04:** 77

Daedalea
   G + C composition of DNA of, table arranged by specie, **04:** 196

Dansyl
   covalent protein conjugates, data, **01:** 208

Danunorubicin reductase
   average hydrophobicity value, **01:** 218

Data, equilibrium, measurement and presentation, **06:** 93-106

Davis's minimal medium, preparation of, **04:** 649

DD-Carboxypeptidase-transpeptidase
   circular dichroism in near-UV region, at room temperature, **07:** 146

Debaryomyces
   G + C composition of DNA of, table arranged by specie, **04:** 196

Decarboxylation
   free energy values for several compounds, **06:** 303

Decarboxylation of α-Keto acids
   yeast decarboxylase, by, **01:** 181

Decoylnine, physicochemical constants, spectral, chemotherapeutic and biological properties, **03:** 312

Deferrichrysin
   proton NMR and suggested conformations, **07:** 567-568

Dehydroalanine
   structure and properties, **01:** 175

ω-Dehydroalloisoleucine
   antagonism to valine, **01:** 180

Dehydroarginine
   structure and properties, **01:** 175

Dehydrocysteine
   structure and properties, **01:** 175

ω-Dehydroisoleucine
   antagonism to isoleucine, **01:** 178

Dehydroleucine
   structure and properties, **01:** 175

trans-4-Dehydrolysine
   antagonism to lysine, **01:** 178

Dehydrophenylalanine
   structure and properties, **01:** 175

Dehydroproline
   structure and properties, **01:** 175

3,4-Dehydroproline
   antagonism to proline, **01:** 179

Dehydroquinic acid synthetase
   Neurospora crassa mutant, **04:** 745

Dehydroretinol, properties of, **08:** 284

Dehydroserine
   structure and properties, **01:** 175

Dehydroshikimic acid reductase
   Neurospora crassa mutant, **04:** 745

Dehydrotryptophan
   structure and properties, **01:** 175

Dehydrovaline
   structure and properties, **01:** 175

Dendaitic cells
   immunological response, **07:** 538

Density
   cesium chloride solution as a function of refractive index, table of values, **06:** 419-423

   coefficients for calculation of, from refractive indexes of solutions at 25°, **06:** 424

   fats and oils, table of values, **05:** 502-503

   fatty acids from C_8 to C_{12}, **05:** 492

   guanidine hydrochloride, aqueous solutions with added reagents, at 25°, **06:** 406

   guanidine·HCl, table of values, 06: 404

   kinetoplast DNA, table, **04:** 375-377

   mitochondrial DNAs, table, **04:** 363-372

   organic solvents, calculations for change with temperature for some, **06:** 540

   polyol esters, table, **05:** 515

   salt solutions used for density gradients, **06:** 425

   solvents, mixed, for use in low temperature biochemistry, **06:** 520

   sucrose in water, tables at varying concentrations and temperatures, **06:** 415-418

   urea, aqueous solutions with added reagents, at 25°, **06:** 406

Density, particle, of biological particles in sucrose solutions, **06:** 429

Density gradient
   salt solutions, values for some at equilibrium, **06:** 424

   viscosity and density of salt solutions used, **06:** 424-425

3-Deoxy-D-arabinoheptulosonate 7-phosphate synthetase-chroismate mutase
   average hydrophobicity value, **01:** 218

(R)-3-(2-Deoxy-β-D-erythro-pentofuranosyl)3,6,7,8-tetrahydroimidazo-[4,5-d] [1,3]diazepin-8-ol, physicochemical constants, spectral, chemotherapeutic and biological properties, **03:** 314

Deoxyadenosine
   physical constants and spectral properties, **03:** 141

3'-Deoxyadenosine, *see* Cordycepin

Deoxyadenosine, N^6-Methyl-
   physical constants and spectral properties, **03:** 141

Deoxyadenosine nucleotide derivatives
   physical constants and spectral properties, index to, **03:** 73

Deoxycycline, origin, structure, and characteristic as protein biosynthesis inhibitor, **04:** 570

Deoxycytidine and nucleoside derivatives
   physical constants and spectral properties, index to, **03:** 70

Deoxycytidine nucleotide derivatives
   physical constants and spectral properties, index to, **03:** 73

Deoxycytidylate deaminase
   average hydrophobicity value, **01:** 218
   subunit, constitution of, **02:** 328

Deoxycytidylate deaminase (T-2 bacteriophage induced)
   subunit, constitution of, **02:** 336

Deoxyguanosine and nucleoside derivatives
physical constants and spectral properties, index to, **03:** 70

Deoxyguanosine nucleotide derivatives
physical constants and spectral properties, index to, **03:** 73

Deoxyhemoglobin, HB
UV and visible absorption spectrum, **07:** 176

Deoxynucleotide polymerizing enzymes
properties, template specificities of, and reactions, **04:** 536-545

1-β-2'-Deoxyribofuranosyl-4-methylamino-2-pyrimidinone
physical constants and spectral properties, **03:** 142

Deoxyribohomopolymer complexes (purine·pyrimidine),
melting temperatures, **03:** 581-582

Deoxyribohomopolymers, melting temperatures, **03:** 581

Deoxyribonuclease
amino acid composition, complete data, **07:** 506
average hydrophobicity value, **01:** 218
carbohydrate content, **02:** 273

Deoxyribonuclease, pancreatic
refractive index increments, **02:** 374

Deoxyribonuclease A, B, C, II, average hydrophobicity
values, **01:** 219

Deoxyribonuclease I
circular dichroism in the UV region, **07:** 93
molar absorptivity and-or absorbance values, **02:** 417
optical rotatory dispersion
UV region, **07:** 54
visible and near UV regions, **07:** 22

Deoxyribonuclease II-B
circular dichroism in near-UV region, at room temperature, **07:** 150

Deoxyribonuclease inhibitor
amino acid composition, complete data, **07:** 506
molar absorptivity and-or absorbance values, **02:** 418

Deoxyribonucleases
characteristics, functional, **04:** 495-507

Deoxyribonucleic acid, *see also* DNA

Deoxyribonucleic acid ligase
average hydrophobicity value, **01:** 218

Deoxyribonucleoside, 6-Methylaminopurine-
physical constants, and spectral properties, **03:** 141

Deoxyribonucleotidase inhibitor II
average hydrophobicity value, **01:** 218

Deoxyribose 5-phosphate aldolase
amino acid composition, incomplete data, **07:** 512

Deoxyuridine and nucleoside derivatives
physical constants and spectral properties, index to, **03:** 70

Deoxyuridine nucleotide derivatives
physical constants and spectral properties, index to, **03:** 73

Dependent dehydrogenases
amino acid sequence, **07:** 314

Derxia
G + C composition of DNA of, table arranged by specie, **04:** 81

Desaminocanavanine
physical and chemical properties, **01:** 133

Desmosine
physical and chemical properties, **01:** 161

Desoxyribonuclease
carbohydrate content, **02:** 274

Desulfotomaculum
G + C composition of DNA of, table arranged by specie, **04:** 167

Desulfovibrio
G + C composition of DNA of, table arranged by specie, **04:** 167

Desulfovibrio C_{553}
amino acid sequence, **07:** 302

Detergent, table of properties, **08:** 216-217

Deuterium oxide
heat of proton ionization, pK, and related thermodynamic quantities, **06:** 261

2-*N*,6-*N*-Di-(2,3-dihydroxybenzoyl)lysine
physical and chemical properties, **01:** 138

N,*N*'-Diacetyl-L-cystine dimethyl ester
UV spectra of, **01:** 199

Dialdoses, nomenclature rules, **05:** 109

α-Dialkylamino transamidase
average hydrophobicity value, **01:** 218

Diamine oxidase
molar absorptivity and-or absorbance values, **02:** 418
table of cofactors, molecular weights, stoichiometry and sources, **02:** 282

L-Diamino, dicarboxylic acids
physical and chemical properties, **01:** 121

2,6-Diamino-4-hexynoic acid
structure and symbols for those incorporated into synthetic polypeptides, **01:** 101

2,6-Diamino-7-hydroxyazelaic acid
physical and chemical properties, **01:** 120

α,ε-Diamino-α-hydroxycaproic acid, *see* α-Hydroxylysine

α,ε-Diamino-δ-hydroxycaproic acid, *see* δ-Hydroxylysine

α,ε-Diamino-β-hydroxypimelic acid, *see* Tabtoxinine

L-Diamino, monocarboxylic acids
physical and chemical properties, **01:** 119-121

α,γ-Diaminobutyric acid
physical and chemical properties, **01:** 120

2,4-Diaminobutyric acid
structure and symbols for those incorporated into synthetic polypeptides, **01:** 101

α,ε-Diaminocaproic acid, *see* Lysine

β,ε-Diaminocaproic acid, *see* β-Lysine

2,6-Diaminoheptanoic acid
antagonism to lysine, **01:** 178

3,5-Diaminohexanoic acid
physical and chemical properties, **01:** 120

3,6-Diaminohexanoic acid
physical and chemical properties, **01:** 121
structure and symbols for those incorporated into synthetic polypeptides, **01:** 101

α,ε-Diaminopimelic acid
antagonists of, **01:** 177
physical and chemical properties, **01:** 122

2,2'-Diaminopimelic acid
structure and symbols for those incorporated into synthetic polypeptides, **01:** 101

α,β-Diaminopropionic acid
physical and chemical properties, **01:** 120

2,3-Diaminopropionic acid
structure and symbols for those incorporated into synthetic polypeptides, **01**: 101

α,α-Diaminosebacic acid
antagonism to α,ε-Diaminopimelic acid, **01**: 177

α,α-Diaminosuberic acid
antagonism to α,ε-Diaminopimelic acid, **01**: 177

Diaminosuccinic acid
antagonism to aspartic acid, 01: 177

2,3-Diaminosuccinic acid
physical and chemical properties, **01**: 122

α,δ-Diaminovaleric acid, *see* Ornithine

Diaphorase, *see* Lipoamide dehydrogenase (NADH)

ε-Diazo
physical and chemical properties, **01**: 135

6-Diazo-5-oxonorleucine
antagonism to glutamine, 01: 177

O-Diazoacetylserine, *see* Azaserine

3,5-Dibromotyrosine
physical and chemical properties, **01**: 159

S-(1,2-Dicarboxy-ethyl)-cysteine
physical and chemical properties, **01**: 154

Dicarboxylic acid, alkyl, diesters, refractive index, **05**: 494

S-(1,2-Dichlorovinyl)-cysteine
antagonism to phenylalanine, 01: 179

Dichrostachinic acid
physical and chemical properties, **01**: 154

Dictyostelium
G + C composition of DNA of, table arranged by specie, **04**: 196

Dictyuchus
G + C composition of DNA of, table arranged by specie, **04**: 197

Dielectric constant
N,N-dimethylformamide-water mixtures, **06**: 528
dimethylsulfoxide-water mixtures, **06**: 527
ethylene glycol-methanol-water mixtures, **06**: 528
ethylene glycol-water mixtures, **06**: 522
glycerol-water mixtures, **06**: 526
methanol-water mixtures, **06**: 523
2-Methyl-2-4-pentanediol-water mixtures, **06**: 524
1-2-Propanediol-water mixtures, **06**: 525

Dielectric constants of some fats, fatty acids, and fatty acid esters, **05**: 494

Diet
animal requirements of vitamins, **08**: 305-308
human, NAS-NRC recommended daily allowances, **08**: 248-249
human, U.S. Government recommended daily allowances of vitamins and minerals, **08**: 310

Diethylalanine, *see* 2-Amino-3-ethylvaleric acid

Diffusion coefficients
proteins
carbohydrates, index to studies containing, **02**: 232
fibrous, index to studies containing, **02**: 229
globular, index to studies containing, **02**: 222-228
organelles, index to studies containing, **02**: 232
particles, index to studies containing, **02**: 232
plasma, human, table of values, **02**: 242-250
virus, index to studies containing, **02**: 232
Tamm-Horsfall mucoprotein, **02**: 304
urokinase, **02**: 302

4-9-Dihydro-4,6-dimethyl-9-oxo-3-β-D-ribofuranosyl-1*H*-imidazo [1,2-a] purine
physical constants and spectral properties, **03**: 139

2,3-Dihydro-3,3-dimethyl-1 *H*-pyrrolo-[1,2-α] indole-9-alanine
physical and chemical properties, **01**: 148

ε(1,4-Dihydro-6-methyl-3-hydroxy-4-oxo-1-pyridyl)-lysine, *see* Pyridosine

2,5-Dihydro-phenylalanine
physical and chemical properties, **01**: 138

Dihydro orotate dehydrogenase
Neurospora crassa mutant, **04**: 748

Dihydroallin
physical and chemical properties, **01**: 154

Dihydrofolate reductase
average hydrophobicity value, **01**: 218
molar absorptivity and-or absorbance values, **02**: 418

N-Dihydrojas-monoylisoleucine
physical and chemical properties, **01**: 138

Dihydrolipoyl transacetylase
molar absorptivity and-or absorbance values, **02**: 419
subunit, constitution of, **02**: 350, 351

Dihydrophenylalanine, *see* β-(1,4-Cyclohexadienyl) alanine

Dihydrorhizobitoxine
physical and chemical properties, **01**: 124

Dihydrostreptomycin; origin, structure, and characteristic as protein biosynthesis inhibitor, **04**: 570

Dihydrouridine
composition in various tRNA's, **04**: 428-441

5,6-Dihydrouridine
isolation and detection of, in RNA, general remarks, **03**: 243
RNA, various, natural occurrence in, **03**: 231-232

Dihydroxy-acid dehydrase
Neurospora crassa mutant, **04**: 751

2,3-Dihydroxy-*N*-berzoylserine
physical and chemical properties, **01**: 129

2,4-Dihydroxy-6-methylphenylalanine
physical and chemical properties, **01**: 130

3,4-Dihydroxy-(α-methyl)phenylalanine
structure and symbols for those incorporated into synthetic polypeptides, **01**: 101

β-(2,6-Dihydroxy-pyrimidin-1-yl) alanine
physical and chemical properties, **01**: 139

4,6-Dihydroxy-quinoline-2-carboxylic acid
physical and chemical properties, **01**: 139

β,γ-Dihydroxyglutamic acid
physical and chemical properties, **01**: 124

β,γ-Dihydroxyisoleucine
physical and chemical properties, **01**: 124

γ,δ-Dihydroxyleucine
physical and chemical properties, **01**: 124

δ,ε-Dihydroxynorleucine
physical and chemical properties, **01**: 124

β-(3,4-Dihydroxyphenyl)-α-methylalanine, *see* 3,4-Dihydroxy-(α-methyl)phenylalanine

3,4-Dihydroxyphenylacetate-2,3-oxygenase
average hydrophobicity value, **01**: 218

3,4-Dihydroxyphenylalanine
physical and chemical properties, **01**: 130

3,4-Dihydroxyphenylalanine *(continued)*
structure and symbols for those incorporated into synthetic polypeptides, **01:** 101
3,5-Dihydroxyphenylglycine
physical and chemical properties, **01:** 130
(3,4-Dihydroxyphenyl)serine
structure and symbols for those incorporated into synthetic polypeptides, **01:** 101
cis-3,4-*trans*-3,4-Dihydroxyproline
physical and chemical properties, **01:** 139
Dihydrozanthurenic acid (8-hydroxy-1,2,3,4-tetrahydro-4-ketoquinaldic acid)
physical and chemical properties, **01:** 139
β-[3,5-Diiodo-4-(3′,5′-diiodo 4′-hydroxyphenoxy)phenyl] acid
properties of , **01:** 182
2,4-Diiodohistidine
physical and chemical properties, **01:** 159
3,3′-Diiodothyronine
physical and chemical properties, **01:** 159
3,5-Diiodotyrosine
physical and chemical properties, **01:** 159
Diketoses, nomenclature rules, **05:** 107-108
Dimers, proposals for abbreviations, **03:** 51-53
Dimethyl 2-amino-4,6-dimethyl-3-oxophenoxazine-1,9-carboxylate
UV spectra, formula, molecular weight, **08:** 165
N^6,N^6-Dimethyladenosine
isolation and detection of, in RNA, general remarks, **03:** 235
RNA, various, natural occurrence in, **03:** 220
2-Dimethylamionoethylphosphonic acid
physical and chemical properties, **01:** 161
N^G,N^G-Dimethylarginine
physical and chemical properties, **01:** 133
N^G,N^{1G}-Dimethylarginine
physical and chemical properties, **01:** 133
N,N-Dimethylaspartic N-oxide
structure and symbols for those incorporated into synthetic polypeptides, **01:** 102
β,β-Dimethylcysteine
structure and symbols for those incorporated into synthetic polypeptides, **01:** 102
N^4,O^2-Dimethylcytidine
isolation and detection of, in RNA, general remarks, **03:** 237
RNA, various, natural occurrence in, **03:** 223
N-N-Dimethylformamide-water mixtures, dielectric constants and freezing points, **06:** 528
N^2,N^2-Dimethylguanosine
composition in various tRNA's, **04:** 428-441
isolation and detection of, in RNA, general remarks, **03:** 238
RNA, various, natural occurrence in, **03:** 225-226
β,N-Dimethylleucine
physical and chemical properties, **01:** 148
threo-N, β-Dimethylleucine
structure and symbols for those incorporated into synthetic polypeptides, **01:** 102
Nε,Nε-Dimethyllysine
physical and chemical properties, **01:** 120

N,N-Dimethylphenylalanine
physical and chemical properties, **01:** 148
Dimethylsulfoxide-water mixtures, dielectric constants and freezing points, **06:** 527
α,3-Dimethyltyrosine
structure and symbols for those incorporated into synthetic polypeptides, **01:** 102
$5,O^{2'}$-Dimethyluridine
isolation and detection of, in RNA, general remarks, **03:** 244
RNA, various, natural occurence in, **03:** 233
2,4-Dinitrophenylhydrazone of α-Keto acids, **01:** 181-182
Dinucleoside monophosphates
mean residue absorptivities, **03:** 597
molar residue ellipticities, **03:** 600
molar residue rotations, **03:** 598
Dinucleoside monophosphates, 2′-O-methylated, circular dichroism parameters, **03:** 471
Dipeptidase
amino acid composition, incomplete data, **07:** 512
enzymatic activity, subcellular fractions, **02:** 698
molar absorptivity and-or absorbance values, **02:** 419
molecular weights, stoichiometry, and sources, **02:** 286
Dipeptidase M
subunit, constitution of, **02:** 332
α,α-Diphenylglycine
structure and symbols for those incorporated into synthetic polypeptides, **01:** 102
Diphosphopyridine nucleosidase
amino acid composition, complete data, **07:** 506
Diplococcus
G + C composition of DNA of, table arranged by specie, **04:** 116
Dipnoans, DNA content per cell, **04:** 293
Dipodascus
G + C composition of DNA of, table arranged by specie, **04:** 197
Dipsacomyces
G + C composition of DNA of, table arranged by specie, **04:** 197
Diptheria toxin; origin, structure, and characteristic as protein biosynthesis inhibitor, **04:** 571
Dipyrimidines, singly bonded, proposal for abbreviations, **03:** 53-55
Dipyrimidines, singly bonded, proposals for abbreviations, **04:** 53-55
Disaccharide units isolated from complex carbohydrates of mammalian origin, structure of, **05:** 278-280
Disaccharides
chemical formula, **05:** 283-297, 327-334
derivatives, **05:** 283-297, 327-334
melting point, **05:** 283-297, 327-334
nomenclature rules, **05:** 133-134
specific rotation, **05:** 283-297, 327-334
synonyms, **05:** 283-297, 327-334
Dispersoids, gas, chart of diameters for various, **08:** 425
Dissociation constant
proteinase inhibitors
animal sources, **02:** 618-641
plant sources, **02:** 588-596, 600
Dissociation constants
glycohydrolases table, **05:** 426-445

Dissociation constants *(continued)*
  prostaglandin metabolizing enzymes, **08:** 364-367
Dissociation constants, acidic
  alkyl bases, **03:** 409-416
  nucleosides, **03:** 409-416
  nucleotides, **03:** 409-416
Disulfide-exchange enzyme
  amino acid composition, incomplete data, **07:** 512
Disulfide protein group, chemical modification of
  reagents used, table of specificities, **02:** 203-204
$\beta\beta'$-Dithiodi-(α-aminopropionic acid), *see* Cystine
Diuretics
  ligands binding to plasma albumin, **02:** 571
Djenkolic acid
  physical and chemical properties, **01:** 154
DNA, *see also* Deoxyribonucleic acid
  base compositions of eucaryotic protists, tables, **04:** 236-239
  cellular, buoyant density values for several, **03:** 565-566
  chloroplast
    buoyant density, table of values, **04:** 356-358
    GC mol %, table of values, **04:** 356-358
  content per cell
    algae from various sources, table, **04:** 286
    amphibians from various sources, table, **04:** 298-299
    animal viruses from various sources, table, **04:** 310
    annelida from various sources, table, **04:** 291
    arthropoda from various sources, table, **04:** 291-293
    bacteriophages from various sources, table, **04:** 307-308
    birds from various sources, table, **04:** 300-301
    chordata from various sources, table, **04:** 293-305
    coelenterata from various sources, table, **04:** 290
    echinodermata from various sources, table, **04:** 290
    fish from various sources, table, **04:** 293-297
    fungi from various sources, table, **04:** 284-285, 289
    mammals from various sources, table, **04:** 302-305
    mollusca from various sources, table, **04:** 291
    nematoda from various sources, table, **04:** 291
    porifera from various sources, table, **04:** 290
    pteropsida from various sources, table, **04:** 287-288
    reptiles from various sources, table, **04:** 298-299
  T-even coliphage, buoyant density values, **03:** 568
  extinction coefficients for double-strand types as a function of A + T content, graph, **03:** 590
  extinction coefficients for single-strand types, **03:** 589
  fluorescent dyes bound to, data tables, **04:** 470
  kinetoplast, properties of, table, **04:** 375-377
  lambda molecule of *Escherichia coli*, genetic and molecular map, **04:** 678
  6-methylaminopurine, content of, **04:** 282-283
  5-methylcytosine, content of, **04:** 282-283
  mitochondrial, properties of, table, **04:** 363-372
  nearest neighbor frequencies in acids from diverse sources, **04:** 312-318
  nuclear
    buoyant density, table of values, **04:** 356-358
    GC mol %, table of values, **04:** 356-358
  oligonucleotides, circular dichroism parameters, **03:** 465-468
  oligonucleotides, optical dispersion parameters, **03:** 459-460

polymerase
    properties, template specificities, tables of, **04:** 538-540
    reactions catalyzed by, **04:** 536
    sources of, **04:** 536
  polynucleotide double helices with Watson-Crick base pairs
    atomic coordinates and molecular conformations for, **04:** 411-412
  purine and pyrimidine, distribution of, in acids from diverse sources, **04:** 241-281
  raman spectral changes, melting calf thymus DNA, **03:** 544
  sequences in eukaryotes, **04:** 319-322
  synthesis; pathways chart, **04:** insert
  viral
    nucleotide sequences, **04:** 350-353
  viral, buoyant densities, melting temperature and GC content, **03:** 560-562
  viral, buoyant density values for several, **03:** 566-567
  viral DNA molecules, content per virion, **03:** 551-556
  viral molecules, composition and physical properties, **03:** 552-556
DNA, range of weights, **08:** 424
DNA polymerase
  amino acid composition, complete data, **07:** 506
  enzymatic activity, subcellular fractions, **02:** 699, 718
DNase, *see* Deoxyribonuclease I
Dog
  MHC designation, **04:** 885
  mitochondrial DNA from, properties, **04:** 371
Domoic acid
  physical and chemical properties, **01:** 139
DOPA, *see* 3,4-Dihydroxyphenylalanine
Dopamine-β-hydroxylase
  average hydrophobicity value, **01:** 219
Double helix
  molecular structure, geometry of, for RNA, **04:** 363-369
  polynucleotide, atomic coordinates and molecular conformations for, **04:** 411-422
  polynucleotide, views perpendicular to helix axis, **04:** 417-418
DPNase
  carbohydrate content, **02:** 273
  molar absorptivity and-or absorbance values, **02:** 419
DPNase inhibitor
  carbohydrate content, **02:** 274
Drosophila, buoyant density and G + C content of satellite DNAs for several strains, table, **04:** 380-382
Drosophila melanogaster
  biochemical mutants
    cuticle pigment, **04:** 853-854
    enzyme and structural protein, **04:** 848-849
    eye pigment and malpighian tubule pigment, **04:** 851-853
    insecticide resistant, **04:** 855
    nutrition, **04:** 855
    protein synthesis, **04:** 849-851
    tumor and melanotic pseudotumor, **04:** 854
  mitochondrial DNA, properties of, **04:** 369
Drude equation
  visible optical rotatory dispersion, discussion, **07:** 3-4
Drugs, ligands binding to plasma albumin, **02:** 568-574

Dunaliella
  G + C composition of DNA of, table arranged by spe-
    cie, **04:** 225
Duomycin, *see* Aureomycin, Chlortetracycline
Dyes
  pK'_a values, **06:** 348
Dyes, fluorescent, bound to nucleic acids, data tables, **04:**
  470
Dyes, visible, ligands binding to plasma albumin, **02:**
  564-568

E

E. coli, see also Escherichia coli
  RNAs from; amino acid sequence, **04:** 333, 335
  5S RNA from, secondary structure model, **04:** 328
Echinine
  physical and chemical properties, **01:** 140
Echinodermata
  deoxyribonucleic acids from, purine and pyrimidine dis-
    tribution in, **04:** 267
  DNA content per cell for various, table, **04:** 290
Edeine; origin, structure, and characteristic as protein bi-
    osynthesis inhibitor, **04:** 571
Edestin
  optical rotatory dispersion in the visible and near UV
    regions, **07:** 22
  refractive index increments, **02:** 374
  subunit, constitution of, **02:** 345
EDTA
  heat of proton ionization, pK, and related thermody-
    namic quantities, **06:** 197
EDTA inhibition of transamitase activity, **02:** 669-673
Egg white cross-reacting protein
  amino acid composition, complete data, **07:** 506
Egg whites, birds
  proteinase inhibitors from, specificities and properties,
    02: 624-629
Eggs
  glycoproteins from carbohydrate content, **02:** 268-269
Eicosapentaenoic acid
  biological and physical properties, **08:** 322-328
  isolation and synthesis of, **08:** 326-327
  occurrence, **08:** 325
Eicosatetraenoic acid
  biological and physical properties, **08:** 322-328
  isolation and synthesis of, **08:** 326-327
  occurrence, **08:** 325
Eicosatrienoic acid
  biological and physical properties, **08:** 322-328
  isolation and synthesis of, **08:** 326-327
  occurrence, **08:** 325
Eidamella
  G + C composition of DNA of, table arranged by spe-
    cie, **04:** 197
Elasmobranchii, DNA content per cell, **04:** 293
Elastase
  circular dichroism
    UV and near-UV region, **07:** 93, 150
  luminescence of, table, **01:** 205
  molar absorptivity and-or absorbance values, **02:** 419

optical rotatory dispersion
  UV region, **07:** 54
  visible and near UV regions, **07:** 22
Elastase-like enzyme
  molar absorptivity and-or absorbance values, **02:** 419
Elastase inhibitor
  legume sources, specificity and properties, **02:** 588-589
  mammalian organs and secretions, specificities and
    properties, **02:** 632-641
Elastin
  average hydrophobicity value, **01:** 219
α-Elastin
  circular dichroism in the UV region, **07:** 93
Electrode measurements, conventional methods for
    presentation, **06:** 103
Electrodes
  use in pH measurement, **06:** 355-356
Electronic charge distribution
  monosaccharides and some of their derivatives, **05:**
    474-477
  polysaccharides, **05:** 478-481
Electrophoretic mobility
  amino sugars, naturally occurring, **05:** 359-370
  proteins
    human plasma, table of values, **02:** 242-250
    urokinase, **02:** 302
Electrophoretic separation, *Escherichia coli* B 236 70 S
    ribosomal proteins, **04:** 474
Eledoisin group, natural and related synthetic oligopep-
    tide
  amino acid sequence, physical and biological properties,
    07: 236-257
Elfvingia
  G + C composition of DNA of, table arranged by spe-
    cie, **04:** 197
Ellipticity, *see* Mean residue ellipticities
Ellipticity, molar residue, *see* Molar residue ellipticity
Elution behavior, ninhydrin-positive compounds, **08:** 122
Elution time
  rapid short column chromatography, amino acids
    related to metabolic diseases, **08:** 128-129
EMB medium for detecting sugar fermentation, prepara-
    tion of, **04:** 650
Emericella
  G + C composition of DNA of, table arranged by spe-
    cie, **04:** 197
Emericellopsis
  G + C composition of DNA of, table arranged by spe-
    cie, **04:** 197
Emetine; origin, structure, and characteristic as protein
    biosynthesis inhibitor, **04:** 572
Enamel proteins
  optical rotatory dispersion in the visible and near UV
    regions, **07:** 22
Enantiomers, definition and nomenclature, **01:** 36-58, **03:**
    28-50, **04:** 28-50, **05:** 33-55, **06:** 35, **08:** 35-40
Enantiomers definition and nomenclature, **02:** 36-58
Encephalitogenic A-1 protein
  average hydrophobicity value, **01:** 219
Encephalitogenic protein
  amino acid composition, complete data, **07:** 506
  circular dichroism in the UV region, **07:** 94

Encephalitogenic protein *(continued)*
  optical rotatory dispersion
    UV region, **07**: 54
    visible and near UV regions, **07**: 22
Endo-β-*N*-Acetylglucosaminidase
  circular dichroism in the UV region, **07**: 94
Endo-γ-Glutamine: ϵ-lysine transferase
  transamilase activity, discussion and data, **02**: 669-683
Endogenous ligands binding to plasma albumin, **02**: 556-557
Endomyces
  G + C composition of DNA of, table arranged by specie, **04**: 197
Endomycopsis
  G + C composition of DNA of, table arranged by specie, **04**: 198
Endonuclease
  luminescence of, table, **01**: 205
Endonucleases, restriction
  characteristics, functional, **04**: 493-494
  cleavage sites, number of, for several, **04**: 532-534
  definition and discussion, **04**: 491-492
  recognition sequences for several, **04**: 532-534
Endopolygalacturonase
  average hydrophobicity value, **01**: 219
  molar absorptivity and-or absorbance values, **02**: 420
Endotoxin-receptor, *see* Lipopolysaccharide-receptor
Enduracididine
  physical and chemical properties, **01**: 140
Energy measurements, standardization of, for equilibrium data, **06**: 101
Enniatin B
  proton NMR and suggested conformations, **07**: 561
Enolase
  amino acid composition, complete data, **07**: 506
  average hydrophobicity value, **01**: 219
  circular dichroism in the UV region, **07**: 94
  enzymatic activity, subcellular fractions, **02**: 698, 715
  molar absorptivity and-or absorbance values, **02**: 420
  optical rotatory dispersion
    UV region, **07**: 54
    visible and near UV regions, **07**: 22
  subunit, constitution of, **02**: 331, 332, 346
3-Enolpyruvylshikimic acid-5PO$_4$ synthetase
  Neurospora crassa mutant, **04**: 745
Enomycin; origin, structure, and chracteristic as protein biosynthesis inhibitor, **04**: 572
Entamoeba
  G + C composition of DNA of, table arranged by specie, **04**: 228
Enterobacteriaceae
  G + C composition of DNA of, table arranged by genera and specie, **04**: 104-114
Enterotoxin A
  average hydrophobicity value, **01**: 220
Enterotoxin A, B, C, E
  molar absorptivity and-or absorbance values, **02**: 420-421
Enterotoxin C
  amino acid composition, complete data, **07**: 506
  average hydrophobicity value, **01**: 220

Enterotoxin E
  average hydrophobicity value, **01**: 220
Enthalpy
  redox in reactions, **06**: 121
Enthalpy of formation
  amino acids, table, **06**: 111-112
  peptides, table, **06**: 112
Entner-Doudoroff pathway; pathways chart, **04**: insert
Entropy
  chemical compounds, table of values, **06**: 153-262
  redox in reactions, **06**: 121
Entropy, absolute
  amino acids, table of values, **06**: 109
  peptides, table of values for several, **06**: 110
  proteins, table of values for several, **06**: 110
Entropy of formation
  amino acids, table of values, **06**: 109
  peptides, values for several, **06**: 110
Envelope protein, *see* Matrix protein
Enzymatic activity
  nonmuscle myosins, data table, **02**: 319
  subcellular fractions, tables, **02**: 697-719
Enzymatic cross-linking
  discussion and data, **02**: 668-683
Enzymatic hydrolysis
  conjugated proteins, table, **02**: 211
  proteins and polypeptides, **02**: 209
Enzymatic incorporation of amines
  proteins serving as substrates, list of, **02**: 680
Enzymatic synthesis of sugar nucleotides, **05**: 446-452
Enzyme, *see also* Enzymes, Isoenzymes, Isozymes
Enzyme, thrombin-like
  molar absorptivity and-or absorbance values, **02**: 421
Enzyme cofactors
  fluorescence of, **07**: 601-602
Enzyme inhibitors
  fluorescent properties, table, **07**: 598-599
Enzyme kinetics
  Michaelis constant, equation and symbols, **02**: 111
  rate constants, definition, **02**: 112
  symbols used in, **02**: 111-114
Enzyme studies, preparation of buffers for, **06**: 370-377
Enzymes, *see also* Coenzyme, Metalloenzyme, Multienzyme
  amino acid sequences of proteins, **07**: 308-313
  classification of, **02**: 93-109
  cleavage sites, number of, for restriction and modification types, **04**: 532-534
  defects in amino acid metabolism errors, **01**: 317-322
  defects in organic acid metabolism errors, **01**: 326
  deoxynucleotide polymerizing
    enzymatic functions of several, **04**: 545
    eucaryotes sources, template specificities and properties for some, **04**: 539-544
    procaryotes sources, template specificity properties, molecular weights, **04**: 538
  dissociation constants, glycohydrolases, table of, **05**: 426-445
  DNA polymerase, sources of and reactions, **04**: 536
  electron-transfer proteins, nomenclature, **02**: 114-121
  genetically variant, nomenclature, **02**: 86
  glycoproteins, carbohydrate content, **02**: 273-274

Enzymes *(continued)*

human disorders demonstrating deficient activity of specific enzymes, list, **04:** 882-883

immobilization of

absorption method, table of supports, **02:** 723

covalent bond method, table of polymeric supports, **02:** 725-734

entrapment method, table of supports, **02:** 724

fixation on solid supports, multifunctional reagents for, **02:** 735

methods used, description, **02:** 722

immobilized, uses of, **02:** 722

isoenzymes, definition and nomenclature of, **02:** 84-86

isozymes, definition and nomenclature of, **02:** 84-86

list of recommended and systematic names, **02:** 121-172

metalloenzymes, table of cofactors, molecular weights, stoichiometry and sources, **02:** 278-286

Michaelis constants, glycohydrolases, table of, **05:** 426-445

molecular turnover in animal tissue, table, **07:** 552-556

multiple forms, list of groups, **02:** 85

names, list of recommended and systematic, **02:** 121-172

nomenclature, multiple forms of, **02:** 84-86

nomenclature, recommendations, **02:** 91-172

pH values (optimum and stable) in glycohydrolase reactions, **05:** 426-445

prostaglandin metabolizing

properties and activity, **08:** 364-367

target sites, diagram, **08:** 320

proteolytic, digestion cross-linked proteins, **02:** 669

reaction rates, parameters for glycohydrolases, **05:** 426-445

restriction and modification enzymes in several strains, recognition sequences for, **04:** 532-534

reverse transcriptase, sources of and reactions, **04:** 536

ribonucleotide polymerizing, subunits, molecular weights, **04:** 549-553

specificity, for glycohydrolases, **05:** 426-445

substrates used in glycohydrolase reactions, **05:** 426-445

susceptibility of poly(α-amino acids) to, **01:** 393-396

terminal transferase, sources of and reactions, **04:** 536

transamidase activity, detection and sources, **02:** 670, 671

urine, normal human, molecules weight of those found in, **02:** 301

velocity of reaction, maximum for glycohydrolases, **05:** 426-445

Enzymic activity

definition of, **02:** 109

units of, defined, **02:** 109-110

Eosin-methylene blue medium for detecting sugar fermentation, preparation of, **04:** 650

Epicoccum

G + C composition of DNA of, table arranged by specie, **04:** 198

Epidermal growth factor

circular dichroism in the UV region, **07:** 94

Epimerase, *see* UDPglucose 4-epimerase

Epimerases

definition and nomenclature, **02:** 98

numbering and classification of, **02:** 108

Epon®, chemical resistance and other properties, **08:** 429

Epoxy, used as prefix in nomenclature, **06:** 68, **08:** 68

Epoxy fatty acids, physical and chemical characteristics, **05:** 488-489

Equilibrium constants

measurement conditions, **06:** 105

standardization of data presentation, **06:** 95-99

Equilibrium data, measurement and presentation, **06:** 93-106

Erabutoxin

amino acid composition, incomplete data, **07:** 512

Erabutoxin a

molar absorptivity and-or absorbance values, **02:** 421

Eremascus

G + C composition of DNA of, table arranged by specie, **04:** 198

Ergocalciferol, properties of, **08:** 286

Ergothionine

physical and chemical properties, **01:** 161

Erwinia

G + C composition of DNA of, table arranged by specie, **04:** 105-109

Erythrocruorin

molar absorptivity and-or absorbance values, **02:** 421

subunit, constitution of, **02:** 351

Erythrocuprein, *see* Superoxide dismutase

average hydrophobicity value, **01:** 220

molar absorptivity and-or absorbance values, **02:** 421, 422

subunit, constitution of, **02:** 328

Erythromycin A; origin, structure, and characteristic as protein biosynthesis inhibitor, **04:** 573

Erythromycin cation

UV spectra, formula, molecular weight, **08:** 182

Erythropoietin

carbohydrate content, **02:** 272-273

molar absorptivity and-or absorbance values, **02:** 422

Escherichia

standard media for growth, **04:** 649

Escherichia coli, see also E. coli

affected phenotypic trait, **04:** 654-659

amino acid composition, ribosomal proteins: 30 S, **04:** 476

amino acid requirements for growth, table, **04:** 633

bacteriophage lambda, genetic and molecular map of, **04:** 678

deoxynucleotide polymerizing enzymes from, enzymatic functions of, **04:** 545

deoxynucleotide polymerizing enzymes from, template specificity properties, **04:** 538

deoxyribonucleases from, functional characteristics, **04:** 497-502

deoxyribonucleic acids from, purine and pyrimidine distribution in, **04:** 247-248, 276

DNA content per cell for various, table, **04:** 285

electrophoretic separation of ribosomal proteins, tracing, **04:** 474

G + C composition of DNA of, table arranged by specie, **04:** 110

gene symbols, **04:** 654-659

genetic markers, list, **04:** 654-659

glycohydrolase from, enzymatic reaction parameters, **05:** 435-436

Escherichia coli (continued)
linkage map, **04:** 651-653
lipopolysaccharides of
  sugar composition for O-type, **05:** 396-399
  sugar sequences, general structures, **05:** 406, 409-411
MRE 600 30 S ribosomal proteins, separation on cellulose phosphate Whatman® P 11, **04:** 475
nearest neighbor frequencies in DNA from various, **04:** 314
physical characteristics of ribosome 70 S, **04:** 472
restriction and modification enzymes present in several strains, recognition sequences for, **04:** 532
restriction endonucleases from, functional characteristics, **04:** 493-494
ribonuclease from, functional characteristics, **04:** 508, 510-511, 513
ribosomal components
  data tables, **04:** 471-486
ribosomal proteins
  50 S, amino acid composition, **04:** 477-478
  amino acid sequence data, **04:** 479-481
  30 S, physical and functional characteristics of, **04:** 482-486
5S-ribosomal RNA from, nucleotide sequences, **04:** 324-327
RNA from, natural occurrence of the modified nucleosides in, **03:** 217-232
RNA molecules from, physical properties, **04:** 406,409
4.5S RNA from, nucleotide sequence model, **04:** 331
6S RNA from, nucleotide sequence model, **04:** 332
Esterase
  average hydrophobicity value, **01:** 220
  enzymatic activity, subcellular fractions, **02:** 698, 706
  molar absorptivity and-or absorbance values, **02:** 422
  subunit, constitution of, **02:** 337
Estradiol dehydrogenase
  average hydrophobicity value, **01:** 220
Estrogens, structures and properties, **05:** 539-540
Etamycin®, *see* Viridogrisein
Ethane derivatives
  heat of proton ionization, pK, and related thermodynamic quantities, **06:** 195-197
Ethanolamine
  free acid in blood plasma of newborn infants and adults, **01:** 328
Ethanolamine deaminase
  amino acid composition, complete data, **07:** 506
Ethers of 3,5-diiodotyrosine
  antagonism to thyroxine, **01:** 179
Ethionine
  antagonism to methionine, **01:** 178
  physical and chemical properties, **01:** 154
  structure and symbols for those incorporated into synthetic polypeptides, **01:** 102
P-Ethyl-γ-phosphonoglutamic acid
  antagonism to glutamic acid, **01:** 177
Ethylasparagine
  physical and chemical properties, **01:** 118
Ethylene glycol-methanol-water mixtures
  dielectric constants and freezing points, **06:** 528
  viscosity table, **06:** 521

Ethylene glycol-water mixtures, dielectric constants and freezing points, **06:** 522
N-Ethylglycine
  structure and symbols for those incorporated into synthetic polypeptides, **01:** 102
*tele*Ethylhistidine
  structure and symbols for those incorporated into synthetic polypeptides, **01:** 102
1-Ethylhistidine, *see tele*Ethylhistidine
O-Ethylhomoserine
  physical and chemical properties, **01:** 124
γ-Ethylidene glutamic acid
  physical and chemical properties, **01:** 118
Euglena
  G + C composition of DNA of, table arranged by specie, **04:** 228
Eukaryotes, DNA sequences, **04:** 319-322
Eukaryotes, multicellular
  nearest neighbor frequencies in DNA from various, **04:** 316-318
Eukaryotes, unicellular
  nearest neighbor frequencies in DNA from various, **04:** 315-316
Eukaryotic cytochromes *c*
  amino acid sequences of protein, tables, **07:** 268-285
  animals, **07:** 268-272, 282-283
  plants, **07:** 273-277, 284-285
Eukaryotic protists, DNA base compositions of, table, **04:** 236-239
Eukaryotic satellite DNAs, properties of selected, **04:** 379-402
Eupenicillium
  G + C composition of DNA of, table arranged by specie, **04:** 198
Eurotium
  G + C composition of, table arranged by specie, **04:** 198
Evolidine
  proton NMR and suggested conformations, **07:** 566
Excelsin
  molar absorptivity and-or absorbance values, **02:** 422
  subunit, constitution of, **02:** 345
Exo-β-D-(1→3)-Glucanase
  amino acid composition, complete data, **07:** 506
exo-3,4-Methanoproline
  physical and chemical properties, **01:** 143
Exogenous ligands binding to plasma albumin, **02:** 558-574
Exonucleases
  definitions, discussion of, **04:** 491
Extinction coefficient
  DNA, double-strand, as a function of A + T content, graph, **03:** 590
  DNA, single-strand, **03:** 589
  oligonucleotides, single-strand, formula for calculating, **03:** 589
  RNA, single-strand, **03:** 589
Extinction coefficients
  heme-base complexes, α bands, **08:** 280
  vitamins, table of data, **08:** 284-300

Ezomycin A_1, A_2, B_1, B_2, physicochemical constants, spectral, chemotherapeutic and biological properties, **03**: 316-319

F

Factor A nucleoside
  physical constants and spectral properties, **03**: 111
Factor I-XIII, *see also* synonyms
  molar absorptivity and-or absorbance values, **02**: 422
  nomenclature, synonyms and symbols, **02**: 195
  subunit, constitution of, **02**: 327
  table of data and characteristics, **02**: 254-255
Factor III lac
  average hydrophobicity value, **01**: 220
Factor R, properties of, **08**: 295
Factor U, properties of, **08**: 295
Factor VIII
  average hydrophobicity value, **01**: 220
Factor X
  amino acid composition, complete data, **07**: 506
Factor X_1
  amino acid sequence of, **07**: 353
Factor X, properties of, **08**: 293
Familial protein intolerance
  characteristics of , **01**: 323
Fats
  density of, **05**: 502-503
  dielectric constants of some, **05**: 494
  fatty acid content of, **05**: 502-503
  iodine value of, **05**: 502-503
  melting points of, **05**: 502-503
  refractive index of, **05**: 502-503
  saponification value of, **05**: 502-503
  solidification points of, **05**: 502-503
  specific gravity of, **05**: 502-503
Fatty acid monolayers
  comparison of surface pressures at transition and collapse, **05**: 518
Fatty acid oxidation and synthesis; pathways chart, **04**: insert
Fatty acid synthetase
  amino acid composition, incomplete data, **07**: 512
  molar absorptivity and-or absorbance values, **02**: 422
  subunit, constitution of, **02**: 348, 350
Fatty acids, *see also* Lipids, Wax fatty acids
  alkyl diesters of dicarboxylic acid, refractive index, **05**: 494
  alkyl esters refractive index and equations for some, **05**: 493
  alkyl monoesters of carboxylic acid, refractive index, **05**: 494
  branched-chain
    chemical characteristics, **05**: 490-491
    chemical formula, **05**: 490-491
    common name, **05**: 490-491
    physical characteristics, **05**: 490-491
  composition in plasma and erythrocyte lipids, effect of dietary fat, **05**: 522
  composition of unesterified, in parts of human skin, **05**: 507

content of, in fats and oils, table of values, **05**: 502-503
cyclo
  chemical characteristics, **05**: 488-489
  chemical formula, **05**: 488-489
  common name, **05**: 488-489
  physical characteristics, **05**: 488-489
density, table, of acids from C_8 to C_{12}, **05**: 492
dielectric constants of some fats, fatty acids and esters, **05**: 494
epoxy
  chemical characteristics, **05**: 488-489
  chemical formula, **05**: 488-489
  common name, **05**: 488-489
  physical characteristics, **05**: 488-489
freezing point, effect of addition of water upon, graph, **05**: 495
human skin surface lipids, type and amount contained, **05**: 508
hydroxy unsaturated
  chemical characteristics, **05**: 488-489
  chemical formula, **05**: 488-489
  common name, **05**: 488-489
  physical characteristics, **05**: 488-489
hydroxyalkanoic
  chemical characteristics, **05**: 488-489
  chemical formula, **05**: 488-489
  common name, **05**: 488-489
  physical characteristics, **05**: 488-489
keto
  chemical characteristics, **05**: 488-489
  chemical formula, **05**: 488-489
  common name, **05**: 488-489
  physical characteristics, **05**: 488-489
linseed oil acids and esters, force-area data, **05**: 497
metabolism, mammalian, outline for unsaturated, **08**: 319
methyl esters, refractive index and equations for some, **05**: 493
methyl esters derived from herring oils and Pacific pilchard oil, weight %, **05**: 523-524
methyl esters of some synthetic alkenyl and alkyl substituted, physical constants, **05**: 516
methyl linoleate in carbon tetrachloride solution, NMR spectrum, **05**: 511
monounsaturated, key fragments in the spectra of pyrrolidides of, **05**: 506
prostaglandin precursors
  biological and physical properties, **08**: 322-328
  isolation and synthesis of, **08**: 326-327
  mammalian diet, metabolism reactions, **08**: 322-323
  nomenclature, **08**: 315-316
  occurrence, **08**: 323
refractive indices and equations for some, **05**: 493
saturated
  chemical characteristics, **05**: 484-485
  chemical formula, **05**: 484
  common name, **05**: 484
  physical characteristics, **05**: 484-485
solubilities of some, in water, table of values, **05**: 495
solubilities of water in saturated fatty acids, table, **05**: 495
specific volume, table, of acids from C_8 to C_{12}, **05**: 492

Fatty acids *(continued)*
  sunflower hull composition, **05:** 511
  temperature coefficients, table, of acids from C_8 to C_{12}, **05:** 492
  triglycerides, mixed triacid, solubility tables, **05:** 497
  triglycerides, simple saturated, solubility table, **05:** 496
  unsaturated
    chemical characteristics, **05:** 484-487
    chemical formula, **05:** 484-487
    common name, **05:** 484-487
    physical characteristics, **05:** 484-487
  wax esters and sterol esters from vernix caseosa and from human skin surface lipid, **05:** 509
Fatty acids, ligands binding to plasma albumin, **02:** 558-562
Feces
  human, porphyrin excretion, normal values, **08:** 279
  laboratory animal, porphyrin excretion, normal values, **08:** 279
Felinine
  physical and chemical properties, **01:** 154
Fermicidin; origin and characteristic as protein biosynthesis inhibitor, **04:** 38
Ferredoxin
  amino acid composition, complete data, **07:** 506
  average hydrophobicity value, **01:** 220
  circular dichroism, **07:** 94
    UV and near-UV region, **07:** 94, 150
  cyanogen bromide cleavage, **02:** 199
  molar absorptivity and-or absorbance values, **02:** 423-424
  nomenclature recommendations, **02:** 89-90, 120
  optical rotatory dispersion in the UV region, **07:** 55
  table of cofactors, molecular weights, stoichiometry and sources, **02:** 279
Ferredoxin hydrogenase
  circular dichroism in the UV region, **07:** 95
Ferredoxin I, II
  average hydrophobicity values, **01:** 220
Ferredoxins, bacterial
  amino acid sequences of some, **07:** 421-424
Ferrichrome
  proton NMR and suggested conformations, **07:** 567
Ferricrocin
  proton NMR and suggested conformations, **07:** 567-568
Ferrihemoglobin
  calorimetric ΔH values accompanying conformational changes, **06:** 270
Ferrihemoglobin, Hi^+
  UV and visible absorption spectrum, **07:** 179
Ferrihemoglobin cyanide, HiCN
  UV and visible absorption spectrum, **07:** 181
Ferrihemoglobin hydroxide, HiOH
  UV and visible absorption spectrum, **07:** 180
Ferrihemoproteins
  heat of proton ionization, pK, and related thermodynamic quantities, **06:** 200
Ferrimyoglobin complex
  heat of proton ionization, pK, and related thermodynamic quantities, **06:** 200
Ferriprotoporphyrin IX-globin
  UV spectra, molecular weight, **08:** 172

Ferritin
  average hydrophobicity value, **01:** 220
  circular dichroism in the UV region, **07:** 95
  molar absorptivity and-or absorbance values, **02:** 425
  molecular weight, stoichiometry, source, function, **02:** 276
  optical rotatory dispersion
    UV region, **07:** 55
    visible and near UV regions, **07:** 22
Ferrodoxyins, plant
  amino acid sequences, **07:** 425-426
Ferrohemoglobin
  UV and visible absorption spectrum, **07:** 176
Fetuin
  amino acid composition, complete data, **07:** 506
  animal sources, amino acid composition, **02:** 653
  circular dichroism, **07:** 95
    UV and near-UV region, **07:** 95, 150
  enzymatic hydrolysis, conjugated proteins, **02:** 211
  mammalian and chicken blood, specificity and properties, **02:** 638-639
  molar absorptivity and-or absorbance values, **02:** 425
  optical rotatory dispersion
    UV region, **07:** 55
    visible and near UV regions, **07:** 22
  plasma, nonhuman
    carbohydrate content, **02:** 259
Fiber protein
  circular dichroism in the UV region, **07:** 95
Fibrin
  calorimetric ΔH values accompanying conformational changes, **06:** 270
  molar absorptivity and-or absorbance values, **02:** 425
Fibrin stabilizing factor
  disc gel electrophoresis, **02:** 678
  measurement of, graph, **02:** 677
  molar absorptivity and-or absorbance values, **02:** 425
  physical data and characteristics, **02:** 254-255
  system in blood plasma, description, **02:** 670
Fibrinogen
  calorimetric Δ values accompanying conformational changes, **06:** 270
  circular dichroism in the UV region, **07:** 95
  molar absorptivity and-or absorbance values, **02:** 425-426
  molecular parameters, **02:** 248
  optical rotatory dispersion
    UV region, **07:** 55
    visible and near UV regions, **07:** 23
  physical data and characteristics, **02:** 254-255
  plasma, human
    carbohydrate content, molecular weights, sedimentation coefficients, **02:** 258
  refractive index increments, **02:** 375
Fibrinogen, iodinated
  refractive index increments, **02:** 375
Fibrinogen B
  average hydrophobicity value, **01:** 220
Fibrinoligase, transamidase activity, **02:** 671-681
Fibrinopeptides A
  amino acid sequences, **07:** 431-433

Fibrinopeptides B
  amino acid sequences, **07**: 433-435
Fibroin
  average hydrophobicity value, **01**: 220
  molar absorptivity and-or absorbance values, **02**: 426
Fibrous protein
  physical-chemical data for, index to ultracentrifuge studies, **02**: 229
Ficin
  amino acid sequence, **07**: 356-357
  molar absorptivity and-or absorbance values, **02**: 426
Ficin II
  average hydrophobicity value, **01**: 221
Ficin III
  average hydrophobicity value, **01**: 221
Filaments of nonmuscle myosins, table of data, **02**: 318
Filter holders, millipore, chemical compatibility, **08**: 431-432
Filters, millipore, chemical compatibility, **08**: 431-432
Filtration media, gel, *see* Gel filtration media
Fischer projection formula, description, **01**: 46, **02**: 46, **04**: 38, **05**: 43, **06**: 45, **08**: 45
Fischer projection in carbohydrate nomenclature, **05**: 100, 100-101
Fish
  DNA content per cell for various, table, **04**: 293-305
Fixation of enzymes, multifunctional reagents for, **02**: 735
Flagellin
  amino acid composition, complete data, **07**: 506
  average hydrophobicity value, **01**: 221
  circular dichroism in the UV region, **07**: 95
  optical rotatory dispersion
    UV region, **07**: 55
    visible and near UV regions, **07**: 23
Flavins, luminescence data table, **08**: 154-158
Flaviolin
  UV spectra, formula, molecular weight, **08**: 163
Flavobacterium
  amino acid requirements for growth, table, **04**: 633-634
  G + C composition of DNA of, table arranged by specie, **04**: 74
Flavodoxin
  amino acid composition, complete data, **07**: 506
  amino acid sequence, **07**: 430
  average hydrophobicity value, **01**: 221
  circular dichroism in the UV region, **07**: 95
  molar absorptivity and-or absorbance values, **02**: 426-427
Flavoprotein
  definition and nomenclature, **02**: 116
  molar absorptivity and-or absorbance values, **02**: 428
Flavoprotein containing FMN, *see* Flavodoxin
Flavoprotein containing riboflavin, *see* Riboflavin flavoprotein
Flexibacter
  G + C composition of DNA of, table arranged by specie, **04**: 104
Flexibacteria
  G + C composition of DNA of, table arranged by specie, **04**: 181

Flexothrix
  G + C composition of DNA of, table arranged by specie, **04**: 182
Flory-Fox equation for size of RNA, **04**: 405
Fluorescamine
  covalent protein conjugates, data, **01**: 208
Fluorescein isothiocyanate
  covalent protein conjugates, data, **01**: 208
Fluorescence
  flavins, table of luminescence data, **08**: 205-209
  porphyrins, maxima in various solvents, **08**: 275
  vitamin B_6 compounds, properties, **08**: 215
Fluorescent dyes bound to nucleic acids, data tables, **04**: 470
Fluorescent parameters, folic acid compounds of biological interest, **08**: 214
Fluorescent polyene probes, absorption, emission, lifetime, quantum yield, **08**: 211-212
Fluorescent probes
  commonly used for membrane studies, properties, **07**: 608-610
  enzyme cofactors, **07**: 601-602
  enzyme inhibitors, **07**: 598-599
  naphthalene sulfonates, protein structure, **07**: 604-606
γ-Fluoroglutamic acid
  antagonism to glutamic acid, **01**: 177
Fluorophenylalanines
  antagonism to phenylalanine, **01**: 179
5-Fluorotryptophan
  antagonism to tryptophan, **01**: 179
Fluorotyrosines
  antagonism to tyrosine, **01**: 180
6-Flurotryptophan
  antagonism to tryptophan, **01**: 179
Folacin
  nomenclature and structures, **08**: 17-18
  properties of, **08**: 295
Folic acid
  biological characteristics, **08**: 303
  nomenclature, journal references for, **02**: 87
  nomenclature and structure, **08**: 17-18
  properties of, **08**: 295
Folic acid compounds, fluorescent parameters, **08**: 214
Folic acid reductase, *see* Tetrahydrofolate dehydrogenase
Folinic acid, properties of, **08**: 295
Follicle-stimulating hormones
  amino acid composition, complete data, **07**: 506
  amino acid sequence of α subunit, **07**: 393-394
  circular dichroism in the UV region, **07**: 96
Follicle stimulating hormone
  average hydrophobicity value, **01**: 221
  molar absorptivity and-or absorbance values, **02**: 428
Fomes
  G + C composition of DNA of, table arranged by specie, **04**: 199
Fomitopsis (Fomes)
  G + C composition of DNA of, table arranged by specie, **04**: 199
Force-area data, linseed oil acids and esters, **05**: 497
Formic acid
  heat of proton ionization, pK, and related thermodynamic quantities, **06**: 200

N-Formimino-L-glutamate iminohydrolase
average hydrophobicity value, 01: 221
Formiminoglutamase
molar absorptivity and-or absorbance values, 02: 428
Formula
molecular
α,β-unsaturated amino acids, table, 01: 175
Formula, chemical
aldaric acids, 05: 168-170
alditols, amino, 05: 148-149
alditols, natural, 05: 139-142
aldonic acids, 05: 153-164
aldoses, natural, 05: 181-217
amino sugar acids, 05: 170-176
disaccharides, 05: 283-297, 327-334
fatty acids, 05: 484-490
heptasaccharides, 05: 318-319, 345-346
hexasaccharides, 05: 316-318, 344-345
inosamines, 05: 148-149
inositols, 05: 142-147
inososes, 05: 147
ketoses, natural, 05: 226-239
octasaccharides, 05: 319-346
oligosaccharides, 05: 283-319, 327-346
pentasaccharides, 05: 315-316, 343-344
tetrasaccharides, 05: 308-314, 340-343
trisaccharides, 05: 297-308, 334-340
uronic acids, 05: 165-168
Formula, empirical
pyridoxine, pyridoxal and pyridoxamine derivatives, 08:
252-266
vitamins, 08: 284-300
Formula, molecular
antibiotics, nucleoside, 03: 271-393
nucleosides, index to table, 03: 69-72
nucleotides, index to table, 03: 72-75
prostaglandin analogs, 08: 397-421
prostaglandin biosynthesis intermediates, thromboxanes
and by-products, 08: 334-340
prostaglandin metabolites, 08: 368-391
prostaglandin precursors, 08: 325
prostaglandins, naturally occurring, 08: 346-358
purines, index to table, 03: 67-69
pyrimides, index to table, 03: 67-69
Formula, molecular, steroids, 05: 531-588
Formula, structural, see Structure, also Structures
amino sugar, naturally occurring, 05: 359-370
chemical compounds, table, 06: 153-262
Formulas, for stereochemistry, use of, 05: 43-45
Formulas for stereochemistry, use of, 01: 46-48, 02: 46-48,
04: 38-40, 06: 45, 08: 45-47
Formycin, physicochemical constants, spectral, chemotherapeutic and biological properties, 03: 320
Formycin B, physicochemical constants, spectral, chemotherapeutic and biological properties, 03: 322
N-Formyl-N-hydroxyaminoacetic acid, see Hadacidin
γ-Formyl-N-methylnorvaline
physical and chemical properties, 01: 148
N-Formyl methionine
physical and chemical properties, 01: 154
Formyltetrahydrofolate synthetase
amino acid composition, incomplete data, 07: 512

Forocidin; origin, structure, and characteristic as protein
biosynthesis inhibitor, 04: 574
Fraction
soluble, enzymatic activity, table, 02: 715-719
subcellular, enzymatic activity, tables, 02: 697-719
Fraction 1 protein
amino acid composition, complete data, 07: 507
Fragment
definition, 02: 181
Free energy
decarboxylation, values for several compounds, 06: 303
hydrolysis
acetic acid esters and related compounds, 06: 300
amides, 06: 301
discussion and sample calculations, 06: 296-299
glycosides, 06: 303
phosphates, 06: 302
thiol esters, 06: 301
redox in reactions, 06: 121
Free energy of formation
amino acids, table, 06: 111-112
amino acids in aqueous solution at 25°C, 06: 118
peptides, table, 06: 112
Free energy of solution
amino acids in aqueous solution at 25°C, 06: 118
Freezing point
N,N-dimethylformamide-water mixtures, 06: 528
dimethylsulfoxide-water mixtures, 06: 527
ethylene glycol-methanol-water mixtures, 06: 528
ethylene glycol-water mixtures, 06: 522
fatty acids, effect of addition of water, graph, 05: 495
glycerol-water mixtures, 06: 526
methanol-water mixtures, 06: 523
2-methyl-2-4-pentanediol-water mixtures, 06: 524
1-2-propanediol-water mixtures, 06: 525
Frequencies, calculated characteristic polypeptide table,
07: 596
Frictional coefficients
proteins
carbohydrate, index to studies containing, 02: 232
globular, index to studies containing, 02: 232
organelles, index to studies containing, 02: 232
particles, index to studies containing, 02: 232
virus, index to studies containing, 02: 232
Frictional ratio
proteins
human plasma, table of values, 02: 242-250
Tamm-Horsfall mucoprotein, 02: 304
Fructosan-specific protein
circular dichroism in the UV region, 07: 96
Fructose
heat of proton ionization, pK, and related thermodynamic quantities, 06: 201
pK'_a values, 06: 317
Fructose-bisphosphate aldolase
amino acid composition, complete date, 07: 507
amino acid sequence, 07: 333-335
circular dichroism in the UV region, 07: 96
optical rotatory dispersion
UV region, 07: 56
visible and near UV regions, 07: 23

Fructose-1,6-diphosphatase, *see* Hexosediphosphatase
average hydrophobicity value, **01:** 221
Fructose 1,6-diphosphate adolase A
amino acid composition, complete data, **07:** 507
Fructose-1,6-diphosphate aldolase, *see* Fructose-
bisphosphate aldolase
Fructose diphosphatase
subunit, constitution of, **02:** 336
Fructose diphosphate aldolase
subunit, constitution of, **02:** 329
Fucose, content of, in glycoproteins, **02:** 258-267, 271-274
α-L-Fucosidase
carbohydrate content, **02:** 274
subunit, constitution of, **02:** 341
Fulgio
G + C composition of DNA of, table arranged by specie, **04:** 199
Fumarase
amino acid composition, complete data, **07:** 507
circular dichroism in near-UV region, at room temperature, **07:** 150
enzymatic activity, subcellular fractions, **02:** 702
molar absorptivity and-or absorbance values, **02:** 429
subunit, constitution of, **02:** 340
Fumarate hydratase
circular dichroism in the UV region, **07:** 97
optical rotatory dispersion
UV region, **07:** 56
visible and near UV regions, **07:** 23
N-Fumarylalanine
physical and chemical properties, **01:** 118
Function $e^{-c^2} \int^c e^{x^2} dx$
numerical values, table, **07:** 14
Fungal Genetics Stock Center
address, **04:** 732
availability of located mutants of *Aspergillus nidulans*,
04: 732-737
Fungi
amino acid requirements for growth, table, **04:** 640
DNA base compositions for, **04:** 237-239
DNA content per cell for various, table, **04:** 284-285
G + C composition of DNA of, table arranged by specie, **04:** 185-224
haploid chromosome numbers in, table of values, **04:**
874-877
Furanomycin
physical and chemical properties, **01:** 140
Furanomycin; origin, structure, and characteristic as
protein biosynthesis inhibitor, **04:** 574
Furosine
physical and chemical properties, **01:** 140
Furostans
names, new standard vs. old, **05:** 69-70
steroid nomenclature, use of term, **05:** 68-69
structures, **05:** 69-70
ε-*N*-(2-Furoyl-methyl)-lypine, *see* Furosine
β-2-Furylalanine
antagonism to phenylalanine, **01:** 179
β-3-Furylalanine
antagonism to phenylalanine, **01:** 179
Fusarenone X; origin, structure, and characteristic as
protein biosynthesis inhibitor, **04:** 574

Fusarinine
physical and chemical properties, **01:** 149
Fusarium
amino acid requirements for growth, table, **04:** 640
G + C composition of DNA of, table arranged by specie, **04:** 199
Fusidic acid; origin, structure, and characteristic as
protein biosynthesis inhibitor, **04:** 575
Fusidin, inhibitor of protein biosynthesis, **04:** 575
Fusobacterium
amino acid requirements for growth, table, **04:** 634
G + C composition of DNA of, table arranged by specie, **04:** 87

G

G + C composition
algae DNA, arranged by genera and specie, **04:** 224-227
bacteria DNA, arranged by family, genera, specie, **04:**
69-183
DNA base composition of eucaryotic protists, table, **04:**
236-239
fungi DNA, arranged by genera and specie, **04:** 185-224
protozoa DNA, arranged by genera and specie, **04:**
228-229
G + C composition of DNA of, table arranged by specie, **04:** 192
G + C content
mitochondrial DNAs, table, **04:** 363-372
satellite DNAs
amphibia, **04:** 389-390
birds, **04:** 390-391
crustaceae, **04:** 384-387
insects, **04:** 380-384
mammals, **04:** 391-399
molluscs, **04:** 387
plants, **04:** 399-402
tunicates, **04:** 388
viral DNA, **03:** 560-562
viral DNA molecules, **03:** 551-556
γG Immunoglobulin kappa chain
amino acid composition, complete data, **07:** 508
Gaffkya
G + C composition of DNA of, table arranged by specie, **04:** 127
Galactokinase
amino acid composition, complete data, **07:** 507
Galactose
heat of proton ionization, p*K*, and related thermodynamic quantities, **06:** 201
pK'_a values, **06:** 317
Galactose 1-phosphate uridylyltransferase
amino acid composition, incomplete data, **07:** 512
Galactose oxidase
amino acid composition, incomplete data, **07:** 512
circular dichroism in the UV region, **07:** 97
UV and near-UV region, **07:** 97, 151
α-Galactosidase
carbohydrate content, **02:** 274
molar absorptivity and-or absorbance values, **02:** 429

β-Galactosidase
  amino acid composition, complete data, **07**: 507
  average hydrophobicity value, **01**: 221
  cyanogen bromide cleavage, **02**: 199
  molar absorptivity and-or absorbance values, **02**: 429
  subunit, constitution of, **02**: 348
α-D-Galactoside galactohydrolase
  enzymatic reactions, velocity and parameters, table, **05**: 440-441
β-D-Galactoside galactohydrolase
  enzymatic reactions, velocity and parameters, table, **05**: 435-438
Ganoderma
  G + C composition of DNA of, table arranged by specie, **04**: 127
Gastricin
  average hydrophobicity value, **01**: 221
Gastrin
  cyanogen bromide cleavage, **02**: 199
  molar absorptivity and-or absorbance values, **02**: 429
Gastrin I
  amino acid composition, incomplete data, **07**: 512
  circular dichroism in the UV region, **07**: 97
Gastrins
  amino acid sequence, **07**: 323
Gaugliodise, generic term usage, **05**: 10
GC composition
  calculation of, from buoyant density, **04**: 356
  DNA
    chloroplast, table of values, **04**: 356-358
    nuclear, table of values, **04**: 356-358
GDP, *see* Guanylic acid
  pK'_a values, **06**: 331
Gel filtration media
  Bio-Gel A$^®$, properties, 08: 130
  Bio-Gel P$^®$, properties, 08: 131-132
  Sephadex$^®$, properties, 08: 133-134
  Sepharose$^®$, properties, 08: 135
Gelasinospora
  G + C composition of DNA of, table arranged by specie, **04**: 199-200
Gelatin
  refractive index increments, **02**: 375
Gene symbols
  Escherichia coli, genetic markers, **04**: 654-659
Generic terms, for lipids, **05**: 9-10
Genes
  bacteriophage T4, map and data, **04**: 665-673
Genetic code, codons, table, **04**: 896
Genetic factors
  immunoglobulins, human, notation for, **02**: 186
Genetic map
  Escherichia coli bacteriophage lambda (λ), **04**: 678
  saccharomyces cerevisiae, **04**: 765-766
Genetic markers, *see also* Morphogenetic markers
  designation of, for *Bacillus subtilis*, **04**: 686-698
  Escherichia coli, **04**: 654-659
  Streptomyces coelicolor, list, **04**: 724-727
  maize (*Zea mays* L.), annotated list, **04**: 835-844
  mouse (Mus musculus), **04**: 857-870
  Saccharomyces cerevisiae, **04**: 767-826
  Salmonella typhimurium, **04**: 705-717

Genetic symbols
  Drosophila melanogaster, biochemical mutants, **04**: 848-855
  located mutants of *Aspergillus nidulans*, **04**: 732-737
  maize (*Zea mays* L.), list, **04**: 835-844
  Neurospora crassa, **04**: 740-757
Genetic variations in man, tables of enzymes and variations in proteins and clotting factors, **04**: 879-883
Gentamycin (C$_1$ and C$_2$); origin, structure, and characteristic as protein biosynthesis inhibitor, **04**: 575
Geotrichum
  G + C composition of DNA of, table arranged by specie, **04**: 200
Gibbs energy, standardization of data presentation, **06**: 95-99
Gigartinine
  physical and chemical properties, **01**: 133
Gilbertella
  G + C composition of, DNA of, table arranged by specie, **04**: 200
Glaucoma
  amino acid requirements for growth, table, **04**: 641
  G + C composition of DNA of, table arranged by specie, **04**: 228
Gliadin
  circular dichroism in the UV region, **07**: 97
  optical rotatory dispersion
    UV region, **07**: 56
    visible and near UV regions, **07**: 23
α-Gliadin
  amino acid composition, incomplete data, **07**: 512
  circular dichroism in the UV region, **07**: 97
  optical rotatory dispersion
    UV region, **07**: 56
    visible and near UV regions, **07**: 23
Gliadin SP 2-2, SP 2-1
  average hydrophobicity values, **01**: 221
Gliocladium
  amino acid requirements for growth, table, **04**: 640
  G + C composition of DNA of, table arranged by specie, **04**: 200
Globin, *see also* Haptoglobin, Hemoglobin listings
  molar absorptivity and-or absorbance values, **02**: 430
  refractive index increments, **02**: 375, 376
  stereo drawings of several, **02**: 761
Globins, metazoan, aligned chains
  amino acid sequence, **07**: 456-458
Globular protein
  physical-chemical data for, index to ultracentrifuge studies, **02**: 222-228
Globulin, *see also* Macroglobulin
  carbohydrate content, **02**: 270
  molar absorptivity and-or absorbance values, **02**: 430
  plasma, human
    carbohydrate content, molecular weights, sedimentation coefficients, **02**: 258
  subunit, constitution of, **02**: 349
α$_2$-Globulin
  refractive index increments, **02**: 376
γ-Globulin, *see* Immunoglobulin
  refractive index increments, **02**: 376

γI-Globulin
  luminescence of, table, **01**: 205
*β*₁-Globulin
  refractive index increments, **02**: 376
Globulin, 0.6 S γ₂
  average hydrophobicity value, **01**: 221
Gloeophyllum (Lenzites)
  G + C composition of DNA of, table arranged by spe-
    cie, **04**: 200
Glu(Asp)-plasminogen, amino-terminus of single chain
  alignment of amino-terminal amino acid sequences
    homologous to, **07**: 341
Glucagon
  amino acid sequence, **07**: 376
  average hydrophobicity value, **01**: 221
  circular dichroism in the UV region, **07**: 97
  luminescence of, table, **01**: 205
  molar absorptivity and-or absorbance values, **02**: 431
  optical rotatory dispersion in the UV region, **07**: 56
S-β-1-(Gluco-pyranosyl)-3-indolylacetothiohydroximyl-
    O-sulfate, *see* Glucobrassicin
Glucobrassicin
  physical and chemical properties, **01**: 154
Gluconobacter
  G + C composition of DNA of, table arranged by spe-
    cie, **04**: 153
Glucose
  p*K′*ₐ values, **06**: 317
Glucose 6-phosphate dehydrogenase, **02**: 336
  Neurospora crassa mutant, **04**: 755
  optical rotatory dispersion
    UV region, **07**: 56
    visible and near UV regions, **07**: 23
Glucose-6-phosphate isomerase, *see* Glucosephosphate,
    isomerase
Glucose derivatives
Glucose oxidase
  carbohydrate content, **02**: 273
  circular dichroism in the UV region, **07**: 97
  molar absorptivity and-or absorbance values, **02**: 431
  optical rotatory dispersion
    UV region, **07**: 56
    visible and near UV region, **07**: 23
Glucosephosphate isomerase
  circular dichroism in the UV region, **07**: 97
  optical rotatory dispersion
    UV region, **07**: 56
    visible and near UV regions, **07**: 23
v-Glucuronidase
  amino acid composition, incomplete data, **07**: 512
β-Glucuronidase
  carbohydrate content, **02**: 274
  molar absorptivity and-or absorbance values, **02**: 432
Glutamate decarboxylase
  average hydrophobicity value, **01**: 221
  molar absorptivity and-or absorbance values, **02**: 432
  subunit, constitution of, **02**: 331, 345
Glutamate decarboxylation pathway; pathways chart, **04**:
    insert
Glutamate dehydrogenase
  amino acid sequence, **07**: 316-318
  average hydrophobicity value, **01**: 221

  luminescence of, table, **01**: 205
  molar absorptivity and-or absorbance values, **02**: 432
  subunit, constitution of, **02**: 344, 345
Glutamate dehydrogenase (NADP⁺)
  circular dichroism in the UV region, **07**: 98
  optical rotatory dispersion
    UV region, **07**: 57
    visible and near UV regions, **07**: 24
Glutamate dehydrogenase³ neurospora (NADP)
  amino acid sequence, **07**: 318-320
Glutamate mutase component
  amino acid composition, incomplete data, **07**: 512
Glutamic acid
  active site peptides, **07**: 188
  antagonists of, **01**: 177
  free acid in amniotic fluid in early pregnancy and at
    term, **01**: 327
  free acid in blood plasma of newborn infants and
    adults, **01**: 328
  heat of proton ionization, pK, and related thermody-
    namic quantities, **06**: 202
  nucleoside composition, tables of values, **04**: 429
  nucleotide sequences of, **04**: 442-443
  p*K′*ₐ values, **06**: 318
  physical and chemical properties, **01**: 118
  requirements of, for growth of various microorganisms,
    table, **04**: 630-643
  specific rotatory dispersion constants, 0.1 *M* solution,
    01: 244
  spectra, far UV, **01**: 184
  symbols for atoms and bonds in side chains, **01**: 70, **02**:
    74
  thumbprint, content in, **08**: 121
Glutamic dehydrogenase
  cofactors, molecular weights, stoichiometry and sources,
    02: 284
  molar absorptivity and-or absorbance values, **02**: 432
  refractive index increments, **02**: 376
Glutaminase-asparaginase
  average hydrophobicity value, **01**: 222
Glutamine
  antagonists of, **01**: 177
  free acid in amniotic fluid in early pregnancy and at
    term, **01**: 327
  free acid in blood plasma of newborn infants and
    adults, **01**: 328
  nucleoside composition, tables of values, **04**: 430
  nucleotide sequences of, **04**: 444-445
  p*K*ₐ values, **06**: 318
  physical and chemical properties, **01**: 118
  requirements of, for growth of various microorganisms,
    table, **04**: 630-643
  symbols for atoms and bonds in side chains, **01**: 70, **02**:
    74
Glutamine-synthetase adenyltransferase, **07**: 98
  circular dichroism in the UV region, **07**: 98
Glutamine synthetase
  average hydrophobicity value, **01**: 222
  circular dichroism in the UV region, **07**: 98
  molar absorptivity and-or absorbance values, **02**: 433
  Neurospora crassa mutant, **04**: 752
  optical rotatory dispersion in the UV region, **07**: 57

Glutamine synthetase *(continued)*
  subunit, constitution of, **02:** 345, 346, 347, 349
γ-Glutaminyl-3,4-benzoquinone
  physical and chemical properties, **01:** 140
γ-Glutaminyl-4-hydroxybenzene
  physical and chemical properties, **01:** 130
γ-Glutamyl-2-amino-4-methyl-hex-4-enoic acid
  physical and chemical properties, **01:** 115
β-N-(γ-Glutamyl)-aminopropionitrile, *see* Lathyrus factor
γ-Glutamyl cyclotransferase
  average hydrophobicity value, **01:** 222
γ-Glutamyl transferase
  carbohydrate content, **02:** 274
γ-Glutamylethylamide
  antagonism to glutamic acid, **01:** 177
γ-Glutamylhydrazide
  antagonism to glutamine, **01:** 177
Glutaric acidemia
  characteristics of, **01:** 326
Glutathione peroxidase
  circular dichroism
    UV and near-UV region, **07:** 98, 151
  molar absorptivity and-or absorbance values, **02:** 433
  molecular weight, stoichiometry and source, **02:** 285
Glutathione reductase
  molar absorptivity and-or absorbance values, **02:** 433
  subunit, constitution of, **02:** 333
Glutathione reductase (NAD(P)H)
  amino acid composition, incomplete data, **07:** 512
  optical rotatory dispersion
    UV region, **07:** 57
    visible and near UV regions, **07:** 24
Gluten
  optical rotatory dispersion in the visible and near UV regions, **07:** 24
Glutenin
  circular dichroism in the UV region, **07:** 98
  optical rotatory dispersion
    UV region, **07:** 57
    visible and near UV regions, **07:** 24
Glyceraldehyde-phosphate dehydrogenase
  circular dichroism in the UV region, **07:** 99
  optical rotatory dispersion
    UV region, **07:** 57
    visible and near UV regions, **07:** 24
D-Glyceraldehyde-3-phosphate dehydrogenase
  refractive index increments, **02:** 376
Glyceraldehyde-3-phosphate dehydrogenase
  amino acid sequence, **07:** 327-329
  circular dichroism in near-UV region, at room temperature, **07:** 151
  molar absorptivity and-or absorbance values, **02:** 434
  subunit, constitution of, **02:** 349
  viscosity, intrinsic, **02:** 721
Glyceroglycolipids, nomenclature and classification, **05:** 416, 421-423
Glycerokinase
  optical rotatory dispersion
    UV region, **07:** 58
    visible and near UV regions, **07:** 25
L-Glycerol 3-phosphate dehydrogenase
  amino acid composition, complete data, **07:** 507

Glycerol-3-phosphate dehydrogenase
  average hydrophobicity value, **01:** 222
  molar absorptivity and-or absorbance values, **02:** 434
Glycerol-water mixtures, dielectric constants and freezing points, **06:** 526
Glycerol derivatives
  heat of proton ionization, pK, and related thermodynamic quantities, **06:** 202
Glycerol derivatives, stereospecific nomenclature, **05:** 10
α-Glycerophosphate dehydrogenase
  optical rotatory dispersion
    UV region, **07:** 58
    visible and near UV regions, **07:** 25
Glycine
  antagonism to α alanine, **01:** 177
  antagonists of, **01:** 177
  free acid in amniotic fluid in early pregnancy and at term, **01:** 327
  free acid in blood plasma of newborn infants and adults, **01:** 328
  hyperglycinemia ketotic (severe infantile), effect of, **01:** 318
  ninhydrin reaction, absorption ratio, **08:** 123
  nucleoside composition, tables of values, **04:** 430-432
  nucleotide sequences of, **04:** 444-445
  pK'_a values, **06:** 318
  physical and chemical properties, **01:** 116
  requirements of, for growth of various microorganisms, table, **04:** 630-643
  thumbprint, content in, **08:** 121
Glycine-HCl buffer, preparation of, **06:** 370
Glycine-NaOH buffer, preparation of, **06:** 376
Glycine betaine, *see* Lycin
Glycine buffers
  protonic activity tables, **06:** 537-539
Glycine derivatives
  heat of proton ionization, pK, and related thermodynamic quantities, **06:** 203-205
Glycine nonketotic
  hyperglycinemia, effect of, **01:** 319
Glycinin
  circular dichroism in the UV region, **07:** 99
  optical rotatory dispersion
    UV region, **07:** 58
    visible and near UV regions, **07:** 25
N⁶-Glycinocarbonyladenosine
  isolation and detection of, in RNA, general remarks, **03:** 234
  RNA, various, natural occurrence in, **03:** 218
Glycocyamine, *see* Guanidinoacetyl
Glycocyamine kinase, *see* Guanidinoacetate, kinase
  average hydrophobicity value, **01:** 222
Glycocyaminekinase
  molar absorptivity and-or absorbance values, **02:** 435
Glycogen phosphorylase
  amino acid composition, incomplete data, **07:** 507
  average hydrophobicity value, **01:** 222
Glycohydrolases
  enzymatic reactions, velocity and parameters, tables, **05:** 426-445
Glycolipids
  classification and nomenclature of, **05:** 416-423

Glycolipids *(continued)*
of bacteria, structures and organisms, **05:** 373-393
Glycolytic enzymes
amino acid sequences, **07:** 324, 337
Glycoprotein
amino acid composition, complete data, **07:** 507
amino acid composition, incomplete data, **07:** 512
circular dichroism in the UV region, **07:** 99
γ-Glycoprotein
average hydrophobicity value, **01:** 222
Glycoprotein, Tamm-Horsfall
circular dichroism in the UV region, **07:** 98
Glycoprotein hormones
amino acid sequences of α subunit, **07:** 393-394
Glycoprotein M-1
amino acid composition, incomplete data, **07:** 513
Glycoproteins
blood group substances
carbohydrate content, **02:** 262-263
body fluids
carbohydrate content, **02:** 267
cell membrane
carbohydrate content, **02:** 266
definition of, **02:** 257
eggs
carbohydrate content, **02:** 268-269
enzymes
carbohydrate content, **02:** 273-274
hormones
carbohydrate content, **02:** 271-272
lectins, purified, table of properties, **02:** 546-551
milk
carbohydrate content, **02:** 268-269
molar absorptivity and-or absorbance values, **02:** 435-436
molecular parameters, **02:** 242
mouse plasma, tumor
molar absorptivity and-or absorbance values, **02:** 435
mucins
carbohydrate content, **02:** 262-263
plants
carbohydrate content, **02:** 270
plasma, human
carbohydrate content, molecular weights, sedimentation coefficients, **02:** 258
plasma, nonhuman
carbohydrate content, **02:** 259-260
Tamm-Horsfall, *see also* Tamm-Horsfall glycoprotein; Tamm-Horsfall mucoprotein
molar absorptivity and-or absorbance values, **02:** 435
Tamm-Horsfall, human urine
Tamm-Horsfall, rabbit urine
molar absorptivity and-or absorbance values, **02:** 435
Tamm-Horsfall, rat intestinal mucosa
molar absorptivity and-or absorbance values, **02:** 435
tissues
carbohydrate content, **02:** 264-265
viruses, enveloped
carbohydrate content, **02:** 267
Glycoproteins, mammalian, carbohydrate-amino acid linkages found in, **05:** 281

Glycosaminoglycans, *see* Mucopolysaccharides
table of data and characteristics, **02:** 686-687
Glycoses, acyl, structures and organisms, **05:** 373-375
Glycoside derivatives of phospholipids, structures and organisms, **05:** 385-387
Glycosides
free energy values of hydrolysis, **06:** 303
Glycosides, nomenclature rules, **05:** 116-117
Glycosidic lipids, miscellaneous, structures and organisms, **05:** 388-390
Glycosphingolipid, generic term usage, **05:** 9
Glycosyl diglycerides, structures and organisms, **05:** 376-385
Glycosyl esters of polyisoprenol phosphate and pyrophosphate, structures and organisms, **05:** 391-393
Glycosyl radicals and glycosylamines, nomenclature rules, **05:** 117-118
Glycosyloxy radicals, nomenclature rules, **05:** 119
Glycylglycine
heat capacity and entropy values, **06:** 110
Glyoxalase
optical rotatory dispersion
UV region, **07:** 58
visible and near UV region, **07:** 25
Glyoxylate cycle; pathways chart, **04:** insert
Glyoxylate reductase
optical rotatory dispersion
UV region, **07:** 58
visible and near UV regions, **07:** 25
Glyoxylic acid, properties of, **01:** 181
Golgi material
enzymatic activity, table, **02:** 714
Gonadotrophin-transporting protein
plasma, nonhuman
carbohydrate content, **02:** 259
Gonadotropin, chorionic, *see* Chorionic gonadotropin
Gougerotin, physicochemical constants, spectral, chemotherapeutic and biological properties, **03:** 324
Gougerotin; origin, structure, and characteristic as protein biosynthesis inhibitor, **04:** 576
Graft rejection
hisocompatibility antigens, presence of, **04:** 884
histocompatibility loci, estimation of, **04:** 885
laws of transplantation, defined, **04:** 884
major histocompatibility complex, role of, **04:** 885
Gramicidin S-A
proton NMR and suggested conformations, **07:** 563
Griseoviridine; origin, structure, and characteristic as protein biosynthesis inhibitor, **04:** 576
Group specific protein
amino acid composition, incomplete data, **07:** 513
Growth hormone
amino acid composition, complete data, **07:** 507
amino acid sequence, **07:** 376, 388-389, 392-393
average hydrophobicity value, **01:** 222
bovine
pituitary gland, constitution of subunit, **02:** 327
circular dichroism
UV and near UV region, **07:** 98, 151
cyanogen bromide cleavage, **02:** 199
luminescence of, table, **01:** 206
molar absorptivity and-or absorbance values, **02:** 437

Growth hormone *(continued)*
  optical rotatory dispersion
    UV regions, **07**: 58
    visible and near UV regions, **07**: 25
Guanidine
  pK'_a values, **06**: 344
Guanidine-1-pyrroline-5-carboxylic acid, *see* Viomycidine
Guanidine hydrochloride
  densities of aqueous solutions with added reagents, at 25°, **06**: 406
  density, summary of data, **06**: 404
  index of refraction, summary of data, **06**: 404
  viscosities of aqueous solutions with added reagents, at 25°, **06**: 407
  viscosity of aqueous solutions at 25°, **06**: 405
Guanidinoacetate kinase
  optical rotatory dispersion in the visible and near UV regions, **07**: 25
Guanidinoacetyl
  structure and symbols for those incorporated into synthetic polypeptides, **01**: 102
β-Guanidinoalanine
  structure and symbols for those incorporated into synthetic polypeptides, **01**: 102
Guanidinomethylarginine, *see* ω-*N*-Methylarginine
5-Guanidinovaleric acid
  structure and symbols for those incorporated into synthetic polypeptides, **01**: 102
Guanidinyl protein group, chemical modification of reagents used, table of specificities, **02**: 203-204
β-Guanido-γ-hydroxyvaline
  physical and chemical properties, **01**: 124
Guanido amino acids
  physical and chemical properties, **01**: 132-134
Guanidotaurine
  physical and chemical properties, **01**: 154
Guanine
  pK'_a values, **06**: 331
Guanine and derivatives
  physical constants and spectral properties, index to, **03**: 67
  UV spectra, **03**: 423-427
  UV spectral characteristics and acid dissociation constants, **03**: 411-412
Guanosine
  bond angles and distances, **08**: 225
  chemical structures and approved numbering schemes, **08**: 224
  composition in various tRNA's, **04**: 428-441
  pK'_a values, **06**: 331
  raman frequencies, table of values, **03**: 538-539
Guanosine and derivatives
  UV spectra, **03**: 436-440
  UV spectral characteristics and acid dissociation constants, **03**: 414
Guanosine and nucleoside derivatives
  physical constants and spectral properties, index to, **03**: 70
Guanosine derivatives
  heat of proton ionization, pK, and related thermodynamic quantities, **06**: 206

Guanosine nucleotide derivatives
  physical constants and spectral properties, index to, **03**: 73-74
Guanylic acid
  derivatives, UV spectral characteristics and acid dissociation constants, **03**: 416
Guanyloribonuclease
  amino acid composition, complete data, **07**: 510
  amino acid sequences, **07**: 311
  circular dichroism
    UV and near UV region, **07**: 99, 161
  optical rotatory dispersion
    UV region, **07**: 58
    visible and near UV regions, **07**: 25
5′-Guanylylmethylene diphosphate; origin, structure, and characteristic as protein biosynthesis inhibitor, **04**: 577
Guinea pig
  inbred strain availability, **04**: 884
  MHC designation, **04**: 885
  mitochondrial DNA from, properties, **04**: 371
  satellite DNAs
    buoyant density and G + C content of, table, **04**: 394
Guvacine
  physical and chemical properties, **01**: 140
Gylceraldehyde-3-phosphate dehydrogenase
  average hydrophobicity value, **01**: 222
  luminescence of, table, **01**: 206
Gymnoascus
  G + C composition of DNA of, table arranged by specie, **04**: 200
Gymnosperms; buoyant density and G + C content of satellite DNAs for several varieties, table, **04**: 399-400

H

Hadacidin
  antagonism to aspartic acid, **01**: 177
  physical and chemical properties, **01**: 135
Haemophilus
  G + C composition of DNA of, table arranged by specie, **04**: 91
Hageman factor
  amino acid composition, incomplete data, **07**: 513
  physical data and characteristics, **02**: 254-255
  plasma, nonhuman
    carbohydrate content, **02**: 260
Halobacterium
  amino acid requirements for growth, table, **04**: 634
  G + C composition of DNA of, table arranged by specie, **04**: 154
L-Halogen-containing amino acids
  physical and chemical properties, **01**: 159-160
Hamster
  deoxynucleotide polymerizing enzymes from, properties of, **04**: 539-544
  mitochondrial DNA from, properties, **04**: 371
Hanseniaspora
  G + C composition of DNA of, table arranged by specie, **04**: 200

Hansenula
G + C composition of DNA of, table arranged by specie, **04:** 200-203

Haploid chromosome numbers in fungi, table of values, **04:** 874-877

Haplosporangium
G + C composition of DNA of, table arranged by specie, **04:** 203

Haptoglobin
amino acid composition, complete data, **07:** 507
circular dichroism in the UV region, **07:** 99
molar absorptivity and-or absorbance values, **02:** 437
optical rotatory dispersion in the visible and near UV regions, **07:** 25
plasma, human
carbohydrate content, molecular weights, sedimentation coefficients, **02:** 258

Haptoglobin, α_{1S}-chain
average hydrophobicity value, **01:** 222

Haptoglobin, α_2-chain
average hydrophobicity value, **01:** 222

Haptoglobin, β-chain
average hydrophobicity value, **01:** 222

Haptoglobin 1-1, human
molar absorptivity and-or absorbance values, **02:** 437
subunit, constitution of, **02:** 331

Haptoglobulin, human
molar absorptivity and-or absorbance values, **02:** 437

Harringtonine; origin, structure, and characteristic as protein biosynthesis inhibitor, **04:** 577

Hartnup disease
characteristics of, **01:** 324

Harvard system in citation of bibliographic references, **01:** 18-19, **02:** 18-19, **03:** 60-61, **04:** 60-61, **05:** 14-16, **06:** 59, **08:** 59-60

Haworth representation in carbohydrate nomenclature, **05:** 100-101

HCl numbers, porphyrins, **08:** 275

Heat capacity
amino acids, table of values, **06:** 109
peptides, table of values for several, **06:** 110
proteins, table of values for several , **06:** 110

Heat of combustion
amino acids, table, **06:** 111-112
peptides, table, **06:** 112

Heat of proton ionization
chemical compounds, table of values, **06:** 153-262

Heat of reaction
macromolecules, conformational changes of, **06:** 270-293

Heat of solution
amino acids in aqueous solution at 25°C, **06:** 116-117

Heavy merromyosin (HMM), *see* Myosin, HMM

Helical complexes, double
molar residue ellipticity, table of values, **03:** 601
molar residue rotation, **03:** 599

Helical content
of some proteins, spectra, **07:** 8-13

Helical segments, nomenclature rules in polypeptides chain, **01:** 72, **02:** 76

Helicoma
G + C composition of DNA of, table arranged by specie, **04:** 203

Helicorubin
definition and nomenclature, **02:** 118

Helicostylium
G + C composition of DNA of, table arranged by specie, **04:** 203

α-Helix content
tropomyosin from nonmuscle values, **02:** 321

Helminthosporium
amino acid requirements for growth, table, **04:** 640
G + C composition of DNA of, table arranged by specie, **04:** 203

Helvella
G + C composition of DNA of, table arranged by specie, **04:** 203

Hemagglutin
average hydrophobicity value, **01:** 222-223

Hemagglutin I and II
average hydrophobicity values, **01:** 222

Hemagglutinin
amino acid composition, complete data, **07:** 507
amino acid composition, incomplete data, **07:** 513
carbohydrate content, **02:** 270
molar absorptivity and-or absorbance values, **02:** 437
subunit, constitution of, **02:** 327

Hematin
absorption maxima in ether, **08:** 279

Heme-base complexes, positions and extinctions of α bands, **08:** 280

Heme proteins
resonance raman spectra, **07:** 589

Hemerythrin
amino acid composition, complete data, **07:** 507
amino acid sequences, **07:** 498
average hydrophobicity value, **01:** 223
circular dichroism
UV and near UV region, **07:** 99, 151
molar absorptivity and-or absorbance values, **02:** 437
molecular weight, stoichiometry, source, function, **02:** 276
optical rotatory dispersion in the UV region, **07:** 58
refractive index increments, **02:** 376
subunit, constitution of, **02:** 327, 334

Hemin
absorption maxima in ether, **08:** 279
R_F value in 2,6-lutidine-water system, **08:** 276

Hemin chloride dimethyl ester
UV and visible absorption spectrum, **07:** 183
UV spectra, formula, molecular weight, **08:** 174

Hemochrome spectra, pyridine, **08:** 280

Hemocuprein, *see* Superoxide dismutase

Hemocyanin
amino acid composition, complete data, **07:** 507
average hydrophobicity value, **01:** 223
circular dichroism
UV and near UV region, **07:** 99, 152
molar absorptivity and-or absorbance values, **02:** 438
molecular weight, stoichiometry, source, function, **02:** 277
subunit, constitution of, **02:** 350

Hemoglobin
amino acid composition, complete data, **07:** 507
average hydrophobicity value, **01:** 223

Hemoglobin *(continued)*
  beef
    molar absorptivity and-or absorbance values, **02:** 443
  bovine
    refractive index increments, **02:** 376
  canine
    refractive index increments, **02:** 376
  α-chain variants, **07:** 461-468
  β-chain variants, **07:** 461-468
  circular dichroism
    UV and near UV region, **07:** 152
  helical number, **07:** 461-468
  horse
    molar absorptivity and-or absorbance values, **02:** 443
  human, *see also* Human hemoglobin
    heat of proton ionization, pK, and related thermody-
      namic quantities, **06:** 206
    molar absorptivity and-or absorbance values, **02:** 444
    pK values, α-amino groups, table, **02:** 693
    pK values, cysteine β 93 SH, **02:** 696
    pK values, histidine, **02:** 690
    pK values, histidine 146 β, **02:** 690
    pK values, tyrosine, **02:** 695
    refractive index increments, **02:** 376
  human Hb, subunits
    molar absorptivity and-or absorbance values, **02:** 447
  known substitutions deletions, index to, **07:** 461-468
  luminescence of, table, **01:** 206
  molar absorptivity and-or absorbance values, **02:**
    439-445
  mouse
    molar absorptivity and-or absorbance values, **02:** 444
  optical rotatory dispersion
    UV region, **07:** 58
    visible and near UV regions, **07:** 25
  oxidation-reduction potentials of, **06:** 137-139
  sheep
    molar absorptivity and-or absorbance values, **02:** 443
  subunit, constitution of, **02:** 328, 351
  viscosity, intrinsic, **02:** 721
Hemoglobin, deoxy(ferro)-
  optical rotatory dispersion in the UV region, **07:** 59
Hemoglobin, met (ferri)-
  circular dichroism in the UV region, **07:** 100
  optical rotatory dispersion in the UV region, **07:** 59
Hemoglobin, oxy (ferro)-
  optical rotatory dispersion in the UV region, **07:** 60
Hemoglobin, vertebrate tetrameric
  amino acid sequence
    α type chains, **07:** 441-447
    β type chains, **07:** 448-455
Hemoglobin A
  circular dichroism in near UV region, at room tempera-
    ture, **07:** 153-154
Hemoglobin carbonyl (ferro)-
  optical rotatory dispersion in the UV region, **07:** 58
Hemoglobin derivatives
  UV and visible absorption spectra from human normal
    adult, **07:** 174-185
Hemoglobin F
  circular dichroism in near UV region, at room tempera-
    ture, **07:** 154

Hemoglobin (Hb) (human)
  circular dichroism in the UV region, **07:** 100
Hemoglobin I
  subunit, constitution of, **02:** 326
Hemoglobin III
  subunit, constitution of, **02:** 329
Hemoglobin Rainier
  circular dichroism in near UV region, at room tempera-
    ture, **07:** 154
Hemoglobin Yakima
  circular dichroism in near UV region, at room tempera-
    ture, **07:** 154
Hemoglobins, synthetic
  molar absorptivity and-or absorbance values, **02:** 446
Hemolysin
  amino acid composition, incomplete data, **07:** 513
Hemopexin
  average hydrophobicity value, **01:** 223
  blood, human
    molar absorptivity and-or absorbance values, **02:** 447
  blood, rabbit
    molar absorptivity and-or absorbance values, **02:** 447
  circular dichroism in the UV regions, **07:** 101
  molecular parameters, **02:** 246
  optical rotatory dispersion in the UV region, **07:** 60
  plasma, human
    carbohydrate content, molecular weight, sedimentation
      coefficient, **02:** 258
Hemophilus
  amino acid requirements for growth, table, **04:** 634
Hemoproteins
  oxidation-reduction potentials, **06:** 132-139
Hemovanadin, source of, **02:** 276
Heparin
  table of data and characteristics, **02:** 686
Heptasaccharides
  chemical formula, **05:** 318-319, 345-346
  derivatives, **05:** 318-319, 345-346
  melting point, **05:** 318-319, 345-346
  specific rotation, **05:** 318-319, 345-346
  synonyms, **05:** 318-319, 345-346
Heptoglobin
  molecular parameters, **02:** 245
Hercynin
  physical and chemical properties, **01:** 161
Herellea
  G + C composition of DNA of, table arranged by spe-
    cie, **04:** 91-92
Heroin
  pK'_a values, **06:** 326
Herpetosiphon
  G + C composition of DNA of, table arranged by spe-
    cie, **04:** 182
Herring oil
  chain length composition, **05:** 525
  isomers in partially hydrogenated, **05:** 513
  properties and weight % composition of derived fatty
    acid methyl esters, **05:** 523-524
  properties of interest, comparisons, **05:** 526-527
L-Heterocyclic amino acids
  physical and chemical properties, **01:** 135-148
Heterograft, definition of, **04:** 884

γ_6-Hexafluorovaline
  structure and symbols for those incorporated into synthetic polypeptides, **01:** 102
Hexahydrophenylalanine, *see* β-(Cyclohexyl)alanine
Hexanoic acid derivatives
  heat of proton ionization, pK, and related thermodynamic quantities, **06:** 207-208
Hexasaccharides
  chemical formula, **05:** 316-318, 344-345
  derivatives, **05:** 316-318, 344-345
  melting point, **05:** 316-318, 344-345
  specific rotation, **05:** 316-318, 344-345
  synonyms, **05:** 316-318, 344-345
Hexokinase
  amino acid composition, incomplete data, **07:** 513
  circular dichroism in the UV region, **07:** 101
  enzymatic activity, subcellular fractions, **02:** 698, 702, 715
  molar absorptivity and-or absorbance values, **02:** 448
  optical rotatory dispersion
    UV region, **07:** 60
    visible and near UV regions, **07:** 26
  subunit, constitution of, **02:** 333
Hexon
  circular dichroism in the UV region, **07:** 101
  optical rotatory dispersion
    UV region, **07:** 60
    visible and near UV regions, **07:** 26
Hexose, content of, in glycoproteins, **02:** 258
Hexosediphosphatase
  amino acid composition, complete data, **07:** 507
  circular dichroism in the UV region, **07:** 101
  optical rotatory dispersion in the UV region, **07:** 60
High-potential iron-sulfur protein
  circular dichroism in near UV region, at room temperature, **07:** 154
High potential, *see* High potential iron protein
High potential iron protein
  molar absorptivity and-or absorbance values, **02:** 448
High potential iron sulfur protein
  average hydrophobicity value, **01:** 224
Hikizimycin, physicochemical constants, spectral, chemotherapeutic and biological properties, **03:** 325
Hiochi bacteria
  amino acid requirements for growth, table, **04:** 634
Hirudin
  amino acid composition, complete data, **07:** 507
  animal sources, amino acid composition, **02:** 649
  lower animal sources, specificity and properties, **02:** 620-621
Histamine
  heat of proton ionization, pK, and related thermodynamic quantities, **06:** 208
  pK'_a values, **06:** 319, 333
Histidine
  active site peptides, **07:** 186-187
  antagonists of, **01:** 178
  bond distances and angles for side chain, **08:** 223
  far ultraviolet absorption spectra
    aqueous solution at pH 5, **01:** 184
    neutral water, table, **01:** 185
    0.1 *M* sodium dodecyl sulfate, table, **01:** 185

  free acid in amniotic fluid in early pregnancy and at term, **01:** 327
  free acid in blood plasma of newborn infants and adults, **01:** 328
  heat of proton ionization, pK, and related thermodynamic quantities, **06:** 209
  histidinemia, effect of, **01:** 319
  metabolism, pathways chart, **04:** insert
  molar extinctions, **01:** 185
  nucleoside composition, tables of values, **04:** 432
  nucleotide sequences of, **04:** 444-445
  pK'_a values, **06:** 319
  physical and chemical properties, **01:** 141
  pK values in various proteins, table, **02:** 689-692
  requirements of, for growth of various microorganisms, table, **04:** 630-643
  spectra, far UV, **01:** 184
  symbols for atoms and bonds in side chains, **01:** 70, **02:** 74
  thumbprint, content in, **08:** 121
  UV spectra of, **01:** 196
D-Histidine
  antagonism to histidine, **01:** 178
Histidine 146 β
  pK value in human hemoglobin, **02:** 690
Histidine-binding protein
  average hydrophobicity value, **01:** 224
Histidine ammonia lyase
  average hydrophobicity value, **01:** 224
  molar absorptivity and-or absorbance values, **02:** 448
Histidine ammonialyase
  amino acid composition, complete data, **07:** 507
  circular dichroism in the UV region, **07:** 102
Histidine betaine, *see* Ergothioneine, Hercynin
Histidine decarboxylase
  amino acid composition, complete data, **07:** 507
  average hydrophobicity value, **01:** 224
  molar absorptivity and-or absorbance values, **02:** 448
  subunit, constitution of, **02:** 334, 340
Histidinemia
  characteristics of, **01:** 319
Histidinol dehydrogenase
  amino acid composition, complete data, **07:** 507
  molar absorptivity and-or absorbance values, **02:** 449
  Neurospora crassa mutant, **04:** 741
  subunit, constitution of, **02:** 331
L-Histidinol phosphate aminotransferase
  average hydrophobicity value, **01:** 224
Histidinol phosphate phosphatase
  Neurospora crassa mutant, **04:** 749
Histidyl-tRNA synthetase
  average hydrophobicity value, **01:** 224
Histidyl tRNA synthetase
  subunit, constitution of, **02:** 331
Histochemical studies, preparation of buffers, **06:** 370-377
Histocompatibility
  genetics of, **04:** 884-887
  graft rejection, basis of, **04:** 884
  loci, estimation of, **04:** 885
  major histocompatibility complex, **04:** 885-888
  tissue grafting terminology, **04:** 884

Histone
circular dichroism in the UV region, **07:** 102
optical rotatory dispersion
UV region, **07:** 60
visible and near UV regions, **07:** 26
Histone III
average hydrophobicity value, **01:** 224
Histone IV
amino acid composition, complete data, **07:** 507
amino acid sequence, **07:** 499
Histones
calf thymus, cyanogen bromide cleavage, **02:** 199
characterization, data table, **02:** 294
molar absorptivity and-or absorbance values, **02:** 449
sequences, table for several, **02:** 295-299
Histoplasma
G + C composition of DNA of, table arranged by specie, **04:** 203
Holostei, DNA content per cell, **04:** 293
Homarine
physical and chemical properties, **01:** 149
Homoarginine
antagonism to arginine, 01: 177
physical and chemical properties, **01:** 133
structure and symbols for those incorporated into synthetic polypeptides, **01:** 102
Homobetaine
physical and chemical properties, **01:** 161
Homocitrulline
physical and chemical properties, **01:** 133
Homocitrullylaminoadenosine, physicochemical constants,
spectral, chemotherapeutic and biological properties, **03:** 326
Homocysteine
physical and chemical properties, **01:** 155
Homocystine
homocystinuria, effect of, **01:** 319
physical and chemical properties, **01:** 155
Homocystinecysteine disulfide
physical and chemical properties, **01:** 155
Homocystinuria
characteristics of, **01:** 319
Homogentisic acid; origin, structure, and characteristic as
protein biosynthesis inhibitor, **04:** 578
Homograft, definition of, **04:** 884
Homoisoleucine, *see* 2-Amino-4-methylhexanoic acid
Homolanthionine
physical and chemical properties, **01:** 155
Homolysine
structure and symbols for those incorporated into synthetic polypeptides, **01:** 102
Homomethionine
physical and chemical properties, **01:** 155
Homooligomers
ribonucleotides, mean residue absorptivities, **03:** 603
Homopolymer complexes, double-stranded
mean residue absorptivity, table of values, **03:** 602
Homopolymers
ribonucleotides, mean residue absorptivities, **03:** 603
Homoserine
antagonism to serine, 01: 179
physical and chemical properties, **01:** 125

Homostachydrine
physical and chemical properties, **01:** 163
Hormone, *see also* Luteinizing hormone
chorionic gonadotropin, human
carbohydrate content, **02:** 271
molar absorptivity and-or absorbance values, **02:** 450
chorionic somatomammotropin, human
molar absorptivity and-or absorbance values, **02:** 450
follicle-stimulating, human
carbohydrate content, **02:** 271
molar absorptivity and-or absorbance values, **02:** 450
subunit, constitution of, **02:** 326
glycoproteins from, carbohydrate content, **02:** 271-272
growth, beef pituitary
molar absorptivity and-or absorbance values, **02:** 450
growth, human pituitary
molar absorptivity and-or absorbance values, **02:** 450
growth, sheep pituitary
molar absorptivity and-or absorbance values, **02:** 450
interstitial cell stimulating
carbohydrate content, **02:** 271
subunit, constitution of, **02:** 326
lactogen (MPL-2)
molar absorptivity and-or absorbance values, **02:** 450
luteinizing
carbohydrate content, **02:** 272-273
molar absorptivity and-or absorbance values, **02:** 468
parathyroid
cyanogen bromide cleavage, **02:** 199
molar absorptivity and-or absorbance values, **02:** 450
parathyroid, pig
molar absorptivity and-or absorbance values, **02:** 450
peptide, list of, **02:** 177-178
peptide, nomenclature recommendations, **02:** 175-178
prolactin, sheep
molar absorptivity and-or absorbance values, **02:** 450
Hormone-binding polypeptide
amino acid composition, complete data, **07:** 507
Hormones
amino acid sequence, **07:** 375-376, 378-381
anterior pituitary
amino acid sequence, **07:** 385-397
neurohypophysial
distribution in vertebrates, table, **07:** 400-401
parathyroid
amino acid sequence, **07:** 399
placenta
amino acid sequence, **07:** 385-397
Human
antigens, red cell, list of, **04:** 880
blood proteins demonstrating quantitative abnormality,
list, **04:** 881
deoxynucleotide polymerizing enzymes from, properties
of, **04:** 539-544
disorders demonstrating deficient activity of specific enzymes, list, **04:** 882-883
DNA content per cell, **04:** 305
genetic variation, data tables relating to, **04:** 879-883
genetically determined structural variations, proteins
demonstrating, list of, **04:** 879
major histocompatibility complex, values of, **04:** 886
MHC designation, **04:** 885

Human *(continued)*
mitochondrial DNA from, properties, **04:** 372
plasma; clotting factors, quantitative variation in, **04:** 881
satellite DNAs; buoyant density and G + C content of, table, **04:** 397-398
Human adults
free amino acid in blood plasma of, **01:** 328
Human globin
chymotryptic hydrolysis of α-chains of, **02:** 213
Human hemoglobin, *see also* Hemoglobin, human
hydrolysis peptides by leucine, **02:** 217
hydrolysis peptides by papain, **02:** 219
Human organs and secretions
proteinase inhibitors from, specificity and properties, **02:** 632-639
Human plasma, *see also* Plasma, human, *also* Blood plasma; Plasma
glycoproteins from, carbohydrate content, **02:** 258
ligand binding
drugs, list of references, **02:** 568-574
endogenous ligands, list of references, **02:** 556-557
fatty acids, list of references, **02:** 558-562
inorganic anions, list of references, **02:** 563
metal ions, list of references, **02:** 563-564
steroids, list of references, **02:** 563-564
visible dyes, list of references, **02:** 564-568
Human plasma proteins, *see also* Plasma proteins, human
content in normal plasma, **02:** 242-250
molecular parameters, table, **02:** 242-250
Human serum, *see also* Serum, human
proteinase inhibitors from, specificity and properties, **02:** 636-641
Human skin
lipid composition of various parts of adult, **05:** 507
Human skin surface
carbohydrate phosphate esters, **05:** 253-258, 262-273
fatty acid type and content in lipids of, **05:** 508
Hydrolysis constant
lipid, fatty acids from wax esters and sterol esters, **05:** 509-510
Human urine, *see* Urine, human
Humicola
G + C composition of DNA of, table arranged by specie, **04:** 204
Hyaluronic acid
table of data and characteristics, **02:** 686
Hyaluronidase
amino acid composition, complete data, **07:** 507
average hydrophobicity value, **01:** 224
bovine testicle
luminescence of, table, **01:** 206
circular dichroism in the UV region, **07:** 103
optical rotatory dispersion in the visible and near UV regions, **07:** 26
Hyaluronoglucosidase, *see* Hyaluronidase
Hydantoic acid
structure and symbols for those incorporated into synthetic polypeptides, **01:** 102
5-Hydantoinacetyl
structure and symbols for those incorporated into synthetic polypeptides, **01:** 103

Hydrazines, pK'_a values, **06:** 344
Hydrochloric acid-potassium chloride buffer, preparation of, **06:** 370
Hydrodictyon
G + C composition of DNA of, table arranged by specie, **04:** 225
Hydrogen
NMR spectral positions, in organic structures, **08:** 247
Hydrogen equivalents, oxidation and reduction reagents, **06:** 352
Hydrogenase
average hydrophobicity value, **01:** 224
molar absorptivity and-or absorbance values, **02:** 451
subunit, constitution of, **02:** 328
table of cofactors, molecular weights, stoichiometry and sources, **02:** 280
Hydrogenase (*C. pasteurianum* W5), *see* Ferredoxin, hydrogenase
Hydrolases
definition and nomenclature, **02:** 97
numbering and classification of, **02:** 107
Hydrolysis, *see also* Peptic hydrolysis
acid, of peptides, relative rate table, **02:** 208
acid, of proteins, data tables, **02:** 206-207
acid, recovery of tryptophan from various proteins, **02:** 207
chymotryptic, of α-chains of human globin, **02:** 213
chymotryptic, proteins, conditions for, **02:** 214
enzymatic, conjugated proteins, table, **02:** 211
enzymatic, of proteins and polypeptides, **02:** 209
free energy of, discussion and sample calculations, **06:** 296-299
free energy values for compounds, tables, **06:** 300-303
peptic, aromatic amino acids in human α- and β-chains, **02:** 216
peptic, leucine in human α- and β-chains, **02:** 217
peptide bonds, specificity of chymotrypsin, **02:** 212
peptide bonds, specificity of papain, **02:** 218
peptide bonds, specificity of pepsin, **02:** 215
peptide bonds, specificity of subtilisin, **02:** 221
peptides from α- and β-chains of human hemoglobin by papain, **02:** 219
peptides in acid solution, table, **02:** 208
thiol esters, kinetic constants, **02:** 682
Hydrolysis of RNA, conditions for limited, **03:** 404
Hydrolysis of RNA, controlled partial, discussion of, **03:** 402-404
7-[(2-Hydroperoxy)-3-(methoxycarbonyl)-3-(methoxyformamido)propyl] wyosine
isolation and detection of, in RNA, general remarks, **03:** 246
RNA, various, natural occurrence in, **03:** 233
Hydrophobic stacking interactions, yeast phenylalanine transfer RNA, **04:** 461
Hydrophobicity
amino acid side chains
calculation of, **01:** 209
table of values, **01:** 209
proteins, average values for selected, **01:** 210-235
Hydroquinine
pK'_a values, **06:** 326

β-Hydroxbutyrate dehydrogenase
  average hydrophobicity value, **01**: 224
α-Hydroxy-ϵ-amino caproic acid
  physical and chemical properties, **01**: 125
1-Hydroxy-2-amino ethylphosphonic acid
  physical and chemical properties, **01**: 161
Hydroxy-β-aminobutyramide; structure and mode of action as protein biosynthesis inhibitor, **04**: 578
α-Hydroxy-γ-aminobutyric acid
  physical and chemical properties, **01**: 125
β-Hydroxy-γ-aminobutyric acid
  physical and chemical properties, **01**: 125
S-(3-Hydroxy-3-carboxy-n-propyl-thio)-homocysteine
  physical and chemical properties, **01**: 156
S-(3-Hydroxy-3-carboxy-n-propyl) cysteine
  physical and chemical properties, **01**: 156
S-(3-Hydroxy-3-carboxy-n-propyl thio)-cysteine
  physical and chemical properties, **01**: 156
S-(β-Hydroxy-β-carboxyethane-sulfonyl methyl) cysteine,
  see Dichrostachinic acid
S-(2-Hydroxy-2-carboxyethyl)-homocysteine
  physical and chemical properties, **01**: 155
S(2-Hydroxy-2-carboxyethylthio)-homocysteine
  physical and chemical properties, **01**: 155
β-Hydroxy-α,ϵ-diaminopimelic acid
  antagonism to α,ϵ-Diaminopimelic acid, **01**: 177
4-Hydroxy-3-hydroxymethylphenylalanine
  physical and chemical properties, **01**: 130
δ-Hydroxy-γ-ketonorvaline
  physical and chemical properties, **01**: 126
δ-N-(cis-5-Hydroxy-3-methylpent-2-enoyl)-f-N-
  hydroxy-ornithine, *see Fusarinine*
4-Hydroxy-N-methylproline
  physical and chemical properties, **01**: 149
4-Hydroxy-4-methylproline
  physical and chemical properties, **01**: 141
5-Hydroxy-piperidazine-3-carboxylic acid
  physical and chemical properties, **01**: 141
β-(5-Hydroxy-2-pyridyl)-alanine
  antagonism to tyrosine, **01**: 180
Hydroxy-substituted amino acids
  physical and chemical properties, **01**: 122-129
Hydroxy amino acids
  physical and chemical properties, **01**: 122-129
Hydroxy unsaturated acids, physical and chemical characteristics, **05**: 488-489
3-Hydroxyacyl coenzyme A dehydrogenase
  average hydrophobicity value, **01**: 224
α-Hydroxyalanine
  physical and chemical properties, **01**: 125
Hydroxyalkanoic acids, physical and chemical characteristics, **05**: 488-489
γ-Hydroxyarginine
  physical and chemical properties, **01**: 133
N⁵-Hydroxyarginine
  physical and chemical properties, **01**: 134
β-Hydroxyasparagine
  physical and chemical properties, **01**: 125
β-Hydroxyaspartic acid
  antagonism to aspartic acid, **01**: 177
  physical and chemical properties, **01**: 125

4-Hydroxybenzoate 3-monooxygenase (p-hydroxybenzoate hydroxylase)
  circular dichroism in near UV region, at room temperature, **07**: 154
  optical rotatory dispersion in the UV region, **07**: 61
p-Hydroxybenzoate hydroxylase, *see* 4-Hydroxybenzoate, 3-monoxygenase
β-6-(4-Hydroxybenzothiazolyl)-alanine
  physical and chemical properties, **01**: 155
α-Hydroxycysteinecysteine disulfide
  physical and chemical properties, **01**: 156
β-Hydroxydecanoyl thioester dehydrase
  amino acid composition, complete data, **07**: 507
N-(2-Hydroxyethyl)-alanine
  physical and chemical properties, **01**: 125
N⁴-(2-Hydroxyethyl)-asparagine
  physical and chemical properties, **01**: 125
N⁵-(2-Hydroxyethyl)-glutamine
  physical and chemical properties, **01**: 125
γ-Hydroxyglutamic acid
  physical and chemical properties, **01**: 126
β-Hydroxyglutamic acid
  antagonism to glutamic acid, **01**: 177
  physical and chemical properties, **01**: 126
γ-Hydroxyglutamine
  physical and chemical properties, **01**: 126
β-Hydroxyhistidine
  physical and chemical properties, **01**: 141
γ-Hydroxyhomoarginine
  physical and chemical properties, **01**: 134
4-Hydroxyisoleucine
  physical and chemical properties, **01**: 126
N⁶-(4-Hydroxyisopentenyl)-2-methylthioadenosine
  isolation and detection of, in RNA, general remarks, **03**: 234
  RNA various, natural occurrence in, **03**: 218
N⁶-(cis-4-Hydroxyisopentenyl) adenosine
  isolation and detection of, in RNA, general remarks, **03**: 234
  RNA, various, natural occurrence in, **03**: 218
β-Hydroxyisovaleric acidemia
  characteristics of, **01**: 326
3-Hydroxykynurenine
  physical and chemical properties, **01**: 130
Hydroxyl protein group, chemical modification of
  reagents used, table of specificities, **02**: 203-204
Hydroxyl value
  polyol esters, table, **05**: 515
Hydroxylamine; structure and characteristic as protein biosynthesis inhibitor, **04**: 578
ϵ-Hydroxylaminonorleucine
  physical and chemical properties, **01**: 126
δ-Hydroxyleucenine
  physical and chemical properties, **01**: 126
δ-Hydroxyleucine
  physical and chemical properties, **01**: 126
β-Hydroxyleucine
  antagonism to isoleucine, **01**: 178
  antagonism to leucine, **01**: 178
  physical and chemical properties, **01**: 126
α-Hydroxylysine
  physical and chemical properties, **01**: 127

δ-Hydroxylysine
  physical and chemical properties, **01:** 127
N^5-(2-Hydroxymethylbutadienyl)-*allo*-γ-hydroxyglutamine,
  see Pinnatanine
p-Hydroxymethylphenylalanine
  physical and chemical properties, **01:** 131
3-Hydroxymethylphenylalanine
  physical and chemical properties, **01:** 130
5-Hydroxymethyluridine
  isolation and detection of, in RNA, general remarks, **03:** 242
  RNA, various, natural occurrence in, **03:** 230
Hydroxyminaline
  physical and chemical properties, **01:** 141
ε-Hydroxynorleucine
  structure and symbols for those incorporated into synthetic polypeptides, **01:** 103
β-Hydroxynorleucine
  antagonism to leucine, 01: 178
  antagonism to threonine, 01: 179
γ-Hydroxynorvaline
  physical and chemical properties, **01:** 127
β-Hydroxynorvaline
  antagonism to threonine, 01: 179
  physical and chemical properties, **01:** 127
γ-Hydroxyornithine
  physical and chemical properties, **01:** 127
m-Hydroxyphenylglycine
  physical and chemical properties, **01:** 131
p-Hydroxyphenylpyruvic acid, properties of, **01:** 182
1-Hydroxypipecolic acid
  structure and symbols for those incorporated into synthetic polypeptides, **01:** 103
4-Hydroxypipecolic acid
  physical and chemical properties, **01:** 141
5-Hydroxypipecolic acid
  physical and chemical properties, **01:** 141
Hydroxyproline
  antagonism to proline, 01: 179
  free acid in amniotic fluid in early pregnancy and at term, **01:** 327
  free acid in blood plasma of newborn infants and adults, **01:** 328
  symbols for atoms and bonds in side chains, **01:** 70, **02:** 74
*Allo*hydroxyproline
  physical and chemical properties, **01:** 135
1-Hydroxyproline
  structure and symbols for those incorporated into synthetic polypeptides, **01:** 103
3-Hydroxyproline
  structure and chemical properties, **01:** 142
  structure and symbols for those incorporated into synthetic polypeptides, **01:** 103
4-Hydroxyproline
  physical and chemical properties, **01:** 142
  structure and symbols for those incorporated into synthetic polypeptides, **01:** 103
3-Hydroxyproline betaine, *see* 3-Hydroxystachydrine
4-Hydroxyproline betaine, *see* Betonicine
3-Hydroxypyrrolidine-2-carboxylic acid, *see* 3-Hydroxyproline

4-Hydroxypyrrolidine-2-carboxylic acid, *see* 4-Hydroxyproline
Hydroxypyruvate reductase
  amino acid composition, incomplete data, **07:** 513
  molar absorptivity and-or absorbance values, **02:** 451
  subunit, constitution of, **02:** 329
β-Hydroxypyruvic acid, properties of, **01:** 182
N-Hydroxysarcosine
  structure and symbols for those incorporated into synthetic polypeptides, **01:** 103
3-Hydroxystachydrine
  physical and chemical properties, **01:** 163
$α^1$-Hydroxysteroid dehydrogenase
  average hydrophobicity value, **01:** 224
17-β-Hydroxysteroid dehydrogenase
  average hydrophobicity value, **01:** 224
20-β-Hydroxysteroid dehydrogenase
  optical rotatory dispersion
    UV region, **07:** 61
    visible and near UV regions, **07:** 26
Hydroxystreptomycin (Reticulin); origin, structure, and characteristic as protein biosynthesis inhibitor, **04:** 579
2-Hydroxytryptophan
  physical and chemical properties, **01:** 142
5-Hydroxytryptophan
  physical and chemical properties, **01:** 142
5-Hydroxyuridine
  isolation and detection of, in RNA, general remarks, **03:** 242
  RNA, various, natural occurrence in, **03:** 230
α-Hydroxyvaline
  physical and chemical properties, **01:** 127
γ-Hydroxyvaline
  physical and chemical properties, **01:** 127
β-Hydroxyvaline
  antagonism to valine, 01: 180
Hygric acid, *see* *N*-Methylproline
Hygromycin B; origin, structure, and characteristic as protein biosynthesis inhibitor, **04:** 579
Hypaphorin
  physical and chemical properties, **01:** 163
Hyperbetaalaninemia
  characteristics of, **01:** 317
Hyperchromicity ratios
  oligonucleotides, at different wavelengths, **03:** 406-407
Hyperglycinemia
  characteristics of, **01:** 319
Hyperglycinemia ketotic (severe infantile)
  characteristics of, **01:** 318
Hyperlysinemia, characteristics of, **01:** 320
Hyperpipecolic acidemia
  characteristics of, **01:** 321
Hyperprolinemia type I
  characteristics of, **01:** 321
Hyperprolinemia type II
  characteristics of, **01:** 321
Hypervalinemia
  characteristics of, **01:** 322
Hypobranchial mucin
  amino acid composition, incomplete data, **07:** 513

Hypocrea
  G + C composition of DNA of, table arranged by specie, **04**: 204
Hypoglycemic agents, ligands binding to plasma albumin, **02**: 572
Hypoglycin A
  physical and chemical properties, **01**: 116
Hypophosphatasia
  characteristics of, **01**: 321
Hypotaurine
  physical and chemical properties, **01**: 156
Hypothalamic factors, nomenclature, **02**: 175-177
Hypoxanthine and derivatives
  physical constants and spectral properties, index to, **03**: 67
  UV spectral characteristics and acid dissociation constants, **03**: 413
Hypusine
  physical and chemical properties, **01**: 127

I

Ibotenic acid
  physical and chemical properties, **01**: 142
IgA
  circular dichroism in the UV region, **07**: 103
  optical rotatory dispersion
    UV region, **07**: 61
    visible and near UV regions, **07**: 27
IgD, myeloma
  circular dichroism in the UV region, **07**: 103
IgG
  circular dichroism in the UV region, **07**: 103
  optical rotatory dispersion
    UV region, **07**: 62
    visible and near UV regions, **07**: 27
IgM
  circular dichroism in the UV region, **07**: 105
  visible and near UV regions, **07**: 27
Ilamycin B
  proton NMR and suggested conformations, **07**: 566
Imidazole
  antagonism to histidine, **01**: 178
  heat of proton ionization, pK, and related thermodynamic quantities, **06**: 212
Imidazole acetol phosphate transaminase
  Neurospora crassa mutant, **04**: 749
Imidazole aminoaciduria
  characteristics of, **01**: 317
Imidazole derivatives excreted in human urine, mg-day, **03**: 252-269
Imidazole glycerol phosphate dehydrase
  Neurospora crassa mutant, **04**: 751
Imidazole protein group, chemical modification of reagents used, table of specificities, **02**: 203-204
4-Imidazoleacetic acid
  physical and chemical properties, **01**: 142
Imidazoles
  IR spectra, chart of characteristic frequencies between ~ 700-300 cm^{-1}, **08**: 243
β-Imidazolylpuruvic acid, properties of, **01**: 181

Imidazoylacetolphosphate: L-glutamate aminotransferase
  amino acid composition, complete data, **07**: 508
2-Imino-4-hydroxyhexahydro-6-pyrimidinyl glycine, *see* Tuberactidine
N^5-Iminoethylornithine
  physical and chemical properties, **01**: 120
Immobilization of enzymes, methods and tables of supports, **02**: 722-734
Immobilized enzymes, uses of, **02**: 722
Immobilizing antigen
  amino acid composition, complete data, **07**: 508
Immunogenic properties
  some low molecular weight compounds, table, **07**: 541
Immunogenic synthetic polypeptides, *see* Polypeptides, synthetic, immunogenic
Immunoglobulin
  beef
    molar absorptivity and-or absorbance values, **02**: 454
  chain structure, table, **07**: 530-531
    constant regions, **07**: 408, 411, 414-419
    variable region, **07**: 403-407, 409-410, 412-413
  chicken
    molar absorptivity and-or absorbance values, **02**: 453
  circular dichroism in the UV region, **07**: 103
  definition, **02**: 179
  disulfide bonding patterns, **07**: 529
  dog
    molar absorptivity and-or absorbance values, **02**: 454
  goat
    molar absorptivity and-or absorbance values, **02**: 453
  guinea pig
    molar absorptivity and-or absorbance values, **02**: 454
  horse
    molar absorptivity and-or absorbance values, **02**: 454
  human
    genetic factors, notation, **02**: 186
    molar absorptivity and-or absorbance values, **02**: 452
    nomenclature recommendations for, **02**: 173-174, 179-195
    subclasses, notation for, **02**: 184
  human allotypes, **07**: 528, 530-531
  mice allotypes, **07**: 532-533
  molecular parameters, **02**: 249
  mouse
    molar absorptivity and-or absorbance values, **02**: 454
  optical rotatory dispersion
    UV region, **07**: 61
    visible and near UV regions, **07**: 26
  pig
    molar absorptivity and-or absorbance values, **02**: 453
  plasma, human
    carbohydrate content, molecular weights, sedimentation coefficients, **02**: 258
  plasma, nonhuman
    carbohydrate content, **02**: 259
  possible amino acid sequence correlations, **07**: 530-531
  rabbit
    molar absorptivity and-or absorbance values, **02**: 454
  rabbit allotypes, chain structures, **07**: 534
  rabbit haplotypes, **07**: 535
  rat
    molar absorptivity and-or absorbance values, **02**: 454

Immunoglobulin *(continued)*
  sheep
    molar absorptivity and-or absorbance values, **02:** 454
Immunoglobulin, Eu heavy chain
  average hydrophobicity value, **01:** 224
Immunoglobulin, newλ- chain
  average hydrophobicity value, **01:** 224
Immunoglobulin, specific
  γ_1-globulin, human
    molar absorptivity and-or absorbance values, **02:** 456
  γ-globulin fraction, chicken
    molar absorptivity and-or absorbance values, **02:** 456
  γ_1, guinea pig
    molar absorptivity and-or absorbance values, **02:** 456
  γ_2, guinea pig
    molar absorptivity and-or absorbance values, **02:** 456
  horse
    molar absorptivity and-or absorbance values, **02:** 456
  γG, horse
    molar absorptivity and-or absorbance values, **02:** 456
  γG, human
    molar absorptivity and-or absorbance values, **02:** 456
  γM, human
    molar absorptivity and-or absorbance values, **02:** 456
  γM, human, subunit
    molar absorptivity and-or absorbance values, **02:** 456
  γG, lemon shark
    molar absorptivity and-or absorbance values, **02:** 456
  γA, rabbit
    molar absorptivity and-or absorbance values, **02:** 456
  γG, rabbit
    molar absorptivity and-or absorbance values, **02:** 456
Immunoglobulin IgG
  human
    cyanogen bromide cleavage, **02:** 199
  rabbit
    cyanogen bromide cleavage, **02:** 199
Immunoglobulin molecules
  formulas for, **02:** 192
  regions, definition of, **02:** 191
Immunological response
  cell types involved in, table, **07:** 536-538
C1-Inactivator
  carbohydrate composition, **02:** 666-667
  molar absorptivity and-or absorbance values, **02:** 399
  molecular parameters, **02:** 244
C_1-Inactivator
  average hydrophobicity value, **01:** 215
Inacton, origin and structure, **04:** 580
Inbred strains, definition of and availability, **04:** 884
Incisor eruption accelerating protein
  amino acid composition, incomplete data, **07:** 513
Index of refraction
  guanidine·HCl, table of values, **06:** 404
Indicators
  acid-base types, pH range and color change table, **06:** 357
  adsorption, applications of several, **06:** 383
  mixed, transition pH and color change, **06:** 382
  oxidation-reduction, transition potential and color change, **06:** 383
  pK'_a values, **06:** 330, 348

pH determination, table of color change, pH range and preparation data, **06:** 380-382
  pH ranges for various, **06:** 378-379
  universal, for approximate pH determination, **06:** 383
  use in pH measurement, **06:** 357
  volumetric work, table of color change, pH range and preparation data, **06:** 380-382
Indole
  antagonism to tryptophan, **01:** 179
Indole-3-acetly-ε-lysine
  physical and chemical properties, **01:** 143
N-(Indole-3-acetyl)-aspartic acid
  physical and chemical properties, **01:** 142
Indole-3-glycerol phosphate synthetase
  amino acid composition, complete data, **07:** 508
Indole protein group, chemical modification of
  reagents used, table of specificities, **02:** 203-204
Indoleacrylic acid
  antagonism to tryptophan, **01:** 179
β-Indolypyruvic acid
  properties of, **01:** 182
Indospicine
  physical and chemical properties, **01:** 134
Infants, newborn
  free amino acid in blood plasma of, **01:** 328
Infared spectra, *see* IR spectra
Infrared, far region, vibrational frequency correlation chart, **08:** 235-236
Infrared correlation charts, **08:** 228-234
Infrared spectra, *see* IR spectra
  characteristic frequencies between ~ 700-300 cm^{-1}, organic and inorganic compounds, **08:** 237-246
  of proteins, **07:** 596-597
Infrared spectral data, *see* IR spectral data
Inheritance, mode of
  blood coagulation proteins, **02:** 255
Inhibition constant
  enzyme kinetics, definition, **02:** 112
Inhibitor, *see also* Repressor
Inhibitor, protease, *see also* Protease inhibitor
Inhibitors
  prostaglandin metabolizing enzymes, **08:** 364-367
Inhibitors, proteinase, *see also* Proteinase inhibitors
Inhibitors of protein biosynthesis; characteristics, origin and structures, **04:** 555-618
Inonotus
  G + C composition of DNA of, table arranged by specie, **04:** 204
Inorganic acids, *see also* individual acids
  pK'_a values, table, **06:** 307
Inorganic anions, ligands binding to plasma albumin, **02:** 563
Inorganic pyrophosphatase
  average hydrophobicity value, **01:** 224
  circular dichroism in the UV region, **07:** 63, 106
  optical rotatory dispersion
    UV region, **07:** 63
    visible and near UV regions, **07:** 27
Inosamines
  chemical formula, **05:** 148-149
  chromatography, **05:** 148-149
  melting point, **05:** 148-149

Inosamines (continued)
  nomenclature rules, **05**: 94
  specific rotation, **05**: 148-149
Inosine
  composition in various tRNA's, **04**: 428-441
  heat of proton ionization, pK, and related thermody-
    namic quantities, **06**: 213
  isolation and detection of, in RNA, general remarks, **03**:
    239-240
  pK'_a values, **06**: 331
  raman frequencies, table of values, **03**: 542-543
  RNA, various, natural occurrence in, **03**: 227
Inosine and derivatives
  molal osmotic coefficients, **03**: 528
  UV spectra, **03**: 446-447
  UV spectral characteristics and acid dissociation con-
    stants, **03**: 415-416
Inosine and nucleoside derivatives
  physical constants and spectral properties, index to, **03**:
    70
Inosine nucleotide derivatives
  physical constants and spectral properties, index to, **03**:
    74
Inositol
  biological characteristics, **08**: 303
  chemical formula, **05**: 142-147
  chromatography, **05**: 142-147
  IUPAC nomenclature recommendations, **05**: 91-92
  melting point, **05**: 142-147
  properties of, **08**: 295
  specific rotation, **05**: 142-147
  systematic nomenclature for, **05**: 94
Inososes
  chemical formula, **05**: 147
  chromatography, **05**: 147
  melting point, **05**: 147
  nomenclature rules, **05**: 95
  specific rotation, **05**: 147
Insects, satellite DNAs; buoyant density and G + C con-
    tent of, table, **04**: 380-384
Insulin
  average hydrophobicity value, **01**: 224
  beef
    molar absorptivity and-or absorbance values, **02**: 457
  bovine
    luminescence of, **01**: 204
  brain, bovine
    subunit, constitution of, **02**: 326
  circular dichroism
    UV and near UV region, **07**: 106, 155
  optical rotatory dispersion
    UV region, **07**: 64
    visible and near UV regions, **07**: 27
  refractive index increments, **02**: 376
  viscosity, intrinsic, **02**: 721
Insulin, iodinated
  heat of proton ionization, pK, and related thermody-
    namic quantities, **06**: 213
Insulin, zinc
  heat capacity and entropy values, **06**: 110
Insulin A chains
  amino acid sequence, **07**: 378

Insulin B chain
  luminescence of, **01**: 204
Insulin B chains
  amino acid sequence, **07**: 379-380
Intermolecular anhydrides, nomenclature rules, **05**: 132
International rotors, construction data for isokinetic su-
    crose and glycerol gradients, **06**: 480-488
International Union of Immunological Sciences
  human immunoglobulin, nomenclature recommenda-
    tions, **02**: 173-174
Interstitial cell-stimulating hormone
  amino acid composition, incomplete data, **07**: 513
Interstitial cell stimulating hormone, see also Luteinizing
    hormone
Intramolecular anhydride, nomenclature rules, **05**:
    130-132
Intramolecular ether, nomenclature rules, **05**: 130-132
Intrasporangium
  G + C composition of DNA of, table arranged by spe-
    cie, **04**: 172
Intrinsic factor
  amino acid composition, incomplete data, **07**: 513
Invertase
  average hydrophobicity value, **01**: 224
  carbohydrate content, **02**: 274
  molar absorptivity and-or absorbance values, **02**: 458
  subunit, constitution of, **02**: 341
Invertase (external)
  amino acid composition, complete data, **07**: 508
Iodine value
  fats and oils, table of values, **05**: 502-503
  fatty acids, **05**: 485-491
  herring oils and Pacific pilchard oils, **05**: 523-524
  vegetable oils, **05**: 512
Iodoacetamide
  inhibition of transamidase activity, **02**: 672
Iodogorgoic acid, see 3,5-Diiodotyrosine
Ion exchangers, cellulosic, properties, **08**: 136-138
Ionization constants
  acids and bases, tables of values, **06**: 307-348
Ions, see also Anions
Ions, common, transmission limits, **08**: 196
β-IPM dehydrogenase
  Neurospora crassa mutant, **04**: 740, 746
IPM isomerase
  Neurospora crassa mutant, **04**: 740
α-IPM synthetase
  Neurospora crassa mutant, **04**: 740
IR spectra
  antibiotics, nucleoside, **03**: 271-393
  polynucleotides, charts, **03**: 605-621
  polynucleotides, table of values, **03**: 622-623
  polysaccharides, fingerprint region, **02**: 686-687
IR spectral data
  mucopolysaccharides, **05**: 356-357
  steroids, table, **05**: 531-588
Iron-sulfur proteins
  resonance raman spectra, **07**: 589
Iron protein, see High potential iron protein
Iron proteins
  classification of, **02**: 90

Iron sulfur proteins, *see also* Proteins, iron-sulfur
  nomenclature recommendations, **02**: 89-90
  table of cofactors, molecular weights, stoichiometry and
    sources, **02**: 278-280
Iron transport proteins
  resonance raman spectra, **07**: 589
Irpex
  G + C composition of DNA of, table arranged by spe-
    cie, **04**: 204
Isoachyla
  G + C composition of DNA of, table arranged by spe-
    cie, **04**: 204
Isoamylase I, II
  average hydrophobicity value, **01**: 225
Isoasparagine
  structure and symbols for those incorporated into syn-
    thetic polypeptides, **01**: 104
Isocitrate dehydrogenase
  amino acid composition, complete data, **07**: 508
  average hydrophobicity value, **01**: 225
  circular dichroism in the UV region, **07**: 106
  molar absorptivity and-or absorbance values, **02**: 458
  optical rotatory dispersion
    UV region, **07**: 64
    visible and near UV regions, **07**: 28
Isocitrate lyase
  amino acid composition, complete data, **07**: 508
  Neurospora crassa mutant, **04**: 752
Isocytosine, 6-Amino-5-*N*-methylformamido
  physical constants and spectral properties, **03**: 82
Isocytosine, 5-*N*-Methylformamido-6-ribosylamino-
  physical constants and spectral properties, **03**: 116
Isodesmosine
  physical and chemical properties, **01**: 163
Isoelectric point
  proteinase inhibitors
    animal sources, **02**: 618-641
    microbial soures, **02**: 661-662
    plant sources, **02**: 586-600
  proteins, human plasma, **02**: 242-250
  retinol-binding protein, **02**: 304
  Escherichia coli ribosomal proteins 30 S, **04**: 482-486
  Tamm-Horsfall mucoprotein, **02**: 304
Isoenzymes
  definition of, **02**: 84
  nomenclature of, **02**: 84-86
Isoglutamine
  structure and symbols for those incorporated into syn-
    thetic polypeptides, **01**: 104
Isograft, definition of, **04**: 884
Isoguanine
  physical constants and spectral properties, **03**: 77
Isoguanosine
  physical constants and spectral properties, **03**: 99
Isolectin content, purified lectins, **02**: 547-551
Isoleucine
  antagonism to leucine, **01**: 178
  antagonism to valine, **01**: 180
  antagonists of, **01**: 178
  free acid in amniotic fluid in early pregnancy and at
    term, **01**: 327

  free acid in blood plasma of newborn infants and
    adults, **01**: 328
  maple syrup urine disease (intermittent form), effect of,
    01: 319
  maple syrup urine disease (severe infantile), effect of,
    01: 319
  nucleoside composition, tables of values, **04**: 432
  nucleotide sequences of, **04**: 446-447
  pK'_a values, **06**: 319
  physical and chemical properties, **01**: 116
  requirements of, for growth of various microorganisms,
    table, **04**: 630-643
  symbols for atoms and bonds in side chains, **01**: 69, **02**:
    73
  thumbprint, content in, **08**: 121
D-*Allo*isoleucine
  physical and chemical properties, **01**: 164
Isolysine, *see* 3,6-Diaminohexanoic acid
Isomerase
  definition and nomeclature, **02**: 98
  molar absorptivity and-or absorbance values, **02**: 458
  numbering and classification of, **02**: 108
Isomerase I, II
  average hydrophobicity value, **01**: 225
Isomerase of histidine biosynthesis
  amino acid composition, complete data, **07**: 508
Isomerism, types of, discussion and nomenclature, **01**:
    21-58, **02**: 21-58, **03**: 13-26, **04**: 13-50, **05**: 18-55, **06**:
    20, **08**: 20-45
Isomers, monoethylenic
  content in partially hydrogenated herring oil, **05**: 513
  content in rat cardiac lipids, **05**: 513
N^6-(Δ^2-Isopentenyl)-2-methylthioadenosine
  isolation and detection of, in RNA, general remarks, **03**:
    234-235
  RNA, various,natural occurrence in, **03**: 219
N^6-(^{2}-Isopentenyl)-2-methylthioadenosine
  composition in various tRNA's, **04**: 428-441
N^6-(Δ^2-Isopentenyl) adenosine
  isolation and detection of, in RNA, general remarks, **03**:
    234
  RNA, various, natural occurrence in, **03**: 219
N^6-(^{2}-Isopentenyl)adenosine
  composition in various tRNA's, **04**: 428-441
N^5-Isopropyl-glutamine
  physical and chemical properties, **01**: 118
Isopropyl malate isomerase
  Neurospora crassa mutant, **04**: 749
2-Isopropylcarbazic acid
  structure and symbols for those incorporated into syn-
    thetic polypeptides, **01**: 104
Isopropylcarboxy-methylcysteine, *see* Isovalthine
β-Isopropylmalate dehydrogenase
  amino acid composition, complete data, **07**: 508
α-Isopropylmalate synthetase
  amino acid composition, complete data, **07**: 508
N^8-Isopropylornithine
  structure and symbols for those incorporated into syn-
    thetic polypeptides, **01**: 104
Isoserine
  antagonism to serine, **01**: 179
  physical and chemical properties, **01**: 127

Isotocin
amino acid sequence, **07:** 195
Isotopic labeling, nomenclature rules, **06:** 62, **08:** 62
Isotopic labeling, nomenclature rules for, **01:** 16, **02:** 16, **03:** 58, **04:** 58, **05:** 13
Isovaleric acidemia
characteristics of, **01:** 326
Isovalthine
physical and chemical properties, **01:** 156
Isozymes
definition of, **02:** 84
nomenclature of, **02:** 84-86
IUPAC
Commission on the Nomenclature of Organic Chemistry rules affecting biochemical nomenclature, **04:** 3-4
IUB Commission on Biochemical Nomenclature
journal citations for locating rules of, **04:** 5
list of rules and recommendations, **04:** 3-4
tentative rules, nomenclature in fundamental stereochemistry, **04:** 13-50
IUPAC-IUB Commission on Biochemical Nomenclature
amino acid derivatives, symbols, recommendations, **01:** 79-88
amino acid sequences, one-letter notation, tentative rules, **01:** 75-78, **02:** 59-62
carotenoids, definitive rules for nomenclature, **06:** 63-90, **08:** 63-90
enzyme nomenclature, recommendations, **02:** 91-172
enzymes, nomenclature of multiple forms of, **02:** 84-86
iron-sulfur proteins, nomenclature recommendations, **02:** 89-90
journal citations for, locating rules of, **08:** 5
journal citations for locating rules of, **01:** 5, **02:** 5, **05:** 5, **06:** 3
list of rules and recommendations, **01:** 3-4, **02:** 3-4, **05:** 3-4, **06:** 3, **08:** 3
peptide hormones, nomenclature recommendations, **02:** 175-178
peptides, natural, rules for naming synthetic modifications of, **02:** 79-83
peptides, symbols for, recommendations, **01:** 88-90
polypeptide chains, abbreviations and symbols, tentative rules, **01:** 59-73, **02:** 63-77
polypeptides, synthetic, abbreviated nomenclature for, **01:** 91-95
IUPAC-IUB Commission on Biochemical Nomenclature, recommendations of, **03:** 3
IUPAC Commission on the Nomenclature of Organic Chemistry
carotenoids, definitive rules for nomenclature, **06:** 63-90, **08:** 63-90
rules affecting biochemical nomenclature, **01:** 3-4, **02:** 3-4, **05:** 3-4, **06:** 3, **08:** 3-4
IUPAC definitive rules, nomenclature of steroids, **05:** 56-88
IUPAC tentative rules, carbohydrate nomenclature, **05:** 100-136
IUPAC tentative rules, nomenclature in fundamental stereochemistry, **01:** 21-58, **02:** 21-58, **03:** 13-50, **05:** 18-55, **06:** 20, **08:** 20-57

J

N-Jasmonoylisoleucine
physical and chemical properties, **01:** 143
Journal references, use of, CEBJ recommendations, **01:** 17-20, **02:** 17-20, **04:** 59-62, **06:** 58, **08:** 58-61
Journals, biochemical, recommendations for citations in, **05:** 14-17

K

Kainic acid
physical and chemical properties, **01:** 143
*Allo*kainic acid
physical and chemical properties, **01:** 135
Kallidin group
amino acid sequence, physical and biological properties, **07:** 222-235
Kallikrein, *see also* Kininogenin
Kallikrein A, B, *see also* Prekallikrein
molar absorptivity and-or absorbance values, **02:** 458-459
Kallikrein inactivator
molar absorptivity and-or absorbance values, **02:** 459
Kallikrein inhibitor
mammalian and chicken blood, specificity and properties, **02:** 638-639
mammalian organs and secretions, specificity and properties, **02:** 630-631
plant sources, amino acid composition, **02:** 606
potato tuber sources, specificity and properties, **02:** 586-587
Kanamycin A, B, and C; origin, structure, and characteristic as protein biosynthesis inhibitor, **04:** 580
Kasugamycin, origin, structure, and characteristic as protein biosynthesis inhibitor, **04:** 581
Katal, unit of enzymic activity, definition, **02:** 109-110
Kel-F®, chemical resistance and other properties, 08: 428
Keratin
amino acid composition, complete data, **07:** 508
α-Keratin
optical rotatory dispersion in the visible and near UV regions, **07:** 28
Keratin, S-S reduced, **07:** 28
circular dichroism in the UV region, **07:** 106
Keratinase
average hydrophobicity value, **01:** 225
molar absorptivity and-or absorbance values, **02:** 459
α-Keratose
refractive index increments, **02:** 377
L-Keto, amino acids
physical and chemical properties, **01:** 122-129
α-Keto-ε-aminocaproic acid
properties of, **01:** 182
α-Keto-δ-aminovaleric acid
properties of, **01:** 182
α-Keto-δ-carbamidovaleric acid
properties of, **01:** 181

2-Keto-3-deoxy-6-phosphogluconate aldolase, *see*
  Phospho-2-keto-3-deoxygluconate, aldolase
α-Keto-γ-ethiolbutyric acid
  properties of, **01**: 181
α-Keto-δ-guanidinovaleric acid
  properties of, **01**: 181
α-Keto-γ-hydroxybutryic acid
  properties of, **01**: 181
DL-α-Keto-β-hydroxybutyric acid
  properties of, **01**: 182
α-Keto-ε-hydroxycaproic acid
  properties of, **01**: 181
α-Keto-γ-methiolbutyric acid
  properties of, **01**: 182
4-Keto-5-methylproline
  physical and chemical properties, **01**: 143
D-α-Keto-β-methylvaleric acid
  properties of, **01**: 181
DL-α-Keto-β-methylvaleric acid
  properties of, **01**: 181
L-α-Keto-β-methylvaleric acid
  properties of, **01**: 181
α-Keto-γ-methysulfonylbutyric acid
  properties of, **01**: 182
α-Keto-δ-nitroguanidinovaleric acid
  properties of, **01**: 182
α-Keto acids
  decarboxylation by yeast decarboxylase, **01**: 69-70
  2,4-Dinitrophenylhydrazone of, **01**: 181-182
  properties of, **01**: 181-182
  reduction by lactic dehydrogenase, **01**: 181-182
Keto fatty acids, physical and chemical characteristics,
  05: 488-489
β-Ketoacyl acyl carrier protein synthetase
  amino acid composition, complete data, **07**: 508
α-Ketoadipamic acid
  properties of, **01**: 181
α-Ketoadipic acid
  properties of, **01**: 181
Ketoaldonic acids, nomenclature rules, **05**: 122-123
α-Ketobutyric acid
  properties of, **01**: 181
α-Ketocaproic acid, properties of, **01**: 182
α-Ketoglutaramic acid
  properties of, **01**: 181
α-Ketoglutaric γ-ethyl ester acid
  properties of, **01**: 181
α-Ketoglutaric acid, properties of, **01**: 181
β-Ketoglutaric dehydrogenase, *see* Oxoglutarate, dehydrogenase
α-Ketoheptylic acid, properties of, **01**: 181
α-Ketoisocaproic acid
  properties of, **01**: 182
α-Ketoisovaleric acid
  properties of, **01**: 182
δ-Ketoleucine, *see* δ-Hydroxyleucenine
δ-Ketonorleucine, *see* ε-Diazo
4-Ketonorleucine
  physical and chemical properties, **01**: 127
α-Ketophenylacetic acid
  properties of, **01**: 181

4-Ketopipecolic acid
  physical and chemical properties, **01**: 143
4-Ketoproline
  physical and chemical properties, **01**: 143
Ketoses, natural
  chemical formula, **05**: 226-239
  chromatography, **05**: 226-239
  melting point, **05**: 226-239
  specific rotation, **05**: 226-239
Ketoses, nomenclature rules, **05**: 106-107
Δ^5-3-Ketosteroid isomerase
  amino acid composition, complete data, **07**: 508
  average hydrophobicity value, **01**: 225
α-Ketosuccinamic acid
  properties of, **01**: 181
α-Ketovaleric acid, properties of, **01**: 182
Kinetoplast DNAs, properties of, **04**: 375-377
Kininogen
  cyanogen bromide cleavage, **02**: 199
  molecular parameters, **02**: 245
Kininogenase, *see* Kininogenin
Kininogenin
  circular dichroism in the UV region, **07**: 107
Kirromycin (Mocimycin), origin, structure, and characteristic as protein biosynthesis inhibitor, **04**: 581
Klebsiella
  G + C composition of DNA of, table arranged by specie, **04**: 111
Kloeckera
  G + C composition of DNA of, table arranged by spe-
  cie, **04**: 204
Kluyveromyces
  G + C composition of DNA of, table arranged by specie, **04**: 204-205
Kunitz inhibitor
  legume sources, specificity and properties, **02**: 588-589
  mammalian organs and secretions, specificity and
  properties, **02**: 630-631
  plant sources, amino acid composition, **02**: 606
Kupffer cells
  immunological response, **07**: 538
Kynurenine
  physical and chemical properties, **01**: 131

L

Labile aggregation stimulating substances, *see* LASS
Labyrinthula
  G + C composition of DNA of, table arranged by specie, **04**: 205
Lac repressor
  circular dichroism, **07**: 107
Laccase B
  circular dichroism
    UV and near UV-region, **07**: 107, 155
α-Lactalbumin
  amino acid sequence, **07**: 499
  average hydrophobicity value, **01**: 225
  circular dichroism
    UV and near UV-region, **07**: 155
  cyanogen bromide cleavage, **02**: 199

Lectin
  carbohydrate content, **02**: 270
  subunit, constitution of, **02**: 334, 337
Lectin, α-D-galactosyl-binding
  average hydrophobicity value, **01**: 225
Lectin, purified, from various sources, *see also* Purified
      lectins
  binding sites, number of, **02**: 547-551
  carbohydrate content, **02**: 546-551
  isolectins, number of, **02**: 547-551
  metal requirement, **02**: 547-551
  mitogenic activity on lymphocytes, **02**: 547-551
  molecular weight, **02**: 546-551
  specificity, **02**: 546-551
  subunits, number of, **02**: 546-551
Leghemoglobin
  molar absorptivity and-or absorbance values, **02**: 464
Leghemoglobin, soybean, aligned chains
  amino acid sequence, **07**: 456-458
Leghemoglobin I, II
  average hemophobicity value, **01**: 225
Legumes, proteinase inhibitors from, specificities and
      properties, **02**: 588-597
Legumin
  molar absorptivity and-or absorbance values, **02**: 466
  refractive index increments, **02**: 378
Leishmania
  G + C composition of DNA of, table arranged by spe-
      cie, **04**: 228
Lenzites
  G + C composition of DNA of, table arranged by spe-
      cie, **04**: 206
Leptosphaeria
  G + C composition of DNA of, table arranged by spe-
      cie, **04**: 206
Leptospira
  amino acid requirements for growth, table, **04**: 636
  G + C composition of DNA of, table arranged by spe-
      cie, **04**: 180
Leptotrichia
  G + C composition of DNA of, table arranged by spe-
      cie, **04**: 95
Leucine
  antagonism to isoleucine, **01**: 178
  antagonism to valine, **01**: 180
  antagonists of, **01**: 178
  far ultraviolet absorption spectra
    aqueous solution at pH 5, **01**: 184
    neutral water, table, **01**: 185
    0.1 *M* sodium dodecyl sulfate, table, **01**: 185
  free acid in amniotic fluid in early pregnancy and at
      term, **01**: 327
  free acid in blood plasma of newborn infants and
      adults, **01**: 328
  heat of proton ionization, pK, and related thermody-
      namic quantities, **06**: 215
  maple syrup urine disease (intermittent form), effect of,
      01: 319
  maple syrup urine disease (severe infantile), effect of,
      01: 319
  methyl and ethyl ester of, as protein biosynthesis inhibi-
      tor, **04**: 584

  nucleoside composition, tables of values, **04**: 433-434
  nucleotide sequences of, **04**: 446-447
  pK'_a values, **06**: 319
  peptic hydrolysis in human α- and β-chains, **02**: 217
  physical and chemical properties, **01**: 116
  requirements of, for growth of various microorganisms,
      table, **04**: 630-643
  specific rotatory dispersion constants, 0.1 *M* solution,
      01: 244
  spectra, far UV, **01**: 184
  symbols for atoms and bonds in side chains, **01**: 69, **02**:
      73
  thumbprint, content in, **08**: 121
D-Leucine
  antagonism to leucine, **01**: 178
Leucine aminopeptidase
  average hydrophobicity value, **01**: 225
  enzymatic hydrolysis of proteins, **02**: 209
  molar absorptivity and-or absorbance values, **02**: 466
  molecular weights, stoichiometry and sources, **02**: 285
  subunit, constitution of, **02**: 344, 345
Leucine aminopeptidase (Zn-LAP), *see* Aminopeptidase,
      (cystosol)
Leucine binding protein
  amino acid composition, complete data, **07**: 508
Leucomycin A$_3$; origin, structure, and characteristic as
      protein biosynthesis inhibitor, **04**: 582
Leuconostoc
  amino acid requirements for growth, table, **04**: 636
  G + C composition of DNA of, table arranged by spe-
      cie, **04**: 122
Leucothrix
  G + C composition of DNA of, table arranged by spe-
      cie, **04**: 126
Leucotrichaceae
  G + C composition of DNA of, table arranged by gen-
      era and specie, **04**: 126-127
Leucyl tRNA synthetase
  Neurospora crassa mutant, **04**: 751
DL-Leucylglycine
  heat capacity and entropy values, **06**: 110
Levansucrase
  amino acid composition, complete data, **07**: 508
Lichtheimia (Absidia)
  G + C composition of DNA of, table arranged by spe-
      cie, **04**: 206
Ligandin (Y protein), **07**: 108
  circular dichroism in the UV region, **07**: 108
Ligands binding to plasma albumin, table, **02**: 556-574
Ligases
  definition and nomenclature, **02**: 98
  numbering and classification of, **02**: 108
Light merromyosin (LMM), *see* Myosin, LMM
Lincomycin; origin, structure, and characteristic as
      protein biosynthesis inhibitor, **04**: 583
Linderina
  G + C composition of DNA of, table arranged by spe-
      cie, **04**: 206
Linkage map
  Aspergillus nidulans, **04**: 729-731
  bacteriophage T4, **04**: 664
  Escherichia coli, **04**: 651-653

Linkage map *(continued)*
  maize, **04:** 833-834
  mouse, **04:** 856
  Neurospora crassa, **04:** 739-757
  Bacillus subtilis, revised map, **04:** 686
  Salmonella typhimurium, **04:** 704
  Streptomyces coelicolor, **04:** 723
Linseed oil acids and esters, force-area data, **05:** 497
Lipase, *see* Triacylglycerol, lipase
  average hydrophobicity value, **01:** 225
  carbohydrate content, **02:** 274
  enzymatic activity, subcellular fractions, **02:** 698, 711,
    714
  molar absorptivity and-or absorbance values, **02:** 466
Lipid metabolism; pathways chart, **04:** insert
Lipids
  adult human skin, composition of various parts, **05:** 507
  animal tissues, content of total, of cholesteryl esters and
    of phospholipids, **05:** 519-520
  beeswax fractions, composition of acids of, **05:** 504
  chain length composition, herring oils and pilchard oils,
    05: 525
  glycolipids
    classification and nomenclature of, **05:** 416-423
    of bacteria, structures and organisms, **05:** 373-393
  glycosidic, miscellaneous, structures and organisms, **05:**
    388-390
  herring oil, monethylenic isomer content in partially hy-
    drogenated, **05:** 513
  human skin surface, fatty acids of wax esters and sterol
    esters, **05:** 509
  human skin surface, type and amount of fatty acid, **05:**
    508
  mass spectra of methyl esters of alkenyl branched chain
    acids, intensities of key fragments, **05:** 517
  mass spectrum of α-toctrienol-TMS derivative, **05:** 520
  methyl octadecadienoates and octadecatrienoates,
    equivalent chain lengths, **05:** 505
  nomenclature, journal references for, **02:** 87
  polyol esters, properties, **05:** 515
  properties of interest, comparison of, for herring oils
    and pilchard oil, **05:** 526-527
  rat cardiac, monoethylenic isomer content, **05:** 513
  solubility of selected, in chlorinated hydrocarbon sol-
    vents, **05:** 514
  solubility of selected, in chlorinated hydrocarbon mix-
    tures with 33% methanol, **05:** 514
  solubility of selected, in organic solvents, **05:** 512
  surface areas for pure methyl esters and triglycerides,
    05: 515
  trivial names, use of, **05:** 9-12
  vegetable oils, % content unsaponifiables, **05:** 512
  vegetable oils, individual tocopherol contents, **05:** 512
Lipoamide dehydrogenase (NADH)
  amino acid composition, complete data, **07:** 508
  circular dichroism in the UV region, **07:** 108
  optical rotatory dispersion
    UV region, **07:** 65
    visible and near UV regions, **07:** 29
Lipoate succinyltransferase
  circular dichroism in the UV region, **07:** 108
  optical rotatory dispersion in the UV region, **07:** 65

γ-Lipolytic hormone
  average hydrophobicity value, **01:** 225
β-Lipolytic hormone
  average hydrophobicity value, **01:** 225
Lipomyces
  G + C composition of DNA of, table arranged by spe-
    cie, **04:** 206
Lipopolysaccharides of gram-negative bacteria
  sugar composition, **05:** 396-402
  sugar sequences, general structure, **05:** 403-412
Lipopolysaccharides receptor
  circular dichroism in the UV region, **07:** 109
Lipoprotein
  amino acid composition, complete data, **07:** 508
  amino acid composition, incomplete data, **07:** 513
  circular dichroism in the UV region, **07:** 109
  optical rotatory dispersion
    UV region, **07:** 65
    visible and near UV regions, **07:** 29
α_1-Lipoprotein
  molecular parameters, **02:** 242
  refractive index increments, **02:** 378
α_2-Lipoprotein
  molecular parameters, **02:** 245
β-Lipoprotein
  molecular parameters, **02:** 247
  refractive index increments, **02:** 378
β_1-Lipoprotein
  refractive index increments, **02:** 378
Lipoprotein, high density
  subunit, constitution of, **02:** 347
Lipoprotein B
  amino acid sequence, **07:** 387, 499
  circular dichroism in the UV region, **07:** 110
  optical rotatory dispersion
    UV region, **07:** 65
    visible and near UV regions, **07:** 29
Lipoprotein HDL_2, human
  molar absorptivity and-or absorbance values, **02:** 467
Lipoprotein very low density, human ApoLP-Val
  molar absorptivity and-or absorbance values, **02:** 467
Lipoprotein very low density, rat serum
  molar absorptivity and-or absorbance values, **02:** 467
Lipovitellin
  circular dichroism in the UV region, **07:** 110
  molar absorptivity and-or absorbance values, **02:** 467
  optical rotatory dispersion in the UV region, **07:** 66
  refractive index increments, **02:** 379
  subunit, constitution of, **02:** 347
α-Lipovitellin
  average hydrophobicity value, **01:** 225
Lipoyl dehydrogenase, *see* Lipoamide, dehydrogenase
    (NADH)
Listeria
  G + C composition of DNA of, table arranged by spe-
    cie, **04:** 103
Liver alcohol dehydrogenase
  amino acid sequence, **07:** 330-332
α-Livetin
  refractive index increments, **02:** 379
γ-Livetin
  refractive index increments, **02:** 379

β-Livetin
  refractive index increments, **02**: 379
Lividomycin; origin, structure, and characteristic as
      protein biosynthesis inhibitor, **04**: 583
Locants, assignment of, in nomenclature, **05**: 92
Lodderomyces
  G + C composition of DNA of, table arranged by spe-
      cie, **04**: 206
Lombricine
  physical and chemical properties, **01**: 161
Lombricine kinase
  circular dichroism, **07**: 110
      UV and near-UV region, **07**: 110, 156
  molar absorptivity and-or absorbance values, **02**: 467
  optical rotatory dispersion
      UV region, **07**: 66
      visible and near UV regions, **07**: 29
Long chain base, generic term usage, **05**: 9
Long neurotoxins, *see* Neurotoxins, long
Lophomonas
  G + C composition of DNA of, table arranged by spe-
      cie, **04**: 154
Lorentz correction factors
  concentration dependence
      2-chloroethanol at several wavelengths, **06**: 400-401
      methanol at several wavelengths, **06**: 396-399
      2-methoxyethanol at several wavelengths, **06**: 402-403
Lowe's syndrome, characteristics of, **01**: 324
Luciferase
  average hydrophobicity values, **01**: 226
  subunit, constitution of, **02**: 330, 332
Luciferase chain α
  amino acid composition, complete data, **07**: 508
Luminescence
  aromatic amino acid derivatives, table, **01**: 201-203
  aromatic amino acids, table, **01**: 200
  flavins, table of values, **08**: 205-209
  proteins containing tryptophan, table, **01**: 205-207
  proteins lacking tryptophan, table, **01**: 204
luminescence of, table, **01**: 206
Luteinizing hormone, *see also* Interstitial cell-stimulating
      hormone, **07**: 30, 66
  amino acid sequence
      α subunit, **07**: 393-394
      β subunit, **07**: 395-397
  carbohydrate content, **02**: 272-273
  circular dichroism
      UV and near-UV region, **07**: 106, 156
  molar absorptivity and-or absorbance values, **02**: 468
Luteinizing hormone-α chain
  average hydrophobicity value, **01**: 226
Luteinizing hormone-β chain
  average hydrophobicity value, **01**: 226
Lyase
  definition and nomenclature, **02**: 98
  numbering and classification of, **02**: 108
Lycin
  physical and chemical properties, **01**: 163
Lycogala
  G + C composition of DNA of, table arranged by spe-
      cie, **04**: 206

Lycopene
  UV spectra, formula, molecular weight, **08**: 189
Lymphocytes
  immunological response, **07**: 536-537
Lyngbya
  G + C composition of DNA of, table arranged by spe-
      cie, **04**: 226
Lysergic acid
  pK'_a values, **06**: 313, 326
Lysin
  molar absorptivity and-or absorbance values, **02**: 468
Lysine
  active site peptides, **07**: 188
  antagonism to arginine, **01**: 177
  antagonists of, **01**: 178
  far ultraviolet absorption spectra
      aqueous solution at pH 5, **01**: 184
      neutral water, table, **01**: 185
      0.1 *M* sodium dodecyl sulfate, table, **01**: 185
  free acid in amniotic fluid in early pregnancy and at
      term, **01**: 327
  free acid in blood plasma in newborn infants and
      adults, **01**: 328
  heat of proton ionization, pK, and related thermody-
      namic quantities, **06**: 215
  hyperlysinemia, effect of, **01**: 320
  nucleoside composition, tables of values, **04**: 434
  nucleotide sequences of, **04**: 446-447
  pK'_a values, **06**: 319
  physical and chemical properties, **01**: 121
  requirements of, for growth of various microorganisms,
      table, **04**: 630-643
  specific rotatory dispersion constants, 0.1 *M* solution,
      01: 244
  spectra, far UV, **01**: 184
  symbols for atoms and bonds in side chains, **01**: 69, **02**:
      73
  thumbprint, content in, **08**: 121
β-Lysine, *see* 3,6-Diaminohexanoic acid
Lysine-vasopressin
  amino acid sequence, physical and biological properties,
      07: 197-198
Lysine decarboxylase
  average hydrophobicity value, **01**: 226
  molar absorptivity and-or absorbance values, **02**: 468
  subunit, constitution of, **02**: 349
Lysine metabolism; pathways chart, **04**: insert
L-Lysine monooxygenase
  amino acid composition, complete data, **07**: 508
  average hydrophobicity value, **01**: 226
β-Lysine mutase
  subunit, constitution of, **02**: 339
Lysine tRNA synthetase
  subunit, constitution of, **02**: 336
Lysopine
  physical and chemical properties, **01**: 121
Lysosomes
  enzymatic activity, table, **02**: 711
  molecular parameters, **02**: 250
Lysostaphin
  amino acid composition, incomplete data, **07**: 513
  average hydrophobicity value, **01**: 226

Lysozyme
  amino acid composition, complete data, **07**: 508
  amino acid sequences of proteins, **07**: 309
  average hydrophobicity values, **01**: 226
  calorimetric ΔH values accompanying conformational
      changes, **06**: 273
  circular dichroism
    UV and near-UV region, **07**: 111, 157
  cyanogen bromide cleavage, **02**: 199
  egg white
    luminescence of, table, **01**: 206
  molar absorptivity and-or absorbance values, **02**: 468,
      469
  optical rotatory dispersion
    UV region, **07**: 66
    visible and near UV regions, **07**: 30
  refractive index increments, **02**: 379
  viscosity, intrinsic, **02**: 721
Lysyl: tRNA ligase
  average hydrophobicity value, **01**: 226
Lysyl tRNA synthetase
  molar absorptivity and-or absorbance values, **02**: 469
Lysylaminoadenosine, physicochemical constants, spec-
    tral, chemotherapeutic and biological properties, **03**:
    328
α-Lytic protease
  average hydrophobicity value, **01**: 226
β-Lytic protease
  average hydrophobicity value, **01**: 226

M

Macroglobulin, *see also* Ovomacroglobulin
  plasma, nonhuman
    carbohydrate content, **02**: 259
α₂-Macroglobulin
  carbohydrate composition, **02**: 666-667
  human
    carbohydrate content, molecular weight, sedimentation
        coefficients, **02**: 258
    molar absorptivity and-or absorbance values, **02**: 470
  molar absorptivity and-or absorbance values, **02**: 469,
      470
  molecular parameters, **02**: 245
  molecular weight, stoichiometry, source, function, **02**:
      277
  optical rotatory dispersion in the visible and near UV
      regions, **07**: 30
Macrolesionus, classification of mutations, **04**: 893
Macromolecules
  calorimetric ΔH values accompanying conformational
      changes, **06**: 270-293
Macromolecules association reactions
  volume changes for some, table, **07**: 593-594
Macrophage
  immunological response, **07**: 538
Magnamycin®, *see* Carbomycin
Maize, *see also* Corn
  linkage map, **04**: 833-834
Maize (*Zea mays* L.)
  availability of sample quantities, **04**: 835

genetic markers, annotated list, **04**: 835-844
Major histocompatibility complex
  definition, **04**: 885
  designation for a variety of mammalian species, **04**: 885
  man, table of values, **04**: 886
  mouse, table of values, **04**: 886-887
  properties associated with differences at the MHC, **04**:
      885
Malate-lactate transhydrogenase
  molar absorptivity and-or absorbance values, **02**: 470
Malate-vitamin k reductase
  average hydrophobicity value, **01**: 226
Malate dehydrogenase
  average hydrophobicity value, **01**: 226
  molar absorptivity and-or absorbance values, **02**: 470
  optical rotatory dispersion
    UV region, **07**: 66
    visible and near UV regions, **07**: 30
  subunit, constitution of, **02**: 328, 329, 330, 338
Malate dehydrogenase, porcine
  structure, illustration, **02**: 766
Malate synthase
  circular dichroism in the UV region, **07**: 111
Malate synthetase, *see* Malate, synthase
Maleate buffer, preparation of, **06**: 373
Maleate isomerase
  amino acid composition, incomplete data, **07**: 513
Malic dehydrogenase, *see* Malate, dehydrogenase
Malic dehydrogenase (mitochondrial)
  amino acid composition, complete data, **07**: 508
Malic enzyme
  molar absorptivity and-or absorbance values, **02**:
      470-471
  subunit, constitution of, **02**: 343, 344
L-Malic enzyme
  average hydrophobicity value, **01**: 226
Malonic acid derivatives
  heat of proton ionization, pK, and related thermody-
      namic quantities, **06**: 216
N-α-Malonyl-D-methionine
  physical and chemical properties, **01**: 165
N-α-Malonyl-D-tryptophan
  physical and chemical properties, **01**: 165
Mammalian organs and secretions
  proteinase inhibitors from, specificity and properties,
      02: 630-635
Mammals
  DNA content per cell for various, table, **04**: 302-305
  satellite DNAs
    buoyant density and G + C content of, table, **04**:
        391-399
β-Mannase
  amino acid composition, incomplete data, **07**: 513
Mannitol
  pK′ₐ values, **06**: 317
Mannose
  heat of proton ionization, pk, and related thermody-
      namic quantities, **06**: 217
  pK′ₐ values, **06**: 317
α-D-Mannoside mannohydrolase
  enzymatic reactions, velocity and parameters, table, **05**:
      426-428

Mannoside streptomycin; origin and characteristic as protein biosynthesis inhibitor, **04:** 584

Map, *see also* Linkage Map
mutants, biochemical, of *Coprinus radiatus*, **04:** 762

Maple syrup urine disease
intermittent form, characteristics, **01:** 319
severe infantile, characteristics, **01:** 319

Mapping, physical
viral DNA molecules, **03:** 551-556

Maquenne fractional notation for cyclitols, **05:** 89

Mass spectra
intensities of key fragments, methyl esters of alkenyl branched chain acids, **05:** 517
methyl linoleate, **05:** 500
methyl linolenate, **05:** 500
methyl oleate, **05:** 500
α tocotrienol-TMS derivative, **05:** 520

Mast cell
immunological response, **07:** 538

Matate-lactate transhydrogenase
average hydrophobicity value, **01:** 226

Matrix protein
circular dichroism in the UV region, **07:** 112

McCasland notation for cyclitols, **05:** 89-90

MDMP; origin, structure, and characteristic as protein biosynthesis inhibitor, **04:** 584

Me$_2$ SO-chymotrypsin
calorimetric ΔH values accompanying conformational changes, **06:** 274

Mean residue absorptivity
dinucleoside monophosphates, table of values, **03:** 597
homopolymer complexes, double-stranded, table of values, **03:** 602
ribonucleotides, homooligomers and homopolymers, table of values, **03:** 603

Mean residue ellipticities
of three conformations based on synthetic polypeptides, table, **07:** 135
of three reference conformations based on five globular proteins, table, **07:** 138-139

Mean residue rotation
of three reference conformations based on five globular proteins, table, **07:** 140

Mean residue rotation, reduced
of three conformations based on poly(L-lysine), **07:** 137
reference values, tables, **07:** 137, 140

β-Melanocyte stimulating hormone
average hydrophobicity value, **01:** 226

Melanotropin
amino acid sequence
α, **07:** 385
natural, **07:** 375
β, **07:** 386

Melilotate hydroxylase
average hydrophobicity value, **01:** 227
molar absorptivity and-or absorbance values, **02:** 471

Melting point
aldaric acids, **05:** 168-170
alditols, amino, **05:** 148-149
alditols, natural, **05:** 139-142
aldonic acids, **05:** 153-164
aldoses, natural, **05:** 181-217

amino acids, naturally occurring, table, **01:** 111-166
amino sugar acids, **05:** 170-176
amino sugars, naturally occurring, **05:** 359-370
antibiotics, nucleoside, **03:** 271-393
carbohydrate phosphate esters, **05:** 253-258, 262-273
disaccharides, **05:** 283-297, 327-334
fats and oils, table of values, **05:** 502-503
fatty acids, **05:** 484-490
heptasaccharides, **05:** 318-319, 345-346
hexasaccharides, **05:** 316-318, 344-345
inosamines, **05:** 148-149
inositols, **05:** 142-147
inososes, **05:** 147
ketoses, natural, **05:** 226-239
menaquinone, properties of, **08:** 291
methyl esters of some synthetic alkenyl and alkyl substituted fatty acids, **05:** 516
nucleosides, index to table of values, **03:** 69-72
nucleotides, index to table of values, **03:** 72-75
octasaccharides, **05:** 319, 346
oligosaccharides, **05:** 283-319, 327-346
pentasaccharides, **05:** 315-316, 343-344
porphyrin methyl esters, **08:** 276
purines, index to table of values, **03:** 67-69
pyridoxine, pyridoxal and pyridoxamine derivatives, **08:** 252-266
pyrimides, index to table of values, **03:** 67-69
steroids, table, **05:** 531-588
tetrasaccharides, **05:** 308-314, 340-343
trisaccharides, **05:** 297-308, 334-340
uronic acids, **05:** 165-168
vitamins, table of data, **08:** 284-300

Melting temperature
copolymers of repeating sequence, **03:** 583-585
deoxyribohomopolymers and complexes, **03:** 581-582
polynucleotides, synthetic, **03:** 575-585
ribohomopolymer deoxyribohomopolymer hybrids, **03:** 582-583
ribohomopolymers and complexes, **03:** 575-580
viral DNA, **03:** 560-562

Membrane protein
circular dichroism in the UV region, **07:** 112

Membrane protein, mitochondria
circular dichroism in the UV region, **07:** 112
optical rotatory dispersion
UV region, **07:** 66
visible and near UV regions, **07:** 30

Membrane protein, mycoplasma
circular dichroism in the UV region, **07:** 112

Membrane protein, purple
circular dichroism in the UV region, **07:** 112

Membrane protein, thylakoid
circular dichroism in the UV region, **07:** 113

Meningococcus
amino acid requirements for growth, table, **04:** 636

Mercaptalbumin
calorimetric ΔH values accompanying conformational changes, **06:** 270

α-Mercaptoalanine
structure and symbols for those incorporated into synthetic polypeptides, **01:** 104

β-Mercaptolactate-cysteine disulfide
   β-mercaptolactate cysteinuria, effect of, **01:** 317
   physical and chemical properties, **01:** 156
β-Mercaptolactate cysteinuria, characteristics of, **01:** 317
Mercaptopyruvate sulfurtransferase
   molar absorptivity and-or absorbance values, **02:** 471
   subunit, constitution of, **02:** 326
β-Mercaptopyruvic acid, properties of, **01:** 181
β-Mercaptovaline, *see* β,β-Dimethylcysteine
Merodesmosine
   physical and chemical properties, **01:** 149
Meruliopsis (Poria)
   G + C composition of DNA of, table arranged by specie, **04:** 206
Mesaconate pathway; pathways chart, **04:** insert
Mesotocin
   amino acid sequence, **07:** 195
Mesoxalic acid, properties of, **01:** 181
Metabolic disease related amino acids, rapid short column chromatography, **08:** 128-129
Metabolic pathways, chart, **04:** insert
Metabolism
   mammalian unsaturated fatty acid, outline, **08:** 319
Metal complexes of amino acids and peptides, circular dichroism spectra, **01:** 245-315
Metal ions, ligands binding to plasma albumin, **02:** 563
Metal requirement, purified lectins, **02:** 547-551
Metalloenzyme
   cofactors, molecular weights, stoichiometry and sources, **02:** 278-286
Metalloporphyrins
   absorption data table, **08:** 279
   methyl esters
      absorption spectra, **08:** 278
      Soret band data using organic solvents, **08:** 278
   oxidation-reduction potentials, **06:** 139-144
Metalloprotein
   molecular weight, source, stoichiometry, function, **02:** 276-277
   nomenclature rules, **02:** 121
Metalloprotein model systems
   resonance raman spectra, **07:** 590
Metallothionein (Cd, Zn-thionein)
   circular dichroism in the UV region, **07:** 113
Metapyrocatechase, *see* Catechol 2,3, -dioxygenase
   molar absorptivity and-or absorbance values, **02:** 472
   table of cofactors, molecular weights, stoichiometry and sources, **02:** 280
Metazoan globins, *see* Globins, metazoan, aligned chains
Methadone, ligands binding to plasma albumin, **02:** 574
Methallylglycine
   antagonism to isoleucine, **01:** 178
   antagonism to leucine, **01:** 178
   antagonism to valine, **01:** 180
Methane derivatives
   heat of proton ionization, pK, and related thermodynamic quantities, **06:** 218
Methanobacterium
   G + C composition of DNA of, table arranged by specie, **04:** 168

Methanol
   heat of proton ionization, pK, and related thermodynamic quantities, **06:** 218
Methanol-water mixtures, dielectric constants and freezing points, **06:** 523
Methemoglobins
   heat of proton ionization, pK, and related thermodynamic quantities, **06:** 217
Methionine
   antagonists of, **01:** 178
   far ultraviolet absorption spectra, **01:** 185
      aqueous solution at pH 5, **01:** 184
      neutral water, table, **01:** 185
      0.1 *M* sodium dodecyl sulfate, table, **01:** 185
   free acid in amniotic fluid in early pregnancy and at term, **01:** 327
   free acid in blood plasma of newborn infants and adults, **01:** 328
   heat of proton ionization, pK, and related thermodynamic quantities, **06:** 218
   molar extinctions, **01:** 185
   nucleoside composition, tables of values, **04:** 434-436
   nucleotide sequences of, **04:** 448-449
   pK'_a values, **06:** 319
   physical and chemical properties, **01:** 157
   requirements of, for growth of various microorganisms, table, **04:** 630-643
   spectra, far UV, **01:** 184
   symbols for atoms and bonds in side chains, **01:** 69, **02:** 73
   thumbprint, content in, **08:** 121
Methionine malabsorption syndrome, characteristics of, **01:** 323
Methionine sulfoxide
   antagonism to glutamic acid, **01:** 177
Methionine sulfoximine
   antagonism to glutamic acid, **01:** 177
   antagonism to methionine, **01:** 178
Methionyl-lysl-bradykinin
   amino acid sequence, physical and biological properties, **07:** 222
Methionyl tRNA synthetase
   average hydrophobicity value, **01:** 227
   molar absorptivity and-or absorbance values, **02:** 472
Methoxinine
   antagonism to methionine, **01:** 178
7-[(3-Methoxycarbonyl)-3-(methoxyformamido)propyl] wyosine
   isolation and detection of, in RNA, general remarks, **03:** 245-246
   RNA, various, natural occurrence in, **03:** 233
5-(Methoxycarbonylmethyl)-2-thiouridine
   composition in various tRNA's, **04:** 428-441
   isolation and detection of, in RNA, general remarks, **03:** 243
   RNA, various, natural occurrence in, **03:** 231
5-(Methoxycarbonylmethyl)uridine
   composition in various tRNA's, **04:** 428-441
β-(*p*-Methoxyphenyl)-alanine, *see* O-Methyltyrosine
1-Methyl-3-(3-amino-3-carboxypropyl) pseudouridine
   isolation and detection of, in RNA, general remarks, **03:** 240

1-Methyl-3-(3-amino-3-carboxypropyl) pseudouridine
(*continued*)
RNA, various, natural occurrence in, **03:** 229
γ-Methyl-α,ε-diaminopimelic acid
antagonism to α,ε-Diaminopimelic acid, **01:** 177
5-Methyl-5,6-dihydrouridine
isolation and detection of, in RNA, general remarks, **03:** 244
RNA, various, natural occurrence in, **03:** 232
3-Methyl-2-hydroazirine carboxylic acid, *see* Azirinomycin
1-Methyl-6-hydroxy-1,2,3,4-tetrahydroisoquinoline-3-carboxylic acid
physical and chemical properties, **01:** 144
α-Methyl-β-hydroxy butyric aciduria
characteristics of, **01:** 326
γ-Methyl-γ-hydroxy glutamic acid
physical and chemical properties, **01:** 128
N-Methyl-D-leucine
physical and chemical properties, **01:** 166
N-Methyl-γ-methyl-*allo*-isoleucine
physical and chemical properties, **01:** 116
β-Methyl-β-(methylene-cyclopropyl) alanine
physical and chemical properties, **01:** 116
N-Methyl-β-methylleucine
physical and chemical properties, **01:** 150
N-Methyl-O-methylserine
physical and chemical properties, **01:** 150
Methyl 10,12-octadecadienoate, NMR spectra, **05:** 498
2-Methyl-2-4-pentanediol-water mixtures, dielectric constants and freezing points, **06:** 524
2-Methyl-3-phytyl-1,4-naphthaquinone, *see also* Vitamin K
UV spectra, formula, molecular weight, **08:** 156
3-Methyl-1,4-thiazane-5-carboxylic acid oxide, *see* Cycloallin
5-Methyl-2-thiouridine
isolation and detection of, in RNA, general remarks, **03:** 243
RNA, various, natural occurrence in, **03:** 231
N^6-Methyl-N^6-threoninocarbonyladenosine
composition in various tRNA's, **04:** 428-441
isolation and detection of, in RNA, general remarks, **03:** 235
RNA, various, natural occurrence in, **03:** 221
N-Methyl-tryptophan, *see* Abrine
Methyl acetoacetic aciduria, characteristics of, **01:** 326
β-Methyl aspartase
average hydrophobicity value, **01:** 227
Methyl esters, unsaturated
NMR spectra of some, **05:** 498
Methyl linoleate
mass spectra, **05:** 500
NMR spectra, **05:** 498
NMR spectrum in carbon tetrachloride solution, **05:** 511
Methyl linolenate, mass spectra, **05:** 500
Methyl oleate
mass spectra, **05:** 500
NMR spectra, **05:** 498
Methyladenosine
composition in various tRNA's, **04:** 428-441

N^6-Methyladenosine
composition in various tRNA's, **04:** 428-441
isolation and detection of, in RNA, general remarks, **03:** 235
RNA, various, natural occurrence in, **03:** 219
O^2-Methyladenosine
isolation and detection of, in RNA, general remarks, **03:** 235-236
RNA, various, natural occurrence in, **03:** 221
1-Methyladenosine
isolation and detection of, in RNA, general remarks, **03:** 233-234
RNA, various, natural occurrence in, **03:** 216-217
2-Methyladenosine
composition in various tRNA's, **04:** 428-441
isolation and detection of, in RNA, general remarks, **03:** 234
RNA, various, natural occurrence in, **03:** 218
α-Methylalanine, *see* 2-Aminoisobutyric acid
N-Methylalanine
physical and chemical properties, **01:** 149
structure and symbols for those incorporated into synthetic polypeptides, **01:** 104
N-Methylalloisoleucine
structure and symbols for those incorporated into synthetic polypeptides, **01:** 104
2-Methylaminoethylphosphonic acid
physical and chemical properties, **01:** 161
5-(Methylaminomethyl)-2-thiouridine
composition in various tRNA's, **04:** 428-441
isolation and detection of, in RNA, general remarks, **03:** 243
RNA, various, natural occurrence in, **03:** 231
6-Methylaminopurine, content in DNA from various sources, **04:** 282-283
ω-N-Methylarginine
physical and chemical properties, **01:** 134
Methylases
cleavage sites, number of, for several, **04:** 532-534
recognition sequences for several, **04:** 532-534
N^4-Methylasparagine
physical and chemical properties, **01:** 118
β-Methylaspartase
amino acid composition, complete data, **07:** 508
molar absorptivity and-or absorbance values, **02:** 472
α-Methylaspartic acid
antagonism to aspartic acid, **01:** 177
β-Methylaspartic acid
antagonism to aspartic acid, **01:** 177
physical and chemical properties, **01:** 118
β-Methylcrotonylcoenzyme A carboxylase
average hydrophobicity value, **01:** 227
β-Methylcrotonylglycinuria, characteristics of, **01:** 326
S-Methylcysteine
physical and chemical properties, **01:** 46
S-Methylcysteine sulfoxide
antagonism to aspartic acid, **01:** 177
physical and chemical properties, **01:** 156
$O^{2'}$-Methylcytidine
composition in various tRNA's, **04:** 428-441
RNA, various, natural occurrence in, **03:** 223

3-Methylcytidine
  composition in various tRNA's, **04:** 428-441
  isolation and detection of, in RNA, general remarks, **03:** 237
  RNA, various, natural occurrence in, **03:** 222
5-Methylcytidine
  composition in various tRNA's, **04:** 428-441
  isolation and detection of, in RNA, general remarks, **03:** 237
  RNA, various, natural occurrence in, **03:** 222-223
5-Methylcytosine
  content in DNA from various sources, **04:** 282-283
  content in DNAs, discussion of hypothesis, **04:** 358
β-Methyldehydroalanine
  structure and properties, **01:** 175
β-(Methylene-cyclopropyl)-β-methylalanine
  physical and chemical properties, **01:** 117
α-(Methylene-cyclopropyl) glycine
  physical and chemical properties, **01:** 116
γ-Methyleneglutamic acid
  physical and chemical properties, **01:** 119
γ-Methyleneglutamine
  physical and chemical properties, **01:** 119
β-Methylenenorleucine
  physical and chemical properties, **01:** 117
4-Methyleneproline
  physical and chemical properties, **01:** 144
6-Methylenetetracycline; origin, structure, and characteristic as protein biosynthesis inhibitor, **04:** 584
3,3'-(2-Methylethylene-1,2-dithio)-dialanine
  physical and chemical properties, **01:** 157
5-N-Methylformamido-6-ribosylaminoisocytosine 3'(2')-phosphate
  physical constants and spectral properties, **03:** 195
α-Methylglutamic acid, **01:** 177
  antagonism to glutamic acid, **01:** 177
γ-Methylglutamic acid
  physical and chemical properties, **01:** 119
N-Methylglycine, see Sarcosine
N^2-Methylguanosine
  composition in various tRNA's, **04:** 428-441
  isolation and detection of, in RNA, general remarks, **03:** 238
  RNA, various, natural occurrence in, **03:** 224-225
$O^{2'}$-Methylguanosine
  composition in various tRNA's, **04:** 428-441
  isolation and detection of, in RNA, general remarks, **03:** 239
  RNA, various, natural occurrence in, **03:** 227
1-Methylguanosine
  composition in various tRNA's, **04:** 428-441
  isolation and detection of, in RNA, general remarks, **03:** 237-238
  RNA, various, natural occurrence in, **03:** 224
7-Methylguanosine
  composition in various tRNA's, **04:** 428-441
  isolation and detection of, in RNA, general remarks, **03:** 238-239
  RNA, various, natural occurrence in, **03:** 226
prosMethylhistidine
  structure and symbols for those incorporated into synthetic polypeptides, **01:** 104

teleMethylhistidine
  structure and symbols for those incorporated into synthetic polypeptides, **01:** 104
1-Methylhistidine, see also teleMethylhistidine
  physical and chemical properties, **01:** 149
3-Methylhistidine, see also prosMethylhistidine
  physical and chemical properties, **01:** 149
1-Methylinosine
  composition in various tRNA's, **04:** 428-441
  isolation and detection of, in RNA, general remarks, **03:** 240
  RNA, various, natural occurrence in, **03:** 2282'O-Methylpentose residue, UV absorbance of oligonucleotides containing, **03:** 448-449
N-Methylisoasparagine
  structure and symbols for those incorporated into synthetic polypeptides, **01:** 104
N-Methylisoleucine
  physical and chemical properties, **01:** 150
β-Methyllanthionine
  physical and chemical properties, **01:** 157
N-Methylleucine
  physical and chemical properties, **01:** 150
ε-N-Methyllysine
  physical and chemical properties, **01:** 121
Methylmalonatesemialdehydedehydrogenase
  average hydrophobicity value, **01:** 227
Methylmalonic acidemia, characteristics of, **01:** 326
S-Methylmethionine
  physical and chemical properties, **01:** 157
Methylococcus
  amino acid requirements for growth, table, **04:** 636
(N-Methyl)phenylalanine
  structure and symbols for those incorporated into synthetic polypeptides, **01:** 104
N-Methylphenylglycine
  physical and chemical properties, **01:** 150
N-Methylpicolinic acid, see Homarine
N-Methylproline
  physical and chemical properties, **01:** 144
4-Methylproline
  physical and chemical properties, **01:** 144
$O^{2'}$-Methylpseudouridine
  composition in various tRNA's, **04:** 428-441
  isolation and detection of, in RNA, general remarks, **03:** 240
  RNA, various, natural occurrence in, **03:** 229
6-Methylpurine
  molal activity coefficients, **03:** 529
  molal osmotic coefficients, **03:** 528
β-Methylselenoalanine
  physical and chemical properties, **01:** 157
β-Methylselenocysteine, see β-Methylselenoalanine
α-Methylserine
  antagonism to serine, **01:** 179
D-α-Methylserine
  physical and chemical properties, **01:** 166
O-Methylserine
  structure and symbols for those incorporated into synthetic polypeptides, **01:** 104
N-Methylstreptolidine
  physical and chemical properties, **01:** 144

5-Methylthionorvaline, *see* Homomethionine

N-Methylthreonine
  physical and chemical properties, **01:** 150

O-Methylthreonine
  antagonism to isoleucine, **01:** 178
  structure and symbols for those incorporated into synthetic polypeptides, **01:** 104

α-Methyltryosine
  structure and symbols for those incorporated into synthetic polypeptides, **01:** 105

Methyltryptophan
  antagonism to tryptophan, **01:** 179

β-Methyltryptophan
  physical and chemical properties, **01:** 144

N-Methyltyrosine
  physical and chemical properties, **01:** 150
  structure and symbols for those incorporated into synthetic polypeptides, **01:** 105

O-Methyltyrosine
  physical and chemical properties, **01:** 131
  structure and symbols for those incorporated into synthetic polypeptides, **01:** 105

$O^{2'}$-Methyluridine
  composition in various tRNA's, **04:** 428-441
  isolation and detection of, in RNA, general remarks, **03:** 244
  RNA, various, natural occurrence in, **03:** 232

3-Methyluridine
  isolation and detection of, in RNA, general remarks, **03:** 240-241
  RNA, various, natural occurrence in, **03:** 229

5-Methyluridine
  composition in various tRNA's, **04:** 428-441
  isolation and detection of, in RNA, general remarks, **03:** 242
  RNA, various, natural occurrence in, **03:** 230-231

N-Methylvaline
  physical and chemical properties, **01:** 150

Methymycin; origin, structure, and characteristic as protein biosynthesis inhibitor, **04:** 585

Metschnikowia
  G + C composition of DNA of, table arranged by specie, **04:** 206

MHC, *see* Major Histocompatibility Complex

Michaelis constant
  equation and symbols used, **02:** 111

Michaelis constants for glycohydrolases, table of, **05:** 426-445

Microbacterium
  G + C composition of DNA of, table arranged by specie, **04:** 103

Microbial metalloenzyme
  amino acid sequence, **07:** 322
  optical rotatory dispersion
    UV region, **07:** 67
    visible and near UV regions, **07:** 30

Microbispora (*Waksmania*)
  G + C composition of DNA of, table arranged by specie, **04:** 149

Microbodies
  enzymatic activity, table, **02:** 710

Micrococcaceae
  G + C composition of DNA of, table arranged by genera and specie, **04:** 127-138

Micrococcin (Micrococcin P); origin, structure, and characteristic as protein biosynthesis inhibitor, **04:** 585

Micrococcus
  amino acid requirements for growth, table, **04:** 636

Micrococcus (*Staphylococcus*)
  G + C composition of DNA of, table arranged by specie, **04:** 128-134

Microcoleus
  G + C composition of DNA of, table arranged by specie, **04:** 226

Microcyclus
  G + C composition of DNA of, table arranged by specie, **04:** 168

Microellobosporia
  G + C composition of DNA of, table arranged by specie, **04:** 77

$β_2$-Microglobulin
  amino acid composition, incomplete data, **07:** 513
  amino acid sequences, **02:** 305
  molar absorptivity and-or absorbance values, **02:** 472
  properties, table, **02:** 305

Micromonospora
  G + C composition of DNA of, table arranged by specie, **04:** 138

Micromonosporaceae
  G + C composition of DNA of, table arranged by genera and specie, **04:** 138

Microorganisms
  amino acid requirements for growth, table, **04:** 630-643
  growth of, standard media for, **04:** 649
  sugar fermentation, preparation of EMB medium for detecting, **04:** 650

Micropolyspora
  G + C composition of DNA of, table arranged by specie, **04:** 149

Microsomes
  enzymatic activity, table, **02:** 706-709

Microtubule protein
  amino acid composition, complete data, **07:** 509

Mikamycin A; origin, structure, and characteristic as protein biosynthesis inhibitor, **04:** 585

Mikamycin B, *see* Ostreogrycin B, Streptogramin B$_1$

Milk
  glycoproteins from, carbohydrate content, **02:** 268-269

Millipore®, filters O-rings, and filter holders, chemical compatibility, **08:** 431-432

Mima
  G + C composition of DNA of, table arranged by specie, **04:** 92

Mimosine
  physical and chemical properties, **01:** 144

Minaline
  physical and chemical properties, **01:** 145

Minerals
  diet, human, NAS-NRC recommended daily allowances, **08:** 249
  diet, human, U.S. Government recommended daily allowances, **08:** 310

Minimycin, physicochemical constants, spectral, chemotherapeutic and biological properties, **03:** 329

Minosin (Minomycin); origin, structure, and characteristic as protein biosynthesis inhibitor, **04:** 586

Miokinine
  physical and chemical properties, **01:** 163

Mitochondria, isolated
  enzymatic activity, table, **02:** 702-704

Mitochondria, range of weights, **08:** 424

Mitochondrial DNAs, properties of, **04:** 363-372

Mitochondrial membrane protein, *see* Membrane, protein, mitochondria

Mitochondrial structural protein
  amino acid composition, complete data, **07:** 509

Mitogen
  carbohydrate content, **02:** 270

Mitogenic activity on lymphocytes, purified lectins, **02:** 547-551

Mitotic apparatus 22S protein
  amino acid composition, incomplete data, **07:** 513

Mo-Fe Protein
  subunit, constitution of, **02:** 340

Mocimycin, *see* Kirromycin

Moffitt equation
  for estimate or content in protein molecule, **07:** 3-4
  optical rotatory dispersion of proteins in visible and near UV regions, **07:** 15-38

Moffitt equation, numerical constants for b_0 calculations, **08:** 198-200

Molal activity coefficients
  amino acids, table of values, **06:** 119-120
  nucleosides, values for several, **03:** 529
  peptides, table of values, **06:** 120

Molal osmotic coefficients
  nucleosides and nucleic acid bases, **03:** 528

Molar absorbance
  compounds used in biochemical studies, **06:** 123-129

Molar absorption coefficient, *see* Molar absorptivity

Molar absorptivity
  β_2 microglobulin, **02:** 305
  nucleoside 2,3-monophosphates, **03:** 597
  polyribonucleotides, calculation of, **03:** 596
  retinol-binding protein, **02:** 304
  Tamm-Horsfall mucoprotein, **02:** 304
  urokinase, **02:** 302

Molar absorptivity, UV and visible region, table of values for proteins, **02:** 383-514

Molar activity
  enzymes, defined, **02:** 109

Molar ellipticity
  polyribonucleotides, calculation of, **03:** 596

Molar extinction coefficient
  circular dichroism calculations, **03:** 470

Molar extinctions
  N-Acetyl methyl esters of aromatic amino acids, cystine and *N*-acetylcysteine, **01:** 186

Molar residue ellipticity
  dinucleoside monophosphates, **03:** 600
  nucleotides, double helical complexes, and double stranded RNA, **03:** 601

Molar residue rotation
  dinucleoside monophosphates, **03:** 598

nucleotides, double helical complexes and double-stranded RNA, table of values, **03:** 599

Molar rotation
  polyribonucleotides, calculation of, **03:** 596

Molecular absorbances of aromatic amino acids, data, **01:** 187-189

Molecular conformations, polynucleotide double helices, **04:** 411-418

Molecular dimensions, long-chain aliphatic acids and related compounds, **05:** 498

Molecular formula, *see* Formula, molecular
  amino acids, naturally occurring, table, **01:** 111-166

Molecular map
  Escherichia coli bacteriophage lambda (λ), **04:** 678

Molecular weight
  amino acids, naturally occurring, table, **01:** 111-166
  antibiotics, nucleoside, **03:** 271-393
  ascorbic acid and ascorbate-2-sulfate, **08:** 281
  blood coagulation proteins, table of values, **02:** 255
  chromosome, circular chloroplast, **04:** 359-360
  compounds of biological interest, **08:** 144-195
  contractile proteins, table of values, **02:** 306
  deoxynucleotide polymerizing enzymes, tables of values, **04:** 538-540
  enzymes found in normal human urine, table, **02:** 301
  fatty acids, **05:** 484-490
  glycoproteins
    plasma, human, table of values, **02:** 258
  histones, table for several, **02:** 294
  lectins, purified, table of values, **02:** 546-551
  linseed oil acids and esters, **05:** 497
  β_2 microglobulin, **02:** 305
  mucopolysaccharides, **05:** 356-357
  myosins, nonmuscle, table of values, **02:** 317
  nonmuscle actin, of monomer, **02:** 314-315
  nucleosides, index to table of values, **03:** 69-72
  nucleotides, index to table of values, **03:** 72-75
  polysaccharides, table of values, **02:** 686-687
  prostaglandin analogs, **08:** 397-421
  prostaglandin biosynthesis intermediates, thromboxanes and by-products, **08:** 334-340
  prostaglandin metabolites, **08:** 368-391
  prostaglandin metabolizing enzymes, **08:** 364-367
  prostaglandin precursors, **08:** 325
  prostaglandins, naturally occurring, **08:** 346-358
  proteinase inhibitors
    animal sources, **02:** 618-641
    microbial sources, **02:** 661-662
    plant sources, **02:** 586-600
  proteins
    carbohydrate, index to studies containing, **02:** 232
    fibrous, index to studies containing, **02:** 229
    globular, index to studies containing, **02:** 222-228
    human plasma, table of values, **02:** 242-250
    organelles, index to studies containing, **02:** 232
    particles, index to studies containing, **02:** 222-228
    subunits of, table, **02:** 326-351
    table of values, **02:** 326-351
    virus, index to studies containing, **02:** 232
  purines, index to table of values, **03:** 67-69
  pyridoxine, pyridoxal and pyridoxamine derivatives, **08:** 252-266

Molecular weight *(continued)*

pyrimides, index to table of values, **03:** 67-69

retinol-binding protein, **02:** 304

ribonucleotide polymerizing enzymes and subunits of, **04:** 550-553

Escherichia coli ribosomal proteins 30 S, **04:** 482-486

ribosomes from various sources, **04:** 472

RNA molecules, tables for several, **04:** 406-408

steroids, table, **05:** 531-588

Tamm-Horsfall mucoprotein, **02:** 304

transamidases, purified, **02:** 681

tropomyosin from nonmuscle cells, of subunits, **02:** 321

α,β-unsaturated amino acids, structure and properties, table, **01:** 175

urokinase, **02:** 302

viral DNA molecules,, **03:** 551-556

vitamins, table of data, **08:** 284-300

Molecular weights

acids, commercial strength, **06:** 384

bases, commercial strength, **06:** 384

macromolecules, values for several, **06:** 270-293

oxidation and reduction reagents, **06:** 352

Mollusca

deoxyribonucleic acids from, purine and pyrimidine distribution in, **04:** 265

DNA content per cell, **04:** 291

Molluscs, satellite DNAs; buoyant density and G + C content of, table, **04:** 387

Molybdenum-iron protein

average hydrophobicity value, **01:** 227

Molybdoproteins

nomenclature rules, **02:** 121

Monellin

average hydrophobicity value, **01:** 227

molar absorptivity and-or absorbance values, **02:** 472

Monkey

deoxynucleotide polymerizing enzymes from, properties of, **04:** 539-544

mitochondrial DNA from, properties, **04:** 371

Monoamine oxidase

amino acid composition, complete data, **07:** 509

carbohydrate content, **02:** 273, 274

molar absorptivity and-or absorbance values, **02:** 473

subunit, constitution of, **02:** 335, 345, 350

table of cofactors, molecular weights, stoichiometry, and sources, **02:** 282

L-Monoamino, dicarboxylic acids

physical and chemical properties, **01:** 116-119

L-Monoamino, monocarboxylic acids

physical and chemical properties, **01:** 112-115

3-Monobromo-5-monochlorotyrosine

physical and chemical properties, **01:** 160

3-Monobromotyrosine

physical and chemical properties, **01:** 160

Monochlorotyrosine

physical and chemical properties, **01:** 160

Monocotyledons; buoyant density and G + C content of satellite DNAs for several species, table, **04:** 402

Monocytes

immunological response, **07:** 538

Monodus

G + C composition of DNA of, table arranged by specie, **04:** 226

2-Monoiodohistidine

physical and chemical properties, **01:** 160

Monoiodotyrosine

physical and chemical properties, **01:** 160

Monomolecular film measurements

linseed oil acids and esters, force-area data, **05:** 497

Mononucleotides

chemical shifts, **03:** 530

coupling constants (Hz) of the H1′ and H2′ protons, **03:** 530

ultraviolet absorbance, **03:** 405-406

ultraviolet absorbance, in 7 M urea, **03:** 407

ultraviolet absorbance in 97% D_2O, **03:** 408

ultraviolet absorbance in 90% v-v ethylene glycol, **03:** 408

Monophenol monooxygenase

amino acid composition, complete data, **07:** 511

circular dichroism in the UV region, **07:** 113

Monophosphates

dinucleoside

mean residue absorptivities, table of values, **03:** 597

molar residue ellipticities, table of values, **03:** 600

molar residue rotations, table of values, **03:** 598

2,3-Monophosphates, nucleoside

molar absorptivity, table of values, **03:** 597

Monosaccharides

anhydrides, nomenclature rules, **05:** 130-132

circular dichroism, table, **05:** 465-468

dimensions, average, of a unit, **05:** 472

electronic charge distribution, **05:** 474-477

nomenclature rules for some, **05:** 102-105, 109-112

optical rotatory dispersion, table, **05:** 459-462

Monosporium

G + C composition of DNA of, table arranged by specie, **04:** 206

Moraxella

G + C composition of DNA of, table arranged by specie, **04:** 92

Moroyamycin, structure, **03:** 331

Morphine

pK'_a values, **06:** 327

Morphogenetic markers, *see also* Genetic markers

Bacillus subtilis, **04:** 699-701

Mortierella

G + C composition of DNA of, table arranged by specie, **04:** 207

Motilin

average hydrophobicity value, **01:** 227

Mouse

buoyant density and G + C content of satellite DNAs for several varieties, table, **04:** 391-393

deoxynucleotide polymerizing enzymes from, properties of, **04:** 539-544

deoxyribonucleic acids from, purine and pyrimidine distribution in, **04:** 270

DNA content per cell, **04:** 302

gene symbol, **04:** 857-870

genetic markers, **04:** 857-870

inbred strain availability, **04:** 884

Mouse *(continued)*
   linkage map, **04:** 856
   major histocompatibility complex, values of, **04:** 886-887
   MHC designation, **04:** 885
   mitochondrial DNA from, properties, **04:** 371
   nearest neighbor frequencies in DNA from various parts of, **04:** 317
   phenotypic expression, **04:** 857-870
   RNA from, natural occurrence of the modified nucleosides in, **03:** 217-232
MSD-125 A, *see* Showdomycin
MSE rotors, construction data for isokinetic sucrose and glycerol gradients, **06:** 489-518
Mucin (major)
   amino acid composition, incomplete data, **07:** 513
Muconolactone isomerase
   average hydrophobicity value, **01:** 227
Mucopolysaccharides
   occurrence, repeating unit and physical data, **05:** 356-357
   table of data and characteristics, **02:** 686-687
Mucoprotein
   Tamm-Horsfall, *see also* Tamm-Horsfall mucoprotein
   Tamm-Horsfall, properties of, **02:** 304
Mucoprotein, Tamm-Horsfall
   amino acid composition, complete data, **07:** 510
Mucor
   G + C composition of DNA of, table arranged by specie, **04:** 207
Multhiomycin; origin, structure, and characteristic as protein biosynthesis inhibitor, **04:** 586
Multienzyme complex in tryptophan pathway
   amino acid composition, complete data, **07:** 509
Muramidase, *see* Lysozyme
Muscazone
   physical and chemical properties, **01:** 145
Muscle contractile proteins
   amino acid sequence, **07:** 490-496
Mutagenesis, causes of, proposed hydrogen-bonding schemes, **04:** 895
Mutagens, chemical
   alkylating, classes of, table, **04:** 891-892
   properties of selected, table, **04:** 888-889
Mutants, biochemical
   Coprinus radiatus
      loci, number of alleles, precursors, characteristics, **04:** 763-764
      map, **04:** 762
   Drosophila melanogaster, list, **04:** 848-855
Mutants, located, *Aspergillus nidulans*, **04:** 732-737
Mutarotase
   average hydrophobicity value, **01:** 227
Mutase
   definition and nomenclature, **02:** 98
Mutations
   classification of, table, **04:** 893
   point, effect of, on coding, **04:** 894
Mycobacteriaceae
   G + C composition of DNA of, table arranged by genera and specie, **04:** 139-141
Mycobacterium
   amino acid requirements for growth, table, **04:** 636

G + C composition of DNA of, table arranged by specie, **04:** 139-141
Mycoplana
   amino acid requirements for growth, table, **04:** 636
Mycoplasma
   amino acid requirements for growth, table, **04:** 636
   G + C composition of DNA of, table arranged by specie, **04:** 141-145
Mycoplasma membrane, *see* Membrane, protein, mycoplasma
Mycoplasmataceae
   G + C composition of DNA of, table arranged by genera and specie, **04:** 141
Mycotypha
   G + C composition of DNA of, table arranged by specie, **04:** 208
Myelin protein
   circular dichroism in the UV region, **07:** 113
   optical rotatory dispersion in the visible and near UV regions, **07:** 31
Myeloma protein, *see* Immunoglobulin
Myeloperoxidase
   amino acid composition, complete data, **07:** 509
   molar absorptivity and-or absorbance values, **02:** 473
Myoglobin
   amino acid sequence, **07:** 437-440
   calorimetric ΔH values accompanying conformational changes, **06:** 270
   circular dichroism
      UV and near-UV region, **07:** 113, 157
   conformation for sperm whale, **02:** 760
   cyanogen bromide cleavage, **02:** 199
   molar absorptivity and-or absorbance values, **02:** 476-479
   optical rotatory dispersion
      UV region, **07:** 67
      visible and near UV regions, **07:** 31
   oxidation-reduction potentials of, **06:** 137-139
   sperm whale
      heat of proton ionization, pK, and related thermodynamic quantities, **06:** 220
   viscosity, intrinsic, **02:** 721
Myoglobin, average hydrophobicity value, **01:** 227
Myoglobin, met (ferri)-
   optical rotatory dispersion in the UV region: extrema between 185 and 250 NM^3, **07:** 67
Myoglobin, metcyano-
   circular dichroism in the UV region: extrema between 185 and 250 NM^3, **07:** 114
Myoglobin, vertebrate
   amino acid sequence, **07:** 437-440
Myohemerythrin, average hydrophobicity value, **01:** 227
Myokinase, *see* Adenylate, kinase
Myosin
   amino acid composition, complete data, **07:** 509
   amino acid sequence, **07:** 493
   average hydrophobicity value, **01:** 227
   circular dichroism in the UV region, **07:** 115
   identification of, in nonmuscle cells, table, **02:** 307-313
   interaction of nonmuscle actin with, **02:** 316
   molar absorptivity and-or absorbance values, **02:** 481
   molecular parameters, **02:** 306

Myosin *(continued)*
  nonmuscle
    enzymatic activity of, **02:** 319
    filament data for several, **02:** 318
    interaction with action, **02:** 320
    physical properties for several, **02:** 317
  optical rotatory dispersion, **07:** 62
    UV region, **07:** 68
    visible and near UV regions, **07:** 31
  rabbit
    luminescence of, table, **01:** 206
  refractive index increments, **02:** 379
  viscosity, intrinsic, **02:** 721
Myosin, HMM
  circular dichroism in the UV region, **07:** 115
  optical rotatory dispersion
    UV region, **07:** 68
    visible and near UV regions, **07:** 31
Myosin, HMM (S-1)
  circular dichroism in the UV region, **07:** 115
Myosin, light chain
  circular dichroism in the UV region, **07:** 115
Myosin, LMM
  circular dichroism in the UV region, **07:** 115
  optical rotatory dispersion
    UV region, **07:** 68
    visible and near UV regions, **07:** 31
Myosin A
  cyanogen bromide cleavage, **02:** 199
Myosmine
  pK'_a values, **06:** 327
Myrothecium
  G + C composition of DNA of, table arranged by spe-
    cie, **04:** 208
Myxobacterium
  G + C composition of DNA of, table arranged by spe-
    cies, **04:** 146
Myxococcaceae
  G + C composition of DNA of, table arranged by gen-
    era and specie, **04:** 145
Myxococcus (Myxobacterium)
  amino acid requirements for growth, table, **04:** 636
  G + C composition of DNA of, table arranged by spe-
    cie, **04:** 146
Myxotrichum
  G + C composition of DNA of, table arranged by spe-
    cie, **04:** 208
Myxovirus hemagglutination inhibitor
  amino acid composition, incomplete data, **07:** 513

N

NAD
  UV spectra, formula, molecular weight, **08:** 167
NADH$_2$ disodium salt
  UV spectra, formula, molecular weight, **08:** 168
NADP-Glutamate dehydrogenase
  Neurospora crassa mutant, **04:** 751
NAD(P)$^+$ transhydrogenase
  circular dichroism in the UV region, **07:** 115
  optical rotatory dispersion in the UV region, **07:** 68

Naegleria
  G + C composition of DNA of, table arranged by spe-
    cie, **04:** 229
Naganishia
  G + C composition of DNA of, table arranged by spe-
    cie, **04:** 208
N-α-Nalonyl-D-alanine
  physical and chemical properties, **01:** 165
Naphthalene derivatives
  heat of proton ionization, pK, and related thermody-
    namic quantities, **06:** 221-223
Naphthalene sulfonates
  fluorescent probes of protein structure, **07:** 604-606
Naphthylacrylic acid
  antagonism to tryptophan, **01:** 179
β-(1-Naphthyl)alanine
  structure and symbols for those incorporated into syn-
    thetic polypeptides, **01:** 105
β-(2-Naphthyl)alanine
  structure and symbols for those incorporated into syn-
    thetic polypeptides, **01:** 105
Naphthylalanines
  antagonism to tryptophan, **01:** 179
Naramycin® B; origin, structure, and characteristic as
    protein biosynthesis inhibitor, **04:** 586
Nariterashin, physicochemical constants, spectral, chemo-
    therapeutic and biological properties, **03:** 332
Naritheracin, physicochemical constants, spectral, chemo-
    therapeutic and biological properties , **03:** 332
Navicula
  G + C composition of DNA of, table arranged by spe-
    cie, **04:** 226
Near-UV region
  circular dichroism for native proteins at maxima, at
    room temperature, table, **07:** 143-163
Nearest neighbor frequencies
  deoxyribonucleic acids from diverse sources, **04:**
    312-318
Nebrancyin, *see* Tobramycin
N-(Nebularin-6-ylcarbamoyl)glycine
  physical constants and spectral properties, **03:** 103
N-(Nebularin-6-ylcarbamoyl)threonine
  physical constants and spectral properties, **03:** 103
Nebularine
  physical and spectral properties, **03:** 122
  physicochemical constants, spectral, chemotherapeutic
    and biological properties, **03:** 334
Neisseria
  amino acid requirements for growth, table, **04:** 637
  G + C composition of DNA of, table arranged by spe-
    cie, **04:** 147-148
Neisseriaceae
  G + C composition of DNA of, table arranged by gen-
    era and specie, **04:** 147-148
Nematoda
  DNA content per cell, **04:** 291
Neocarzinostatin
  circular dichroism in the UV region, **07:** 115
  optical rotatory dispersion in the UV region, **07:** 68
Neocarzinostatin, average hydrophobicity value, **01:** 227
Neoglucobrassicin
  physical and chemical properties, **01:** 157

Neomycin A, B, and C; origin, structure, and characteristic as protein biosynthesis inhibitor, **04:** 587

Neospiramycin; origin, structure, and characteristic as protein biosynthesis inhibitor, **04:** 588

Nerve growth factor
molar absorptivity and-or absorbance values, **02:** 482
subunit, constitution of, **02:** 326

Nerve growth factor fraction A
amino acid composition, incomplete data, **07:** 513

Neuraminic acid, generic term usage, **05:** 10

Neurohypophysial hormones, *see* Hormones, neurohypophysial

Neurophysin
circular dichroism in near-UV region, at room temperature, **07:** 158

Neurophysin I, II, III, average hydrophobicity values, **01:** 227

Neurospora
G + C composition of DNA of, table arranged by specie, **04:** 208
RNA from, natural occurrence of the modified nucleosides in, **03:** 217-232

Neurospora crassa
deoxyribonucleic acids from, purine and pyrimidine distribution in, **04:** 242
DNA base composition, **04:** 239
G + C composition, **04:** 208
genetic symbol, **04:** 740-757
glycohydrolase from, enzymatic reaction, parameters, **05:** 437
linkage maps, **04:** 739-757
mitochondrial DNA, properties of, **04:** 368
mitochondrial nuclease, functional characteristics, **04:** 518
nuclease, functional characteristics, **04:** 518
phenotypic expression, **04;** 740-757
ribonuclease from, functional characteristics, **04:** 513-514

Neurotoxin, *see also* Toxin
molar absorptivity and-or absorbance values, **02:** 482

Neurotoxin α
amino acid composition, complete data, **07:** 509
amino acid sequence, **07:** 499

Neurotoxin I
optical rotatory dispersion in the UV region, **07:** 68

Neurotoxin I, II, III, IV, V
average hydrophobicity values, **01:** 227,228

Neurotoxin II
amino acid composition, complete data, **07:** 509
circular dichroism in the UV region, **07:** 115
optical rotatory dispersion in the UV region, **07:** 68

Neurotoxin III
optical rotatory dispersion in the UV region, **07:** 68

Neurotoxins, long
amino acid sequences, **07:** 366-369
from venom of various snakes, **07:** 366-369

Neurotoxins, short
amino acid sequence, **07:** 360-365
from venom of various snakes, **07:** 360-365

Neutral proteinase, *see* Microbial metalloenzyme

Neutralization value, fatty acids, **05:** 485-491

Newman projection formula, description, **01:** 46-47, **02:** 46-47, **04:** 38-39, **05:** 43-44, **06:** 45, **08:** 45-46

α-NH$_2$-n-Butyric acid
free acid in blood plasma of newborn infants and adults, **01:** 328

Niacin
nomenclature, preferred usage, **08:** 19
properties of, **08:** 296

Nicotianamine
physical and chemical properties, **01:** 145

Nicotianine
physical and chemical properties, **01:** 163

Nicotinamide, properties of, **08:** 296

β-Nicotinamide adenine dinucleotide
UV spectra, formula, molecular weight, **08:** 167

Nicotinamide deamidase
amino acid composition, complete data, **07:** 509

Nicotine
pK'_a values, **06:** 327

Nicotinic acid
biological characteristics, **08:** 303
properties of, **08:** 296

Niddamycin; origin, structure, and characteristic as protein biosynthesis inhibitor, **04:** 588

Nigrospora
G + C composition of DNA of, table arranged by specie, **04:** 209

Ninhydrin positive compounds, elution behavior, **08:** 122

Ninhydrin positive constituents
urine, resolution of, by ion exchange chromatography, **08:** 114-119

Ninhydrin reaction
amino acids, absorption ratios and product color constants, **08:** 123-124

Ninhydrin reactive substances, chromatographic positions, **08:** 126

Niromycin A and B; origin of protein biosynthesis inhibitor, **04:** 588

Nitella
G + C composition of DNA of, table arranged by specie, **04:** 226

Nitrate reductase
cofactors, molecular weights, stoichiometry and sources, **02:** 285
molar absorptivity and-or absorbance values, **02:** 484
Neurospora crassa mutant, **04:** 740, 749, 750
subunit, constitution of, **02:** 349

Nitric acid
heat of proton ionization, pK, and related thermodynamic quantities, **06:** 223

Nitrobacter
G + C composition of DNA of, table arranged by specie, **04:** 148

Nitrobacteraceae
G + C composition of DNA of, table arranged by genera and specie, **04:** 148

Nitrogen compounds, pK'_a values, **06:** 322-345

Nitrogenase
circular dichroism in the UV region, **07:** 116
molar absorptivity and-or absorbance values, **02:** 484
subunit, constitution of, **02:** 344, 345

Nitroguanidinoacetyl
structure and symbols for those incorporated into synthetic polypeptides, **01:** 105
p-Nitrophenylalanine
antagonism to phenylalanine, **01:** 179
Nitrosomonas
G + C composition of DNA of, table arranged by specie, **04:** 148
m-Nitrotyrosine
antagonism to tyrosine, **01:** 180
Nitrous acid
heat of proton ionization, pK, and related thermodynamic quantities, **06:** 224
Nitzschia
G + C composition of DNA of, table arranged by specie, **04:** 226
Nivalenol; origin, structure, and characteristic as protein biosynthesis inhibitor, **04:** 589
NMR spectra
hydrogen in organic structures, characteristic positions, **08:** 247
methyl l0,12-octadecadienoate, **05:** 498
methyl linoleate, **05:** 498
methyl linoleate in carbon tetrachloride solution, **05:** 511
methyl oleate, **05:** 498
steroids table, **05:** 531-588
Nocardia
G + C composition of DNA of, table arranged by specie, **04:** 149-150
Nocardiaceae
G + C composition of DNA of, table arranged by genera and specie, **04:** 149-150
Nodularia
G + C composition of DNA of, table arranged by specie, **04:** 226
Nomenclature
abbreviations, use of, **03:** 6, 7
amino acid derivatives, symbols for, rules, **01:** 79-88
amino acid sequences, one-letter symbols, rules, **01:** 75-78, **02:** 59-62
amino acids, synthetic, structure and symbols for those incorporated into synthetic polypeptides, **01:** 96
biochemical
abbreviations, use of, **01:** 6,7, **08:** 6-7
list of rules and recommendations affecting, **04:** 3-4
locations of rules in the literature, **04:** 5
rules, location in the literature, **08:** 5
rules, location of in literature, **01:** 5
rules and recommendations, list, **08:** 3-4
rules and recommendations affecting, list of, **01:** 3-4
use of abbreviations in, **04:** 6,7
use of symbols in, **04:** 7-12
biochemical, list of rules and recommendations affecting, **02:** 3-4, **05:** 3-4, **06:** 3
biochemical, location of rules in the literature, **02:** 5, **06:** 3
biochemical, locations of rules in the literature, **05:** 5
biochemical, use of abbreviations, **06:** 6
biochemical, use of abbreviations in, **02:** 6-7, **05:** 6, 7
biochemical, use of symbols in, **05:** 7-9, 12
blood coagulation factors, **02:** 195

carbohydrate, references for rules, **02:** 87
carbohydrates, IUPAC tentative rules for, **05:** 100-136
carotenoids, IUPAC rules, **06:** 63-90, **08:** 63-90
CBN recommendations, bibliographic citations for, **03:** 5
coenzymes, references for rules, **02:** 87
coenzymes, trivial names and preferred usages, **08:** 8-19
conformational map, typical, **01:** 67, **02:** 71
corrinoids, **08:** 12-17
corrinoids, references for rules, **02:** 87
cyclitols, IUPAC recommendations, **05:** 89-98
cyclitols, references for rules, **02:** 87
cytochromes, **02:** 116-120
electron-transfer proteins, **02:** 114-121
enzymes, multiple forms of, **02:** 84-86
enzymes, names, list of recommended and systematic, **02:** 121-172
enzymes, recommendations, **02:** 91-172
enzymes genetically variant, **02:** 86
equilibrium data, terminology and units, **06:** 99-106
folic acid, references for rules, **02:** 87
glycolipids, table of, **05:** 416-423
immunoglobulins, genetic factors, **02:** 186
immunoglobulins, human, recommendations for, **02:** 173-174, 179-195
iron-sulfur proteins, recommendations, **02:** 89-90, 120
isotopically labeled compounds, CEBJ rules for, **01:** 16, **02:** 16, **03:** 58, **04:** 58, **06:** 62, **08:** 62
isotopically labeled compounds, CEBS rules, **05:** 13
IUPAC tentative rules for fundamental stereochemistry, **03:** 13-50
LASS, suggested use of term in prostaglandin studies, **08:** 314
lipids
list of generic terms, **05:** 9-10
stereospecific, use of, **05:** 10
use of trivial names, **05:** 9-12
lipids, references for rules, **02:** 87
peptide hormones, recommendations, **02:** 175-178
peptides
prepared by solid phase peptide synthesis, table of, **01:** 374-390
symbols for, rules, **01:** 88-90
peptides, natural, rules for naming synthetic modifications of, **02:** 79-83
polypeptide chains, rules for abbreviations and symbols,, **01:** 59-73, **02:** 63-77
polypeptides, synthetic, abbreviated style, rules, **01:** 91-95
porphyrins, **08:** 268-269
prostaglandin biosynthesis intermediates, thromboxanes and by-products, **08:** 334-340
prostaglandins, naturally occurring, **08:** 346-358
prostaglandins and precursors, **08:** 313-316
purines and pyrimidines, numbering schemes, **08:** 224
pyrimidine photoproducts, proposals for abbreviations, **03:** 51-57
quinones, references for rules, **02:** 87
RCS, suggested use of term in prostaglandin studies, **08:** 314
rules and recommendations affecting, list, **03:** 3, 4

Nomenclature *(continued)*
  sequence-rule procedure in fundamental stereochemistry, **02:** 50-58, **03:** 42-50, **04:** 42-50, **05:** 47-55, **06:** 49, **08:** 49-57
  sequence-rule procedure in fundamental stereochemistry, **01:** 50-58
  sequence rule, use of, **01:** 61-63, **02:** 65-67
  stereochemistry, fundamental, IUPAČ rules, **06:** 20, **08:** 20-57
  stereochemistry, fundamental, IUPAC rules for, **05:** 18-55
  stereochemistry, fundamental, IUPAC rules for nomenclature, **01:** 21-58, **02:** 21-58, **04:** 13-50
  steroids, IUPAC definitive rules for, **05:** 56-88
  steroids, references for rules, **02:** 87
  symbols, use of, **03:** 7-12
  abeo system, usage for steroids, **05:** 81-83
  torsion angle, choice of, **01:** 62-63, **02:** 66-67
  vitamins, references for rules, **02:** 87
  vitamins, trivial names and preferred usages, **08:** 8-19
Non-human primates
  satellite DNAs
    buoyant density and G + C content of, table, **04:** 398-399
Nonmuscle actins
  interaction of, with myosin, **02:** 316
  physical and chemical properties of, **02:** 314-315
Nonmuscle cells
  proteins in identification of several, **02:** 307-313
  tropomyosin from, properties of, **02:** 361
Nonmuscle myosins
  enzymatic activity of, **02:** data table 319
  filaments of, **02:** data table 318
  interaction with actin, **02:** data table 320
  physical properties of, **02:** 317
Nonsaponifiables
  herring oils and Pacific pilchard oil, **05:** 523-524
N-Nor-amicetin, *see* Bamicetin
Norleucine
  antagonism to leucine, **01:** 178
  antagonism to methionine, **01:** 178
  structure and symbols for those incorporated into synthetic polypeptides, **01:** 105
Norvaline
  antagonism to leucine, **01:** 178
  antagonism to valine, **01:** 180
  pK'_a values, **06:** 319
  structure and symbols for those incorporated into synthetic polypeptides, **01:** 105
Noryl, chemical and physical properties, **08:** 427
Nostoc
  G + C composition of DNA of, table arranged by specie, **04:** 226
Novobiocin
  UV spectra, formula, molecular weight, **08:** 183
Nuclear magnetic resonance spectra, *see* NMR spectra
Nuclease
  amino acid composition, complete data, **07:** 509
  average hydrophobicity value, **01:** 227
  cyanogen bromide cleavage, **02:** 199
  molar absorptivity and-or absorbance values, **02:** 485

optical rotatory dispersion
  UV region, **07:** 69
  visible and near UV regions, **07:** 32
Nuclease-T
  amino acid sequences of protein, **07:** 310
Nuclease (extracellular)
  circular dichroism at maxima in near-UV region, at room temperature, **07:** 158
Nucleases
  nonspecific for the sugar moiety, functional characteristics, **04:** 518-523
Nuclei
  enzymatic activity, subcellular fraction, **02:** 698-700
Nucleic acids, *see also* DNA, RNA
  abbreviations, use of, **08:** 7
  abbreviations for, use of, **01:** 7, **02:** 7, **04:** 7, **05:** 7, **06:** 7
  chloroplast, quantitative data tables, **04:** 356-362
  fluorescent dyes bound to, data tables, **04:** 470
Nucleocidin, physicochemical constants, spectral, chemotherapeutic and biological properties, **03:** 336
Nucleocidin; origin, structure, and characteristic as protein biosynthesis inhibitor, **04:** 589
Nucleoli
  enzymatic activity for several, table, **02:** 701
Nucleophosphodi esterases, functional characterization of, **04:** 491
Nucleoproteins
  circular dichroic spectra, graph, **06:** 393
Nucleoside 2,3-monophosphates
  molar absorptivity, table of values, **03:** 597
Nucleoside antibiotics, *see also* Antibiotics, nucleoside
  physicochemical constants, spectral, chemotherapeutic and biological properties, **03:** 271-393
Nucleoside diphosphokinase
  average hydrophobicity value, **01:** 228
  subunit, constitution of, **02:** 333, 336
Nucleoside phosphorothioates, symbols for, use of, **03:** 12, **04:** 12
Nucleoside phosphorylase
  optical rotatory dispersion
    UV region, **07:** 69
    visible and near UV regions, **07:** 32
Nucleoside phosphotransferase-A-chain
  average hydrophobicity value, **01:** 228
Nucleoside phosphotransferase-B-chain
  average hydrophobicity value, **01:** 228
Nucleosides
  dissociation constants, acidic, **03:** 409-416
  osmometry coefficients, vapor phase, **03:** 528-529
  pK'_a values, **06:** 330-331
  physical constants and spectral properties, **03:** 69-72
  proton chemical shifts, **03:** 530-533
  symbols for, use of, **03:** 8, **04:** 8
  tRNA, content in, tables of values, **04:** 428-441
  tRNA secondary structure; identification, location, distribution, **04:** 427
  UV spectra of some, including their alkyl derivatives, **03:** 420-447
  UV spectral characteristics, **03:** 409-416
Nucleosides, modified
  isolation and detection of, in RNA, general remarks about several compounds, **03:** 233-246

Nucleosides, modified *(continued)*

RNA, natural occurrence in, tables, **03:** 216-233

5′-Nucleotidase

amino acid composition, incomplete data, **07:** 513

average hydrophobicity value, **01:** 228

Nucleotide

abbreviations for, use of, **04:** 6

composition in high molecular weight ribosomal RNA, **04:** 409

composition in viral RNA, **04:** 410

sequence data

phenylanine transfer RNA, **04:** 458

ribosomal RNA, **04:** 473

transfer RNA, tables, **04:** 442-453

sequences and models for several RNAs and DNAs, **04:** 324-353

Nucleotides

abbreviations, use of, **08:** 6

abbreviations for, use of, **01:** 6, **02:** 6, **03:** 6, **05:** 6, **06:** 6

dissociation constants, acidic, **03:** 409-416

molar residue ellipticity, table of values, **03:** 601

molar residue rotation, table of values, **03:** 599

pK'_a values, **06:** 330-331

physical constants and spectral properties, index to, **03:** 72-75

sugar, isolation and enzymatic synthesis of, **05:** 446-452

UV spectral characteristics, **03:** 409-416

Nutrition

animal requirements of vitamins, **08:** 305-308

animals, laboratory, levels of nutrients to meet requirements, **08:** 251

human, recommended daily dietary allowances, **08:** 248-249,310

Nystatin

UV spectra, formula, molecular weight, **08:** 185

O

Ochromonas

amino acid requirements for growth, table, **04:** 642

G + C composition of DNA of, table arranged by specie, **04:** 226

Octadecadienoates, methyl, equivalent chain lengths, **05:** 505

Octadecatrienoate, methyl, equivalent chain lengths, **05:** 505

Octasaccharides

chemical formula, **05:** 319, 346

derivatives, **05:** 319, 346

melting point, **05:** 319, 346

specific rotation, **05:** 319, 346

synonyms, **05:** 319, 346

D-Octopine

physical and chemical properties, **01:** 166

Octopine dehydrogenase

circular dichroism in the UV region, **07:** 116

optical rotatory dispersion

UV region, **07:** 69

visible and near UV regions, **07:** 32

Octosyl acids A, B and C as nucleoside antibiotics, **03:** 337

Oerskovia

G + C composition of DNA of, table arranged by specie, **04:** 75-76

Oils

density of, **05:** 502-503

fatty acid content of, **05:** 502-503

herring, properties, *see* Herring oil

iodine value of, **05:** 502-503

melting points of, **05:** 502-503

pilchard oil, Pacific, *see* Pilchard oil, Pacific

refractive index of, **05:** 502-503

saponification value of, **05:** 502-503

solidification points of, **05:** 502-503

specific gravity of, **05:** 502-503

vegetable, unsaponifiables content, **05:** 512

Old yellow enzyme

amino acid composition, incomplete data, **07:** 513

Oleandomycin; origin, structure, and characteristic of protein biosynthesis inhibitor, **04:** 590

Oligonucleotide digests, guide for producing, **03:** 404

Oligonucleotides

chemical shifts of dinucleoside monophosphates and dinucleotides, **03:** 531-532

coupling constants of dinucleoside monophosphates and dinucleotides, **03:** 531-532

DNA, circular dichroism parameters, **03:** 465-468

DNA, optical rotatory dispersion parameters, **03:** 459-460

extinction coefficients for single-strand types, formula for calculating, **03:** 589

hyperchromicity ratios at different wavelengths, **03:** 406-407

RNA, circular dichroism parameters, **03:** 461-465

RNA, optical rotatory dispersion parameters, **03:** 450-458

ultraviolet absorbance, **03:** 405-406

ultraviolet absorbance of, with 2′O-methylpentose residue content, **03:** 448-449

Oligopeptides, natural, and related synthetic amino acid sequence, physical and biological properties

bradykinin group, **07:** 222-235

eledoisin group, **07:** 236-257

kallidin group, **07:** 222-235

oxytocins, **07:** 192-220

physaleamin group, **07:** 258-260

vasopressins, **07:** 192-220

Oligoribonucleotides

circular dichroism extrema and crossovers for 15 double-helical, **03:** 595

Oligosaccharides

chemical formula, **05:** 283-319, 327-346

circular dichroism, table, **05:** 465-468

derivatives, **05:** 283-319, 327-346

melting point, **05:** 283-319, 327-346

nomenclature rules, **05:** 133-136

optical rotatory dispersion, table, **05:** 459-462

specific rotation, **05:** 283-319, 327-346

synonyms, **05:** 283-319, 327-346

One-letter symbols

amino-acid sequences, journal references, **02:** 87

amino acid sequences, tentative rules, **01:** 75-78, **02:** 59-62

One-letter symbols *(continued)*
    amino acids, table of, **01:** 78, **02:** 62
    purines, pyrimidines, nucleosides, and nucleotides index
        to table, **03:** 67-75
    use of, in nomenclature, **01:** 8, 15, **03:** 8, **04:** 8
    use of in nomenclature, **02:** 8, 15
Ophiobolus
    amino acid requirements for growth, table, **04:** 641
Optical instruments
    calibration techniques, **06:** 390-392
Optical measurements, determination of path length of
        cells used in, **06:** 391
Optical parameters
    polyribonucleotides, calculation of, **03:** 596
Optical properties
    absorption and circular dichroism spectra, nucleic acids,
        03: 589-595
Optical rotation
    amino acids, naturally occurring, table, **01:** 111-116
    antibiotics, nucleoside, **03:** 271-393
Optical rotatory dispersion
    mono- and oligosaccharides, table, **05:** 459-462
    polyribonucleotides, use of tables in calculation of, **03:**
        596
    polysaccharides, table, **05:** 463-464
    water, calculations of the refractive index, **06:** 385
Optical rotatory dispersion (ORD)
    definition and formula, **07:** 3-4
    references, table 2, **07:** 39-43
    references, table 3, **07:** 79-81
    spectra of various proteins, **07:** 8-11
    UV region: extrema between 185 and 250 NM, table,
        07: 44-78
    visible and near UV regions: table, **07:** 15-38
Optical rotatory dispersion parameters
    oligonucleotides of RNA, **03:** 450-458
    oligonucleotides ofDNA, **03:** 459-460
ORD, *see* Optical rotatory dispersion
Organelles, protein
    physical-chemical data for, index to ultracentrifuge
        studies, **02:** 232
Organic acid metabolism, errors of, table, **01:** 326
Ornithine
    antagonism to arginine, **01:** 177
    antagonists of, **01:** 178
    free acid in amniotic fluid in early pregnancy and at
        term, **01:** 327
    free acid in blood plasma of newborn infants and
        adults, **01:** 328
    ornithinemia type I, effect of, **01:** 320
    ornithinemia type II, effect of, **01:** 320
    physical and chemical properties, **01:** 121
    specific rotatory dispersion constants, 0.1 *M* solution,
        01: 244
    thumbprint, content in, **08:** 121
Ornithine aminotransferase
    amino acid composition, complete data, **07:** 509
Ornithine betaine, *see* Miokinine
Ornithine transcarbamylase
    average hydrophobicity value, **01:** 228
    molar absorptivity and-or absorbance values, **02:** 485
    Neurospora crassa mutant, **04:** 745

    subunit, constitution of, **02:** 334
Ornithinemia type I, characteristics of, **01:** 320
Ornithinemia type II, characteristics of, **01:** 320
Orosomucoid
    molar absorptivity and-or absorbance values, **02:** 485
    molecular parameters, **02:** 242
Orotic acid
    physical constants and spectral properties, **03:** 93
Orotidine
    physical constants and spectral properties, **03:** 134
Orotidine 5'-phosphate
    physical constants and spectral properties, **03:** 195
Osmometry coefficients, vapor phase
    nucleic acid bases and nucleosides, **03:** 528-529
Ostreogrycin A, B, B$_1$, B$_2$, B$_3$, *see also* PA 114A, Sta-
        phylomycin M$_1$, Virginiamycin M$_1$; origin, struc-
        ture, and characteristic as protein biosynthesis in-
        hibitor, **04:** 590-592
Ovalbumin
    average hydrophobicity value, **01:** 228
    calorimetric ΔH values accompanying conformational
        changes, **06:** 274
    carbohydrate content, **02:** 268
    circular dichroism
        UV and near-UV region, at room temperature, **07:**
        116, 158
    enzymatic hydrolysis, conjugated proteins, **02:** 211
    luminescence of, table, **01:** 206
    molar absorptivity and-or absorbance values, **02:** 485
    optical rotatory dispersion
        UV region, **07:** 69
        visible and near UV regions, **07:** 32
    refractive index increments, **02:** 379
Ovalbumin A$_1$
    viscosity, intrinsic, **02:** 721
Ovoglycoprotein
    carbohydrate content, **02:** 268
    molar absorptivity and-or absorbance values, **02:** 486
Ovoinhibitor
    amino acid composition, incomplete data, **07:** 513
    bird egg whites, specificities and properties, **02:** 628-629
    carbohydrate composition, **02:** 666-667
    molar absorptivity and-or absorbance values, **02:** 486
Ovomacroglobulin, *see also* Macroglobulin
    average hydrophobicity value, **01:** 228
    molar absorptivity and-or absorbance values, **02:** 486
    subunit, constitution of, **02:** 349
Ovomucin
    average hydrophobicity value, **01:** 228
    carbohydrate content, **02:** 268
    molar absorptivity and-or absorbance values, **02:** 486
    viscosity, intrinsic, **02:** 721
Ovomucoid
    animal sources, amino acid composition, **02:** 650
    average hydrophobicity value, **01:** 228
    bird egg whites, specificities and properties, **02:** 624-629
    carbohydrate composition, **02:** 666-667
    carbohydrate content, **02:** 268
    circular dichroism, **07:** 116
        UV and near-UV region, **07:** 158
    molar absorptivity and-or absorbance values, **02:** 486

Ovomucoid *(continued)*

optical rotatory dispersion
UV region, **07:** 69
visible and near UV region, **07:** 32
viscosity, intrinsic, **02:** 721

Ovorubin
lower animal sources, specificity and properties, **02:**
620-621
molar absorptivity and-or absorbance values, **02:** 486

Ovotransferrin
average hydrophobicity value, **01:** 228
circular dichroism
UV and near-UV region, at room temperature, **07:**
116, 158
molar absorptivity and-or absorbance values, **02:** 486
optical rotatory dispersion
UV region, **07:** 69
visible and near UV regions, **07:** 32

Oxalacetic acid
properties of, **01:** 181

Oxalic acid
heat of proton ionization, pK, and related thermodynamic quantities, **06:** 224-225
pK'_a values, **06:** 310, 312

Oxaloglycolate reductive decarboxylase
amino acid composition, incomplete data, **07:** 513

DL-Oxalosuccinic acid
properties of, **01:** 181

β-N-Oxalyl-α,β-diaminopropionic acid
physical and chemical properties, **01:** 121

Oxalysine
antagonism to lysine, **01:** 178

4-Oxalysine
physical and chemical properties, **01:** 121

Oxalysine, structure and mode of action as protein biosynthesis inhibitor, **04:** 593

Oxamicetin, physiochemical constants, spectral, chemotherapeutic and biological properties, **03:** 338

Oxamycin, D-4-amino-3-isoxazolinone, *see* D-Cycloserine

Oxazinomycin, physicochemical constants, spectral,
chemotherapeutic and biological properties, **03:** 339

Oxidation-reduction indicators, transition potential and
color change, **06:** 383

Oxidation-reduction potentials
compounds used in biochemical studies, **06:** 123-129
cytochromes, **06:** 132-137
hemoglobins, **06:** 137-139
hemoproteins, **06:** 132-139
metalloporphyrins, **06:** 139-144
myoglobins, **06:** 137-139

Oxidation-reduction reactions, enthalpy, entropy and free
energy values, **06:** 121

Oxidation and reduction reagents, deci-normal solutions,
table of data, **06:** 352

Oxidoreductases
definition and nomenclature of, **02:** 96
intramolecular, numbering and classification, **02:** 108
numbering and classification of, **02:** 104-106

β-3-Oxindolylalanine
physical and chemical properties, **01:** 145

Oxoglutarate dehydrogenase
circular dichroism in the UV region, **07:** 117

optical rotatory dispersion in the UV region, **07:** 69

2-Oxoglutarate dehydrogenase
average hydrophobicity value, **01:** 228

5-Oxoproline, *see* Pyrrolidone carboxylic acid

Δ5→4 3-Oxosteroid isomerase, *see* Steroid, Δ-isomerase

Oxyferrohemoglobin, HbO$_2$
UV and visible absorption spectrum, **07:** 177

Oxyglutarate dehydrase
Neurospora crassa mutant, **04:** 749

Oxytetracycline, structure and characteristic as protein biosynthesis inhibitor, *see also* Terramycin and Tetracycline, **04:** 593

Oxytocin
average hydrophobicity value, **01:** 228
circular dichroism at maxima in near-UV region, at
room temperature, **07:** 158
luminescence of, **01:** 204
proton NMR and suggested conformations, **07:** 570-572

Oxytocins, natural and related synthetic oligopeptides
amino acid sequence, physical and biological properties,
07: 193-218

Oyamvcid, physicochemical constants, spectral, chemotherapeutic and biological properties, **03:** 340

P

pK'_a
alcohols and other oxygen acids, **06:** 315-317
alkaloids and derivatives, **06:** 326-327
amine buffers, table of values, **06:** 368-369
amines, **06:** 322-326
amino acids, **06:** 318-320
anilines, **06:** 327-330
antibiotics, **06:** 348
bile pigments, **06:** 348
carbon acids, **06:** 347
carboxylic acids, **06:** 309-313
dyes, **06:** 348
indicators, **06:** 348
inorganic acids, **06:** 307
nitrogen compounds, **06:** 322-345
peptides, **06:** 321
phenols, **06:** 314
phosphates, **06:** 308
phosphonates, **06:** 308
porphyrins, **06:** 348
steroids, **06:** 348
thiols, **06:** 346
vitamins, **06:** 348

PA 114-B; origin, structure, and characteristic as protein
biosynthesis inhibitor, **04:** 594

PA 114A, *see also* Osteogrycin A, Staphylomycin
M$_1$, Virginiamycin M$_1$; origin and mode of action as
protein biosynthesis inhibitor, **04:** 594

PABA, properties of, **08:** 293

Pachysolen
G + C composition of DNA of, table arranged by specie, **04:** 209

Pactamycin; origin, structure, and characteristic as
protein biosynthesis inhibitor, **04:** 593

(Pentafluorophenyl)alanine
structure and symbols for those incorporated into synthetic polypeptides, **01**: 105
2,4-Pentanedione
heat of proton ionization, pK, and related thermodynamic quantities, **06**: 226-227
Pentanoic acid derivatives
heat of proton ionization, pK, and related thermodynamic quantities, **06**: 227-228
Pentasaccharides
chemical formula, **05**: 315-316, 343-344
derivatives, **05**: 315-316, 343-344
melting point, **05**: 315-316, 343-344
specific rotation, **05**: 315-316, 343-344
synonyms, **05**: 315-316, 343-344
2-*tert*-Pentenyl-5,7-diisopentenyltryptophan, *see* Echinine
Penton protein
circular dichroism in the UV region, **07**: 117
Pentopyranine A, B, C, D
physicochemical constants, spectral, chemotherapeutic and biological properties, **03**: 341-344
Pentose cycle; pathways chart, **04**: insert
Pentose interconversion; pathways chart, **04**: insert
Pepsin, *see also* Pepsin A
average hydrophobicity value, **01**: 229
calorimetric ΔH values accompanying conformational changes, **06**: 270
enzymatic hydrolysis, conjugated proteins, **02**: 211
enzymatic hydrolysis of proteins, **02**: 209
luminescence of, table, **01**: 206
molar absorptivity and-or absorbance values, **02**: 489
refractive index increments, **02**: 380
specificity for hydrolysis of peptide bonds, **02**: 215
Pepsin, porcine
amino acid sequence, **07**: 358
Pepsin A
circular dichroism, **07**: 118
UV and near-UV region, **07**: 158
optical rotatory dispersion
UV region, **07**: 70
visible and near UV regions, **07**: 32
Pepsin I, II, average hydrophobicity values, **01**: 229
Pepsin inhibitors
animal sources, amino acid composition, **02**: 649
lower animal sources, specificity and properties, **02**: 618-619
Pepsinogen
amino acid composition, complete data, **07**: 509
carbohydrate content, **02**: 274
circular dichroism
UV and near-UV region, **07**: 118, 158
molar absorptivity and-or absorbance values, **02**: 489
optical rotatory dispersion
UV region, **07**: 70
visible and near UV regions, **07**: 33
viscosity, intrinsic, **02**: 721
Pepsinogen A and C
average hydrophobicity value, **01**: 229
Peptic hydrolysis, *see also* Hydrolysis
aromatic amino acids in human α- and β-chains, **02**: 216
leucine in human α- and β-chains, **02**: 217

Peptidase
subunit, constitution of, **02**: 346
Peptide bonds
hydrolysis, specificity of chymotrypsin, **02**: 212
hydrolysis, specificity of papain, **02**: 218
hydrolysis, specificity of pepsin, **02**: 215
hydrolysis, specificity of subtilisin, **02**: 221
Peptide hormones
list of, **02**: 177-178
nomenclature recommendations, **02**: 175-178
Peptide linkage
dimensions of, **02**: 742-758
Peptide peptidohydrolase
optical rotatory dispersion in the visible and near UV regions, **07**: 33
Peptide synthesis, pathways chart, **04**: insert
Peptides
bond angles and distances for the grouping, **08**: 222
chromatography, gas-liquid, references, **08**: 111
circular dichroism spectra of metal complexes of, **01**: 245-315
cyanogen bromide cleavage of, table, **02**: 199-202
enthalpy of formation, table of values, **06**: 112
entropies, absolute, for several, **06**: 110
entropies of formation for several, **06**: 110
free energy of formation, table of values, **06**: 112
heat capacities for several, **06**: 110
heat of combustion, table of values, **06**: 112
hydrolysis from α- and β-chains of human hemoglobin, **02**: 219
hydrolysis in acid solution, relative rates, **02**: 208
molal activity coefficients, table of values, **06**: 120
natural
abbreviations, use of, for synthetic modification, **01**: 14, **02**: 14-15
rules for naming synthetic modifications of, **02**: 79-83
semitrivial names for variants, **02**: 79
nomenclature for those prepared by solid phase peptide synthesis, table, **01**: 374-375
pK'_a values, **06**: 321
prepared by solid phase peptide synthesis, table of characteristics, **01**: 374-390
symbols for, rules, **01**: 88-90
symbols for, use of, **01**: 8-15, **02**: 8-15
Peptides, active site, **07**: 186-191
Peptides and their derivatives, immunogenic, **07**: 549-550
Peroxidase
carbohydrate content, **02**: 273
circular dichroism
UV and near UV-region, **07**: 118, 159
molar absorptivity and-or absorbance values, **02**: 489, 492
optical rotatory dispersion
UV region, **07**: 70
visible and near UV regions, **07**: 33
subunit, constitution of, **02**: 340
Peroxidase B
amino acid composition, complete data, **07**: 509
Peroxisomes
enzymatic activity, table, **02**: 710
Peroxy Y base
physical constants and spectral properties, **03**: 95

Peroxywybutosine, *see* 7-[2-(Hydroperoxy)-3-(methoxycarbonyl)-3-(methoxyformamido)propyl] wyosine
  composition in various tRNA's, **04:** 428-441
  isolation and detection of, in RNA, general remarks, **03:** 240
Pestalotiopsis
  G + C composition of DNA of, table arranged by species, **04:** 212
Petalosporus
  G + C composition of DNA of, table arranged by specie, **04:** 212
PG, *see* Prostaglandins
pH
  buffer solutions, data for preparation of, **06:** 358-359
  buffer solutions, primary standard
    pH values, **06:** 354
    preparation of, **06:** 355
  buffer solutions, ranges for various, **06:** 362-363
  buffer solutions, values for varying temperatures, **06:** 360-361
  definitions, **06:** 353
  determination, indicators for, **06:** 380-383
  electrodes, use in measurement, **06:** 355
  indicators, ranges for various, **06:** 378-379
  indicators, use in pH measurement, **06:** 357
  measurement techniques, **06:** 355-357
  recommended values for measuring equilibrium data, **06:** 94
pH values for glycohydrolases reactions, **05:** 426-445
Phaeocoriolellus (Lenzites)
  G + C composition of DNA of, table arranged by specie, **04:** 212
Phaeolus (Polyporus)
  G + C composition of DNA of, table arranged by specie, **04:** 212
Phage protein, *see* Bacteriophage protein
Phalloidin
  circular dichroism at maxima in near-UV region, at room temperature, **07:** 159
  proton NMR and suggested conformations, **07:** 569
Phellinus
  G + C composition of DNA of, table arranged by specie, **04:** 212
Phenanthrene derivatives
  heat of proton ionization, pK, and related thermodynamic quantities, **06:** 228-229
Phenobarbital, heat of proton ionization, pK, and related thermodynamic quantities, **06:** 172
Phenol protein group, chemical modification of
  reagents used, table of specificities, **02:** 203-204
Phenols
  heat of proton ionization, pK, and related thermodynamic quantities, **06:** 230-232
  pK'_a values, **06:** 314
Phenomycin; origin, structure, and characteristic as protein biosynthesis inhibitor, **04:** 595
Phenotype
  Aspergillus nidulans, located mutants of, **04:** 732-737
Phenotypic expression, mutants
  mouse, **04:** 857-870

Phenoxymethylpenicillin
  UV spectra, formula, molecular weight, **08:** 158
Phenylalanine
  N-acetyl-DL- -phenylalanine methyl ester, UV spectra of, **01:** 193
  acid vs. neutral difference spectra, **01:** 191
  alkaline vs. neutral difference spectra, **01:** 190-191
  antagonists of, **01:** 179
  far ultraviolet absorption spectra
    aqueous solution at pH 5, **01:** 184
    neutral water, table, **01:** 185
    0.1 *M* sodium dodecyl sulfate, table, **01:** 185
  free acid in amniotic fluid in early pregnancy and at term, **01:** 327
  free acid in blood plasma of newborn infants and adults, **01:** 328
  luminescence of, table, **01:** 200
  luminescence of derivatives of, table, **01:** 203
  molar extinctions, **01:** 185
  molecular absorbances of, table, **01:** 189
  nucleoside composition, tables of values, **04:** 437
  nucleotide sequences of, **04:** 448-449
  pK'_a values, **06:** 319
  phenylketonuria
    atypical, effect of, **01:** 320
    classical, effect of, **01:** 320
  physical and chemical properties, **01:** 131
  requirements of, for growth of various microorganisms, table, **04:** 630-643
  spectra, far UV, **01:** 184
  symbols for atoms and bonds in side chains, **01:** 70, **02:** 74
  thumbprint, content in, **08:** 121
  UV absorption characteristics, **01:** 186
Phenylalanine ammonia lyase
  average hydrophobicity value, **01:** 229
L-Phenylalanine ammonia lyase
  molar absorptivity and-or absorbance values, **02:** 492
Phenylalanine hydroxylase
  average hydrophobicity value, **01:** 229
Phenylalanyl model compounds
  near-UV circular dichroism intensities, **07:** 168
Phenylglycine
  pK'_a values, **06:** 319
  structure and symbols for those incorporated into synthetic polypeptides, **01:** 106
Phenylketonuria
  atypical
    characteristics of, **01:** 320
  classical
    characteristics of, **01:** 320
Phenylpyruvate tautomerase
  amino acid composition, incomplete data, **07:** 513
Phenylpyruvic acid
  properties of, **01:** 182
(α-Phenylsarcosine), *see* *N*-Methylphenylglycine
β-Phenylserine
  antagonism to phenylalanine, **01:** 179
Threo-β-phenylserine
  physical and chemical properties, **01:** 128

Phialophora
  G + C composition of DNA of, table arranged by specie, **04**: 213
Phoma
  amino acid requirements for growth, table, **04**: 641
  G + C composition of DNA of, table arranged by specie, **04**: 213
Phosphatase
  molar absorptivity and-or absorbance values, **02**: 493
  subunit, constitution of, **02**: 334
Phosphate acetyltransferase
  optical rotatory dispersion
    UV region, **07**: 70
    visible and near UV regions, **07**: 33
Phosphate buffer
  preparation of, **06**: 374
  protonic activity tables, **06**: 529-539
Phosphates and phosphonates, pK'_a values, **06**: 308
Phosphatidic acid, generic term usage, **05**: 9
Phosphatidyl serine decarboxylase
  average hydrophobicity value, **01**: 229
3-*sn*-phosphatidylcholine, generic term usage, **05**: 9
Phospho-2-keto-3-deoxygluconate aldolase
  optical rotatory dispersion
    UV region, **07**: 71
    visible and near UV regions, **07**: 33
Phosphocreatine kinase
Phosphoenol pyruvate carboxykinase
  average hydrophobicity value, **01**: 229
Phosphoenolpyruvate carboxykinase
  amino acid composition, complete data, **07**: 509
Phosphoenolpyruvate carboxylase
Phosphoethanolamine
  hypophosphatasia, effect of, **01**: 321
Phosphofructokinase
  amino acid composition, complete data, **07**: 509
  average hydrophobicity value, **01**: 229
  molar absorptivity and-or absorbance values, **02**: 494
  subunit, constitution of, **02**: 349
Phosphoglucoisomerase
  molar absorptivity and-or absorbance values, **02**: 494
Phosphoglucomutase
  amino acid composition, complete data, **07**: 509
  average hydrophobicity value, **01**: 229
  molar absorptivity and-or absorbance values, **02**: 494
  Neurospora crassa mutant, **04**: 741
  optical rotatory dispersion
    UV region, **07**: 70
    visible and near UV regions, **07**: 33
6-Phosphogluconate dehydrogenase, *see* Phosphogluconate, dehydrogenase (decarboxylating)
  molar absorptivity and-or absorbance values, **02**: 494
  Neurospora crassa mutant, **04**: 755
  subunit, constitution of, **02**: 332, 333
Phosphogluconate dehydrogenase (decarboxylating)
  amino acid composition, complete data, **07**: 509
  optical rotatory dispersion in the UV region, **07**: 71
Phosphoglucose isomerase, *see* Glucosephosphate, isomerase
  molar absorptivity and-or absorbance values, **02**: 495
Phosphoglycerate dehydrogenase
  amino acid composition, complete data, **07**: 509

Phosphoglycerate kinase
  average hydrophobicity value, **01**: 229
  circular dichroism in the UV region, **07**: 118
3-Phosphoglycerate kinase
  optical rotatory dispersion in the UV region: extrema between 185 and 250 NM³, **07**: 71
Phosphoglycerate mutase, *see* Phosphoglyceromutase
Phosphoglyceric acid mutase, *see* Phosphoglyceromutase
Phosphoglyceride, generic term usage, **05**: 9
Phosphoglyceromutase
  amino acid composition, complete data, **07**: 509
  optical rotatory dispersion
    UV region, **07**: 71
    visible and near UV regions, **07**: 33
O-Phosphohomoserine
  physical and chemical properties, **01**: 161
Phosphoinositide, generic term usage, **05**: 9
Phospholipase A
  amino acid composition, complete data, **07**: 509
  circular dichroism in the UV region, **07**: 118
  prostaglandin biosynthesis, importance, **08**: 320
Phospholipase A$_2$
  circular dichroism, **07**: 119
    UV and near-UV region, **07**: 159
  molar absorptivity and-or absorbance values, **02**: 495
Phospholipase A, A$_1$, A$_2$
  average hydrophobicity value, **01**: 229
Phospholipid, generic term usage, **05**: 9
Phospholipids
  composition in parts of human skin, **05**: 507
  content in different animal tissues, **05**: 519-520
  prostaglandins, pathways diagram, **08**: 317
  stereoconfiguration of PGF$_{1\beta}$, **08**: 318
Phospholipids, glycoside derivatives of, structures and organisms, **05**: 385-387
γ-Phosphonoglutamic acid
  antagonism to glutamic acid, **01**: 177
Phospho*enol*pyruvate carboxykinase
  molar absorptivity and-or absorbance values, **02**: 494
Phospho*enol*pyruvate carboxylase
  molar absorptivity and-or absorbance values, **02**: 494
Phosphoribosyl-ATP-dephosphorylase
  Neurospora crassa mutant, **04**: 741
N-1-(5'-Phosphoribosyl) adenosine triphosphate pyrophosphate phosphoribosyl transferase
  amino acid composition, incomplete data, **07**: 513
Phosphoribosyl transferase
  viscosity, intrinsic, **02**: 721
Phosphoric acid
  heat of proton ionization, pK, and related thermodynamic quantities, **06**: 232-233
Phosphorylase
  average hydrophobicity value, **01**: 229
  enzymatic hydrolysis, conjugated proteins, **02**: 211
  molar absorptivity and-or absorbance values, **02**: 496
  subunit, constitution of, **02**: 347
α-Phosphorylase
  optical rotatory dispersion
    UV region, **07**: 71
    visible and near UV regions, **07**: 34
Phosphorylase, purine-nucleoside
  molar absorptivity and-or absorbance values, **02**: 497

Phosphorylase b (muscle), *see* α-Phosphorylase
Phosphorylase kinase
   molar absorptivity and-or absorbance values, **02:** 497
   subunit, constitution of, **02:** 350
Phosphorylated compounds
   symbols for, use of, **01:** 8, **02:** 8, **04:** 8
Phosphorylated compounds, use of symbols for, **03:** 8, **05:** 8
O-Phosphoserine
   physical and chemical properties, **01:** 161
Phosphotransacetylase, *see* Phosphate, acetyltransferase
Phosvitin
   circular dichroism in the UV region, **07:** 119
   optical rotatory dispersion in the visible and near UV regions, **07:** 34
Phosvitin fraction II
   amino acid composition, complete data, **07:** 509
Photobacterium
   amino acid requirements for growth, table, **04:** 637
Photoelastic modulator, circular dichroism spectrophotometer design, **08:** 201-202
Photosynthesis; pathways chart, **04:** insert
Phthalate-hydrochloric acid buffer, preparation of, **06:** 371
Phthalate-sodium hydroxide buffer, preparation of, **06:** 373
Phthalic acid
   heat of proton ionization, pK, and related thermodynamic quantities, **06:** 174
   pK'_a values, **06:** 313
Phthalocyanine
   UV spectra, formula, molecular weight, **08:** 177
Phycocyanin
   amino acid composition, incomplete data, **07:** 513
   average hydrophobicity value, **01:** 229
   molar absorptivity and-or absorbance values, **02:** 497
   subunit, constitution of, **02:** 327, 346
C-Phycocyanin
   molar absorptivity and-or absorbance values, **02:** 498
Phycocyanin, anacystis
   molar absorptivity and-or absorbance values, **02:** 498
Phycoerythrin
   average hydrophobicity value, **01:** 230
   molar absorptivity and-or absorbance values, **02:** 498
Phycomyces ᐸ
   amino acid requirements for growth, table, **04:** 641
   G + C composition of DNA of, table arranged by specie, **04:** 213
Physalaemin group, natural and related synthetic oligopeptide
   amino acid sequence, physical and biological properties, **07:** 258-260
Physarum
   G + C composition of DNA of, table arranged by specie, **04:** 213
A-9145, physicochemical constants, spectral, chemotherapeutic and biological properties, **03:** 273
Phytochrome
   amino acid composition, incomplete data, **07:** 514
   average hydrophobicity value, **01:** 230
   circular dichroism intensities at maxima in near-UV region, at room temperature, **07:** 159

molar absorptivity and-or absorbance values, **02:** 498
   subunit, constitution of, **02:** 344
Phytohemagglutinin
   circular dichroism in the UV region, **07:** 119
   optical rotatory dispersion in the UV region, **07:** 72
Phytolacca americana peptide (PAP); origin, structure, and characteristic as protein biosynthesis inhibitor, **04:** 595
Phytophthora
   amino acid requirements for growth, table, **04:** 641
   G + C composition of DNA of, table arranged by specie, **04:** 213
Phytylmenaquinone, properties of, **08:** 290
Pichia
   G + C composition of DNA of, table arranged by specie, **04:** 214
Pigeon droppings
   molar absorptivity and-or absorbance values, **02:** 498
Pigment
   molar absorptivity and-or absorbance values, **02:** 498
Pilaira
   G + C composition of DNA of, table arranged by specie, **04:** 214
Pilchard oil, Pacific
   chain length composition, **05:** 525
   properties and weight % composition of derived fatty acid methyl esters, **05:** 523-524
   properties of interest, comparisons, **05:** 526-527
Pinnatanine
   physical and chemical properties, **01:** 128
Pipecolic acid
   hyperpipecolic acidemia, effect of, **01:** 321
   physical and chemical properties, **01:** 145
   structure and symbols for those incorporated into synthetic polypeptides, **01:** 106
Pipecolic acid betaine, *see* Homostachydrine
Piperidazine-3-carboxylic acid
   physical and chemical properties, **01:** 145
Piperidine
   heat of proton ionization, pK, and related thermodynamic quantities, **06:** 234-235
Piperidinic acid, *see* γ-Aminobutyric acid
Piperine
   pK'_a values, **06:** 327
Piptoporus (Polyporus)
   G + C composition of DNA of, table arranged by specie, **04:** 214
Pituitary, anterior, hormones
   amino acid sequences, **07:** 385-397
Pituitary hormones, nomenclature, **02:** 176-178
pK
   α-amino groups in proteins, table of values, **02:** 693
   ε-amino groups in proteins, table of values, **02:** 694
   antibiotics, nucleoside, **03:** 271-393
   carboxyl side chain, values estimated in lysozyme, **02:** 696
   chemical compounds, table of values, **06:** 153-262
   cysteine β93 SH in human hemoglobin, **02:** 696
   histidine in
      carbonic anhydrase, values for residues, **02:** 691
      cytochrome *c* specific values, **02:** 691
      hemoglobin, human, table of values, **02:** 690

pK *(continued)*
    hemoglobin human, values for His 146β, **02:** 690
    myoglobin, values for residues, **02:** 690
    nuclease, table of values, **02:** 691
    proteins, various, table of values, **02:** 692
    ribonuclease A, nonspecific values, table, **02:** 689
    ribonuclease A, specific values, table, **02:** 689
    nucleosides, index to table of values, **03:** 69-72
    nucleotides, index to table of values, **03:** 72-75
    proteins, techniques for determining values in, **02:** 689
    purines, index to table of values, **03:** 67-69
    pyrimides, index to table of values, **03:** 67-69
    tyrosine, table of values, **02:** 694
    tyrosine in
        hemoglobin, table of values, **02:** 695
        myoglobin, table of values, **02:** 695
pK_a
    amino acids, naturally occurring, table, **01:** 111-166
pKa
    alkyl bases, table of values, **03:** 409-416
    nucleosides, table of values, **03:** 409-416
    nucleotides, table of values, **03:** 409-416
Placenta, hormones
    amino acid sequence, **07:** 385-397
Placental lactogen, human
    amino acid sequence compared with human growth hormone and human prolactin, **07:** 392-393
Planobispora
    G + C composition of DNA of, table arranged by specie, **04:** 77
Plants
    glycoproteins from, carbohydrate content, **02:** 270
Plants, satellite DNAs; buoyant density and G + C content of, table, **04:** 399-402
Plasma, *see also* Blood plasma; Human plasma
    human, basic B_2
    molar absorptivity and-or absorbance values, **02:** 498
Plasma, human, quantitative variation in clotting factors, **04:** 881
Plasma albumin, *see also* Albumin, plasma; Human plasma albumin
Plasma cell
    immunological response, **07:** 537
Plasma concentration
    blood coagulation proteins, table of values, **02:** 255
Plasma membrane, *see* Membrane protein, plasma
    enzymatic activity, table, **02:** 713
Plasma proteins
    human, *see also* Human plasma proteins
    refractive index increments, **02:** 380
Plasmin
    human
    molar absorptivity and-or absorbance values, **02:** 498
    human, urokinase activated
    molar absorptivity and-or absorbance values, **02:** 498
    molecular parameters, **02:** 246
Plasminogen
    general building plan, **07:** 353
    human
    molar absorptivity and-or absorbance values, **02:** 499
    human, A
    molar absorptivity and-or absorbance values, **02:** 499

    human, B
    molar absorptivity and-or absorbance values, **02:** 499
    molecular parameters, **02:** 245
    physical data and characteristics, **02:** 254-255
    plasma, human
        carbohydrate content, molecular weights, sedimentation coefficients, **02:** 258
    sequence of the 69 residue amino-terminal peptide released from, upon activation with urokinase, **07:** 354
Plasmodium
    amino acid requirements for growth, table, **04:** 642
    G + C composition of DNA of, table arranged by specie, **04:** 229
Plastics, commercial
    chemical and physical properties, **08:** 427
    chemical compatibility of Millipore® filters, O-rings and filter holders, **08:** 431-432
    chemical resistance of those used in ultracentrifuge, **08:** 428-429
    ultracentrifuge tubes, chemical resistance, **08:** 434
Plastocyanin
    average hydrophobicity value, **01:** 230
    molar absorptivity and-or absorbance values, **02:** 499
    molecular weights, stoichiometry and sources, **02:** 282
Plectonema
    G + C composition of DNA of, table arranged by specie, **04:** 226
Pleurotus
    G + C composition of DNA of, table arranged by specie, **04:** 214
Plicacetin, physicochemical constants, spectral chemotherapeutic and biological properties, **03:** 345
Plicacetin; origin, structure, and characteristic as protein biosynthesis inhibitor, **04:** 596
PMR spectra
    antibiotics, nucleoside, **03:** 271-393
Pneumococcus
    amino acid requirements for growth, table, **04:** 637
Pockels cell, circular dichroism spectrophotometer design, **08:** 201-202
Poly (β-benzyl-L-aspartate)
    calorimetric ΔH values accompanying conformational changes, **06:** 275-276
Poly (γ-benzyl-L-glutamate)
    calorimetric ΔH values accompanying conformational changes, **06:** 276-280
Poly (N-γ-carbobenzoxy-L-α,γ-(diaminobutric acid)
    calorimetric ΔH values accompanying conformational changes, **06:** 280
Poly(ε-carbobenzoxy-L-lysine)
    calorimetric ΔH values accompanying conformational changes, **06:** 280
Poly(N-δ-carbobenzoxy-L-ornithine)
    calorimetric ΔH values accompanying conformational changes, **06:** 280
Poly(γ-ethyl-L-glutamate)
    calorimetric ΔH values accompanying conformational changes, **06:** 280
Poly A
    calorimetric ΔH values accompanying conformational changes, **06:** 291

Poly C
  calorimetric ΔH values accompanying conformational
    changes, **06:** 293
Poly (L-glutamic acid)
  calorimetric ΔH values accompanying conformational
    changes, **06:** 280
Poly (L-lysine)
  calorimetric ΔH values accompanying conformational
    changes, **06:** 280
Polyallomer, chemical and physical properties, **08:** 427
Polyangiaceae
  G + C composition of DNA of, table arranged by gen-
    era and specie, **04:** 150-151
Polyangium
  G + C composition of DNA of, table arranged by spe-
    cie, **04:** 151
Poly(A·U)
  calorimetric ΔH values accompanying conformational
    changes, **06:** 284-290
Polycarbonate, chemical and physical properties, **08:** 427
Poly(dA·dT)
  calorimetric ΔH values accompanying conformational
    changes, **06:** 291
Polydextran sulfate, characteristics as protein biosynthesis
    inhibitor, **04:** 596
Polyene probes, fluorescent, absorption data, **08:** 211-212
Polyethylene, chemical and physical properties, **08:** 427
Poly(I)
  calorimetric ΔH values accompanying conformational
    changes, **06:** 292
Poly(I·C)
  calorimetric ΔH values accompanying conformational
    changes, **06:** 292
Polyides
  G + C composition of DNA of, table arranged by spe-
    cie, **04:** 226
Polymerization of product, determination for sequential
    polypeptides, **01:** 332
Polymerized amino acids, *see* Amino acids, polymerized,
    Amino acids, polymerized
Polymethylpentene, chemical and physical properties, **08:**
    427
Polymorphonuclear leukocytes
  immunological response, **07:** 537
Polymyxin
  proton NMR and suggested conformations, **07:** 564
Polynucleotide phosphorylase
  molar absorptivity and-or absorbance values, **02:** 499
  subunit, constitution of, **02:** 340
Polynucleotides
  chemical shifts, **03:** 533
  circular dichroism extrema and crossovers for synthetic
    types, **03:** 592-595
  coupling constants of the H1' and H2' protons, **03:** 533
  IR spectra, charts, **03:** 605-621
  IR spectra, table of values, **03:** 622-623
  melting temperatures, for synthetic types, **03:** 575-585
  symbols for, use of, **03:** 10-11, **04:** 10-11
Polynucleotides, synthetic
  buoyant density, values, **03:** 571-573
Polyol dehydrogenase
  amino acid composition, incomplete data, **07:** 514

Polyol esters, acid value, density, hydroxyl value, **05:** 515
Polyoxin A, B, C, D, E, F, G, H, I, J, K, L
  physicochemical constants, spectral, chemotherapeutic
    and biological properties, **03:** 347-370
Polypaecilum
  G + C composition of DNA of, table arranged by spe-
    cie, **04:** 214
Polypeptide chain
  nomenclature rules, **01:** 59-73
  primary structure of a segment, definition, **01:** 73
  secondary structure of a segment, definition, **01:** 73
Polypeptide chains
  blood coagulation proteins, table of values, **02:** 255
  immunoglobulin molecules, notation for, **02:** 180
  nomenclature rules, **02:** 63-77
  primary structure of a segment, definition, **02:** 77
  secondary structure of a segment, definition, **02:** 77
Polypeptides
  cyclic
    symbols for, use of, **01:** 11
  enzymatic hydrolysis of, **02:** 209
  nomenclature, abbreviated, of synthetic, **01:** 91-95
  sequential
    abbreviations, **01:** 333
    polymerization, determination of degree of, **01:** 332
    preparation and product analysis, index to table, **01:**
      334-339
    racemization, determination of degree of, **01:** 332
  symbols for, rules, **01:** 88-90
  symbols for, use of, **01:** 10-11, **02:** 10-11
  synthetic
    symbols for, use of, **01:** 13
Polypeptides, cyclic
  symbols for, use of, **02:** 11
Polypeptides, synthetic
  symbols for, use of, **02:** 13-14
Polypeptides, synthetic immunogenic, **07:** 546-547
Polypropylene, chemical and physical properties, **08:** 427
Polyribonucleotide
  optical parameter, calculation of, **03:** 596
Polysaccharide depolymerase
  molar absorptivity and-or absorbance values, **02:** 500
  subunit, constitution of, **02:** 347
Polysaccharides
  connective tissues, table of data and characteristics, **02:**
    686-687
Polysaccharides, electronic charge distribution, **05:**
    478-481
Polysphondylium
  G + C composition of DNA of, table arranged by spe-
    cie, **04:** 214
Polystyrene, chemical and physical properties, **08:** 427
Polytoma
  G + C composition of DNA of, table arranged by spe-
    cie, **04:** 227
Polytomella
  G + C composition of DNA of, table arranged by spe-
    cie, **04:** 227
Polyvinyl chloride, chemical and physical properties, **08:**
    427
Polyvinyl sulfate, mode of action as protein biosynthesis
    inhibitor, **04:** 596

Protein, M-
circular dichroism in the UV region, **07:** 111
optical rotatory dispersion in the UV region, **07:** 66
Y-Protein, *see* Ligandin, (y-protein)
Z-protein, **07:** 129
circular dichroism in the UV region, **07:** 129
Protein, S-100 brain-
amino acid composition, incomplete data, **07:** 514
Protein, high density
subunit, constitution of, **02:** 341
Protein, R17 coat-
amino acid composition, complete data, **07:** 510
Protein, Red-
amino acid composition, complete data, **07:** 510
Protein biosynthesis, inhibitors of; characteristics, origin
and structures, table, **04:** 555-618
Protein chemical data on *Escherichia coli* ribosomes, **04:**
471-486
Protein composition
Tamm-Horsfall glycoprotein, **02:** 303
Protein kinase
subunit, constitution of, **02:** 344
Protein kinase modulator
average hydrophobicity value, **01:** 230
Protein P11
subunit, constitution of, **02:** 329
Protein phosphokinase
subunit, constitution of, **02:** 337
Protein toxin B
subunit, constitution of, **02:** 335
Proteinase--alkaline, *Aspergillus, see Aspergillus* alkaline--
proteinase
Proteinase, neutral, *see* Microbial metalloenzyme
Proteinase A and B--alkaline, thermophilic, *Streptomyces,*
see Trypsin, thermophilic Streptomyces
Clostridium histolyticum proteinase B
optical rotatory dispersion
UV region, **07:** 52
visible and near UV regions, **07:** 21
Proteinase B, alkaline
circular dichroism intensities at maxima in near UV region, at room temperature, **07:** 159
Proteinase inhibitor I
subunit, constitution of, **02:** 327
Proteinase inhibitors
animal sources
amino acid composition, table, **02:** 649-653
amino acid sequences, table, **02:** 656-659
carbohydrate content, **02:** 618-628
dissociation constant, **02:** 618-641
isoelectric point, **02:** 618-641
molecular weight, **02:** 618-641
specificity, **02:** 618-641
carbohydrate composition of selected, **02:** 666-667
microbial sources
amino acid composition, **02:** 664
amino acid sequence, **02:** 665
isoelectric point, **02:** 661-662
molecular weight, **02:** 661-662
specificity, **02:** 661-662
plant sources
amino acid composition, table, **02:** 605-610

amino acid sequences, **02:** 611-617
carbohydrate content, **02:** 598-599
dissociation constant, **02:** 588-596, 600
isoelectric point, **02:** 586-600
molecular weight, **02:** 586-600
specificity, **02:** 586-600
Proteinase zymogen
amino acid composition, complete data, **07:** 509
Proteins, *see also* Bacteriophage Flavoproteins, Matrix
protein, *also* Protein, individual proteins, Molybdoproteins
absorbance, UV and visible region, table of values, **02:**
383-514
average hydrophobicity values for selected, table, **01:**
210-235
blood coagulation, table of data and characteristics, **02:**
254-255
carbohydrate content tables for glycoproteins from various sources, **02:** 257-274
carbohydrate linkages, types of, **02:** 257
carbohydrates
physical-chemical data for, index to ultracentrifuge
studies, **02:** 232
chymotryptic hydrolysis, conditions for, **02:** 214
concentration determination in short-wavelength UV region, **08:** 197
conjugated, *see also* Conjugated proteins
contractile, molecular parameters, **02:** 306
covalent conjugates, *see also* Conjugated proteins;
Covalent protein conjugates
covalent conjugates, table of data, **01:** 208
cyanogen bromide cleavage of, table, **02:** 199-202
electron-transfer, nomenclature, **02:** 114-121
entropies, absolute, for several, **06:** 110
enzymatic cross-linking, **02:** 669-683
enzymatic hydrolysis of, **02:** 209
fibrous, physical-chemical data for, index to ultracentrifuge studies, **02:** 229
globular, physical-chemical data for, index to ultracentrifuge studies, **02:** 222-228
heat capacities for several, **06:** 110
histones, sequence and characterization tables, **02:**
294-299
human plasma, molecular parameters, table, **02:** 242-250
hydrolysis of, tables of data for several, **02:** 206-221
iron, classification of, **02:** 90
iron-sulfur, *see also* Iron sulfur proteins
iron-sulfur, nomenclature recommendations, **02:** 89-90,
120
luminescence of some containing tryptophan, table, **01:**
205-207
luminescence of some lacking tryptophan, table, **01:** 204
metalloproteins, table of molecular weights, sources,
stoichiometry and function, **02:** 276-277
modification of, specificities of reagents used, **02:**
203-204
molar absorptivity, UV and visible region, table of
values, **02:** 383-514
nonmuscle cells, identification of several in, **02:** 307-313
organelles
physical-chemical data for, index to ultacentrifuge
studies, **02:** 232

Proteins (continued)

oxidation-reduction potentials of hemoproteins and metalloporphyrins, **06**: 132-144

particles, physical-chemical data for, index to ultracentrifuge studies, **02**: 232

pK values for several amino acids in, **02**: 689-696

refractive index increments, table, **02**: 372-380

retinol-binding protein, properties, **02**: 304

serum vertebrate

sedimentation coefficients for, **02**: 230-231

structures, drawings of several, **02**: 760-766

substrates for enzymatic incorporation of amines, **02**: 680

subunit constitution of, table, **02**: 326-351

symbols for, use of, **01**: 8-15, **02**: 8-15

techniques for determining pK values in, **02**: 689

viruses, physical-chemical data for, index to ultracentrifuge studies, **02**: 232

viscosity, intrinsic, table for several in native and denatured states, **02**: 721

M-proteins

molecular parameters, **02**: 306

Proteins, iron-sulfur primary structures

amino acid sequences, **07**: 425-427

Proteins, ribosomal

amino acid composition of *Escherichia coli* 30 S, **04**: 476

amino acid composition of *Escherichia coli* 50 S, **04**: 477-478

Escherichia coli derivation, amino acid sequence data, **04**: 479-481

electrophoretic separation, tracing, **04**: 474

Escherichia coli MRE 600 30 S, separation on cellulose phosphate Whatman® P11, **04**: 475

Escherichia coli 30S, physical and functional characteristics, **04**: 482-486

Proteins demonstrating genetically-determined structural variation in man, **04**: 879

Proteoglycan

circular dichroism in the UV region, **07**: 120

Proteus

amino acid requirements for growth, table, **04**: 637

G + C composition of DNA of, table arranged by specie, **04**: 112-113

Prothrombin

amino acid sequence, **07**: 351-352

average hydrophobicity value, **01**: 230

beef

molar absorptivity and-or absorbance values, **02**: 503

circular dichroism intensities at maxima in near UV region, at room temperature, **07**: 160

general building plan, **07**: 350

human

molar absorptivity and-or absorbance values, **02**: 503

optical rotatory dispersion in the UV region, **07**: 73

physical data and characteristics, **02**: 254-255

plasma, human

carbohydrate content, molecular weights, sedimentation coefficients, **02**: 258

plasma, nonhuman

carbohydrate content, **02**: 260

Protoachlya

G + C composition of DNA of, table arranged by specie, **04**: 215

Protocatechuate 3,4-dioxygenase

amino acid composition, complete data, **07**: 509

Protomycin®, origin and mode of action as protein biosynthesis inhibitor, **04**: 597

Proton chemical shifts, nucleosides, **03**: 530-533

Proton chemical shifts (τ), table of values, **05**: 499-500

Proton NMR data, suggested conformations

biologically active cyclic peptides, **07**: 561-573

Protonic activity of some usual buffers, tables, **06**: 529-539

Protoporphyrin IX dimethyl ester

UV and visible absorption spectrum, **07**: 184

UV spectra, formula, molecular weight, **08**: 175

Protoporphyrin IX dimethyl ester dication

UV and visible absorption spectrum, **07**: 185

UV spectra, formula, molecular weight, **08**: 176

Protostelium

G + C composition of DNA of, table arranged by specie, **04**: 215

ϵ-Protoxin

optical rotatory dispersion in the UV region, **07**: 73

Protozoa

amino acid requirements for growth, table, **04**: 641

deoxyribonucleic acids from, purine and pyrimidine distribution in, **04**: 263

DNA base compositions for, **04**: 236

DNA content per cell for various, table, **04**: 289

G + C composition of DNA of, table arranged by genera and specie, **04**: 228-229

Protyrosinase

average hydrophobicity value, **01**: 230

Providencia

G + C composition of DNA of, table arranged by specie, **04**: 113

Prymnesium

G + C composition of DNA of, table arranged by specie, **04**: 227

Psalliota

G + C composition of DNA of, table arranged by specie, **04**: 215

Pseudeurotium

G + C composition of DNA of, table arranged by specie, **04**: 215

Pseudoacetyl cholinesterase

human

luminescence of, table, **01**: 206

Pseudoarachniotus

G + C composition of DNA of, table arranged by specie, **04**: 215

Pseudogymnoascus

G + C composition of DNA of, table arranged by specie, **04**: 215

Pseudomonadaceae

G + C composition of DNA of, table arranged by genera and species, **04**: 152-162

Pseudomonas

amino acid requirements for growth, table, **04**: 637

G + C composition of DNA of, table arranged by specie, **04**: 154-160

Pseudomonas cytochrome c_{551}
amino acid sequence, 07: 292-294
Pseudonocardia
G + C composition of DNA of, table arranged by specie, 04: 150
Pseudouridine
composition in various tRNA's, 04: 428-441
RNA, various, natural occurrence in, 03: 228-229
β-f-Pseudouridine 5'-diphosphate
physical constants and spectral properties, 03: 194
Pseudouridine 5'-diphosphate
physical constants and spectral properties, 03: 194
β-f-Pseudouridine 3'(2')-phosphate
physical constants and spectral properties, 03: 193
β-f-Pseudouridine 5'-phosphate
physical constants and spectral properties, 03: 194
Pseudouridine 3'(2')-phosphate
physical constants and spectral properties, 03: 193
Pseudouridine 5'-phosphate
physical constants and spectral properties, 03: 194
Pseudouridine and nucleoside derivatives
physical constants and spectral properties, index to, 03:
70-71
Pseudouridine C 3'(2')-phosphate
physical constants and spectral properties, 03: 193
Pseudouridine C 5'-phosphate
physical constants and spectral properties, 03: 194
Pseudovitamin B_{12} nucleoside
physical constants and spectral properties, 03: 110
Psicofuranine, physicochemical constants, spectral chemo-
therapeutic and biological properties, 03: 371
Psoriatic scale protein
amino acid composition, complete data, 07: 509
Pteropsida
DNA content per cell for various, table, 04: 287-288
Purified lectins, *see also* Lectin, purified
Purine
heat of proton ionization, pK, and related thermodynamic quantities, 06: 240
pK'_a values, 06: 331, 337
Purine biosynthesis; pathways chart, 04: insert
Purine derivatives excreted in human urine, mg-day, 03:
252-269
Purine nucleoside phosphorylase
amino acid composition, complete data, 07: 509
Purines
bond angles and distances, 08: 224-227
distribution of, in deoxyribonucleic acids from diverse
sources, 04: 241-281
IR spectra, chart of characteristic frequencies between
~ 700 - 300 cm^{-1}, 08: 243
molal activity coefficients, 03: 529
molal osmotic coefficients, 03: 528
physical constants and spectral properties, index to, 03:
67-69
Puromycin, physicochemical constants, spectral, chemotherapeutic and biological properties, 03: 373
Puromycin; origin, structure, and characteristic as protein
biosynthesis inhibitor, 04: 597
Purothionin
circular dichroism in the UV region, 07: 120
Purple membrane, *see* Membrane protein, purple

Putidaredoxin
average hydrophobicity value, 01: 230
Putidaredoxin, bacterial
amino acid sequence, 07: 428
β-Putreanine
physical and chemical properties, 01: 121
Putrescine oxidase
average hydrophobicity value, 01: 230
molar absorptivity and-or absorbance values, 02: 504
Pycnidiophora
G + C composition of DNA of, table arranged by specie, 04: 215
Pycnoporus
G + C composition of DNA of, table arranged by specie, 04: 215
Pyocyanine
UV spectra, formula, molecular weight, 08: 186
Pyostacin A, B, *see* Pristinamycin II
Pyrazofuran, *see* Pyrazomycin
Pyrazofurin B, *see* Pyrazomycin B
β-Pyrazol-1-ylalanine
physical and chemical properties, 01: 146
β-(1-Pyrazolyl)alanine
structure and symbols for those incorporated into synthetic polypeptides, 01: 106
β-(3-Pyrazolyl)alanine
structure and symbols for those incorporated into synthetic polypeptides, 01: 106
β-(4-Pyrazolyl)alanine
antagonism to phenylalanine, 01: 179
structure and symbols for those incorporated into synthetic polypeptides, 01: 106
Pyrazomycin, physicochemical constants, spectral, chemotherapeutic and biological properties, 03: 375
Pyrazomycin B, physicochemical constants, spectral,
chemotherapeutic and biological properties, 03: 377
Pyrenebutyrate
covalent protein conjugates, data, 01: 208
Pyridazine
pK'_a values, 06: 331
Pyridine
infrared correlation chart, 08: 231, 234
IR spectra, chart of characteristic frequencies between
~ 700 - 300 cm^{-1}, 08: 243
pK'_a values, 06: 331, 338-339
Pyridine derivatives
heat of proton ionization, pK, and related thermody-
namic quantities, 06: 240-243
Pyridine derivatives excreted in human urine, mg-day, 03:
252-269
Pyridine hemochrome spectra, 08: 280
Pyridine hemochromogen
UV and visible absorption spectrum, 07: 182
UV spectra, formula, molecular weight, 08: 173
Pyridine nucleotide
amino acid sequence, 07: 314
Pyridine nucleotide transhydrogenase, *see* NAD(P)⁺,
trans-hydrogenase
Pyridosine
physical and chemical properties, 01: 146
Pyridoxal
properties of, 08: 298

Pyridoxal derivatives
   structure, melting point, UV absorption data, **08:** 256-261
Pyridoxamine, properties of, **08:** 299
Pyridoxamine derivatives
   structure, melting point, UV absorption data, **08:** 261-263
Pyridoxine
   biological characteristics, **08:** 304
   nomenclature recommendations, **08:** 12
Pyridoxine derivatives
   structure, melting point, UV absorption data, **08:** 252-256
Pyridoxine hydrochloride, properties, **08:** 298
Pyridoxol
   nomenclature recommendations, **08:** 12
β-2-Pyridylalanine
   antagonism to phenylalanine, **01:** 179
β-4-Pyridylalanine
   antagonism to phenylalanine, **01:** 179
Pyrimidine
   bond angles and distances, **08:** 224-227
   infrared correlation chart, **08:** 234
   IR spectra, chart of characteristic frequencies between ~ 700 - 300 cm^{-1}, **08:** 243
Pyrimidine-specific carbamyl phosphate synthetase; aspartate transcarbamylase
   Neurospora crassa mutant, **04:** 748
Pyrimidine deoxyribonucleosidase
   Neurospora crassa mutant, **04:** 744
Pyrimidine derivatives excreted in human urine, mg-day, **03:** 252-269
Pyrimidine photobyproducts, proposed abbreviations for, **03:** 51-57
Pyrimidines
   distribution of, in deoxyribonucleic acids from diverse sources, **04:** 241-281
   pK'_a values, **06:** 331, 339-341
   photoproducts, proposed abbreviations for, **04:** 51-57
   physical constants and spectral properties, index to, **03:** 67-69
Pyro-2-aminoadipic acid
   structure and symbols for those incorporated into synthetic polypeptides, **01:** 106
Pyrocatechase, *see* Catechol 1,2, -dioxygenase (pyrocatechase)
   molar absorptivity and-or absorbance values, **02:** 504
   table of cofactors, molecular weights, stoichiometry and sources, **02:** 278
Pyrocatechol violet; origin, structure, and characteristic as protein biosynthesis inhibitor, **04:** 598
Pyroglutamic acid
   structure and symbols for those incorporated into synthetic polypeptides, **01:** 106
Pyroglutamic aciduria
   characteristics of, **01:** 326
Pyrolidine-2-carboxylic acid, *see* Proline
Pyrophosphatase
   amino acid composition, incomplete data, **07:** 514
Pyrrole-2-carboxylic acid, *see* Minaline
β-2-Pyrrolealanine
   antagonism to phenylalanine, **01:** 179

5-Pyrrolidone-2-carboxylic acid, *see* Pyroglutamic acid
Pyrrolidone carboxylic acid
   physical and chemical properties, **01:** 146
Pyrroline-5-carboxylate reductase
   Neurospora crassa mutant, **04:** 746
Pyruvate carboxylase
   Neurospora crassa mutant, **04:** 740
   subunit, constitution of, **02:** 341, 348, 349
Pyruvate carboxylase deficiency
   characteristics of, **01:** 326
Pyruvate decarboxylase
   circular dichroism intensities at maxima in near-UV region, at room temperature, **07:** 160
Pyruvate decarboxylase (cytoplasmic)
   optical rotatory dispersion
      UV region, **07:** 73
      visible and near UV regions, **07:** 34
Pyruvate dehydrogenase
   molar absorptivity and-or absorbance values, **02:** 504
   subunit, constitution of, **02:** 332, 338
Pyruvate dehydrogenase complex
   subunit, constitution of, **02:** 351
Pyruvate dehydrogenase deficiency
   characteristics of, **01:** 326
Pyruvate dehydrogenase multiple-enzyme complex
   circular dichroism in the UV region, **07:** 121
Pyruvate kinase
   amino acid composition, complete data, **07:** 510
   average hydrophobicity value, **01:** 230
   circular dichroism
      UV and near UV region, **07:** 121, 160
   molar absorptivity and-or absorbance values, **02:** 504
   optical rotatory dispersion
      UV region, **07:** 73
      visible and near UV regions, **07:** 34
   rabbit
      luminescence of, table, **01:** 206
   subunit, constitution of, **02:** 340, 341, 342, 343
Pyruvic acid
   properties of, **01:** 181
Pyruvic acidosis
   characteristics of, **01:** 326
Pythium
   G + C composition of DNA of, table arranged by specie, **04:** 215

Q

Quercitols, generic name abandoned, **05:** 92
Quinine
   pK'_a values, **06:** 327
Quinoline, derivatives
   heat of proton ionization, pK, and related thermodynamic quantities, **06:** 245-247
Quinones
   nomenclature, journal references for, **02:** 87
Quinones with isoprenoid side chains, nomenclature, **08:** 10-11
Quinonoid dihydropterin reductase
   average hydrophobicity value, **01:** 230

R

Rabbit
  deoxynucleotide polymerizing enzymes from, properties of, **04:** 539-544
  inbred strain availability, **04:** 884
  MHC designation, **04:** 885
  mitochondrial DNA from, properties, **04:** 371
Rabbit aorta contracting substance, *see* RCS
Racemases
  definition and nomenclature, **02:** 98
  numbering and classification of, **02:** 108
Racemic forms, in carbohydrate nomenclature, **05:** 103
Racemization of product, determination for sequential polypeptides, **01:** 332
Radii
  covalent and Van der Waals', of common elements, **08:** 221
Radio-opaque agents, ligands binding to plasma albumin, **02:** 572
Radiomyces
  G + C composition of DNA of, table arranged by specie, **04:** 216
Raman frequencies
  adenosine, table of values, **03:** 534-535
  cytidine, table of values, **03:** 540-541
  guanosine, table of values, **03:** 538-539
  inosine, table of values, **03:** 542-543
  uridine, tables of values, **03:** 536-537
Raman lines, conformationally sensitive
  histogram, **07:** 580
  proteins, **07:** 584-587
Raman spectral changes, melting of calf thymus DNA, **03:** 544
Raman spectral changes, melting of ribonucleic acids, **03:** 545
Raman spectroscopy
  introduction, **07:** 575
  proteins, **07:** 576-578
Raman spectrum
  α-casein, **07:** 583
  β-lactoglobulin, native and denatured, **07:** 582
  Lys$_n$, **07:** 579
  tropomyosin, native and denatured, **07:** 581
Ramibacterium
  G + C composition of DNA of, table arranged by specie, **04:** 123
Rat
  deoxynucleotide polymerizing enzymes from, properties of , **04:** 539-544
  DNA content per cell, **04:** 302
  inbred strain availability, **04:** 884
  MHC designation, **04:** 885
Rat cardiac lipids, isomers in, **05:** 513
RCS
  biological activity of, **08:** 332
  prostaglandin nomenclature, suggested use of term, **08:** 314
C-Reactive protein
  molar absorptivity and-or absorbance values, **02:** 409
  subunit, constitution of, **02:** 337
Reagents
  protein modification, table of specificities for those in common use, **02:** 203-204
Reduction-oxidation indicators, transition potential and color change, **06:** 383
Reduction-oxidation potentials, *see* Oxidation-reduction potentials
Reduction-oxidation reactions, enthalpy, entropy and free energy values, **06:** 121
Reduction and oxidation reagents, deci-normal solutions, table of data, **06:** 352
Reference carbon atom in carbohydrate nomenclature, **05:** 101
Refractive index
  alkyl esters of some fatty acids, **05:** 493
  calculations, constants for several solvent systems, **06:** 389
  concentration dependence
    Lorentz correction factors, values for several compounds, **06:** 396-403
    Sellmeier constants, values for several compounds, **06:** 395
  density of cesium chloride solution as function, table of values, **06:** 419-423
  dispersion of, for various solvents, tables, **06:** 388
  ethyl alcohol, equation for change with temperature, **06:** 540
  fats and oils, table of values, **05:** 502-503
  fatty acids, **05:** 485-491
  fatty acids, values for some, **05:** 493
  herring oils and Pacific pilchard oil, **05:** 523-524
  linseed oil acids and esters, **05:** 497
  liquids, table of values, **06:** 408-410
  lithium bromide versus concentration, **06:** 387
  methyl esters of some fatty acids, **05:** 493
  methyl esters of some synthetic alkenyl and alkyl substituted fatty acids, **05:** 516
  sodium chloride versus concentration, **06:** 387
  solvents, various, calculations of, **06:** 386
  urea solutions versus concentration, **06:** 387
  water, optical rotatory dispersion calculations, **06:** 385
  water, variation with temperature, **06:** 386
Refractive index increments, table for proteins, **02:** 372-380
Relaxing protein
  molar absorptivity and-or absorbance values, **02:** 505
Relomycin; origin, structure, and characteristic as protein biosynthesis inhibitor, **04:** 598
Rennin, *see* Chymosin
Repressor, *see also* Inhibitor
Lac repressor
  molar absorptivity and-or absorbance values, **02:** 460
  subunit, constitution of, **02:** 338
Reptiles
  DNA content per cell for various, table, **04:** 298-299
Resonance raman spectra
  proteins, discussion, **07:** 588
  table, **07:** 589-591

Respiratory proteins--nonheme
  resonance raman spectra, 07: 589
Restriction-modification system, definition, 04: 491
Restriction endonucleases, *see* Endonucleases, restriction
Restriction enzymes, *see* Endonucleases, restriction
Retinaldehyde, properties of, 08: 284
Retinochrome
  circular dichroism in the UV region, 07: 121
Retinoic acid, properties of, 08: 285
Retinol-binding protein
  average hydrophobicity value, 01: 230
  circular dichroism
    UV and near UV region, 07: 121, 160
  human, amino acid composition, 02: 303
  molar absorptivity and-or absorbance values, 02: 505
  optical rotatory dispersion in the UV region, 07: 121
  properties of, 02: 304
Retinol, properties of, 08: 284
Retinol alcohol, *see also* Vitamin A
  UV spectra, formula, molecular weight, 08: 151
Retinyl acetate, properties of, 08: 285
Retinyl palmitate, properties of, 08: 285
Retro, used as prefix in nomenclature, 06: 70, 08: 70
Rhabdonema
  G + C composition of DNA of, table arranged by spe-
    cie, 04: 227
Rhesus monkey
  MHC designation, 04: 885
Rheumatoid factor
  plasma, human
    carbohydrate content, molecular weights, sedimenta-
      tion coefficients, 02: 258
Rhizobiaceae
  G + C composition of DNA of, table arranged by gen-
    era and specie, 04: 162-165
Rhizobitoxine
  physical and chemical properties, 01: 128
Rhizobium
  G + C composition of DNA of, table arranged by spe-
    cie, 04: 164-165
Rhizoclonium
  G + C composition of DNA of, table arranged by spe-
    cie, 04: 227
Rhizophlyctis
  G + C composition of DNA of, table arranged by spe-
    cie, 04: 216
Rhizophydium
  G + C composition of DNA of, table arranged by spe-
    cie, 04: 216
Rhizopus
  G + C composition of DNA of, table arranged by spe-
    cie, 04: 216
Rhodamine B isothiocyanate
  covalent protein conjugates, data, 01: 208
Rhodanese
  molar absorptivity and-or absorbance values, 02: 505
  subunit, constitution of, 02: 327
Rhodopseudomonas
  G + C composition of DNA of, table arranged by spe-
    cie, 04: 78-79
Rhodopsin
  amino acid composition, incomplete data, 07: 514
  average hydrophobicity value, 01: 231

  circular dichroism in the UV region, 07: 121
  molar absorptivity and-or absorbance values, 02: 505
  optical rotatory dispersion in the visible and near UV
    regions, 07: 35
  optical rotatory dispersion in the UV region: extrema
    between 185 and 250 NM^3, 07: 74
Rhodospirillum
  amino acid requirements for growth, table, 04: 637
  G + C composition of DNA of, table arranged by spe-
    cie, 04: 80
Rhodotorula
  G + C composition of DNA of, table arranged by spe-
    cie, 04: 216-217
Rhodymenia
  G + C composition of DNA of, table arranged by spe-
    cie, 04: 227
Ribitol dehydrogenase
  molar absorptivity and-or absorbance values, 02: 505
  subunit, constitution of, 02: 334
Riboflavin, *see also* Flavins
  biological characteristics, 08: 304
  heat of proton ionization, pK, and related thermody-
    namic quantities, 06: 249
  luminescence data, 08: 206-207
  pK'_a values, 06: 348
  properties of, 08: 299
  UV spectra formula, molecular weight, 08: 148, 162
Riboflavin-binding protein
  average hydrophobicity value, 01: 231
Riboflavin anion
  UV spectra, formula, molecular weight, 08: 161
Riboflavin cation
  UV spectra, formula, molecular weight, 08: 160
Riboflavin flavoprotein
  circular dichroism in the UV region: extrema between
    185 and 250 NM^3, 07: 122
  optical rotatory dispersion in the visible and near UV
    regions, 07: 35
  optical rotatory dispersion in the UV region: extrema
    between 185 and 250 NM^3, 07: 74
1-β-D-Ribofuranosyl-4-acetylamino-2-pyrimidinone
  physical constants and spectral properties, 03: 113
1-β-D-Ribofuranosyl-4-methylamino-2-pyrimidinone
  physical constants and spectral properties, 03: 113
7-α-D-Ribofuranosyladenine
  physical constants and spectral properties, 03: 110
7-α-D-Ribofuranosyladenine, 2-Methyl-
  physical constants and spectral properties, 03: 111
N-[(9-β-D-Ribofuranosylpurin-6-yl)-N-
    methylcarbamoyl] threonine 5'-phosphate
  physical constants and spectral properites, 03: 158
N-[(9-β-D-Ribofuranosylpurin-6-yl)carbamoyl] threo-
    nine 3'(2')-phosphate
  physical constants and spectral properties, 03: 156
N-[(9-β-D-Ribofuranosylpurin-6-yl)carbamoyl] threo-
    nine 5'-phosphate
  physical constants and spectral properties,
    03: 157
9-β-D-Ribofuranosylpurine, and nucleoside derivatives
  physical constants and spectral properties, index to, 03:
    71

9-β-D-Ribofuranosylpurine 5'-diphosphate,
6-Dimethylamino-
physical constants and spectral properties, **03**: 155
9-β-D-Ribofuranosylpurine 5'-diphosphate,
6-Methylamino-
physical constants and spectral properties, **03**: 154
9-β-D-Ribofuranosylpurine-6-one 3'(2')-phosphate derivatives
physical constants and spectral properties, index to, **03**:
74
9-β-D-Ribofuranosylpurine 5'-phosphate derivatives
physical constants and spectral properties, index to, **03**:
74
1-β-Ribofuranosylthymine
physical constants and spectral properties, **03**: 131
5-α-D-Ribofuranosyluracil
physical constants and spectral properties, **03**: 136
5-β-D-Ribofuranosyluracil
physical constants and spectral properties, **03**: 136
Ribohomopolymer complexes (purine·purine) (purine
·pyrimidine), melting temperatures, **03**: 578-580
Ribohomopolymer deoxyribohomopolymer hybrids, melting temperatures, **03**: 582-583
Ribohomopolymers, melting temperatures, **03**: 575-578
Ribonuclease
amino acid composition, complete data, **07**: 510
average hydrophobicity value, **01**: 231
bovine
cyanogen bromide cleavage, **02**: 199
luminescence of, **01**: 204
bovine pancreatic
cyanogen bromide cleavage, **02**: 199
calorimetric ΔH values accompanying conformational
changes, **06**: 271-272
carbohydrate content, **02**: 273, 274
circular dichroism at maxima in near UV region, at
room temperature, **07**: 160
cross-linked bovine pancreatic
cyanogen bromide cleavage, **02**: 199
enzymatic activity, subcellular fractions, **02**: 701
heat of proton ionization, pK, and related thermodynamic quantities, **06**: 248
molar absorptivity and-or absorbance values, **02**: 505,
506
refractive index increments, **02**: 380
viscosity, intrinsic, **02**: 721
Ribonuclease, pancreatic
amino acid sequences of proteins, **07**: 311
Ribonuclease A, *see* Ribonuclease I
cyanogen bromide cleavage, **02**: 199
Ribonuclease B
circular dichroism in the UV region, **07**: 122
optical rotatory dispersion in the UV region, **07**: 74
Ribonuclease B' (a glycosylated RNase A)
circular dichroism at maxima in near UV region, at
room temperature, **07**: 160
Ribonuclease I
circular dichroism
UV and near-UV region, **07**: 122, 160
optical rotatory dispersion
UV region, **07**: 74
visible and near UV regions, **07**: 35

Ribonuclease II
circular dichroism in the UV region, **07**: 122
optical rotatory dispersion
UV region, **07**: 74
visible and near UV regions, **07**: 35
Ribonuclease P (des-121-124 RNase A)
circular dichroism in the UV region, **07**: 122
Ribonuclease S
circular dichroism, **07**: 123
UV and near-UV region, **07**: 160
optical rotatory dispersion in the UV region, **07**: 74
Ribonuclease St (extracellular)
circular dichroism at maxima in near UV region, at
room temperature, **07**: 161
Ribonuclease T$_1$, *see* Guanyloribonuclease
Ribonuclease V$_{s^1}$
circular dichroism in the UV region, **07**: 123
Ribonucleic acid, *see* RNA, Transfer RNA, TRNA
(TRNA)
Ribonucleotide
homooligomers of, mean residue absorptivities, **03**: 603
homopolymers of, mean residue absorptivities, **03**: 603
spectrophotometric constants, **03**: 405-406
Ribonucleotide-diphosphate reductase
molar absorptivity and-or absorbance values, **02**: 506
Ribonucleotide polymerizing enzymes
subunits, molecular weights, tables of, **04**: 550-553
Ribonucleotide reductase
amino acid composition, incomplete data, **07**: 514
average hydrophobicity value, **01**: 231
subunit, constitution of, **02**: 347
5-α-D-Ribopyranosyluracil
physical constants and spectral properties, **03**: 137
5-β-D-Ribopyranosyluracil
physical constants and spectral properties, **03**: 137
Ribose
heat of proton ionization, pK, and related thermodynamic quantities, **06**: 248
pK'_a values, **06**: 317
Ribosomal components, *Escherichia coli*, data, **04**: 471-486
Ribosomal proteins, *see* Proteins, ribosomal, **04**: 474
Ribosomal RNA, *see* RNA, ribosomal
Ribosome binding sites, sequences, **04**: 354
Ribosomes
physical characteristics of ribosomes from various
sources, **04**: 472
Ribosomes, range of weights, **08**: 424
O_2' (3')-Ribosyladenosine
isolation and detection of, in RNA, general remarks, **03**:
236
RNA, various, natural occurrence in, **03**: 221
6-Ribosylaminoisocytosine, 5-*N*-methylformamido-
physical constants and spectral properties, **03**: 116
6-Ribosylaminoisocytosine 3'(2')-phosphate derivatives
physical constants and spectral properties, index to, **03**:
74
6-Ribosylaminopyrimidine, 2-Amino-4-hydroxy-5-*N*-
methylformamido
physical constants and spectral properties, **03**: 116
Ribosylpurine
molal osmotic coefficients, **03**: 528

Ribosylthymine 5'-diphosphate
physical constants and spectral properties, **03**: 192
Ribosylthymine 3'(2')-phosphate
physical constants and spectral properties, **03**: 191
Ribosylthymine 5'-phosphate
physical constants and spectral properties, **03**: 192
Ribosylthymine and nucleoside derivatives
physical constants and spectral properties, index to, **03**: 71
5-Ribosyluracil
physical constants and spectral properties, **03**: 136
5-Ribosyluracil 5'-diphosphate
physical constants and spectral properties, **03**: 194
5-Ribosyluracil 3'(2')-phosphate
physical constants and spectral properties, **03**: 193
5-Ribosyluracil 5'-phosphate
physical constants and spectral properties, **03**: 194
Ribosylzeatin
physical constants and spectral properties, **03**: 140
Ribothymidine
physical constants and spectral properties, **03**: 131
Ribothymidine, O_2'-Methyl-
physical constants and spectral properties, **03**: 134
L-Ribulokinase
amino acid composition, incomplete data, **07**: 514
molar absorptivity and-or absorbance values, **02**: 506
subunit, constitution of, **02**: 333
Ribulose 1,5-diphosphate carboxylase
amino acid composition, complete data, **07**: 510
L-Ribulose 5-phosphate 4-epimerase
amino acid composition, complete data, **07**: 510
Ribulose diphosphate carboxylase
average hydrophobicity value, **01**: 231
Ricin; origin, structure, and characteristic as protein biosynthesis inhibitor, **04**: 598
Rickettsia (Coxiella)
G + C composition of DNA of, table arranged by specie, **04**: 165
Rickettsiaceae
G + C composition of DNA of, table arranged by genera and specie, **04**: 165
O-rings, millipore, chemical compatibility, **08**: 431-432
RNA, *see* Nucleic acids, Transfer RNA, TRNA (TRNA)
chain termini in partially hydrolyzed, discussion of, **03**: 403
content in subunits of ribosomes from various sources, **04**: 472
controlled partial hydrolysis of, discussion, **03**: 402-404
double-stranded, molar residue ellipticity, **03**: 601
double-stranded, molar residue rotation, **03**: 599
double helices at atomic resolution, geometry of, **04**: 463-469
extinction coefficients for single-strand types, **03**: 589
fluorescent dyes bound to, data tables, **04**: 470
hydrolysis, limited, conditions for, **03**: 404
molecular weights for several, **04**: 406-408
nucleosides, modified, natural occurrence in various, **03**: 216-233
nucleotide sequences and models for several, **04**: 324-349
oligonucleotides, circular dichroism parameters, **03**: 461-465
oligonucleotides, optical rotatory dispersion parameters, **03**: 450-458
physical properties, of, **04**: 405-410
polynucleotide double helices with Watson-Crick base pairs
atomic coordinates and molecular conformations for, **04**: 411-422
protein (wt %) in ribosomes from various sources, **04**: 472
raman spectral changes observed on melting, **03**: 545
ribosomal
chloroplast, base composition, **04**: 361-362
cytoplasmic, base composition, **04**: 361-362
molecular weights of some, **04**: 408
nucleotide composition of high molecular weight types, **04**: 409
nucleotide sequence data 5 S RNA from *Escherichia coli*, **04**: 473
5S type, nucleotide sequences for several, **04**: 324-327
5S type from *E. coli*, secondary structure model, **04**: 328
5.85 type from yeast, nucleotide sequence model, **04**: 330
ribosome binding sites, sequences, **04**: 354
sedimentation coefficient for several, **04**: 406-407
size of, Flory-Fox equation for, **04**: 405
structure, secondary, for *E. coli* 5S type, **04**: 328
synthesis; pathways chart, **04**: insert
transfer type, *see also* Transfer RNA, TRNA (TRNA)
classes of sequences, **04**: 424-425
"cloverleaf" secondary configuration, generalized representation, **04**: 423
comparison of homology from prokaryotic and eukaryotic origins, **04**: 426
nucleoside composition of tables of values, **04**: 428-441
nucleoside in secondary structure; indentification, location, distribution, **04**: 427
nucleotide sequences, tables, **04**: 442-453
structure, three-dimensional, yeast phenylalanine transfer RNA, **04**: 457-461
viral
bacteriophage types, nucleotide sequences and models, **04**: 337-344
code word table for the coat protein gene, **04**: 340
nucleotide composition of some, **04**: 410
viral, buoyant density values, $Cs_2 SO_4$ gradient, **03**: 569
virus-induced
nucleotide sequences and models, **04**: 346-349
RNA nucleotidyltransferase
amino acid composition, complete data, **07**: 510
circular dichroism in the UV region, **07**: 123
optical rotatory dispersion
UV region, **07**: 75
visible and near UV regions, **07**: 35
RNA polymerase, *see* RNA, nucleotidyltransferase
enzymatic activity, subcellular fractions, **02**: 700-701
molar absorptivity and-or absorbance values, **02**: 504
subunit, constitution of, **02**: 347-350
RNase A, *see* Ribonuclease I

RNase B
optical rotatory dispersion in the visible and near UV
regions, **07**: 35
RNase M, *see* Ribonuclease II
RNase S, *see* Ribonuclease S
RNase T, *see* Guanyloribonuclease
Roseanine
physical and chemical properties, **01**: 146
Rotation, mean residue, *see* Mean residue rotation
Rotation, molar, *see* Molar rotation
Rotation, molar residue, *see* Molar residue rotation
Rothia
G + C composition of DNA of, table arranged by specie, **04**: 76
Rotors for density gradient centrifugation, centrifugal
force chart, **08**: 433
Rubradirin; origin, structure, and characteristic as protein
biosynthesis inhibitor, **04**: 599
Rubredoxin
amino acid composition, complete data, **07**: 510
amino acid sequence, **07**: 429
average hydrophobicity value, **01**: 231
circular dichroism in the UV region, **07**: 123
molar absorptivity and-or absorbance values, **02**: 506
nomenclature recommendations, **02**: 89-90, 120
optical rotatory dispersion in the UV region, **07**: 75
table of cofactors, molecular weights, stoichiometry and
sources, **02**: 278
Rubredoxin reductase
molar absorptivity and-or absorbance values, **02**: 507

S

30S Ribosomal protein
amino acid composition, incomplete data, **07**: 514
Saccharin
pK'_a values, **06**: 347
Saccharin, ligands binding to plasma albumin, **02**: 574
Saccharomyces
amino acid requirements for growth, table, **04**: 643
G + C composition of DNA of, table arranged by specie, **04**: 217-218
Saccharomyces cerevisiae
amino acid requirements for growth, table, **04**: 643
DNA base composition, **04**: 239
DNA content per cell for various, table, **04**: 284
G + C composition of, **04**: 217
genetic map, **04**: 765-766
genetic markers, **04**: 771-826
genetic markers, table, index by gene, **04**: 767-770
haploid chromosome numbers, **04**: 874
mitochondrial DNA, properties, **04**: 367
Saccharopine
physical and chemical properties, **01**: 151
saccharopinuria, effect of, **01**: 321
Saccharopinuria
characteristics of, **01**: 321
Sacromycin, physicochemical constants, spectral, chemotherapeutic and biological properties, **03**: 379
Salmonella
amino acid requirements for growth, table, **04**: 638

G + C composition of DNA of, table arranged by specie, **04**: 113
lipopolysaccharides of
sugar composition for O-group, **05**: 396-399
sugar sequences, general structures, **05**: 403-406, 409,
412
standard media for growth of, **04**: 649
Salmonella typhimurium
deoxyribonucleic acids from, purine and pyrimidine distribution in, **04**: 247
DNA content per cell, **04**: 285
G + C composition of, **04**: 113
genetic markers, list of, **04**: 705-717
linkage map, **04**: 704
Salt solutions
density calculation, coefficients for, from refractive indexes, **06**: 424
density gradient at equilibrium for some, **06**: 424
density values for some used for density gradients, **06**:
425
viscosities for some used for density gradients, **06**: 425
Sangivamycin, physicochemical constants, spectral,
chemotherapeutic and biological properties, **03**: 381
Saponification value
fats and oils, table of values, **05**: 502-503
vegetable oils, **05**: 512
Saprolegnia
G + C composition of DNA of, table arranged by specie, **04**: 219
Sapromyces
G + C composition of DNA of, table arranged by specie, **04**: 219
Saprospira
G + C composition of DNA of, table arranged by specie, **04**: 171
Sarcina
G + C composition of DNA of, table arranged by spe-
cie, **04**: 134-135
Sarcosine
pK'_a values, **06**: 319
physical and chemical properties, **01**: 151
sarcosinemia, effect of, **01**: 321
structure and symbols for those incorporated into syn-
thetic polypeptides, **01**: 107
Sarcosinemia
characteristics of, **01**: 321
Sarkomycin origin, structure, and characteristic as protein
biosynthesis inhibitor, **04**: 599
Sartorya
G + C composition of DNA of, table arranged by spe-
cie, **04**: 219
Satellite DNA, *see* DNA
Scenedesmus
G + C composition of DNA of, table arranged by spe-
cie, **04**: 227
Scheraga-Mandelkern equation for sedimentation-
viscosity molecular weights, **04**: 405
Schizomycetes
DNA content per cell for various, table, **04**: 284
Schizophyllum
G + C composition for DNA of, table arranged by
specie, **04**: 219

Schizosaccharomyces
  G + C composition of DNA of, table arranged by specie, **04:** 219
Schwanniomyces
  G + C composition of DNA of, table arranged by specie, **04:** 219
Sclerotinia
  G + C composition of DNA of, table arranged by specie, **04:** 219
Scopolamine
  pK'_a values, **06:** 327
Scopulariopsis
  G + C composition of DNA of, table arranged by specie, **04:** 219-220
Secretin
  amino acid sequence, **07:** 376
Sedimentation coefficient
  calculation of, and use of gradient methods for data, **06:** 426-431
  glycoproteins
    plasma, human, table of values, **02:** 258
  intrinsic, contractile proteins, **02:** 306
  β_2 microglobulin, **02:** 305
  myosins, nonmuscle, table of values, **02:** 317
  proteins
    carbohydrates, index to studies containing, **02:** 232
    fibrous, index to studies containing, **02:** 229
    globular, index to studies containing, **02:** 222-228
    organelles, index to studies containing, **02:** 232
    particles, index to studies containing, **02:** 232
    plasma, human, table of values, **02:** 242-250
    serum, vertebrate, table of values, **02:** 230-231
    virus, index to studies containing, **02:** 232
  retinol-binding protein, **02:** 304
  Tamm-Horsfall mucoprotein, **02:** 304
  urokinase, **02:** 302
Sedimentation coefficient of some RNA molecules, **04:** 406-407
Sedimentation velocity
  discussion and calculations, **06:** 426-427
Selenocystathionine
  physical and chemical properties, **01:** 158
Selenocystine
  physical and chemical properties, **01:** 158
Selenomethionine
  antagonism to methionine, **01:** 178
  physical and chemical properties, **01:** 158
Selenomethylselenocysteine
  physical and chemical properties, **01:** 158
Sellmeier constants, concentration dependence values for several compounds, **06:** 395
Sephadex® filtration media, table of properties, **08:** 133-134
Sepharose® filtration media, table of properties, **08:** 135
Sequence-rule procedure in nomenclature of fundamental stereochemistry, **01:** 50-63, **02:** 50-58, **03:** 42-50, **04:** 42-50, **05:** 47-55, **06:** 49, **08:** 49-57
Sequence data
  histones, table for several, **02:** 295-299
Sequence rule, use of in nomenclature, **02:** 65-67
Sequential polypeptides, *see* Polypeptides, sequential

Ser, Ile oxytocin
  amino acid sequence, **07:** 194-195
Serine
  active site peptides, **07:** 186
  antagonism to α alanine, **01:** 177
  antagonism to threonine, **01:** 179
  antagonists of, **01:** 179
  destruction of, during acid hydrolysis, **02:** 206
  far ultraviolet absorption spectra
    aqueous solution at pH 5, **01:** 184
    neutral water, table, **01:** 185
    0.1 *M* sodium dodecyl sulfate, table, **01:** 185
  free acid in amniotic fluid in early pregnancy and at term, **01:** 327
  free acid in blood plasma of newborn infants and adults, **01:** 328
  nucleoside composition, tables of values, **04:** 438-439
  nucleotide sequences of, **04:** 450-451
  pK'_a values, **06:** 319
  physical and chemical properties, **01:** 128
  requirements of, for growth of various microorganisms, table, **04:** 630-643
  specific rotatory dispersion constants, 0.1 *M* solution, **01:** 244
  spectra, far UV, **01:** 184
  symbols for atoms and bonds in side chains, **01:** 69, **02:** 73
  thumbprint, content in, **08:** 121
D-Serine
  antagonism to β-Alanine, **01:** 177
Serine dehydratase
  molar absorptivity and-or absorbance values, **02:** 507
  subunit, constitution of, **02:** 328
D-Serine dehydratase
  average hydrophobicity value, **01:** 231
  molar absorptivity and-or absorbance values, **02:** 507
L-Serine hydroxamate, characteristic as protein biosynthesis inhibitor, **04:** 599
Serine proteases, trypsin-related
  amino acid sequence data, index to
    blood clotting factors, **07:** 350-354
    explanation of tables, **07:** 340-341
    sequence alignments, **07:** 341-349
Serine proteases active, bearing the active site serine
  alignments of the chains of, **07:** 344-349
Serine transacetylase
  amino acid composition, incomplete data, **07:** 514
Serotypic antigen 51A
  amino acid composition, incomplete data, **07:** 514
Serratamolide
  proton NMR and suggested conformations, **07:** 563
Serratia
  G + C composition of DNA of, table arranged by specie, **04:** 114
Serum, human, *see also* Human serum
Serum albumin
  amino acid composition, complete data, **07:** 510
  amino acid sequence, **07:** 497
  heat capacity and entropy values, **06:** 110
  viscosity, intrinsic, **02:** 721
Serum antibodies
  methods for detection, **07:** 543-544

Serum content
  retinol-binding protein, **02:** 304
Serum proteins
  vertebrate, sedimentation coefficients, table, **02:** 230-231
Shape, Tamm-Horsfall mucoprotein, **02:** 304
Sheep
  mitochondrial DNA from, properties, **04:** 371
Shethna flavoprotein
  circular dichroism at maxima in near UV region, at
    room temperature, **07:** 161
Shigella
  amino acid requirements for growth, table, **04:** 638
  G + C composition of DNA of, table arranged by spe-
    cie, **04:** 114
Shikimic acid kinase
  Neurospora crassa mutant, **04:** 745
Short neurotoxins, *see* Neurotoxins short
Showdomycin, physicochemical constants, spectral,
  chemotherapeutic and biological properties, **03:** 383
Showdomycin; origin, structure, and characteristic as
  protein biosynthesis inhibitor, **04:** 599
SI units and their symbols, **06:** 106
Sialic acid, content of, in glycoproteins, **02:** 258-269,
  271-274
Sialic acid, generic term usage, **05:** 10
Side chains, *see also* Chains
Siderophilin
  molar absorptivity and-or absorbance values, **02:** 507
Silk fibroin
  circular dichroism in the UV region, **07:** 123
  optical rotatory dispersion
    UV region, **07:** 75
    visible and near UV regions, **07:** 35
Simian virus 40, nucleotide sequences, **04:** 351-353
Siomycin; origin, structure, and characteristic as protein
  biosynthesis inhibitor, **04:** 600
Siromycin, *see* Toyocamycin
Snake venom toxins, *see* Toxins, snake venom
Sodium benzylpenicillin
  UV spectra, formula, molecular weight, **08:** 157
Sodium fluoride; structure and characteristic as protein
  biosynthesis inhibitor, **04:** 600
Solidification point
  fats and oils, table of values, **05:** 502-503
Solubility
  amino acids in water, equations and coefficient values
    for several, **06:** 107-108
  amino acids in water at various temperatures, **06:** 115
  antibiotics, nucleoside, **03:** 271-393
  fatty acids, **05:** 485-491
  fatty acids in water, table of values, **05:** 495
  lipids in chlorinated hydrocarbon mixtures with 33%
    methanol, **05:** 514
  lipids in chlorinated hydrocarbon solvents, **05:** 514
  lipids in organic solvents, **05:** 512
  poly(α-amino acids), table, **01:** 393-396
  triglycerides, mixed triacid, table of values, **05:** 497
  triglycerides, simple saturated, table of values, **05:** 496
  water in saturated fatty acids, table of values, **05:** 495
Solubilizers, table of detergent properties, **08:** 216
Solvents, mixed, for use in low temperature biochemistry
  density table for several, **06:** 520

dielectric constants and freezing points
  N,N-dimethylformamide-water mixtures, **06:** 528
  dimethylsulfoxide-water mixtures, **06:** 527
  ethylene glycol-methanol-water mixtures, **06:** 528
  ethylene glycol-water mixtures, **06:** 522
  glycerol-water mixtures, **06:** 526
  methanol-water mixtures, **06:** 523
  2-methyl-2-4-pentanediol-water mixtures, **06:** 524
  1-2-propanediol-water mixtures, **06:** 525
  ethylene glycol-methanol-water mixtures, viscosity, **06:**
    521
Sorangiaceae
  G + C composition of DNA of, table arranged by spe-
    cie, **04:** 166
Sorangium
  G + C composition of DNA of, table arranged by spe-
    cie, **04:** 166
Sordaria
  G + C composition of DNA of, table arranged by spe-
    cie, **04:** 220
Soret band data
  hemin and hematin spectra in ether, **08:** 279
  metalloporphyrins, **08:** 279
  metalloporphyrins in organic solvents, **08:** 278
  porphyrin dications in aqueous HCl, **08:** 269-271
  porphyrins in organic solvents, **08:** 273-274
  pyridine hemochrome spectra, **08:** 280
Soybean leghemoglobin, *see* Leghemoglobin, soybean,
  aligned chains
Soybean 7S globulin, *see* γ-Conglycinin
Soybean 11S globulin, *see* Glycinin
Soybean trypsin inhibitor
  refractive index increments, **02:** 380
Soybean trypsin inhibitor F_3
  amino acid composition, complete data, **07:** 510
Spadicoides
  G + C composition of DNA of, table arranged by spe-
    cie, **04:** 220
Sparsomycin, A, physicochemical constants, spectral,
  chemotherapeutic and biological properties, **03:** 385
Sparsomycin; origin, structure, and characteristic as
  protein biosynthesis inhibitor, **04:** 600
Specific activity
  enzymes, defined, **02:** 109
Specific gravity
  acids, commercial strength, **06:** 384
  bases, commercial strength, **06:** 384
  fats and oils, table of values, **05:** 502-503
  fatty acids, **05:** 485-491
  liquids, table of values, **06:** 411-414
  plastics, commercial, **08:** 427
Specific rotation
  aldaric acids, **05:** 168-170
  alditols, amino, **05:** 148-149
  alditols, natural, **05:** 139-142
  aldonic acids, **05:** 153-164
  aldoses, natural, **05:** 181-217
  amino sugar acids, **05:** 170-176
  amino sugars, naturally occurring, **05:** 359-370
  carbohydrate phosphate esters, **05:** 253-258, 262-273
  disaccharides, **05:** 283-297, 327-334
  heptasaccharides, **05:** 318-319, 345-346

Specific rotation *(continued)*
   hexasaccharides, **05**: 316-318, 344-345
   inosamines, **05**: 148-149
   inositols, **05**: 142-147
   inososes, **05**: 147
   ketoses, natural, **05**: 226-239
   mucopolysaccharides, **05**: 356-357
   nucleosides, index to table of values, **03**: 69-72
   nucleotides, index to table of values, **03**: 72-75
   octasaccharides, **05**: 319, 346
   oligosaccharides, **05**: 283-319, 327-346
   pentasaccharides, **05**: 315-316, 343-344
   polysaccharides, table of values, **02**: 686-687
   purines, index to table of values, **03**: 67-69
   pyrimides, index to table of values, **03**: 67-69
   steroids, table, **05**: 531-588
   tetrasaccharides, **05**: 308-314, 340-343
   trisaccharides, **05**: 297-308, 334-340
   uronic acids, **05**: 165-168
Specific rotatory dispersion constants
   0.1 *M* amino acid solutions, table, **01**: 244
Specific volume
   fatty acids from C_8 to C_{12}, **05**: 492
Specificity
   lectins, purified, table of values, **02**: 546-551
   protein modification, table for reagents used in, **02**: 203-204
   proteinase inhibitors
     animal sources, **02**: 618-641
     microbial sources, **02**: 661-662
     plant sources, **02**: 586-600
   trypsin toward synthetic substrates, **02**: 211
Specificity, for glycohydrolase reactions, table, **05**: 426-445
Spectinomycin; origin, structure, and characteristic as protein biosynthesis inhibitor, **04**: 601
Spectra
   difference
     acid vs. neutral of tyrosine, tryptophan and phenylalanine, **01**: 191
     alkaline vs. neutral of tyrosine, tryptophan and phenylalanine, **01**: 190
   pyrrolidides of monosaturated fatty acids, key fragments, **05**: 506
   transmission limits of common ions, **08**: 196
Spectral data, *see also* IR spectra, PMR spectra, UV spectra, Circular dichroism
   acidic
     nucleosides, index to table of values, **03**: 69-72
     nucleotides, index to table of values, **03**: 72-75
     purines, index to table of values, **03**: 67-69
     pyrimides, index to table of values, **03**: 67-69
   alkaline
     nucleosides, index to table of values, **03**: 69-72
     nucleotides, index to table of values, **03**: 72-75
     purines, index to table of values, **03**: 67-69
     pyrimides, index to table of values, **03**: 67-69
   circular dichroism, of representative naturally occurring nucleic acids, **03**: 591
   neutral
     nucleosides, index to table of values, **03**: 69-72
     nucleotides, index to table of values, **03**: 72-75
     purines, index to table of values, **03**: 67-69
     pyrimides, index to table of values, **03**: 67-69
Spectrin, human erythrocytes
   molar absorptivity and-or absorbance values, **02**: 508
Spectrophotometers
   circular dichroism, modern design of, **08**: 201-202
Spectrophotometers, calibration techniques for, **06**: 390
Spectrophotometric determination, protein concentration, short-wavelength UV, **08**: 197
Spectropolarimeters, calibration techniques for, **06**: 390
Sperm whale myoglobin
   conformation, three-dimensional, **02**: 760
Sphaerophorus
   G + C composition of DNA of, table arranged by specie, **04**: 87
Sphaerotilus
   G + C composition of DNA of, table arranged by specie, **04**: 95
Sphingoglycolipids, nomenclature and classification, **05**: 416-421
Sphingolipid, generic term usage, **05**: 9
Sphingolipids, stereospecific nomenclature, **05**: 10
Sphingomyelin, generic term usage, **05**: 10
Spiramycin I, II, and III; origin, structure, and characteristic asprotein biosynthesis inhibitor, **04**: 601
Spirillaceae
   G + C composition of DNA of, table arranged by genera and specie, **04**: 166-171
Spirillospora
   G + C composition of DNA of, table arranged by specie, **04**: 77
Spirilloxanthin
   UV spectra, formula, molecular weight, **08**: 193
Spirillum
   G + C composition of DNA of, table arranged by specie, **04**: 168-169
Spirochaeta
   G + C composition of DNA of, table arranged by specie, **04**: 172
Spirochaetaceae
   G + C composition of DNA of, table arranged by genera and specie, **04**: 171-172
Spirogyra
   G + C composition of DNA of, table arranged by specie, **04**: 227
Spirosoma
   G + C composition of DNA of, table arranged by specie, **04**: 182
Spirostans
   names, new standard vs. old, **05**: 69-70
   steroid nomenclature, use of term, **05**: 66-68
   structures, **05**: 67, 70
Spizizen's minimal salts, preparation of, **04**: 649
Spleen acid DNase B, *see* Deoxyribonuclease II-B
Spondylocladium
   G + C composition of DNA of, table arranged by specie, **04**: 220
Spongipellis (Polyporus)
   G + C composition of DNA of, table arranged by specie, **04**: 220
Sporangiomycin; origin, structure, and charateristic as protein biosynthesis inhibitor, **04**: 602

Sporobolomyces
  G + C composition of DNA of, table arranged by specie, **04:** 220-221
Sporocytophaga
  G + C composition of DNA of, table arranged by specie, **04:** 146
Sporomia
  G + C composition of DNA of, table arranged by specie, **04:** 221
Sporotrichum
  G + C composition of DNA of, table arranged by specie, **04:** 221
Stachybotrys
  G + C composition of DNA of, table arranged by specie, **04:** 221
Stachydrine
  physical and chemical properties, **01:** 164
Staphylococci
  amino acid requirements for growth, table, **04:** 638
Staphylococcus
  G + C composition of DNA of, table arranged by specie, **04:** 128-134
Staphylococcus aureus nuclease
  luminescence of, table, **01:** 206
Staphylomycin M$_1$ (PA114A), *see* Osteogrycin A, Virginiamycin M$_1$, **04:** 602
Staphylomycin® S; origin, structure and characteristic as protein biosynthesis inhibitor, **04:** 602
Stellacyanin
  amino acid composition, incomplete data, **07:** 514
  carbohydrate content, **02:** 270
  molar absorptivity and-or absorbance values, **02:** 508
Stem bromelain, *see* Bromelain (stem)
Stem names in carbohydrate nomenclature, **05:** 103
Stemphylium
  G + C composition of DNA of, table arranged by specie, **04:** 221
Stendomycidine
  physical and chemical properties, **01:** 146
Stendomycin
  proton NMR and suggested conformations, **07:** 564
Stereo drawings of several proteins, **02:** 761, 763, 766
Stereochemistry, carotenoid nomenclature, **06:** 71-73, **08:** 72-73
Stereochemistry, fundamental, IUPAC rules for, nomenclature, **08:** 20-57
Stereochemistry, fundamental, IUPAC rules for nomenclature, **01:** 21-58, **02:** 21-58, **03:** 13-50, **05:** 18-55, **06:** 20
Stereochemistry, fundamental; IUPAC rules for nomenclature, **04:** 13-50
Stereoformulas, use of, **01:** 46-48, **02:** 46-48, **04:** 38-40, **05:** 43-45, **06:** 45, **08:** 45-47
Stereospecific nomenclature, lipids, **05:** 10
Steroid Δ-isomerase
  circular dichroism in the UV region, **07:** 123
Steroid alkaloids, nomenclature rules, **05:** 83-85
Steroid derivatives, nomenclature rules, **05:** 71-73
Steroids
  ligands binding to plasma albumin, **02:** 563
  nomenclature, IUPAC rules for, **05:** 56-88
  nomenclature, journal references for, **02:** 87

pK'_a values, **06:** 348
  structures and properties, **05:** 531-558
Sterol, structures and properties, **05:** 544-558
Stizolobic acid
  physical and chemical properties, **01:** 147
Stizolobinic acid
  physical and chemical properties, **01:** 147
Stokes radius
  myosins, nonmuscle, table of values, **02:** 317
Strand separation
  mitochondrial DNAs, table, **04:** 363-372
Strand separation in viral DNA molecules, **03:** 551-556
Streptavidin
  circular dichroism at maxima in near-UV region, at room temperature, **07:** 161
  circular dichroism in the UV region, **07:** 124
  optical rotatory dispersion in the UV region, **07:** 75
Streptimidone; origin, structure, and characteristic as protein biosynthesis inhibitor, **04:** 602
Streptobacillus
  G + C composition of DNA of, table arranged by specie, **04:** 87
Streptococcal proteinase
  amino acid sequence, **07:** 356-357
Streptococci
  amino acid requirements for growth, table, **04:** 638
Streptococcus
  G + C composition of DNA of, table arranged by specie, **04:** 123-126
Streptogramin A; origin, structure, and characteristic as protein biosynthesis inhibitor, **04:** 603
Streptogramin B$_1$; origin, structure, and characteristic as protein biosynthesis inhibitor, **04:** 603
Streptokinase
  amino acid composition, complete data, **07:** 510
  average hydrophobicity value, **01:** 231
  circular dichroism in the UV region, **07:** 124
  cyanogen bromide cleavage, **02:** 199
  molar absorptivity and-or absorbance values, **02:** 508
Streptolidine
  physical and chemical properties, **01:** 147
Streptomyces
  G + C composition of DNA of, table arranged by specie, **04:** 172-177
Streptomyces coelicolor
  G + C composition coelicolor, **04:** 173
  genetic markers, list, **04:** 724-727
  linkage map, **04:** 723
Streptomycetaceae
  G + C composition of DNA of, table arranged by genera and specie, **04:** 172-177
Streptomycin; origin, structure, and characteristic as protein biosynthesis inhibitor, **04:** 604
Streptonigrin; origin, structure, and characteristic as protein biosynthesis inhibitor, **04:** 604
Streptosporangium
  G + C composition of DNA of, table arranged by specie, **04:** 78
Streptoverticillium
  G + C composition of DNA of, table arranged by specie, **04:** 177

Streptovitacin A; origin, structure, and characteristic as protein biosynthesis inhibitor, **04:** 605

Structural formula
amino acids, naturally occurring, table, **01:** 111-166

Structure
antibiotics, nucleoside, **03:** 271-393
ascorbic acid and ascorbate-2-sulfate, **08:** 281
biologically interesting compounds, **08:** 144-195
nucleosides, index to table of values, **03:** 69-72
nucleotides, index to table of values, **03:** 72-75
porphyrins, **08:** 268-269
prostaglandin analogs, **08:** 396-421
prostaglandin biosynthesis intermediates, thromboxanes and by-products, **08:** 334-340
prostaglandin metabolites, **08:** 368-391
prostaglandin precursors, **08:** 325
prostaglandins, naturally occurring, **08:** 346-358
purines, index to table of values, **03:** 67-69
pyridoxine, pyridoxal and pyridoxamine derivatives, **08:** 252-266
pyrimides, index to table of values, **03:** 67-69
thymine, homodimers, **03:** 52
α,β-unsaturated amino acids, structure and properties, table, **01:** 175
vitamins, **08:** 284-300

Structures
carbohydrates, IUPAC rules for nomenclature, **05:** 100-136
cyclitols, IUPAC rules for nomenclature, **05:** 91-98
glycolipids of bacteria, **05:** 373-393
physical data and characteristics, **02:** 254-255
proteins, drawings of several, **02:** 760-766
stereochemistry, fundamental, IUPAC rules, **05:** 18-55
steroids, IUPAC rules for nomenclature, **05:** 56-88
steroids, table, **05:** 531-588

Strychnine
pK'_a values, **06:** 327

Styrene-acronitrile, chemical and physical properties, **08:** 427

Styrylacetic acid
antagonism to trypotophan, **01:** 179

Substrate concentration
enzyme kinetics, definition, **02:** 112

Substrate constant
enzyme kinetics, definition, **02:** 112

Substrate specificity
myosins, nonmuscle, table of values, **02:** 319

Substrates used in glycohydrolase reactions, **05:** 426-445

Subtilisin
amino acid composition, complete data, **07:** 510
amino acid sequences of proteins, **07:** 312
circular dichroism
UV and near-UV region, **07:** 124, 161
conformation, stereo pair illustrating, **02:** 763
enzymatic hydrolysis, conjugated proteins, **02:** 211
enzymatic hydrolysis of proteins, **02:** 209
molar absorptivity and-or absorbance values, **02:** 508
optical rotatory dispersion in the UV region: extrema between 185 and 250 NM^3, **07:** 75
specificity for hydrolysis of peptide bonds, **02:** 221

Subtilisin, Thiol-
molar absorptivity and-or absorbance values, **02:** 508

Subtilisin BPN'
circular dichroism in the UV region, **07:** 124
molar absorptivity and-or absorbance values, **02:** 508
optical rotatory dispersion
UV region, **07:** 75
visible and near UV regions, **07:** 36

Subtilisin BPN, average hydrophobicity value, **01:** 231

Subtilisin carlsberg
luminescence of, table, **01:** 207

Subtilopeptidase A, *see* Subtilisin

Subunit composition
myosins, nonmuscle, table of values, **02:** 317

Subunit constitution, proteins
index, alphabetical, to table, **02:** 352-360
table of data, **02:** 326-351

Subunit content
lectins, purified, **02:** 546-551

Subunit size
Tamm-Horsfall mucoprotein, **02:** 304

Subunit structures
dogfish lactate dehydrogenase, illustration, **02:** 766
porcine malate dehydrogenase, illustration, **02:** 766
transamidase, purified, **02:** 681

Succinamic acid
structure and symbols for those incorporated into synthetic polypeptides, **01:** 107

Succinate buffer, preparation of, **06:** 373

Succinic acid
heat of proton ionization, pK, and related thermodynamic quantities, **06:** 250-251

N-Succinyl-α-amino-ϵ-ketopimelic (15) acid
properties of, **01:** 182

Succinyl-CoA synthetase
molar absorptivity and-or absorbance values, **02:** 508
subunit, constitution of, **02:** 337

Succinyl-CoA synthetase (ADP-forming)
circular dichroism in the UV region, **07:** 124

Succinyl coenzyme A synthetase
average hydrophobicity value, **01:** 231

O-Succinylhomoserine
physical and chemical properties, **01:** 128

Sucrose
pK'_a values, **06:** 317
standard solution for calibrating spectropolarimeters, **06:** 390
viral DNA molecules, relative content in, **03:** 551-556
water solutions, viscosity and density tables, **06:** 415-418

Sucrose synthetase
average hydrophobicity value, **01:** 231

Sugar, *see also* Amino sugar

Sugar, neutral, content of in glycoproteins, **02:** 259-274

Sugar and sugar derivatives, use of symbols for, **05:** 8-9

Sugar composition
lipopolysaccharides of gram-negative bacteria, **05:** 396-402

Sugar fermentation, EMB medium for detection of, **04:** 650

Sugar nucleotide
isolation and enzymatic synthesis of, **05:** 446-452

Sugar sequences
lipopolysaccharides of gram-negative bacteria, **05:** 403-412

Sugar unit
  bond lengths and angles, average, **05:** 472
  dimensions, average, **05:** 472
Sulfatase A
  amino acid composition, incomplete data, **07:** 514
Sulfate-binding protein
  amino acid composition, complete data, **07:** 510
Sulfate permease
  Neurospora crassa mutant, **04:** 744
Sulfhydryl protein group, chemical modification of
  reagents used, table of specificities, **02:** 203-204
β-Sulfinyl-α-aminopropionic acid, *see* Cysteine sulfinic
    acid
Sulfite oxidase deficiency
  characteristics of, **01:** 322
Sulfite reductase
  Neurospora crassa mutant, **04:** 748, 750, 753, 755
β-Sulfo-α-amino-propionic acid, *see* Cysteic acid
S-Sulfo-L-cysteine
  sulfite oxidase deficiency, effect of, **01:** 322
Sulfonamides
  ligands binding to plasma albumin, **02:** 568
S-Sulfopepsin
  cyanogen bromide cleavage, **02:** 199
β-Sulfopyruvic acid
  properties of, **01:** 181
Sulfur, *see also* Sulphur
Sulfur metabolism; pathways chart, **04:** wall chart
Sulfur permease-I, conidial type
  Neurospora crassa mutant, **04:** 741
Sulfur permease II
  Neurospora crassa mutant, **04:** 750
Sulfuric acid
  heat of proton ionization, pK, and related thermody-
    namic quantities, **06:** 252
Sulfurous acid
  heat of proton ionization, pK, and related thermody-
    namic quantities, **06:** 252
Sulphur, *see also* Sulfur
Sunflower hull, wax fatty acids composition, **05:** 511
Superoxide dismutase
  amino acid composition, complete data, **07:** 506
  average hydrophobicity value, **01:** 231
  circular dichroism in the UV region: extrema between
    185 and 250 NM³, **07:** 124
    UV and near-UV region, **07:** 94, 124, 161
  optical rotatory dispersion in the UV region, **07:** 55
  subunit, constitution of, **02:** 326, 327
Supports, tables of, used in immobilization of enzymes,
    02: 723-734
Surface areas, pure methyl esters and triglycerides, **05:**
    515
Surface pressures
  fatty acid monolayers, comparison at transition and col-
    lapse, **05:** 518
Surinamine, *see* N-Methyltyrosine
Sweet-sensitive protein
  amino acid composition, incomplete data, **07:** 514
Swine
  MHC designation, **04:** 885
Symbols
  amino acid derivatives, rules, **01:** 79-88

L-amino acids, side chains of, **02:** 73-75
  chemical names, journal reference to rules, **02:** 87
  distinguished from abbreviations, **01:** 7, **02:** 7, **04:** 7, **05:**
    7, **06:** 7, **08:** 7
  enzyme kinetics, description of, **02:** 111-114
  1-letter
    nucleosides, index to table of values, **03:** 67-69
    nucleotides, index to table, **03:** 72-75
    purines, index to table, **03:** 67-69
    pyrimidine photoproducts, proposals for use, **03:** 52,
      53
    pyrimidines, index to table, **03:** 67-69
    use of, **03:** 65
  3-letter
    nucleosides, index to table, **03:** 69-72
    nucleotides, index to table, **03:** 72-75
    purines, index to table, **03:** 67-69
    pyrimidine photoproducts, proposals for use, **03:** 52,
      53
    pyrimidines, index to table, **03:** 67-69
    use of, **03:** 65
    use of, in biochemical nomenclature, **03:** 7-12
  nucleic acids, journal reference to, **02:** 87
  peptides, rules, **01:** 88-90
  polynucleotides, journal references to, **02:** 87
  polypeptide chains, conformation, journal reference, **02:**
    87
  polypeptide chains, nomenclature rules, **01:** 59-73, **02:**
    63-77
  side chains of, L-amino acids, **01:** 69
  thermodynamic, for equilibrium data, **06:** 104-105
  use of, in biochemical nomenclature, **01:** 7-15, **02:** 7-15,
    04: 7-12, **05:** 7-9, 12, **08:** 7
  use of in biochemical nomenclature, **06:** 7
Syncephalastrum
  G + C composition of DNA of, table arranged by spe-
    cie, **04:** 221
Syndrome of ketoacidosis
  characteristics of, **01:** 326
Synergistin® A-1 (PA114-A-1); origin, structure, and
    characteristic as protein biosynthesis inhibitor, **04:**
    605
Synergistin B-1, B-3; origin, structure, and charateristic as
    protein biosynthesis inhibitor, **04:** 606
Synonyms
  disaccharides, **05:** 283-297, 327-334
  heptasaccharides, **05:** 318-319, 345-346
  hexasaccharides, **05:** 316-318, 344-345
  octasaccharides, **05:** 319, 346
  oligosaccharides, **05:** 283-319, 327-346
  pentasaccharides, **05:** 315-316, 343-344
  tetrasaccharides, **05:** 308-314, 340-343
  trisaccharides, **05:** 297-308, 334-340
Synthesis
  peptides by solid phase method, table of characteristics,
    01: 374-390
Synthetases
  definition and nomenclature, **02:** 98
  numbering and classification of, **02:** 108
Synthetic dehydroquinase
  Neurospora crassa mutant, **04:** 745

Synthetic polypeptides, *see* Polypeptides, synthetic, Polypeptides, synthetic

abeo System, nomenclature usage for steroids, **05:** 81-83

Systematic names vs. trivial names, steroid derivatives, **05:** 73

Systematic nomenclature
acyclic aldoses, **05:** 105
carbohydrates, **05:** 102
cyclitols, rules for, **05:** 95-97
steroids, table, **05:** 531-588

T

T2 Toxin; origin, structure, and characteristic as protein biosynthesis inhibitor, **04:** 613

Tabtoxinine
physical and chemical properties, **01:** 129

T-2 Tail sheath
refractive index increments, **02:** 380

Taka-amylase A, *see* α-Amylase
carbohydrate content, **02:** 247

Talaromyces
G + C composition of DNA of, table arranged by specie, **04:** 221-222

Tamm-Horsfall glycoprotein, *see also* Glycoproteins Tamm-Horsfall
amino acid composition, **02:** 303
carbohydrate composition, **02:** 303
carbohydrate content, **02:** 267
protein composition, **02:** 303

Tamm-Horsfall mucoprotein, *see also* Mucoprotein, Tamm-Horsfall

Tamm-Horsfall urinary glycoprotein, *see also* Glycoprotein, Tamm-Horsfall

Tartrate dehydrogenase
amino acid composition, complete data, **07:** 510

Tartrate epoxidase
amino acid composition, complete data, **07:** 510

Tartronic semialdehyde reductase
amino acid composition, complete data, **07:** 510
molar absorptivity and-or absorbance values, **02:** 509

Taurine
free acid in amniotic fluid in early pregnancy and at term, **01:** 327
free acid in blood plasma of newborn infants and adults, **01:** 328
physical and chemical properties, **01:** 158
structure and symbols for those incorporated into synthetic polypeptides, **01:** 107
thumbprint, content in, **08:** 121

Taurocyamine kinase
circular dichroism, **07:** 124
UV and near-UV region, **07:** 161
molar absorptivity and-or absorbance values, **02:** 509
optical rotatory dispersion
UV region, **07:** 75
visible and near UV regions, **07:** 36
subunit, constitution of, **02:** 331

Tautomerases
definition and nomenclature, **02:** 98

Teflon FEP, chemical and physical properties, **08:** 427

Telomycin® (Antibiotic A-128-OP); origin, structure, and characteristic as protein biosynthesis inhibitor, **04:** 607

Telostei
DNA content per cell for various, table, **04:** 293-297

Temperature
data, standardization of, for equilibrium data, **06:** 101
recommended values for measuring equilibrium data, **06:** 94

Temperature coefficient
fatty acids from C_8 to C_{12}, **05:** 492

Temperature midpoint
kinetoplast DNAs, table, **04:** 375-377
mitochondrial DNAs, table, **04:** 363-372

Tenuazonic acid; origin, structure, and characteristic as protein biosynthesis inhibitor, **04:** 607

Terracin, *see* Tetracycline

Terramycin®; origin, structure, and characteristic as protein biosynthesis inhibitor, **04:** 608

Tetanus toxin
molar absorptivity and-or absorbance values, **02:** 509

Tetracycline hydrochloride
UV spectra, formula, molecular weight, **08:** 180

Tetracycline; origin, structure, and characteristic as protein biosynthesis inhibitor, **04:** 608

Tetrahydrofolate dehydrogenase
circular dichroism in the UV region, **07:** 124

1,2,3,6-Tetrahydropyridine-α-carboxylic acid, *see* Baikiain

Tetrahymena
amino acid requirements for growth, table, **04:** 642
G + C composition of DNA of, table arranged by specie, **04:** 229

Tetrapyrrole tables, **08:** 268-280

Tetrasaccharides
chemical formula, **05:** 308-314, 340-343
derivatives, **05:** 308-314, 340-343
melting point, **05:** 308-314, 340-343
specific rotation, **05:** 308-314, 340-343
synonyms, **05:** 308-314, 340-343

Thalassiosira
G + C composition of DNA of, table arranged by specie, **04:** 227

Thallophyta; algae
deoxyribonucleic acids from, purine and pyrimidine distributionin, **04:** 256-257

Thallophyta; fungi
deoxyribonucleic acids from, purine and pyrimidine distribution in, **04:** 242-253

THAM
heat of proton ionization, pK, and related thermodynamic quantities, **06:** 236

Thamnidium
G + C composition of DNA of, table arranged by specie, **04:** 222

Theanine
physical and chemical properties, **01:** 119

Theo-α,β-diaminobutyric acid
physical and chemical properties, **01:** 120

Thermoactinomyces
G + C composition of DNA of, table arranged by specie, **04:** 150

4-Thiouridine disulphide
physical constants and spectral properties, **03:** 128
2-Thiouridine nucleotide derivatives
physical constants and spectral properties, index to, **03:** 74-75
Thraustomycin, physicochemical constants, spectral, chemotherapeutic and biological properties, **03:** 387
Thraustotheca
G + C composition of DNA of, table arranged by specie, **04:** 222
Three-letter symbols
amino acids, table of, **01:** 78, **02:** 62
purines, pyrimidines, nucleosides, and nucleotides, index to table, **03:** 67-65
use of, in nomenclature, **01:** 8, **02:** 8, **03:** 8, **04:** 8
Threo-α-amino-β,$\gamma\gamma$ihydroxybutyric acid
physical and chemical properties, **01:** 122
Threo-β-hydroxyleucine
physical and chemical properties, **01:** 127
Threonine
antagonism to methionine, **01:** 178
antagonism to serine, **01:** 179
antagonists of, **01:** 179
destruction of, during acid hydrolysis, **02:** 206
far ultraviolet absorption spectra
aqueous solution at pH 5, **01:** 184
neutral water, table, **01:** 185
0.1 M sodium dodecyl sulfate, table, **01:** 185
free acid in amniotic fluid in early pregnancy and at term, **01:** 327
free acid in blood plasma of newborn infants and adults, **01:** 328
nucleoside composition, tables of values, **04:** 439
nucleotide sequences of, **04:** 450-451
pK'_a values, **06:** 319
physical and chemical properties, **01:** 129
requirements of, for growth of various microorganisms, table, **04:** 630-643
spectra, far UV, **01:** 184
symbols for atoms and bonds in side chains, **01:** 69, **02:** 73
thumbprint, content in, **08:** 121
Threonine deaminase
amino acid composition, complete data, **07:** 510
molar absorptivity and-or absorbance values, **02:** 509
subunit, constitution of, **02:** 338, 340, 341
Threonine derivatives
heat of proton ionization, pK, and related thermodynamic quantities, **06:** 254-255
N^6-Threoninocarbonyladenosine
composition in various tRNA's, **04:** 428-441
isolation and detection of in RNA, general remarks, **03:** 235
RNA, various, natural occurrence in, **03:** 220
Thrombin
beef
molar absorptivity and-or absorbance values, **02:** 510
human
molar absorptivity and-or absorbance values, **02:** 510
zymogen conversion during coagulation of plasma, **02:** 670

Thrombon
average hydrophobicity value, **01:** 232
Thromboplastin
physical data and characteristics, **02:** 254-255
Thromboxane A
isolation, biological effects, stability, **08:** 337-339
occurrence, structure, molecular weight, **08:** 336,338
Thromboxane B
isolation, biological effects, stability, **08:** 337, 339
occurrence, structure, molecular weight, **08:** 336, 338
Thumbprint, amino acid content, **08:** 121
Thylakoid membrane protein, *see* Membrane protein, thylakoid
Thymidine
chemical structures and approved numbering schemes, **08:** 224
molal osmotic coefficients, **03:** 528
pK'_a values, **06:** 331, 339
Thymidine and derivatives
UV spectra, **03:** 445-446
UV spectral characteristics and acid dissociation constants, **03:** 415
Thymidine and nucleoside derivatives
physical constants and spectral properties, index to, **03:** 72
Thymidine nucleotide derivatives
physical constants and spectral properties, index to, **03:** 75
Thymidylate synthetase
average hydrophobicity value, **01:** 232
circular dichroism in the UV region, **07:** 124
Thymidylic acid
derivatives, UV spectral characteristics and acid dissociation constants, **03:** 416
Thymine
pK'_a values, **06:** 331, 339
Thymine, homodimers of, structures and symbolic representations, **04:** 52-53
Thymine and derivatives
homodimers, structure, **03:** 52
physical constants and spectral properties, index to, **03:** 68
UV spectra, **03:** 431
UV spectral characteristics and acid dissociation constants, **03:** 413
Thymocytes
immunological response, **07:** 536
Thyrocalcitonin
circular dichroism at maxima in near-UV region, at room temperature, **07:** 161
cyanogen bromide cleavage, **02:** 199
Thyroglobulin
amino acid composition, incomplete data, **07:** 514
average hydrophobicity value, **01:** 232
carbohydrate content, **02:** 271-272
cyanogen bromide cleavage, **02:** 199
molar absorptivity and-or absorbance values, **02:** 510
refractive index increments, **02:** 380
subunit, constitution of, **02:** 349
viscosity, intrinsic, **02:** 721

Thyroglobulin (19S)
  optical rotatory dispersion in the visible and near UV regions, **07:** 36
Thyroid stimulating hormone
  amino acid sequence, **07:** 393-397
  beef
    molar absorptivity and-or absorbance values, **02:** 510
  human
    molar absorptivity and-or absorbance values, **02:** 510
Thyroid stimulating hormone-α-chain
  average hydrophobicity value, **01:** 232
Thyroid stimulating hormone-β-chain
  average hydrophobicity value, **01:** 232
Thyrotrophin
  carbohydrate content, **02:** 271-272
Thyrotropin
  circular dichroism at maxima in near-UV region, at room temperature, **07:** 162
  optical rotatory dispersion
    UV region, **07:** 76
    visible and near UV regions, **07:** 36
Thyroxine
  antagonists of, **01:** 179
  physical and chemical properties, **01:** 160
Thyroxine-binding globulin
  amino acid composition, incomplete data, **07:** 514
Thyroxine-binding prealbumin, *see* Prealbumin (thyroxine-binding prealbumin)
Tingitanine, *see* Lathytine
TMV, *see* Tobacco mosaic virus
Tobacco mosaic virus
  amino acid composition, complete data, **07:** 510
  amino acid sequence of coat proteins, **07:** 261-262
  circular dichroism in the UV region, **07:** 125
  location of some amino acid replacements in naturally occurring andchemical induced mutants of, **07:** 266-267
Tobacco mosaic virus, A protein
  circular dichroism in the UV region, **07:** 125
Tobacco mosaic virus protein
  depolymerized, luminescence of, table, **01:** 206
  polymerized, luminescence of, table, **01:** 206
Tobacco mosaic virus protein subunit
  optical rotatory dispersion
    UV region, **07:** 76
    visible and near UV regions, **07:** 36
Tobramycin; origin, structure, and characteristic as protein biosynthesis inhibitor, **04:** 610
Tocinamide
  proton NMR and suggested conformations, **07:** 572
DL-α-Tocopherol, *see also* Vitamin E
  properties, **08:** 289
  UV spectra, formula, molecular weight, **08:** 153-154
DL-α-Tocopheryl acetate, *see also* Vitamin E
  UV spectra, formula, molecular weight, **08:** 155
d-α-Tocopheryl acetate, properties of, **08:** 289
d-α-Tocopheryl acid succinate, properties of, **08:** 290
Toluene derivatives
  heat of proton ionization, pK, and related thermodynamic quantities, **06:** 255-256
Torsion angle
  choice of, in nomenclature, **01:** 62-63, **02:** 66-67

  designation of, **01:** 71, **02:** 75
  peptides of L-amino acids, table of, **01:** 65, **02:** 69
  principal, use of, **02:** 68-75
  principal use of, **01:** 64-71
  regular structures, table, **01:** 66, **02:** 70
Torula
  amino acid requirements for growth, table, **04:** 643
  G + C composition of DNA of, table arranged by specie, **04:** 222
Torulopsis
  G + C composition of DNA of, table arranged by specie, **04:** 223
L-l-Tosylamido-2-phenylethyl choloromethyl ketone (TPCK), origin, structure, and characteristic as protein biosynthesis inhibitor, **04:** 611
Toxicity
  antibiotics, nucleoside, **03:** 271-393
Toxin, *see also* Neurotoxin
  amino acid composition, complete data, **07:** 510
  animal sources, amino acid composition, **02:** 650
  average hydrophobicity values, **01:** 232
  lower animal sources, specificity and properties, **02:** 622-623
  optical rotatory dispersion
    UV region, **07:** 76
    visible and near UV regions, **07:** 36
ε-Toxin
  circular dichroism in the UV region, **07:** 125
  optical rotatory dispersion
    UV region, **07:** 76
    visible and near UV regions, **07:** 36
α-Toxin A
  average hydrophobicity value, **01:** 233
α-Toxin B
  average hydrophobicity value, **01:** 233
Toxin (type A)
  amino acid composition, complete data, **07:** 510
Toxins, angusticeps-type
  from venom of various snakes, amino acid sequence, **07:** 365
Toxins, snake venom, **07:** 360-373
Toxoplasma
  G + C composition of DNA of, table arranged by specie, **04:** 229
Toxotrichum
  G + C composition of DNA of, table arranged by specie, **04:** 223
Toyocamycin, physiocochemical constants, spectral, chemotherapeutic and biological properties, **03:** 390
Tracheophyta
  deoxyribonucleic acids from, purine and pyrimidine distribution in, **04:** 258-261
Tranquilizers
  ligands binding to plasma albumin, **02:** 571
(trans)-α-(Carboxycyclopropyl) glycine
  physical and chemical properties, **01:** 115
Transamidase
  molecular weight, subunit structure, **02:** 681
Transamidase activity
  detection of, **02:** 670
  inhibition of, **02:** 669-674
  sources of, **02:** 671

Transamidase activity *(continued)*
  tissues, list of references, **02:** 680
Transaminase B
  average hydrophobicity value, **01:** 233
Transcortin
  amino acid composition, incomplete data, **07:** 514
  average hydrophobicity value, **01:** 233
  molecular parameters, **02:** 242
  plasma, human
    carbohydrate content, molecular weight, sedimentation coefficients, **02:** 258
    molecular absorptivity and-or absorbance values, **02:** 510
Transfer RNA, *see also* RNA, transfer type; TRNA (TRNA)
Transferase
  definition and nomenclature of, **02:** 96-97
  intramolecular, numbering and classification of, **02:** 108
  numbering and classification of, **02:** 106
Transferrin, *see also* Ovotransferrin
  amino acid composition, complete data, **07:** 510
  average hydrophobicity value, **01:** 233
  carbohydrate content, **02:** 268
  circular dichroism
    UV and near-UV region, **07:** 125, 162
  molecular parameters, **02:** 246
  molecular weight, stoichiometry, source, function, **02:** 276
  optical rotatory dispersion
    UV region, **07:** 76
    visible and near UV regions, **07:** 36
  plasma, human
    carbohydrate content, molecular weights, sedimentation coefficients, **02:** 258
    molar absorptivity and-or absorbance values, **02:** 510
  plasma, nonhuman
    carbohydrate content, **02:** 260
Transglutaminase
  amino acid composition, complete data, **07:** 510
Transketolase
  circular dichroism in the UV region, **07:** 125
  optical rotatory dispersion
    UV region, **07:** 76
    visible and near UV regions, **07:** 36
Translational control RNA; origin, structure, and characteristic as protein biosynthesis inhibitor, **04:** 611
Transplantation laws defined, **04:** 884
Trehalase
  Neurospora crassa mutant, **04:** 742
Tremella
  G + C composition of DNA of, table arranged by specie, **04:** 223
Treponema
  amino acid requirements for growth, table, **04:** 639
  G + C composition of DNA of, table arranged by specie, **04:** 181
Treponemataceae
  G + C composition of DNA of, table arranged by genera and specie, **04:** 180-181
Triacanthine
  physical constants and spectral properties, **03:** 78

Triacylglycerol lipase
  circular dichroism in the UV region, **07:** 125
  optical rotatory dispersion
    UV region, **07:** 76
    visible and near UV regions, **07:** 36
1,2,4-Triazolealanine
  antagonism to histidine, **01:** 178
Trichithecium
  G + C composition of DNA of, table arranged by specie, **04:** 223
Trichoderma
  G + C composition of DNA of, table arranged by specie, **04:** 223
Trichodermin; origin, structure, and characteristic as protein biosynthesis inhibitor, **04:** 611
Trichodermol; origin, structure, and characteristic as protein biosynthesis inhibitor, **04:** 612
Tricholomic acid
  physical and chemical properties, **01:** 147
Trichomonas
  amino acid requirements for growth, table, **04:** 642
  G + C composition of DNA of, table arranged by specie, **04:** 229
Trichophyton
  amino acid requirements for growth, table, **04:** 641
Trichosporon
  G + C composition of DNA of, table arranged by specie, **04:** 223
Trichothecin; origin, structure, and characteristic as protein biosynthesis inhibitor, **04:** 612
Tri(di)acylglycerol, generic term usage, **05:** 9
5',5',5'-Trifluoroleucine
  antagonism to leucine, **01:** 178
Triglycerides, mixed triacid, solubility values, **05:** 497
Triglycerides, simple saturated, solubility values, **05:** 496
Trigonelline
  physical and chemical properties, **01:** 164
Trigonopsis
  G + C composition of DNA of, table arranged by specie, **04:** 223
3,5,3-Triiodothyronine
  physical and chemical properties, **01:** 160
Trimers, proposal for use of abbreviations, **03:** 57
ϵ-N-Trimethyl-ϵ-hydroxylysine betaine
  physical and chemical properties, **01:** 164
2-Trimethylaminoethyl-betaine phosphonic acid
  physical and chemical properties, **01:** 161
(ϵ-Trimethylammonio)caproic acid, *see* ϵ-(Trimethylammonio)hexanoic acid
ϵ-(Trimethylammonio)hexanoic acid
  structure and symbols for those incorporated into synthetic polypeptides, **01:** 107
$N^2,N^2,7$-Trimethylguanosine
  isolation and detection of, in RNA, general remarks, **03:** 239
  RNA, various, natural occurrence in, **03:** 226
ϵ-N-Trimethyllysine betaine
  physical and chemical properties, **01:** 164
Trimethylpyruvic acid
  properties of, **01:** 182
Triosephosphate dehydrogenase
  average hydrophobicity value, **01:** 233

Triosephosphate isomerase
  amino acid composition, complete data, **07:** 510
  amino acid sequences, **07:** 324-326
  average hydrophobicity value, **01:** 233
  optical rotatory dispersion in the visible and near UV
      regions, **07:** 36
Triosephosphate isomerase-I, average hydrophobicity
      values, **01:** 233
Triosephosphate isomerase-III, average hydrophobicity
      values, **01:** 233
Tripeptide synthetase
  amino acid composition, complete data, **07:** 510
TRIS
  heat of proton ionization, pK, and related thermody-
      namic quantities, **06:** 236
Tris buffer
  protonic activity tables, **06:** 529-539
Trisaccharides
  chemical formula, **05:** 297-308, 334-340
  derivatives, **05:** 297-308, 334-340
  melting point, **05:** 297-308, 334-340
  nomenclature rules, **05:** 134-135
  specific rotation, **05:** 297-308, 334-340
  synonyms, **05:** 297-308, 334-340
Tris(hydroxymethyl)-amino methane-maleate (trismaleate)
      buffer, preparation of, **06:** 374
Tris(hydroxymethyl)-aminomethane (tris) buffer, prepara-
      tion of, **06:** 375
Trivial names
  acyclic aldoses, **05:** 103, 105
  carbohydrate nomenclature, **05:** 102-103
  carotenoids, naturally occurring, **08:** 74-90
  coenzymes, **08:** 8-19
  linolenic acid isomers, usage, **08:** 316
  lipids, **05:** 9-12
  porphyrins, **08:** 269
  prostaglandin analogs, **08:** 396-421
  prostaglandin biosynthesis intermediates, thromboxanes
      and by-products, **08:** 334-340
  prostaglandin precursors, **08:** 325
  prostaglandins, naturally occurring, **08:** 346-358
  vitamins, **08:** 8-19
Trivial names, naturally-occurring carotenoids, **06:** 74-90
Trivial names vs. systematic names, steroid derivatives,
      05: 73
tRNA, *see also* RNA, transfer type
Tropine
  pK'_a values, **06:** 327
Tropocollagen
  calorimetric ΔH values accompanying conformational
      changes, **06:** 273
  circular dichroism in the UV region, **07:** 126
Tropoelastin
  circular dichroism in the UV region, **07:** 26
Tropomyosin
  amino acid sequence, **07:** 492
  circular dichroism in the UV region, **07:** 126
  molecular parameters, **02:** 306
  nonmuscle cells, properties, **02:** 321
  optical rotatory dispersion
      UV region, **07:** 76
      visible and near UV regions, **07:** 37

refractive index increments, **02:** 380
  viscosity, intrinsic, **02:** 721
Tropomyosin B
  molar absorptivity and-or absorbance values, **02:** 510
  refractive index increments, **02:** 380
  subunit, constitution of, **02:** 329
Troponin
  circular dichroism in the UV region, **07:** 126
  molar absorptivity and-or absorbance values, **02:** 510
  molecular parameters, **02:** 306
  optical rotatory dispersion
      UV region, **07:** 76
      visible and near UV regions, **07:** 37
  subunit, constitution of, **02:** 331
Troponin-C
  average hydrophobicity value, **01:** 233
Troponin-T
  average hydrophobicity value, **01:** 233
Troponin A, *see* Troponin C
Troponin B, *see* Troponin I and Troponin T
Troponin C
  circular dichroism
      UV and near-UV region, **07:** 126, 162
  optical rotatory dispersion in the visible and near UV
      regions, **07:** 37
Troponin Ca^{++}-binding protein (Tn-C) rabbit skeletal
  amino acid sequence, **07:** 495
Troponin I
  circular dichroism in the UV region, **07:** 127
  optical rotatory dispersion in the visible and near UV
      regions, **07:** 37
Troponin inhibitor (Tn-I), rabbit skeletal
  amino acid sequence, **07:** 494
Troponin T
  circular dichroism in the UV region, **07:** 127
  optical rotatory dispersion in the visible and near UV
      regions, **07:** 37
Trypanosoma
  G + C composition of DNA of, table arranged by spe-
      cie, **04:** 229
Trypsin
  average hydrophobicity value, **01:** 233-234
  bovine
      luminescence of, table, **01:** 206
  calorimetric ΔH values accompanying conformational
      changes, **06:** 270
  circular dichroism, **07:** 127
      UV and near-UV region, **07:** 162
  enzymatic hydrolysis, conjugated proteins, **02:** 211
  enzymatic hydrolysis of proteins, **02:** 209
  molar absorptivity and-or absorbance values, **02:** 510
  optical rotatory dispersion
      UV region, **07:** 77
      visible and near UV regions, **07:** 37
  refractive index increments, **02:** 380
  specificity toward synthetic substrates, **02:** 211
α-Trypsin
  circular dichroism in the UV region, **07:** 127
  optical rotatory dispersion in the UV region, **07:** 77
β-Trypsin
  circular dichroism in the UV region, **07:** 127
  optical rotatory dispersion in the UV region, **07:** 77

Trypsin-kallikrein inhibitor, *see* Trypsin-kininogenin inhibitor

Trypsin-kininogenin inhibitor
circular dichroism in the UV region, **07:** 128

Trypsin, thermophilic *Streptomyces*
circular dichroism in the UV region, **07:** 127
optical rotatory dispersion
UV region, **07:** 77
visible and near UV regions, **07:** 37

Trypsin-Trypsin inhibitor complex
molar absorptivity and-or absorbance values, **02:** 511

Trypsin inhibitor, *see also* Trypsin inhibitors
amino acid composition, complete data, **07:** 510
amino acid sequence, **07:** 500
animal sources, amino acid composition, **02:** 649
average hydrophobicity value, **01:** 234
beef pancreas
molar absorptivity and-or absorbance values, **02:** 511
circular dichroism in the UV region, **07:** 128
inter-α, human
molar absorptivity and-or absorbance values, **02:** 511
legume and grain sources, specificity and properties, **02:** 590-600
lower animal sources, specificity and properties, **02:** 618-621
mammalian organs and secretions, specificities and properties, **02:** 632-641
optical rotatory dispersion
UV region, **07:** 77
visible and near UV regions, **07:** 37
pig pancreas
molar absorptivity and-or absorbance values, **02:** 511
plant sources, amino acid composition, **02:** 607-609
soybean
molar absorptivity and-or absorbance values, **02:** 511

Trypsin inhibitor, basic (kallikrein inactivator)
amino acid composition, complete data, **07:** 510
circular dichroism at maxima in near-UV region, **07:** 163

Trypsin inhibitor, Bowman-Birk
circular dichroism at maxima in near-UV region, at room temperature, **07:** 163

Trypsin inhibitor, Kunitz
circular dichroism at maxima in near-UV region, at room temperature, **07:** 163

Trypsin inhibitor (acidic)
amino acid composition, complete data, **07:** 510

Trypsin inhibitor I, II
average hydrophobicity value, **01:** 234

Trypsin inhibitors, *see also* Trypsin inhibitor
carbohydrate composition, **02:** 666-667

Trypsinogen
amino acid composition, complete data, **07:** 510
anionic, average hydrophobicity value, **01:** 234
average hydrophobicity value, **01:** 234
bovine pancreatic
cyanogen bromide cleavage, **02:** 199
circular dichroism in the UV region, **07:** 128
luminescence of, table, **01:** 206
molar absorptivity and-or absorbance values, **02:** 511
optical rotatory dispersion in the UV region, **07:** 78
refractive index increments, **02:** 380

Tryptophan
N-acetyl-DL-tryptophan methyl ester, UV spectra of, **01:** 192
acid vs. neutral difference spectra, **01:** 191
alkaline vs. neutral difference spectra, **01:** 190-191
antagonism to phenylalanine, **01:** 179
antagonists of, **01:** 179
bond distances and angles for side chain, **08:** 223
far ultraviolet absorption spectra
aqueous solution at pH 5, **01:** 184
neutral water, table, **01:** 185
0.1 *M* sodium dodecyl sulfate, table, **01:** 185
free acid in amniotic fluid in early pregnancy and at term, **01:** 327
free acid in blood plasma of newborn infants and adults, **01:** 328
luminescence of, table, **01:** 200
luminescence of derivatives of, table, **01:** 201-202
molar extinctions, **01:** 185
molecular absorbances of, table, **01:** 188
nucleoside composition, tables of values, **04:** 439
nucleotide sequences of, **04:** 450-451
pK'_a values, **06:** 319
physical and chemical properties, **01:** 147
recovery from various proteins after acid hydrolysis, **02:** 207
requirements of, for growth of various microorganisms, table, **04:** 630-643
spectra, far UV, **01:** 184
symbols for atoms and bonds in side chains, **01:** 71, **02:** 75
tryptophanemia, effect of, **01:** 322
UV absorption characteristics, **01:** 186

Tryptophan betaine, *see* Hypaphorin

Tryptophan oxygenase
amino acid composition, complete data, **07:** 510
molar absorptivity and-or absorbance values, **02:** 511
subunit constitution of, **02:** 335, 339

Tryptophan synthetase
average hydrophobicity values, **01:** 234
cyanogen bromide cleavage, **02:** 199
molar absorptivity and-or absorbance values, **02:** 512
Neurospora crassa mutant, **04:** 745
subunit, constitution of, **02:** 337, 338

Tryptophan synthetase A protein
amino acid composition, complete data, **07:** 510
amino acid sequences of proteins, **07:** 313

Tryptophanase
amino acid composition, complete data, **07:** 510
average hydrophobicity value, **01:** 234
molar absorptivity and-or absorbance values, **02:** 512
subunit, constitution of, **02:** 341, 342

Tryptophanemia
characteristics of, **01:** 322

Tryptophanyl model compounds
near-UV circular dichroism intensities, **07:** 169

Tryptophanyl residues
homology in sequences adjoining active center aspartyl residues and, in pepsin, **07:** 359

Tryptophanyl tRNA synthetase
amino acid composition, complete data, **07:** 510
luminescence of, table, **01:** 206

Tryptophanyl tRNA synthetase *(continued)*
 molar absorptivity and-or absorbance values, **02:** 512
 Neurospora crassa mutant, **04:** 753
 subunit, constitution of, **02:** 330, 334
Tryptozan, *see* α-Amino-β-3 (indazole)-propionic acid
Tuberactidine
 physical and chemical properties, **01:** 147
Tubercidin, physicochemical constants, spectral, chemo-
  therapeutic and biological properties, **03:** 388
Tuberculosis
 G + C composition of DNA of, table arranged by spe-
  cie, **04:** 94
Tubulin (6S microtubule protein)
 circular dichroism in the UV region, **07:** 128
Tubulosine; origin, structure, and characteristic as protein
  biosynthesis inhibitor, **04:** 613
Tunicates
 DNA content per cell, **04:** 293
 satellite DNAs
  buoyant density and G + C content of, table, **04:** 388
Turcine
 physical and chemical properties, **01:** 166
Turnip yellow mosaic virus
 amino acid sequences of virus coat proteins, **07:** 263-265
Turnover number
 deoxynucleotide polymerizing enzymes, tables of values,
  04: 538-540
Tylocrebrine; origin, structure, and characteristic as
  protein biosynthesis inhibitor, **04:** 614
Tylophorine; origin, structure, and characteristic as
  protein biosynthesis inhibitor, **04:** 614
Tylosin; origin, structure, and characteristic as protein bi-
  osynthesis inhibitor, **04:** 615
TYM, *see* Turnip yellow mosaic virus
Tyramine; structure and characteristic as protein biosynthesis inhibitor, **04:** 615
Tyrocidin A
 proton NMR and suggested conformations, **07:** 563
Tyrosinase, *see* Monophenol, monooxygenase
 molecular weights, stoichiometry and sources, **02:** 282
Tyrosinate model compounds
 near-UV circular dichroism intensities, **07:** 171-172
Tyrosine
 N-acetyl-L-tyrosine ethyl ester, UV spectra of, **01:** 194
 N-acetyl-L-tyrosine ethyl ester anion, UV spectra of, **01:**
  195
 acid vs. neutral difference spectra, **01:** 191
 active site peptides, **07:** 187
 alkaline vs. neutral difference spectra, **01:** 190-191
 antagonism to phenylalanine, **01:** 179
 antagonists of, **01:** 180
 destruction of, during acid hydrolysis, **02:** 206
 far ultraviolet absorption spectra
  aqueous solution at pH 5, **01:** 184
  neutral water, table, **01:** 185
  0.1 *M* sodium dodecyl sulfate, table, **01:** 185
 free acid in amniotic fluid in early pregnancy and at
  term, **01:** 327
 free acid in blood plasma of newborn infants and
  adults, **01:** 328
 luminescence of, table, **01:** 200
 luminescence of derivatives of, table, **01:** 202-203

 molar extinctions, **01:** 184
 molecular absorbances of, table, **01:** 187
 nucleoside composition, tables of values, **04:** 440
 nucleotide sequences of, **04:** 452-453
 pK'_a values, **06:** 319
 pK values in various proteins, tables, **02:** 694-695
 requirements of, for growth of various micro-organisms,
  table, **04:** 630-643
 spectra, far UV, **01:** 184
 symbols for atoms and bonds in side chains, **01:** 71, **02:**
  75
 thumbprint, content in, **08:** 121
 tyrosinemia, effect of, **01:** 322
 UV absorption characteristics, **01:** 186
m-Tyrosine
 physical and chemical properties, **01:** 132
 structure and symbols for those incorporated into synthetic polypeptides, **01:** 107
o-Tyrosine
 structure and symbols for those incorporated into synthetic polypeptides, **01:** 107
β-Tyrosine
 physical and chemical properties, **01:** 131
Tyrosine-*O*-sulfate
 physical and chemical properties, **01:** 158
Tyrosine aminotransferase
 amino acid composition, complete data, **07:** 511
Tyrosine derivatives
 heat of proton ionization, pK, and related thermodynamic quantities, **06:** 258
Tyrosine hydroxyphenyl
 physical and chemical properties, **01:** 131
Tyrosinemia
 characteristics of, **01:** 322
Tyrosyl-tRNA synthetase
 average hydrophobicity value, **01:** 234
Tyrosyl model compounds
 near-UV circular dichroism intensities, **07:** 170

U

UDP, *see* Uridylic acid
 pK'_a values, **06:** 331
UDP-D-glucose dehydrogenase, *see* UDPglucose, dehy-
  drogenase
UDPglucose 4-epimerase
 circular dichroism in the UV region, **07:** 128
UDPglucose dehydrogenase, **07:** 128
Ulothrix
 G + C composition of DNA of, table arranged by spe-
  cie, **04:** 227
Ultracentrifuge centerpiece materials
 chemical resistance and other properties, **08:** 428-430
Ultracentrifuge tubes, chemical resistance of plastics used,
  08: 434
Ultraviolet, *see* UV absorption spectra
Ultraviolet spectra, *see* UV spectra, UV spectra, UV spec-
  tra
Umecyanin
 circular dichroism, **07:** 128
  UV and near-UV region, **07:** 163

Umecyanin *(continued)*
  molar absorptivity and-or absorbance values, **02:** 512
  molecular weights, stoichiometry and sources, **02:** 282
UMP
  pK'_a values, **06:** 331
Unamycin B, physicochemical constants, spectral, chemotherapeutic and biological properties, **03:** 392
Units
  SI,- and their symbols, **06:** 106
  thermodynamic, for equilibrium data, **06:** 104-105
Unsaponifiables in vegetable oils, % content, **05:** 512
Uracil
  heat of proton ionization, pK, and related thermodynamic quantities, **06:** 258
  pK'_a values, **06:** 331, 339
Uracil and derivatives
  physical constants and spectral properties, index to, **03:** 68-69
  UV spectra, **03:** 430
  UV spectral characteristics and acid dissociation constants, **03:** 413
Uracil phosphorylase
  Neurospora crassa mutant, **04:** 744
3-(1-Uracyl)-alanine, *see* Willardine
Urea
  densities of aqueous solutions with added reagents, at 25°, **06:** 406
  enthalpy and free energy of formation, **06:** 112
  free acid in blood plasma of newborn infants and adults, **01:** 328
  heat capacity and entropy values, **06:** 110
  heat of combustion, **06:** 112
  pK'_a values, **06:** 345
  refractive index of solutions at varying concentration, **06:** 387
  thumbprint, content in, **08:** 121
  viscosities of aqueous solutions with added reagents, at 25°, **06:** 407
  viscosity of aqueous solutions at 25°, **06:** 405
Urea cycle; pathways chart, **04:** insert
Urease
  amino acid composition, incomplete data, **07:** 514
  average hydrophobicity value, **01:** 235
  molar absorptivity and-or absorbance values, **02:** 513
  subunit, constitution of, **02:** 348
Uric acid
  pK'_a values, **06:** 331
Uricase
  enzymatic activity, subcellular fractions, **02:** 699
  molar absorptivity and-or absorbance values, **02:** 513
  molecular weights, stoichiometry and sources, **02:** 282
  subunit, constitution of, **02:** 336
Uridine
  bond angles and distances, **08:** 225
  chemical structures and approved numbering schemes, **08:** 224
  composition in various tRNA's, **04:** 428-441
  heat of proton ionization, pK, and related thermodynamic quantities, **06:** 259
  pK'_a values, **06:** 331, 339
  raman frequencies, table of values, **03:** 536-537

Uridine and derivatives
  molal activity coefficients, **03:** 529
  molal osmotic coefficients, **03:** 528
  UV spectra, **03:** 444-445
  UV spectral characteristics and acid dissociation constants, **03:** 415
Uridine and nucleoside derivatives
  physical constants and spectral properties, index to, **03:** 72
Uridine diphosphate galactose 4-epimerase
  amino acid composition, complete data, **07:** 511
Uridine diphosphate galactose: lipopolysaccharide α-3-galactosyl transferase
  amino acid composition, incomplete data, **07:** 514
Uridine nucleotide derivatives
  physical constants and spectral properties, index to, **03:** 75
Uridylic acid
  derivatives, UV spectral characteristics and acid dissociation constants, **03:** 416
Urine
  chromatography of, resolution of ninhydrin positive constituents, **08:** 114-119
  human
    enzymes found in, molecular weights, **02:** 301
  human, porphyrin excretion, normal values, **08:** 279
  laboratory animal, porphyrin excretion, normal values, **08:** 279
Urine, human, purine, pyrimidine, pyridine and imidazole derivatives excreted mg-day, **03:** 252-269
Urine disease, maple syrup, characteristics of, **01:** 319
Urocanase
  molar absorptivity and-or absorbance values, **02:** 513
  subunit, constitution of, **02:** 334
Urokinase
  amino acid composition, **02:** 302
  amino acid composition, incomplete data, **07:** 514
  human placenta
    molar absorptivity and-or absorbance values, **02:** 513
  human urine
    molar absorptivity and-or absorbance values, **02:** 513
  properties, **02:** 302
Urokinase inhibitor
  mammalian organs and secretions, specificities and properties, **02:** 632-641
Urokinase S-1, S-2
  average hydrophobicity value, **01:** 235
Uronic acids
  chemical formula, **05:** 165-168
  chromatography, **05:** 165-168
  melting point, **05:** 165-168
  nomenclature rules, **05:** 123-125
  specific rotation, **05:** 165-168
UTP
  pK'_a values, **06:** 331
UV absorbance
  mono- and oligonucleotides, **03:** 405-406
  mononucleotides in 97% D_2O, **03:** 408
  mononucleotides in 7 M urea, **03:** 407
  mononucleotides in 90% v-v ethylene glycol, **03:** 408

UV absorbance *(continued)*
oligonucleotides containing $2'O$-methylpentose residues, 03: 448-449
UV absorption characteristics
N-acetyl methyl esters of aromatic amino acids, cystine and of N-acetylcysteine, 01: 186
UV absorption spectra
circular dichroism of proteins in, extrema between 185 and 250 NM, table, 07: 82-129
human normal adult hemoglobin derivatives, 07: 174-185
optical rotatory dispersion of proteins
extrema between 185 and 250 NM^3, table, 07: 44
visible, table, 07: 15-38
UV spectra
N-acetyl-DL-β-phenylalanine methyl ester, 01: 193
Nacetyl-DL-tryptophan methyl ester, 01: 192
N-acetyl-L-tyrosine ethyl ester, 01: 194
N-acetyl-L-tyrosine ethyl ester anion, 01: 195
amino acids, far absorption spectra, 01: 185
aqueous solution at pH 5, 01: 184
neutral water, table, 01: 185
0.1 M sodium dodecyl sulfate, table, 01: 185
antibiotics, nucleoside, 03: 271-393
compounds of biological interest, 08: 144-195
cysteine, 01: 197
cystine, 01: 198
N,N'-diacetyl-L-cystine dimethyl ester, 01: 199
histidine, 01: 196
nucleosides and some of their alkyl derivatives, 03: 420-447
protein concentration determination in short-wavelength region, 08: 197
unmodified bases and some of their alkyl derivatives, 03: 420-447
vitamins, maximum values, 08: 284-300
UV spectral characteristics
alkyl bases, 03: 409-416
nucleosides, 03: 409-416
nucleotides, 03: 409-416
UV spectral data
steroids, table, 05: 531-588

V

Valine
antagonism to leucine, 01: 178
antagonists of, 01: 180
free acid in amniotic fluid in early pregnancy and at term, 01: 327
free acid in blood plasma of newborn infants and adults, 01: 328
heat of proton ionization, pK, and related thermodynamic quantities, 06: 259-260
hypervalinemia, effect of, 01: 322
maple syrup urine disease
intermittent form, effect of, 01: 319
severe infantile, effect of, 01: 319
nucleoside composition, tables of values, 04: 441
nucleotide sequences of, 04: 452-453
pK'_a values, 06: 319

physical and chemical properties, 01: 117
requirements of, for growth of various microorganisms, table, 04: 630-643
specific rotatory dispersion constants, 0.1 M solution, 01: 244
symbols for atoms and bonds in side chains, 01: 69, 02: 73
thumbprint, content in, 08: 121
Valine:tRNA ligase
average hydrophobicity value, 01: 235
Valinomycin
proton NMR and suggested conformations, 07: 561-563
Van der Waals' radii of common elements, 08: 221
Vasopressin
proton NMR and suggested conformations, 07: 572-573
Vasopressin, lysine
average hydrophobicity value, 01: 235
Vasopressin, natural and related synthetic oligopeptides
amino acid sequence, physical and biological properties, 07: 195-218
Vegetable oils
tocopherol contents, individual, 05: 521
unsaponifiables, % content, 05: 512
Veillonella
G + C composition of DNA of, table arranged by specie, 04: 148
Vengicide, physicochemical constants, spectral, chemotherapeutic and biological properties, 03: 393
Veramycin B$_a$
proton NMR and suggested conformations, 07: 565
Vernamycin A; origin, structure, and characteristic as protein biosynthesis inhibitor, 04: 615
Vernamycin Ba, mode of action of protein biosynthesis inhibitor, 04: 615
Vernix caseosa
lipid, fatty acids from wax esters and sterol esters, 05: 509-510
Verruacarins; origin, structure, and characteristic as protein biosynthesis inhibitor, 04: 616
Verrucarol; origin, structure, and characteristic as protein biosynthesis inhibitor, 04: 616
Vertebrate myoglobins, *see* Myoglobin, vertebrate
Vertebrate tetrameric hemoglobins, *see* Hemoglobins, vertebrate tetrameric
Verticillium
G + C composition of DNA of, table arranged by specie, 04: 224
Vibrio
amino acid requirements for growth, table, 04: 640
G + C composition of DNA of, table arranged by specie, 04: 169-171
Violacein
UV spectra, formula, molecular weight, 08: 187
Viomycidine
physical and chemical properties, 01: 147
Viomycin; origin, structure, and characteristic as protein biosynthesis inhibitor, 04: 617
Viosterol, properties of, 08: 286
Viral DNA, buoyant densities, melting temperatures and GC content, 03: 560-562
Viral DNA molecules, composition and physical properties, 03: 551-556

Viral RNA, *see* RNA, viral

Virginiamycin M$_1$, *see also* Osteogrycin A, PA 114A, Staphylomycin M$_1$; origin, structure, and characteristic as protein biosynthesis inhibitor, **04:** 617

Viridogrisein; origin, structure, and characteristic as protein biosynthesis inhibitor, **04:** 618

Virus, definition, **03:** 549

Virus, protein
  molar absorptivity and-or absorbance values, **02:** 514
  physical-chemical data for, index to ultracentrifuge studies, **02:** 232

Virus, tobacco mosaic, *see* Tobacco mosaic virus

Virus coat protein

Viruses
  chordate
    deoxyribonucleic acids from, purine and pyrimidine distribution in, **04:** 281
  insect
    deoxyribonucleic acids from, purine and pyrimidine distribution in, **04:** 280
    nearest neighbor frequencies in DNA from various, **04:** 313-314
  plant DNA
    deoxyribonucleic acids from purine and pyrimidine distribution in, **04:** 280

Viruses, range of weights, **08:** 424

Viscosity
  ethylene glycol-methanol-water mixtures, **06:** 521
  guanidine hydrochloride, aqueous solutions at 25°, **06:** 405
  guanidine hydrochloride, aqueous solutions with added reagents, at 25°, **06:** 407
  intrinsic
    contractile proteins, **02:** 306
    polysaccharides, table of values, **02:** 686-687
    proteins, human plasma, **02:** 242-250
    proteins in native and denatured states, **02:** 721
    Tamm-Horsfall mucoprotein, **02:** 304
  salt solutions used for density gradients, **06:** 425
  sucrose in water, tables at varying concentrations and temperatures, **06:** 415-418
  urea, aqueous solutions at 25°, **06:** 405
  urea, aqueous solutions with added reagents, at 25°, **06:** 407

Viscosity, intrinsic, mucopolysaccharides, **05:** 356-357

Viscotoxin A3
  amino acid sequence, **07:** 500

Visible absorption spectra
  human normal adult hemoglobin derivatives, **07:** 178-185
  optical rotatory dispersion of proteins in near UV and, table, **07:** 15-38

Visual pigment
  molar absorptivity and-or absorbance values, **02:** 514

Visual pigment$_{500}$
  amino acid composition, complete data, **07:** 511

Vitamin A
  biological characteristics, **08:** 301
  nomenclature, preferred usage, **08:** 8
  properties, formulas, **08:** 284-286
  UV spectra, formula, molecular weight, **08:** 151

Vitamin A$_1$, properties of, **08:** 284

Vitamin A$_2$, properties of, **08:** 284

Vitamin B$_1$, *see also* Thiamine
  properties, **08:** 300
  UV spectra, formula, molecular weight, **08:** 145-147

Vitamin B$_{12}$, *see also* Cyanocobalamin
  nomenclature and structures, **08:** 12-17
  properties of, **08:** 294

Vitamin B$_2$, *see also* Riboflavin
  properties, formulas, **08:** 299
  UV spectra, formula, molecular weight, **08:** 148, 162

Vitamin B$_6$
  fluorescence properties of compounds, **08:** 215
  nomenclature recommendations, **08:** 12
  properties, formulas, **08:** 298-299

Vitamin B$_c$, properties of, **08:** 295

Vitamin B$_x$, properties of, **08:** 296

Vitamin B$_{10}$, properties of, **08:** 295

Vitamin B$_{11}$, properties of, **08:** 295

Vitamin B$_3$, properties of, **08:** 296

Vitamin B$_5$, properties of, **08:** 296

Vitamin C, *see also* Ascorbic acid
  nomenclature, preferred usage, **08:** 19
  properties, formula, **08:** 293
  structure and properties, **08:** 281
  UV spectra, formula, molecular weight, **08:** 149-150

Vitamin C$_2$
  structure and properties, **08:** 281

Vitamin D
  biological characteristics, **08:** 301
  nomenclature, preferred usage, **08:** 9
  properties, formulas, **08:** 286-288

Vitamin D$_2$
  properties, **08:** 286
  UV spectra, formula, molecular weight, **08:** 152

Vitamin D$_3$, properties of, **08:** 287

Vitamin E
  biological characteristics, **08:** 301
  nomenclature recommendations, **08:** 9-11
  properties, formulas, **08:** 288-290
  UV spectra, formula, molecular weight, **08:** 153-155

Vitamin G, properties of, **08:** 299

Vitamin H, properties of, **08:** 293

Vitamin K
  biological characteristics, **08:** 301
  nomenclature recommendations, **08:** 9-11
  properties, formulas, **08:** 290-292
  UV spectra, formula, molecular weight, **08:** 156

Vitamin K$_1$, properties of, **08:** 290

Vitamin K$_2$, properties of, **08:** 291

Vitamin K$_3$, properties of, **08:** 291

Vitamin M, properties of, **08:** 295

Vitamin PP, properties of, **08:** 296

Vitamins
  abbreviations, use of, **08:** 6
  abbreviations for, use of, **01:** 6, **02:** 6, **03:** 6, **04:** 6, **06:** 6
  alternate names, list, **08:** 311
  animal requirements, table, **08:** 305-308
  animals, laboratory, levels needed, **08:** 251
  corrinoids, nomenclature and structures, **08:** 12-17
  diet, human, NAS-NRC recommended daily allowances, **08:** 248-249

Vitamins *(continued)*

diet, human, U.S. Government recommended daily allowances, **08:** 310

nomenclature, journal references for, **02:** 87

pK'_a values, **06:** 348

properties, solubility, stability, formula, **08:** 284-300

quinones with isoprenoid side chains, nomenclature, **08:** 10-11

Vitamins, use of abbreviations for, **05:** 6

Vitreoscilla

G + C composition of DNA of, table arranged by specie, **04:** 181

Vitreoscillaceae

G + C composition of DNA of, table arranged by genera and specie, **04:** 181

Vogel and Bonner minimal medium, preparation of, **04:** 649

Volume, partial specific, *see* Partial specific volume

Volumetric work, indicators for, **06:** 380-382

W

Warfarin, ligands binding to plasma albumin, **02:** 572

Water

heat of proton ionization, pK, and related thermodynamic quantities, **06:** 260-261

refractive index, optical rotatory dispersion calculations, **06:** 385

refractive index, variation with temperature, **06:** 386

Water, deuterated

heat of proton ionization, pK, and related thermodynamics quantities, **06:** 261

Watson-Crick duplexes, viral DNA molecules, **03:** 549

Watson-Crick pairs

base stacking in standard models, diagrams, **04:** 414

standard polynucleotide double helices, values for constrained hydrogen bonds, **04:** 413

weights, range of, **08:** 424

Wickerhamia

G + C composition of DNA of, table arranged by specie, **04:** 224

Willardine

physical and chemical properties, **01:** 148

D-Win-5094; origin, structure, and characteristic as protein biosynthesis inhibitor, **04:** 571

Wolbachia

G + C composition of DNA of, table arranged by specie, **04:** 165

Wybutine

physical constants and spectral properties, **03:** 94

Wybutine, Peroxy-

physical constants and spectral properties, **03:** 95

Wyosine, 7-[3-(Methoxycarbonyl-3-(methoxyformamido)propyl]

composition in various tRNA's, **04:** 428-441

Wye and derivatives

physical constants and spectral properties, index to, **03:** 69

Wyosine

isolation and detection of, in RNA, general remarks, **03:** 244-245

physical constants and spectral properties, **03:** 139

RNA, various, natural occurrence in, **03:** 233

Wybutosine, *see* 7[3-(Methoxycarbonyl)-3-(methoxyformamido)propyl] wyosine

physical constants and spectral properties, **03:** 139

X

X-Ray crystal structure data

dimensions, average, of a sugar unit, **05:** 472

Xanthine

pK'_a values, **06:** 331, 337

physical constants and spectral properties, **03:** 96

Xanthine, 7-Methyl-

physical constants and spectral properties, **03:** 96

Xanthine and derivatives

UV spectra, **03:** 428-429

UV spectral characteristics and acid dissociation constants, **03:** 412

Xanthine oxidase

amino acid composition, complete data, **07:** 511

circular dichroism

UV and near-UV region, **07:** 128, 163

molar absorptivity and-or absorbance values, **02:** 514

optical rotatory dispersion

UV region, **07:** 78

visible and near UV regions, **07:** 38

table of cofactors, molecular weights, stoichiometry, and sources, **02:** 278

Xanthomonas

amino acid requirements for growth, table, **04:** 640

G + C composition of DNA of, table arranged by specie, **04:** 161-162

Xanthosine

derivatives, UV spectral characteristics and acid dissociation constants, **03:** 416

pK'_a values, **06:** 331

physical constants and spectral properties, **03:** 140

Y

Y

physical constants and spectral properties, **03:** 139

Y base or Y^+

physical constants and spectral properties, **03:** 94

Yeast

amino acid requirements for growth, table, **04:** 642

Yeast phenylalanine transfer RNA

hydrophobic stacking interactions, **04:** 461

interactions, diagram of secondary and tertiary, **04:** 460

molecule, side views of, **04:** 459

nucleotide sequence, **04:** 458

Yohimbine

pK'_a values, **06:** 327

Yr base

physical constants and spectral properties, **03:** 95

Yt

physical constants and spectral properties, **03:** 139

Yt base or Yt^+

physical constants and spectral properties, **03:** 93

Yw base or Yw^+

physical constants and spectral properties, **03:** 95

Z

Zeatin
  physical constants and spectral properties, **03:** 97
Zeatosine and derivatives
  physical constants and spectral properties, index to, **03:** 72

Zenograft, definition of, **04:** 884
Zygorhynchus
  G + C composition of DNA of, table arranged by specie, **04:** 224
Zygosaccharomyces
  amino acid requirements for growth, table, **04:** 643
Zymogen
  conversion during coagulation of plasma, **02:** 670

Part II: Chemical Substances Entries

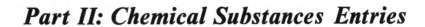

A

α
  Melanotropin; amino acid sequence; •, 07: 385
α- and β-
  peptic hydrolysis, *see also* Hydrolysis; leucine in human
    •chains, 02: 217
γA
  immunoglobulin, specific; •, rabbit
    molar absorptivity and-or absorbance values, 02: 456
A + T
  extinction coefficient; DNA, double-strand, as a func-
    tion of • content, graph, 03: 590
A-9145
  physicochemical constants, spectral, chemotherapeutic
    and biological properties, 03: 273
Abrin
  origin, structure, and characteristics as protein biosyn-
    thesis inhibitor, 04: 555
Abrine
  physical and chemical properties, 01: 148
Acetals
  nomenclature rules, 05: 126-130, 132
β-Acetamido-L-alanine, *see* β-N-Acetyl-α-,
    β-diaminopropionic acid
3'-Acetamido-3'-deoxyadenosine
  physicochemical constants, spectral, chemotherapeutic
    and biological properties, 03: 274
2-Acetamidoacrylic acid
  structure and symbols for those incorporated into syn-
    thetic polypeptides, 01: 97
Acetate
  buffer
    preparation of, 06: 372
    protonic activity tables, 06: 529-539
Acetic acid
  free energy; hydrolysis; • esters and related compounds,
    06: 300
Acetic acid derivatives
  heat of proton ionization, pK, and related thermody-
    namic quantities, 06: 153-157
α Aceto-acid reductoisomerase
  Neurospora crassa mutant, 04: 751
Acetoacetate
  decarboxylase
    amino acid composition, complete data, 07: 505
    circular dichroism
      in near UV region, 07: 143
      in the UV region, 07: 82
    molar absorptivity and-or absorbance values, 02: 383
    optical rotatory dispersion
      in UV region, 07: 44
      in visible and near UV region, 07: 15
Acetoacetic acid
  decarboxylase
    average hydrophobicity value, 01: 210
Acetonic acid
  heat of proton ionization, pK, and related thermody-
    namic quantities, 06: 157
Acetophenone
  heat of proton ionization, pK, and related thermody-

namic quantities, 06: 157
Acetoxy-cycloheximide
  origin, structure, and characteristic as protein biosynthe-
    sis inhibitor, 04: 555
β-N-Acetyl-α,β-diaminopropionic acid
  physical and chemical properties, 01: 119
Nα-Acetyl-2-fluorophenylalanine
  structure and symbols for those incorporated into syn-
    thetic polypeptides, 01: 97
N-Acetyl-β-D-glucosaminidase
  average hydrophobicity value, 01: 210
N-Acetyl-β-D-glucosaminidase-A
  average hydrophobicity value, 01: 210
N-Acetyl-β-D-glucosaminidase-B
  average hydrophobicity value, 01: 210
N-Acetyl-DL- -phenylalanine
  phenylalanine; • methyl ester, UV spectra of, 01: 193
N-Acetyl-DL-β-phenylalanine
  methyl ester
    UV spectra of, 01: 193
N-Acetyl-DL-tryptophan
  methyl ester UV spectra, 01: 192
  tryptophan; • methyl ester, UV spectra of, 01: 192
N-Acetyl-L-tyrosine
  ethyl ester, UV spectra, 01: 194
  ethyl ester anion, UV spectra, 01: 195
Acetyl CoA synthetase
  Neurospora crassa mutant, 04: 744
Acetyl hexosamine
  content of, in glyco-proteins, 02: 258-274
  molar extinctions; • of aromatic amino acids,
    cystine and N-acetylcysteine, 01: 186
N-acetyl methyl esters
  amino acids; UV absorption characteristics, • of
    aromatic types, cystine and N-acetylcysteine,
    01: 186
Acetyl ornithine transferase
  Neurospora crassa mutant, 04: 745
N-Acetylalanine
  physical and chemical properties, 01: 148
β-2-Acetylamino-2-deoxy-D-glucoside acetylamino-
    deoxyglucohydrolase
  enzymatic reactions, velocity and parameters, table, 05:
    430-433
N-Acetylarginine
  physical and chemical properties, 01: 132
N-Acetylaspartic acid
  physical and chemical properties, 01: 148
Acetylcholine
  receptor
    average hydrophobicity value, 01: 210
  receptor protein
    circular dichroism in the UV region, 07: 82
Acetylcholinesterase
  amino acid composition, incomplete data, 07: 512
  average hydrophobicity value, 01: 210
  molar absorptivity and-or absorbance values, 02: 383
  optical rotatory dispersion
    in the UV region, 07: 44
    in the visible and near UV regions, 07: 15
  subunit, constitution of, 02: 344

N-Acetylcysteine
  molar extinctions; N-Acetyl methyl esters of aromatic amino acids, cystine and •, 01: 186
  UV absorption characteristics, 01: 186
N⁴-Acetylcytidine
  composition in various tRNA's, 04: 428-441
  isolation and detection of, in RNA, general remarks, 03: 237
  RNA, various, natural occurrence in, 03: 222
N-Acetyldjenkolic acid
  physical and chemical properties, 01: 151
Acetylenic dicarboxylic acid diamide
  physical and chemical properties, 01: 121
N-Acetylglutamic acid
  physical and chemical properties, 01: 148
O-Acetylhomoserine
  physical and chemical properties, 01: 122
Nᵅ-Acetyllysine-N-methylamide
  structure and symbols for those incorporated into synthetic polypeptides, 01: 97
Acetylornithine
  γ-transaminase
    average hydrophobicity value, 01: 210
N-Acetylornithine
  physical and chemical properties, 01: 119
Acetylsalicylic acid
  heat of proton ionization, pK, and related thermodynamic quantities, 06: 179
O-Acetylserine
  sulfhydrylase A
    amino acid composition, complete data, 07: 505
    average hydrophobicity value, 01: 210
Acetyltransferase
  carnitine •
    optical rotatory dispersion
      UV region, 07: 50
      visible and near UV regions, 07: 19
  phosphate •
    optical rotatory dispersion
      UV region, 07: 70
      visible and near UV regions, 07: 33
Achromycin, see Tetracycline
Achromycin 260, see Puromycin
Acid, see also Acids
  adenine and derivatives; UV spectral characteristics and • dissociation constants, 03: 409-410
  alanine; free • in amniotic fluid in early pregnancy and at term, 01: 327
  alanine; free • in blood plasma of newborn infants and adults, 01: 328
  β-alanine; free • in blood plasma of newborn infants and adults, 01: 328
  amino acids, see also Aromatic amino acids, also specific acids; free • in blood plasma of newborn infants and adults, table, 01: 328
  α-aminobutyric acid; free • in amniotic fluid in early pregnancy and at term, 01: 327
  arginine; free • in amniotic fluid in early pregnancy and at term, 01: 327
  arginine; free • in blood plasma of newborn infants and adults, 01: 328

asparagine; free • in amniotic fluid in early pregnancy and at term, 01: 327
asparagine; free • in blood plasma of newborn infants and adults, 01: 328
aspartic acid; free • in amniotic fluid in early pregnancy and at term, 01: 327
aspartic acid; free • in blood plasma of newborn infants and adults, 01: 328
citrulline; free • in amniotic fluid in early pregnancy and at term, 01: 327
citrulline; free • in blood plasma of newborn infants and adults, 01: 328
cysteic acid; free • in amniotic fluid in early pregnancy and at term, 01: 327
cystine; destruction of, during • hydrolysis, 02: 206
cystine; free • in amniotic fluid in early pregnancy and at term, 01: 327
cystine; free • in blood plasma of newborn infants and adults, 01: 328
cytidine and derivatives; UV spectral characteristics and • dissociation constants, 03: 414-415
cytidylic acid; derivatives, UV spectral characteristics and • dissociation constants, 03: 416
cytosine and derivatives; UV spectral characteristics and • dissociation constants, 03: 412
ethanolamine; free • in blood plasma of newborn infants and adults, 01: 328
glutamic acid; free • in amniotic fluid in early pregnancy and at term, 01: 327
glutamic acid; free • in blood plasma of newborn infants and adults, 01: 328
glutamine; free • in amniotic fluid in early pregnancy and at term, 01: 327
glutamine; free • in blood plasma of newborn infants and adults, 01: 328
glycine; free • in amniotic fluid in early pregnancy and at term, 01: 327
glycine; free • in blood plasma of newborn infants and adults, 01: 328
guanine and derivatives; UV spectral characteristics and • dissociation constants, 03: 411-412
histidine; free • in amniotic fluid in early pregnancy and at term, 01: 327
histidine; free • in blood plasma of newborn infants and adults, 01: 328
hydrolysis, see also Peptic hydrolysis; •, of peptides, relative rate table, 02: 208
hydrolysis, see also Peptic hydrolysis; •, of proteins, data tables, 02: 206-207
hydrolysis, see also Peptic hydrolysis; •, recovery of tryptophan from various proteins, 02: 207
hydrolysis, see also Peptic hydrolysis; peptides in • solution, table, 02: 208
hydroxyproline; free • in amniotic fluid in early pregnancy and at term, 01: 327
hydroxyproline; free • in blood plasma of newborn infants and adults, 01: 328
hypoxanthine and derivatives; UV spectral characteristics and • dissociation constants, 03: 413
inosine and derivatives; UV spectral characteristics and • dissociation constants, 03: 415-416

Acid *(continued)*

isoleucine; free • in amniotic fluid in early pregnancy and at term, **01:** 327

isoleucine; free • in blood plasma of newborn infants and adults, **01:** 328

leucine; free • in amniotic fluid in early pregnancy and at term, **01:** 327

leucine; free • in blood plasma of newborn infants and adults, **01:** 328

lysine; free • in amniotic fluid in early pregnancy and at term, **01:** 327

lysine; free • in blood plasma in newborn infants and adults, **01:** 328

methionine; free • in amniotic fluid in early pregnancy and at term, **01:** 327

methionine; free • in blood plasma of newborn infants and adults, **01:** 328

α-NH₂-n-butyric acid; free • in blood plasma of newborn infants and adults, **01:** 328

ornithine; free • in amniotic fluid in early pregnancy and at term, **01:** 327

ornithine; free • in blood plasma of newborn infants and adults, **01:** 328

peptides; hydrolysis in • solution, relative rates, **02:** 208

phenylalanine; • vs. neutral difference spectra, **01:** 191

phenylalanine; free • in amniotic fluid in early pregnancy and at term, **01:** 327

phenylalanine; free • in blood plasma of newborn infants and adults, **01:** 328

phosphatase
  wheat bran
    luminescence of, table, **01:** 206

polyol esters, • value, density, hydroxyl value, **05:** 515

proline; free • in amniotic fluid in early pregnancy and at term, **01:** 327

proline; free • in blood plasma of newborn infants and adults, **01:** 328

serine; destruction of, during • hydrolysis, **02:** 206

serine; free • in amniotic fluid in early pregnancy and at term, **01:** 327

serine; free • in blood plasma of newborn infants and adults, **01:** 328

taurine; free • in amniotic fluid in early pregnancy and at term, **01:** 327

taurine; free • in blood plasma of newborn infants and adults, **01:** 328

threonine; destruction of, during • hydrolysis, **02:** 206

threonine; free • in amniotic fluid in early pregnancy and at term, **01:** 327

threonine; free • in blood plasma of newborn infants and adults, **01:** 328

thymidine and derivatives; UV spectral characteristics and • dissociation constants, **03:** 415

thymidylic acid; derivatives, UV spectral characteristics and • dissociation constants, **03:** 416

thymine and derivatives; UV spectral characteristics and • dissociation constants, **03:** 413

tryptophan; • vs. neutral difference spectra, **01:** 191

tryptophan; free • in amniotic fluid in early pregnancy and at term, **01:** 327

tryptophan; free • in blood plasma of newborn infants and adults, **01:** 328

tryptophan; recovery from various proteins after • hydrolysis, **02:** 207

tyrosine; • vs. neutral difference spectra, **01:** 191

tyrosine; destruction of, during • hydrolysis, **02:** 206

tyrosine; free • in amniotic fluid in early pregnancy and at term, **01:** 327

tyrosine; free • in blood plasma of newborn infants and adults, **01:** 328

uracil and derivatives; UV spectral characteristics and • dissociation constants, **03:** 413

urea; free • in blood plasma of newborn infants and adults, **01:** 328

uridylic acid; derivatives, UV spectral characteristics and • dissociation constants, **03:** 416

valine; free • in amniotic fluid in early pregnancy and at term, **01:** 327

valine; free • in blood plasma of newborn infants and adults, **01:** 328

value
  polyol esters table, **05:** 515

xanthine and derivatives; UV spectral characteristics and • dissociation constants, **03:** 412

xanthosine; derivatives, UV spectral characteristics and • dissociation constants, **03:** 416

α₁-Acid
  glycoprotein
    amino acid composition, incomplete data, **07:** 512
    optical rotatory dispersion
      UV region, **07:** 44
      visible and near UV regions, **07:** 15

α₁-Acid
  glycoprotein
    average hydrophobicity value, **01:** 210

Acid-base
  indicators; • types, pH range and color change table, **06:** 357

Acid DNase, *see* Deoxyribonuclease I

Acid proteinase, *Aspergillus, see Aspergillus* acid, proteinase
  optical rotatory dispersion
    UV region, **07:** 48
    visible and near UV regions, **07:** 18

Acidic
  glycoprotein
    circular dichroism in the UV region, **07:** 82

Acidic brain
  protein
    amino acid composition, incomplete data, **07:** 512

Acids, *see also* Acid
  alcohols and other oxygen •, pK'_a values, **06:** 315-317
  amino sugar •
    chemical formula, **05:** 170-176
    chromatography, **05:** 170-176
    melting point, **05:** 170-176
    specific rotation, **05:** 170-176
  beeswax fractions, composition of • of, **05:** 504
  commercial strength, table of concentration data, **06:** 384
  pK'_a values, table, **06:** 307-348
  DNA, *see also* Deoxyribonucleic acid; nearest neighbor frequencies in • from diverse sources, **04:** 312-318

Acids *(continued)*

DNA, *see also* Deoxyribonucleic acid; purine and pyrimidine, distribution of, in • from diverse sources, **04:** 241-281

fatty acids, *see also* Lipids, Wax fatty acids; density, table, of • from C_8 to C_{12}, **05:** 492

fatty acids, *see also* Lipids, Wax fatty acids; linseed oil • and esters, force-area data, **05:** 497

fatty acids, *see also* Lipids, Wax fatty acids; specific volume, table, of • from C_8 to C_{12}, **05:** 492

fatty acids, *see also* Lipids, Wax fatty acids; temperature coefficients, table, of • from C_8 to C_{12}, **05:** 492

force-area data, linseed oil • and esters, **05:** 497

formula, chemical; uronic •, **05:** 165-168

ionization constants; • and bases, tables of values, **06:** 307-348

linseed oil • and esters, force-area data, **05:** 497

lipids; beeswax fractions, composition of • of, **05:** 504

molecular weights; •, commercial strength, **06:** 384

natural, derived from carbohydrates
chemical formula, **05:** 153-176
chromatography, **05:** 153-176
melting point, **05:** 153-176
specific rotation, **05:** 153-176

pK'_a; inorganic •, **06:** 307

specific gravity; •, commercial strength, **06:** 384

Aconitate
buffer, preparation of, **06:** 371

Acridine
heat of proton ionization, pK, and related thermodynamic quantities, **06:** 158

Actin
amino acid composition, complete data, **07:** 505
amino acid sequence, **07:** 490-491
average hydrophobicity value, **01:** 210, 211
identification of, in nonmuscle cells, table, **02:** 307-313
molar absorptivity and-or absorbance values, **02:** 384
molecular weight; nonmuscle •, of monomer, **02:** 314-315
myosin; interaction of nonmuscle • with, **02:** 316
myosins, nonmuscle, interaction, **02:** 320
nonmuscle, interaction of several with myosin, **02:** 316
nonmuscle, physical chemical properties of several, **02:** 314-315
optical rotatory dispersion in the UV region, **07:** 44
refractive index increments, **02:** 372

F-Actin
luminescence of, table, **01:** 205
molar absorptivity and-or absorbance values, **02:** 384

G-Actin
molar absorptivity and-or absorbance values, **02:** 384
molecular parameters, **02:** 306

α-Actinin
circular dichroism in the UV region, **07:** 82
molecular parameters, **02:** 306

β-Actinin
optical rotatory dispersion in the visible and near UV regions, **07:** 15

Actinobolin
origin, structure, and characteristic as protein biosynthesis inhibitor, **04:** 556

Actinomycin-D
proton NMR and suggested conformations, **07:** 569

Actinomycin C_3
UV spectra, formula, molecular weight, **08:** 166

Actinospectacin, *see* Spectinomycin

Actinphenol
origin, structure, and characteristic as protein biosynthesis inhibitor, **04:** 556

Active site peptides, *see* Peptides, active site

Actomyosin
identification of, in nonmuscle cells, table, **02:** 307-313
luminescence of, table, **01:** 205
refractive index increments, **02:** 372

Acyclic aldoses
systematic nomenclature; •, **05:** 105
trivial names; •, **05:** 103, 105

Acyclic forms
in carbohydrate nomenclature, **05:** 113

Acyl
phosphatase
amino acid composition, incomplete data, **07:** 512
average hydrophobicity value, **01:** 211
molar absorptivity and-or absorbance values, **02:** 384

Acyl carrier
protein
amino acid composition, complete data, **07:** 505
amino acid sequence, **07:** 498
average hydrophobicity value, **01:** 211
cyanogen bromide cleavage, **02:** 199
molar absorptivity and-or absorbance values, **02:** 384
optical rotatory dispersion
UV region, **07:** 44
visible and near UV regions, **07:** 15

Acylcholine acylhydrolase, *see* Cholinesterase

Adducts
abbreviations for pyrimidine photoproducts, **03:** 53-55

Adenine
and derivatives
physical constants and spectral properties, index to, **03:** 67
UV spectra, **03:** 420-423
UV spectral characteristics and acid dissociation constants, **03:** 409-410
heat of proton ionization, pK, and related thermodynamic quantities, **06:** 158
pK'_a values, **06:** 330
phosphoribosyltransferase
erythrocyte, human
subunit, constitution of, **02:** 326

Adenosine
and derivatives
molal osmotic coefficients, **03:** 528
UV spectra, **03:** 432-435
UV spectral characteristics and acid dissociation constants, **03:** 413-414
and nucleoside derivatives
physical constants and spectral properties, index to, **03:** 69
average hydrophobicity value, **01:** 211
bond angles and distances, **08:** 224
chemical structures and approved numbering schemes, **08:** 224

Aldolase *(continued)*
optical rotatory dispersion
UV region, **07**: 56
visible and near UV regions, **07**: 23
fructose diphosphate •
subunit, constitution of, **02**: 329
luminescence of, table, **01**: 205
molar absorptivity and-or absorbance values, **02**: 389
phospho-2-keto-3-deoxygluconate •
optical rotatory dispersion
UV region, **07**: 71
visible and near UV regions, **07**: 33
subunit, constitution of, **02**: 331, 335, 338, 377
viscosity, intrinsic, **02**: 721
Aldolase, 3-deoxy-2-keto-6-phosphogluconate
molar absorptivity and-or absorbance values, **02**: 390
Aldolase, fructose-1,6-diphosphate
average hydrophobicity values, **01**: 212
Aldolase, fructose diphosphate
average hydrophobicity value, **01**: 212
Aldolase, L-rhamnulose 1-phosphate
molar absorptivity and-or absorbance values, **02**: 390
Aldolase C
average hydrophobicity value, **01**: 212
subunit, constitution of, **02**: 338
Aldonic acids
chemical formula, **05**: 153-176
chromatography, **05**: 153-164
melting point, **05**: 153-164
nomenclature rules, **05**: 121-122
specific rotation, **05**: 153-164
Aldose
l-epimerase
molar absorptivity and-or absorbance values, **02**: 390
Aldoses
natural
chemical formula, **05**: 181-217
chromatography, **05**: 181-217
melting point, **05**: 181-217
specific rotation, **05**: 181-217
Aliphatic acids, long-chain
and related compounds, molecular dimensions, **05**: 498
Alkaline
phosphatase
amino acid composition, complete data, **07**: 505
average hydrophobicity value, **01**: 213
carbohydrate content, **02**: 274
circular dichroism in the UV region, **07**: 83
molecular weights, stoichiometry and sources, **02**: 284
optical rotatory dispersion
UV region, **07**: 45
visible and near UV regions, **07**: 16
subunit, constitution of, **02**: 331, 335, 337
proteinase B
average hydrophobicity value, **01**: 213
Alkaline proteinase A and B, thermophilic, *Streptomyces*,
see Trypsin, thermophilic Streptomyces
Alkaloids
and derivatives, pK'_a, **06**: 326-327
steroid •, nomenclature rules, **05**: 83-85

Alkenyl
fatty acids, *see also* Lipids, Wax fatty acids; methyl esters of some synthetic • and alkyl substituted, physical constants, **05**: 516
melting point; methyl esters of some synthetic • and alkyl substituted fatty acids, **05**: 516
refractive index; methyl esters of some synthetic • and alkyl substituted fatty acids, **05**: 516
Alkenyl branched chain acids
lipids; mass spectra of methyl esters of •, intensities of key fragments, **05**: 517
mass spectra; intensities of key fragments, methyl esters of •, **05**: 517
Alkyl
dicarboxylic acid, •, diesters, refractive index, **05**: 494
fatty acids, *see also* Lipids, Wax fatty acids; • diesters of dicarboxylic acid, refractive index, **05**: 494
fatty acids, *see also* Lipids, Wax fatty acids; • esters refractive index and equations for some, **05**: 493
fatty acids, *see also* Lipids, Wax fatty acids; • monoesters of carboxylic acid, refractive index, **05**: 494
fatty acids, *see also* Lipids, Wax fatty acids; methyl esters of some synthetic alkenyl and • substituted, physical constants, **05**: 516
Alkyl bases
dissociation constants, acidic; •, **03**: 409-416
pKa; •, table of values, **03**: 409-416
UV spectral characteristics; •, **03**: 409-416
Alkyl derivatives
of unmodified bases and nucleosides, UV spectra of some, **03**: 420-447
UV spectra; unmodified bases and some of their •, **03**: 420-447
Alkyl mono
carboxylic acid, •esters, refractive index, **05**: 494
Alkyl substituted fatty acids
melting point; methyl esters of some synthetic alkenyl and •, **05**: 516
refractive index; methyl esters of some synthetic alkenyl and •, **05**: 516
Allantoicase
circular dichroism
in UV and near UV region, **07**: 83, 143
optical rotatory dispersion
UV region, **07**: 46
visible and near UV regions, **07**: 16
Allergen
(antigen K)
amino acid composition, complete data, **07**: 505
Allergen 1-B
amino acid composition, complete data, **07**: 505
Alliin
physical and chemical properties, **01**: 151
D-Alloenduracididine
physical and chemical properties, **01**: 164
D-Allohydroxyproline betaine, *see* Turcine
Alloisoleucine
structure and symbols for those incorporated into synthetic polypeptides, **01**: 97
Allomycin
origin, structure, and characteristic as protein biosynthesis inhibitor, **04**: 557

Allomycin *(continued)*
 physicochemical constants, spectral, chemotherapeutic
  and biological properties, **03:** 276
D-Allothreonine
 physical and chemical properties, **01:** 164
Allyglycine
 antagonism to cysteine, **01:** 177
S-Allylcysteine
 physical and chemical properties, **01:** 151
S-Allylmercaptocysteine
 physical and chemical properties, **01:** 151
Althiomycin
 origin, structure, and characteristic as protein biosynthesis inhibitor, **04:** 557
Aluminichrome
 proton NMR and suggested conformations, **07:** 567
Aluminichrysin
 proton NMR and suggested conformations, **07:** 568
Aluminicrocin
 proton NMR and suggested conformations, **07:** 568
Aluminum
 chemical resistance as used in ultracentrifuge centerpieces, **08:** 429-430
Amandin
 molar absorptivity and-or absorbance values, **02:** 392
 refractive index increments, **02:** 373
Amicetin, *see also* Sacromycin
 origin, structure, and characteristic as protein biosynthesis inhibitor, **04:** 558
 physicochemical constants, spectral, chemotherapeutic
  and biological properties, **03:** 277
Amicetin B, *see also* Plicacetin
 physicochemical constants, spectral, chemotherapeutic
  and biological properties, **03:** 278
Amidase
 β-D-*N*-acetylhexose •
 placenta, human
  subunit, constitution of, **02:** 333
ω-Amidase
 average hydrophobicity value, **01:** 213
Amide I
 and amide II components,[a] cm^{-1} (solid state)
  prominent, table, **07:** 597
Amide II
 amide I and • components,[a] cm^{-1} (solid state)
  prominent, table, **07:** 597
Amides
 absorption data in water and in cyclohexane, **08:**
  141-143
 far ultraviolet absorption spectra
  aqueous solution at pH 5, **01:** 184
  neutral water, table, **01:** 185
  0.1 *M* sodium dodecyl sulfate, table, **01:** 185
 free energy; hydrolysis; •, **06:** 301
N-Amidinoglycyl, *see* Guanidinoacetyl
Amine
 buffers, structures and pK_a values, **06:** 368-369
 derivatives
  heat of proton ionization, pK, and related thermodynamics quantities, **06:** 162-164
 oxidase
  molar absorptivity and-or absorbance values, **02:** 392

table of cofactors, molecular weights, stoichiometry
 and sources, **02:** 282
Amines
 enzymatic incorporation of •
 proteins serving as substrates, list of, **02:** 680
 pK_a values, **06:** 322-326
 proteins, *see also* Bacteriophage Flavoproteins, Matrix
  protein, *also* Protein, individual proteins, Molybdoproteins; substrates for enzymatic incorporation of
  •, **02:** 680
α-Amino
 hemoglobin; human, *see also* Human hemoglobin; pK
  values, • groups, table, **02:** 693
α-Amino-γ-*N*-acetylaminobutyric acid
 physical and chemical properties, **01:** 119
Amino-acid, *see also* Amino acid
 one-letter symbols; • sequences, journal references, **02:**
  87
D-Amino-acid, *see also* D-Amino acid; D-Amino acids
 oxidase
  molar absorptivity and-or absorbance values, **02:** 392
  subunit, constitution of, **02:** 333
L-Amino-acid, *see also* L-Amino acid; L-Amino acids
 oxidase
  molar absorptivity and, **02:** or absorbance values, **02:**
   392
  subunit, constitution of, **02:** 336
α-Amino-actanoic acid
 physical and chemical properties, **01:** 115
α-Amino-ϵ-amidino caproic acid, *see* Indospicine
α-Amino-β-(2-amino-2-carboxyethylmercaptobutyric acid)
 physical and chemical properties, **01:** 151
2-Amino-4-(2-amino-3-hydroxypropoxy)-but-3-enoic acid,
  see Rhizobitoxine
3-Amino-2-benzylpropionic acid
 structure and symbols for those incorporated into synthetic polypeptides, **01:** 97
3-Amino-3-benzylpropionic acid
 structure and symbols for those incorporated into synthetic polypeptides, **01:** 97
α-Amino-*n*-butyric acid
 thumbprint, content in, **08:** 121
N-(3-Amino-3-carboxy-propyl)-β-carboxypyridinium betaine, *see also* Nicotianine
 physical and chemical properties, **01:** 161
3-Amino-(3-carboxy-propyldimethylsulfonium)
 physical and chemical properties, **01:** 151
3-Amino-3-carboxy-pyrrolidine, *see* Cucurbitine
α-Amino-γ-[2-(4-carboxy)-thiazolyl butyric acid]
 physical and chemical properties, **01:** 152
2-Amino-2-carboxyethane-sulfonamide
 antagonism to asparagine, **01:** 177
2-Amino-2-carboxyethyl-2-guanidineethyl hydrogen phosphate, *see* Lombricine
N-ϵ-(2-Amino-2-carboxyethyl)-lysine
 physical and chemical properties, **01:** 119
N-δ-(2-Amino-2-carboxyethyl)-ornithine
 physical and chemical properties, **01:** 119
3-Amino-3-carboxypropane-sulfonamide
 antagonism to glutamine, **01:** 177
3-(3-Amino-3-carboxypropyl)uridine
 composition in various tRNA's, **04:** 428-441

α-Amino-β-methylaminopropionic acid
 physical and chemical properties, 01: 120
γ-Amino-α-methylene butyric acid
 physical and chemical properties, 01: 114
α-Amino-β-(2-methylene cyclopropyl)-propionic acid, *see*
  Hypoglycin A
2-Amino-4-methylhexenoic acid
 antagonism to leucine, 01: 178
α-Amino-γ-methylthiobutyric acid, *see* Methionine
α-Amino-β-methylvaleric acid, *see* Isoleucine
1-Amino-2-nitrocyclopentane carboxylic acid
 physical and chemical properties, 01: 136
2-Amino-3-(*N*-nitrosohydroxyamino) propionic acid, *see*
  Alanosine
α-Amino-β-oxalylaminopropionic acid
 physical and chemical properties, 01: 120
α-Amino-β-phenylbutyric acid
 physical and chemical properties, 01: 129
3-Amino-4-phenylbutyric acid
 structure and symbols for those incorporated into synthetic polypeptides, 01: 99
α-Amino-β-phenylethanesulfonic acid
 antagonism to phenylalanine, 01: 179
β-Amino-β-phenylpropionic acid
 physical and chemical properties, 01: 129
α-Amino-β-phosphonopropionic acid
 physical and chemical properties, 01: 161
2-Amino-4-pontynoic acid
 physical and chemical properties, 01: 115
1-Amino-D-proline
 physical and chemical properties, 01: 165
α-Amino-β-propionic acid, *see* Tyrosine hydroxyphenyl
2-Amino-3-(2-pyridyl)propionic acid
 structure and symbols for those incorporated into synthetic polypeptides, 01: 99
2-Amino-3-(2-pyrimidyl)propionic acid
 structure and symbols for those incorporated into synthetic polypeptides, 01: 99
Amino-terminal
 plasminogen; sequence of the 69 residue • peptide
  released from, upon activation with urokinase, 07:
  354
Amino-terminal amino acid
 glu(Asp)-plasminogen, amino-terminus of single chain;
  alignment of • sequences homologous to, 07: 341
Amino-terminus
 glu(Asp)-plasminogen, • of single chain
  alignment of amino-terminal amino acid sequences
  homologous to, 07: 341
α-Amino-ε-Trimethylamino adipic acid, *see* Laminine
2-Amino-6-(trimethylammonio)hexanoic acid
 structure and symbols for those incorporated into synthetic polypeptides, 01: 99
2-Amino-3-ureidopropionic acid, *see* Albizzine
Amino acid, *see also* Amino-acid; Amino acids
 abbreviations; • derivatives, journal reference to rules,
  02: 87
 Acanthamoeba; • requirements for growth, table, 04: 641
 acetoacetate decarboxylase; • composition, complete
  data, 07: 505
 Acetobacter; • requirements for growth, table, 04: 630

acetylcholinesterase; • composition, incomplete data,
 07: 512
o-acetylserine sulfhydrylase A; • composition, complete
 data, 07: 505
α-acid glycoprotein; • composition, incomplete data,
 07: 512
Acidaminococcus; • requirements for growth, table, 04:
 630
acidic brain protein; • composition, incomplete data,
 07: 512
actin; • composition, complete data, 07: 505
actin; • sequence, 07: 490-491
Actinomyces; • requirements for growth, table, 04: 630
acyl carrier protein; • composition, complete data, 07:
 505
acyl carrier protein; • sequence, 07: 498
acyl phosphatase; • composition, incomplete data, 07:
 512
adenosine deaminase; • composition, complete data, 07:
 505
adenylate kinase; • composition, complete data, 07: 505
adenylosuccinase; • composition, complete data, 07: 505
adrenal iron-sulfur protein; • composition, complete
 data, 07: 505
adrenocorticotropins, natural; • sequence, 07: 375
adrenodoxin; • sequence, 07: 428
aequorin; • composition, complete data, 07: 505
Aerobacter; • requirements for growth, table, 04: 630
Agrobacterium; • requirements for growth, table, 04: 630
alanine amino transferase; • composition, complete
 data, 07: 505
alcohol dehydrogenase; • sequence, 07: 314-315
aldehyde dehydrogenase; • composition, complete data,
 07: 505
algae; • requirements for growth, table, 04: 630
alkaline phosphatase; • composition, complete data, 07:
 505
allergen 1-B; • composition, complete data, 07: 505
allergen (antigen K); • composition, complete data, 07:
 505
d-amino acid oxidase; • composition, complete data,
 07: 505
l-amino acid oxidase; • composition, complete data, 07:
 505
aminopeptidase (cytosol); • composition, complete data,
 07: 508
Amoeba; • requirements for growth, table, 04: 641
α-amylase; • composition, complete data, 07: 505
angiotensin I; • sequence, 07: 375
angiotensin II; • sequence, 07: 375
angiotensinogen; • sequence, 07: 375
antigen NN; • composition, incomplete data, 07: 512
antithrombin III; animal sources, • composition, 02:
 653
α¹-antitrypsin; animal sources, • composition, 02: 653
apoferritin; • composition, complete data, 07: 505
l-arabinose isomerase; • composition, complete data,
 07: 505
arginase; • composition, incomplete data, 07: 512
arginine decarboxylase; • composition, complete data,
 07: 505
arginine kinase; • composition, complete data, 07: 505

Amino acid *(continued)*

arginine vasopressin; • sequence, physical and biological properties, **07**: 197-198

arginine vasotocin; • sequence, biological properties, **07**: 195-196

ascorbic acid oxidase; • composition, incomplete data, **07**: 512

asparaginase; • composition, complete data, **07**: 505

l-aspartate β-decarboxylase; • composition, complete data, **07**: 505

aspartate carbamoyltransferase; • composition, complete data
catalytic subunit, **07**: 505
regulatory subunit, **07**: 505

aspartate carbamoyltransferase; • sequences, **07**: 308

aspartokinase I--homoserine dehydrogenase I; • composition, complete data, **07**: 505

Aspergillus; • requirements for growth, table, **04**: 640

azurin; • composition, complete data, **07**: 505

azurin; • sequence, **07**: 498

Bacillus; • requirements for growth, table, **04**: 631-632

bacteria; • requirements for growth, table, **04**: 630

bacteriochlorophyll-protein complex; • composition, complete data, **07**: 505

bacteriophage protein; • sequence of coat proteins, **07**: 261-262

Bacterium; • requirements for growth, table, **04**: 632

Bacteroides; • requirements for growth, table, **04**: 632

basic brain protein; • composition, incomplete data, **07**: 512

basic plasma protein; • composition, complete data, **07**: 505

Basidiobolus; • requirements for growth, table, **04**: 640

bee venom protein; • sequences, **07**: 498

Blastocladiales; • requirements for growth, table, **04**: 640

blood clotting factors; • sequences, **07**: 350-354

bond angles; • side chains, amino acid group, peptide linkage, **02**: 742-758

bond angles and distances; • side chains values for several, **08**: 222-223

bond lengths; • side chains, amino acid group, peptide linkage, **02**: 742-758

bond lengths; amino acid side chains, • group, peptide linkage, **02**: 742-758

Bordetella; • requirements for growth, table, **04**: 632

bovine α thrombin A chain; alignment of • sequences homologous to, **07**: 342-343

bowman-Birk inhibitor; plant sources, • composition, **02**: 606

bradykinin group; • sequence, physical and biological properties, **07**: 222-235

bradykininogen; • composition, incomplete data, **07**: 512

bromelain; • sequence, **07**: 356-357

Brucella; • requirements for growth, table, **04**: 632

butyric acid; • requirements for growth, table, **04**: 632

calcitonins; • sequence, **07**: 383

calcium-binding protein (high affinity); • composition, incomplete data, **07**: 512

carbamate kinase; • composition, complete data, **07**: 505

carbonic dehydratase B; • composition, complete data, **07**: 505

carboxypeptidase A; • composition, complete data, **07**: 505

carboxypeptidase A; • sequence, **07**: 338-339

carboxypeptidase B; • sequence, **07**: 338-339

carcinogen-binding protein; • composition, incomplete data, **07**: 512

k-casein component A; • composition, complete data, **07**: 505

catalase; • composition, complete data, **07**: 506

catalase; • sequences of proteins, **07**: 308

catechol 2,3-dioxygenase; • composition, complete data, **07**: 508

catechol 1,2-dioxygenase (pyrocatechase); • composition, complete data, **07**: 509

cellulase; • composition, complete data, **07**: 506

Cercospora; • requirements for growth, table, **04**: 640

ceruloplasmin; • composition, complete data, **07**: 506

Chlorella; • requirements for growth, table, **04**: 630

chlorobium, C_{555}; • sequence, **07**: 303

chloroperoxidase; • composition, incomplete data, **07**: 512

chorionic gonadotropin; • composition, complete data, **07**: 506

chorionic gonadotropin; • sequence
α subunit, **07**: 393-394, 402
β subunit, **07**: 402

chymopapain-B[5]; • sequence, **07**: 356-357

cilia protein, outer fibers; • composition, complete data, **07**: 506

citrate oxaloacetate lyase; • composition, incomplete data, **07**: 512

Cladosporium; • requirements for growth, table, **04**: 640

Clostridium; • requirements for growth, table, **04**: 633

clupeine, Pacific herring; • sequences, **07**: 498

coat proteins; • sequences, **07**: 261

cobramine B; • composition, complete data, **07**: 506

collagen; • composition, complete data, **07**: 506

collagen; selected • analysis, **07**: 520-521

collagen chains; • sequences, **07**: 474-488

Collectotrichum; • requirements for growth, table, **04**: 640

composition
proteinase inhibitors
animal sources, table, **02**: 649-653
microbial sources, **02**: 664
plant sources, table, **02**: 605-610
retinol-binding protein human, **02**: 303
Tamm-Horsfall glycoprotein, **02**: 303
urokinase, **02**: 302

composition, complete data, **07**: 509
circular dichroism in the UV region, **07**: 118
optical rotatory dispersion in the UV region, **07**: 70

compositions
discussion, complete data, **07**: 504
references, complete data, **07**: 515-519
selected proteins, complete data, **07**: 504
tables, complete data, **07**: 505-514

concanavalin A; • composition, complete data, **07**: 506

Coprinus; • requirements for growth, table, **04**: 640

Amino acid *(continued)*

corticosteroid-binding globulin; • composition, complete data, **07:** 506

corticotropin; • sequence, **07:** 385

cortisol metabolites binding large protein; • composition, incomplete data, **07:** 512

Corynebacterium; • requirements for growth, table, **04:** 633

Crithidia; • requirements for growth, table, **04:** 641

crotonase; • composition, complete data, **07:** 506

β-crustacyanin; • composition, complete data, 07: 506

β-crystallin; • composition, complete data. 07: 506

Curvularia; • requirements for growth, table, **04:** 640

cystathionase; • composition, complete data, **07:** 506

cystathionine γ-synthetase; • composition, complete data, **07:** 506

cysteamine to hypotaurine enzyme; • composition, complete data, **07:** 506

cytochrome *b*; • composition, complete data, **07:** 506

cytochrome *c*, *see also* Eukaryotic cytochromes *c*; • composition, complete data, **07:** 506

cytochrome *c*, *see also* Eukaryotic cytochromes *c*; • sequence, **07:** 304-306

cytochrome c_2; • sequence, **07:** 294-298

cytochrome c_3; • sequence, **07:** 299-301

cytochrome c_4; • sequence, **07:** 301

cytochrome c_5; • sequence, **07:** 302

cytochrome c_7; • sequence, **07:** 299-301

cytochrome *f*; • sequence, **07:** 304

cytotoxins; • sequences, **07:** 370-373

decarboxylase, aromatic
average hydrophobicity value, **01:** 213

deoxyribonuclease; • composition, complete data, **07:** 506

deoxyribonuclease inhibitor; • composition, complete data, **07:** 506

deoxyribose 5-phosphate aldolase; • composition, incomplete data, **07:** 512

dependent dehydrogenases; • sequence, **07:** 314

desulfovibrio C_{553}; • sequence, **07:** 302

dipeptidase; • composition, incomplete data, **07:** 512

diphosphopyridine nucleosidase; • composition, complete data, **07:** 506

disulfide-exchange enzyme; • composition, incomplete data, **07:** 512

DNA polymerase; • composition, complete data, **07:** 506

E. coli, *see also Escherichia coli*; RNAs from; • sequence, **04:** 333, 335

egg white cross-reacting protein; • composition, complete data, **07:** 506

eledoisin group, natural and related synthetic oligopeptide; • sequence, physical and biological properties, **07:** 236-257

encephalitogenic protein; • composition, complete data, **07:** 506

enolase; • composition, complete data, **07:** 506

enterotoxin C; • composition, complete data, **07:** 506

enzymes, *see also* Coenzyme, Metalloenzyme, Multienzyme; • sequences of proteins, **07:** 308-313

erabutoxin; • composition, incomplete data, **07:** 512

Escherichia coli, *see also E. coli*; • requirements for growth, table, **04:** 633

Escherichia coli ribosomal proteins: 30 S, composition, **04:** 476

Escherichia coli ribosomal proteins: 50 S, composition, **04:** 477-478

ethanolamine deaminase; • composition, complete data, **07:** 506

eukaryotic cytochromes *c*; • sequences of protein, tables, **07:** 268-285

exo-β-D-(1→3)-glucanase; • composition, complete data, **07:** 506

factor X; • composition, complete data, **07:** 506

factor X_1; • sequence of, **07:** 353

fatty acid synthetase; • composition, incomplete data, **07:** 512

ferredoxin; • composition, complete data, **07:** 506

ferredoxins, bacterial; • sequences of some, **07:** 421-424

ferrodoxyins, plant; • sequences, **07:** 425-426

fetuin; • composition, complete data, **07:** 506

fetuin; animal sources, • composition, **02:** 653

fibrinopeptides A; • sequences, **07:** 431-433

fibrinopeptides B; • sequences, **07:** 433-435

ficin; • sequence, **07:** 356-357

flagellin; • composition, complete data, **07:** 506

Flavobacterium; • requirements for growth, table, **04:** 633-634

flavodoxin; • composition, complete data, **07:** 506

flavodoxin; • sequence, **07:** 430

follicle-stimulating hormones; • composition, complete data, **07:** 506

follicle-stimulating hormones; • sequence of α subunit, **07:** 393-394

formyltetrahydrofolate synthetase; • composition, incomplete data, **07:** 512

fraction 1 protein; • composition, complete data, **07:** 507

fructose-bisphosphate aldolase; • composition, complete date, **07:** 507

fructose-bisphosphate aldolase; • sequence, **07:** 333-335

fructose 1,6-diphosphate adolase A; • composition, complete data, **07:** 507

fumarase; • composition, complete data, **07:** 507

fungi; • requirements for growth, table, **04:** 640

Fusarium; • requirements for growth, table, **04:** 640

Fusobacterium; • requirements for growth, table, **04:** 634

γG immunoglobulin kappa chain; • composition, complete data, **07:** 508

galactokinase; • composition, complete data, **07:** 507

galactose 1-phosphate uridylyltransferase; • composition, incomplete data, **07:** 512

galactose oxidase; • composition, incomplete data, **07:** 512

β-galactosidase; • composition, complete data, 07: 507

gastrin I; • composition, incomplete data, **07:** 512

gastrins; • sequence, **07:** 323

Glaucoma; • requirements for growth, table, **04:** 641

α-gliadin; • composition, incomplete data, 07: 512

Gliocladium; • requirements for growth, table, **04:** 640

globins, metazoan, aligned chains; • sequence, **07:** 456-458

glucagon; • sequence, **07:** 376

ν-glucuronidase; • composition, incomplete data, 07: 512

glutamate dehydrogenase; • sequence, **07:** 316-318

Amino acid *(continued)*

glutamate dehydrogenase[3] neurospora (NADP); • sequence, 07: 318-320

glutamate mutase component; • composition, incomplete data, 07: 512

glutathione reductase (NAD(P)H); • composition, incomplete data, 07: 512

glyceraldehyde-3-phosphate dehydrogenase; • sequence, 07: 327-329

l-glycerol 3-phosphate dehydrogenase; • composition, complete data, 07: 507

glycogen phosphorylase; • composition, incomplete data, 07: 507

glycolytic enzymes; • sequences, 07: 324, 337

glycoprotein; • composition, complete data, 07: 507

glycoprotein; • composition, incomplete data, 07: 512

glycoprotein hormones; • sequences of α subunit, 07: 393-394

glycoprotein M-1; • composition, incomplete data, 07: 513

group
dimensions of, 02: 742-758

group specific protein; • composition, incomplete data, 07: 513

growth hormone; • composition, complete data, 07: 507

growth hormone; • sequence, 07: 376, 388-389, 392-393

guanyloribonuclease; • composition, complete data, 07: 510

guanyloribonuclease; • sequences, 07: 311

hageman factor; • composition, incomplete data, 07: 513

Halobacterium; • requirements for growth, table, 04: 634

haptoglobin; • composition, complete data, 07: 507

Helminthosporium; • requirements for growth, table, 04: 640

hemagglutinin; • composition, complete data, 07: 507

hemagglutinin; • composition, incomplete data, 07: 513

hemerythrin; • composition, complete data, 07: 507

hemerythrin; • sequences, 07: 498

hemocyanin; • composition, complete data, 07: 507

hemoglobin; • composition, complete data, 07: 507

hemoglobin, vertebrate tetrameric; • sequence
α type chains, 07: 441-447
β type chains, 07: 448-455

hemolysin; • composition, incomplete data, 07: 513

Hemophilus; • requirements for growth, table, 04: 634

hexokinase; • composition, incomplete data, 07: 513

hexosediphosphatase; • composition, complete data, 07: 507

Hiochi bacteria; • requirements for growth, table, 04: 634

hirudin; • composition, complete data, 07: 507

hirudin; animal sources, • composition, 02: 649

histidine ammonialyase; • composition, complete data, 07: 507

histidine decarboxylase; • composition, complete data, 07: 507

histidinol dehydrogenase; • composition, complete data, 07: 507

histone IV; • composition, complete data, 07: 507

histone IV; • sequence, 07: 499

hormone-binding polypeptide; • composition, complete data, 07: 507

hormones; • sequence, 07: 375-376, 378-381

hormones; anterior pituitary; • sequence, 07: 385-397

hormones; parathyroid; • sequence, 07: 399

hormones; placenta; • sequence, 07: 385-397

hyaluronidase; • composition, complete data, 07: 507

hydrophobicity; • side chains
calculation of, 01: 209
table of values, 01: 209

β-hydroxydecanoyl thioester dehydrase; • composition, complete data, 07: 507

hydroxypyruvate reductase; • composition, incomplete data, 07: 513

hypobranchial mucin; • composition, incomplete data, 07: 513

imidazoylacetolphosphate: L-glutamate aminotransferase; • composition, complete data, 07: 508

immobilizing antigen; • composition, complete data, 07: 508

immunoglobulin; possible • sequence correlations, 07: 530-531

incisor eruption accelerating protein; • composition, incomplete data, 07: 513

indole-3-glycerol phosphate synthetase; • composition, complete data, 07: 508

insulin A chains; • sequence, 07: 378

insulin B chains; • sequence, 07: 379-380

interstitial cell-stimulating hormone; • composition, incomplete data, 07: 513

intrinsic factor; • composition, incomplete data, 07: 513

invertase (external); • composition, complete data, 07: 508

isocitrate dehydrogenase; • composition, complete data, 07: 508

isocitrate lyase; • composition, complete data, 07: 508

isomerase of histidine biosynthesis; • composition, complete data, 07: 508

β-isopropylmalate dehydrogenase; • composition, complete data, 07: 508

α-isopropylmalate synthetase; • composition, complete data, 07: 508

isotocin; • sequence, 07: 195

kallidin group; • sequence, physical and biological properties, 07: 222-235

kallikrein inhibitor; plant sources, • composition, 02: 606

keratin; • composition, complete data, 07: 508

β-ketoacyl acyl carrier protein synthetase; • composition, complete data, 07: 508

Δ[5]-3-ketosteroid isomerase; • composition, complete data, 07: 508

kunitz inhibitor; plant sources, • composition, 02: 606

α-lactalbumin; • sequence, 07: 499

lactate dehydrogenase; • sequence, 07: 320-321, 336-337

d-lactate dehydrogenase; • composition, complete data, 07: 508

Lactobacillus; • requirements for growth, table, 04: 634-635

lactogenic hormone; • sequence, 07: 390-392

β-lactoglobulin; • composition, complete data, 07: 508

lactollin; • composition, complete data, 07: 508

Amino acid *(continued)*

lactoperoxidase; • composition, complete data, 07: 508

leghemoglobin, soybean, aligned chains; • sequence, 07: 456-458

Leptospira; • requirements for growth, table, 04: 636

leucine binding protein; • composition, complete data, 07: 508

Leuconostoc; • requirements for growth, table, 04: 636

levansucrase; • composition, complete data, 07: 508

lipoamide dehydrogenase (NADH); • composition, complete data, 07: 508

lipoprotein; • composition, complete data, 07: 508

lipoprotein; • composition, incomplete data, 07: 513

lipoprotein B; • sequence, 07: 387, 499

liver alcohol dehydrogenase; • sequence, 07: 330-332

luciferase chain α; • composition, complete data, 07: 508

luteinizing hormone, *see also* Interstitial cell-stimulating hormone, 07: 30, 66; • sequence

α subunit, 07: 393-394

β subunit, 07: 395-397

lysine-vasopressin; • sequence, physical and biological properties, 07: 197-198

l-lysine monooxygenase; • composition, complete data, 07: 508

lysostaphin; • composition, incomplete data, 07: 513

lysozyme; • composition, complete data, 07: 508

lysozyme; • sequences of proteins, 07: 309

maleate isomerase; • composition, incomplete data, 07: 513

malic dehydrogenase (mitochondrial); • composition, complete data, 07: 508

β-mannase; • composition, incomplete data, 07: 513

melanotropin; • sequence

α, 07: 385

natural, 07: 375

β, 07: 386

Meningococcus; • requirements for growth, table, 04: 636

mesotocin; • sequence, 07: 195

methionyl-lysl-bradykinin; • sequence, physical and biological properties, 07: 222

β-methylaspartase; • composition, complete data, 07: 508

Methylococcus; • requirements for growth, table, 04: 636

microbial metalloenzyme; • sequence, 07: 322

Micrococcus; • requirements for growth, table, 04: 636

β₂-microglobulin; • composition, incomplete data, 07: 513

microorganisms; • requirements for growth, table, 04: 630-643

microtubule protein; • composition, complete data, 07: 509

mitochondrial structural protein; • composition, complete data, 07: 509

mitotic apparatus 22S protein; • composition, incomplete data, 07: 513

monoamine oxidase; • composition, complete data, 07: 509

monophenol monooxygenase; • composition, complete data, 07: 511

mucin (major); • composition, incomplete data, 07: 513

mucoprotein, Tamm-Horsfall; • composition, complete data, 07: 510

multienzyme complex in tryptophan pathway; • composition, complete data, 07: 509

muscle contractile proteins; • sequence, 07: 490-496

Mycobacterium; • requirements for growth, table, 04: 636

Mycoplana; • requirements for growth, table, 04: 636

Mycoplasma; • requirements for growth, table, 04: 636

myeloperoxidase; • composition, complete data, 07: 509

myoglobin; • sequence, 07: 437-440

myoglobin, vertebrate; • sequence, 07: 437-440

myosin; • composition, complete data, 07: 509

myosin; • sequence, 07: 493

Myxococcus (Myxobacterium); • requirements for growth, table, 04: 636

myxovirus hemagglutination inhibitor; • composition, incomplete data, 07: 513

Neisseria; • requirements for growth, table, 04: 637

nerve growth factor fraction A; • composition, incomplete data, 07: 513

neurotoxin α; • composition, complete data, 07: 509

neurotoxin α; • sequence, 07: 499

neurotoxin II; • composition, complete data, 07: 509

neurotoxins, long; • sequences, 07: 366-369

neurotoxins, short; • sequence, 07: 360-365

nicotinamide deamidase; • composition, complete data, 07: 509

nomenclature; • derivatives, symbols for, rules, 01: 79-88

nuclease; • composition, complete data, 07: 509

nuclease-T; • sequences of protein, 07: 310

5'-nucleotidase; • composition, incomplete data, 07: 513

Ochromonas; • requirements for growth, table, 04: 642

old yellow enzyme; • composition, incomplete data, 07: 513

oligopeptides, natural, and related synthetic • sequence, physical and biological properties

bradykinin group, 07: 222-235

eledoisin group, 07: 236-257

kallidin group, 07: 222-235

oxytocins, 07: 192-220

physaleamin group, 07: 258-260

vasopressins, 07: 192-220

Ophiobolus; • requirements for growth, table, 04: 641

ornithine aminotransferase; • composition, complete data, 07: 509

ovoinhibitor; • composition, incomplete data, 07: 513

ovomucoid; animal sources, • composition, 02: 650

oxaloglycolate reductive decarboxylase; • composition, incomplete data, 07: 513

oxytocins, natural and related synthetic oligopeptides; • sequence, physical and biological properties, 07: 193-218

papain; • sequence, 07: 356-357

Paramecium; • requirements for growth, table, 04: 642

parathyroid hormone; • composition, complete data, 07: 509

parathyroid polypeptide; • composition, complete data, 07: 509

parvalbumins; • sequence, 07: 496

Amino acid *(continued)*

Pasteurella; • requirements for growth, table, **04**: 637
Pediococcus; • requirements for growth, table, **04**: 637
penicillinase; • composition, complete data, **07**: 509
penicillinase; • composition, incomplete data, **07**: 513
penicillinase; • sequences of proteins, **07**: 310
Penicillium; • requirements for growth, table, **04**: 641
pepsin, porcine; • sequence, **07**: 358
pepsin inhibitors; animal sources, • composition, **02**: 649
pepsinogen; • composition, complete data, **07**: 509
peroxidase B; • composition, complete data, **07**: 509
phenylpyruvate tautomerase; • composition, incomplete data, **07**: 513
Phoma; • requirements for growth, table, **04**: 641
phosphoenolpyruvate carboxykinase; • composition, complete data, **07**: 509
phosphofructokinase; • composition, complete data, **07**: 509
phosphoglucomutase; • composition, complete data, **07**: 509
phosphogluconate dehydrogenase (decarboxylating); • composition, complete data, **07**: 509
phosphoglycerate dehydrogenase; • composition, complete data, **07**: 509
phosphoglyceromutase; • composition, complete data, **07**: 509
phospholipase A; • composition, complete data, **07**: 509
n-1-(5′-phosphoribosyl) adenosine triphosphate pyrophosphate phosphoribosyl transferase; • composition, incomplete data, **07**: 513
phosvitin fraction II; • composition, complete data, **07**: 509
Photobacterium; • requirements for growth, table, **04**: 637
phycocyanin; • composition, incomplete data, **07**: 513
Phycomyces; • requirements for growth, table, **04**: 641
physalaemin group, natural and related synthetic oligopeptide; • sequence, physical and biological properties, **07**: 258-260
phytochrome; • composition, incomplete data, **07**: 514
Phytophthora; • requirements for growth, table, **04**: 641
pituitary, anterior, hormones; • sequences, **07**: 385-397
placenta, hormones; • sequence, **07**: 385-397
placental lactogen, human; • sequence compared with human growth hormone and human prolactin, **07**: 392-393
Plasmodium; • requirements for growth, table, **04**: 642
Pneumococcus; • requirements for growth, table, **04**: 637
polyol dehydrogenase; • composition, incomplete data, **07**: 514
poricin; • composition, incomplete data, **07**: 514
prealbumin; • composition, complete data, **07**: 509
proinsulin; • composition, complete data, **07**: 509
proinsulin; • sequence, **07**: 381
prokaryotic cytochromes *b*; • sequence, **07**: 280-281
prokaryotic cytochromes *c*; • sequence, **07**: 292-306
Propionibacterium; • requirements for growth, table, **04**: 637

propionyl coenzyme A carboxylase; • composition, incomplete data, **07**: 514
protein, S-100 brain-; • composition, incomplete data, **07**: 514
protein, R17 coat-; • composition, complete data, **07**: 510
protein, red-; • composition, complete data, **07**: 510
proteinase zymogen; • composition, complete data, **07**: 509
proteins, iron-sulfur primary structures; • sequences, **07**: 425-427
Proteus; • requirements for growth, table, **04**: 637
prothrombin; • sequence, **07**: 351-352
protocatechuate 3,4-dioxygenase; • composition, complete data, **07**: 509
protozoa; • requirements for growth, table, **04**: 641
Pseudomonas; • requirements for growth, table, **04**: 637
pseudomonas cytochrome c_{551}; • sequence, **07**: 292-294
psoriatic scale protein; • composition, complete data, **07**: 509
purine nucleoside phosphorylase; • composition, complete data, **07**: 509
putidaredoxin, bacterial; • sequence, **07**: 428
pyridine nucleotide; • sequence, **07**: 314
pyrophosphatase; • composition, incomplete data, **07**: 514
pyruvate kinase; • composition, complete data, **07**: 510
replacements in naturally occurring (NM) and chemically induced (CM) mutants of TMV, location of some, **07**: 266-267
rhodopsin; • composition, incomplete data, **07**: 514
Rhodospirillum; • requirements for growth, table, **04**: 637
ribonuclease; • composition, complete data, **07**: 510
ribonuclease, pancreatic; • sequences of proteins, **07**: 311
ribonucleotide reductase; • composition, incomplete data, **07**: 514
1-ribulokinase; • composition, incomplete data, **07**: 514
ribulose 1,5-diphosphate carboxylase; • composition, complete data, **07**: 510
1-ribulose 5-phosphate 4-epimerase; • composition, complete data, **07**: 510
RNA nucleotidyltransferase; • composition, complete data, **07**: 510
rubredoxin; • composition, complete data, **07**: 510
rubredoxin; • sequence, **07**: 429
30S ribosomal protein; • composition, incomplete data, **07**: 514
Saccharomyces; • requirements for growth, table, **04**: 643
Saccharomyces cerevisiae; • requirements for growth, table, **04**: 643
salmonella; • requirements for growth, table, **04**: 638
secretin; • sequence, **07**: 376
sequence data, ribosomal proteins from *Escherichia coli*, **04**: 479-481
sequence for selected proteins, **07**: 192-339
sequences
  β_2 microglobulin, **02**: 305

Amino acid *(continued)*

  proteinase inhibitors
    animal sources, table, 02: 656-659
    microbial source, 02: 665
    plant sources, 02: 611-617
  rules for one-letter notation, 02: 59-62
  sequences, tables, 07: 341-349
ser, Ile oxytocin; • sequence, 07: 194-195
serine proteases, trypsin-related; • sequence data, index
  to
  blood clotting factors, 07: 350-354
  explanation of tables, 07: 340-341
  sequence alignments, 07: 341-349
serine transacetylase; • composition, incomplete data,
  07: 514
serotypic antigen 51A; • composition, incomplete data,
  07: 514
serum albumin; • composition, complete data, 07: 510
serum albumin; • sequence, 07: 497
Shigella; • requirements for growth, table, 04: 638
side chains
  dimensions of, 02: 742-758
soybean trypsin inhibitor F$_3$; • composition, complete
  data, 07: 510
Staphylococci; • requirements for growth, table, 04: 638
stellacyanin; • composition, incomplete data, 07: 514
streptococcal proteinase; • sequence, 07: 356-357
Streptococci; • requirements for growth, table, 04: 638
streptokinase; • composition, complete data, 07: 510
subtilisin; • composition, complete data, 07: 510
subtilisin; • sequences of proteins, 07: 312
sulfatase A; • composition, incomplete data, 07: 514
sulfate-binding protein; • composition, complete data,
  07: 510
superoxide dismutase; • composition, complete data, 07:
  506
sweet-sensitive protein; • composition, incomplete data,
  07: 514
tartrate dehydrogenase; • composition, complete data,
  07: 510
tartrate epoxidase; • composition, complete data, 07:
  510
tartronic semialdehyde reductase; • composition, complete data, 07: 510
Tetrahymena; • requirements for growth, table, 04: 642
thiogalactoside transacetylase; • composition, complete
  data, 07: 510
thioredoxin; • composition, complete data, 07: 510
thioredoxin; • sequence, 07: 500
thioredoxin reductase; • composition, complete data,
  07: 510
threonine deaminase; • composition, complete data, 07:
  510
thumbprint, • content, 08: 121
thyroglobulin; • composition, incomplete data, 07: 514
thyroid stimulating hormone; • sequence, 07: 393-397
thyroxine-binding globulin; • composition, incomplete
  data, 07: 514
tobacco mosaic virus; • composition, complete data, 07:
  510
tobacco mosaic virus; • sequence of coat proteins, 07:
  261-262

tobacco mosaic virus; location of some • replacements
  in naturally occurring andchemical induced mutants
  of, 07: 266-267
Torula; • requirements for growth, table, 04: 643
toxin, *see also* Neurotoxin; • composition, complete
  data, 07: 510
toxin, *see also* Neurotoxin; animal sources, • composition, 02: 650
toxin (type A); • composition, complete data, 07: 510
toxins, angusticeps-type; from venom of various snakes,
  • sequence, 07: 365
transcortin; • composition, incomplete data, 07: 514
transferrin, *see also* Ovotransferrin; • composition, complete data, 07: 510
transglutaminase; • composition, complete data, 07: 510
Treponema; • requirements for growth, table, 04: 639
Trichomonas; • requirements for growth, table, 04: 642
Trichophyton; • requirements for growth, table, 04: 641
triosephosphate isomerase; • composition, complete
  data, 07: 510
triosephosphate isomerase; • sequences, 07: 324-326
tripeptide synthetase; • composition, complete data, 07:
  510
tropomyosin; • sequence, 07: 492
troponin Ca^{++}-binding protein (Tn-C) rabbit skeletal; •
  sequence, 07: 495
troponin inhibitor (Tn-I), rabbit skeletal; • sequence,
  07: 494
trypsin inhibitor, *see also* Trypsin inhibitors; • composition, complete data, 07: 510
trypsin inhibitor, *see also* Trypsin inhibitors; • sequence,
  07: 500
trypsin inhibitor, *see also* Trypsin inhibitors; animal
  sources, • composition, 02: 649
trypsin inhibitor, *see also* Trypsin inhibitors; plant
  sources, • composition, 02: 607-609
trypsin inhibitor, basic (kallikrein inactivator); • composition, complete data, 07: 510
trypsin inhibitor (acidic); • composition, complete data,
  07: 510
trypsinogen; • composition, complete data, 07: 510
tryptophan oxygenase; • composition, complete data,
  07: 510
tryptophan synthetase A protein; • composition, complete data, 07: 510
tryptophan synthetase A protein; • sequences of
  proteins, 07: 313
tryptophanase; • composition, complete data, 07: 510
tryptophanyl tRNA synthetase; • composition, complete
  data, 07: 510
turnip yellow mosaic virus; • sequences of virus coat
  proteins, 07: 263-265
tyrosine aminotransferase; • composition, complete
  data, 07: 511
urease; • composition, incomplete data, 07: 514
uridine diphosphate galactose 4-epimerase; • composition, complete data, 07: 511
uridine diphosphate galactose: lipopolysaccharide
  α-3-galactosyl transferase; • composition, incomplete
  data, 07: 514
urokinase; • composition, incomplete data, 07: 514

Amniotic fluid *(continued)*
  citrulline; free acid in • in early pregnancy and at term, **01:** 327
  cysteic acid; free acid in • in early pregnancy and at term, **01:** 327
  cystine; free acid in • in early pregnancy and at term, **01:** 327
  glutamic acid; free acid in • in early pregnancy and at term, **01:** 327
  glutamine; free acid in • in early pregnancy and at term, **01:** 327
  glycine; free acid in • in early pregnancy and at term, **01:** 327
  histidine; free acid in • in early pregnancy and at term, **01:** 327
  hydroxyproline; free acid in • in early pregnancy and at term, **01:** 327
  isoleucine; free acid in • in early pregnancy and at term, **01:** 327
  leucine; free acid in • in early pregnancy and at term, **01:** 327
  lysine; free acid in • in early pregnancy and at term, **01:** 327
  methionine; free acid in • in early pregnancy and at term, **01:** 327
  ornithine; free acid in • in early pregnancy and at term, **01:** 327
  phenylalanine; free acid in • in early pregnancy and at term, **01:** 327
  proline; free acid in • in early pregnancy and at term, **01:** 327
  serine; free acid in • in early pregnancy and at term, **01:** 327
  taurine; free acid in • in early pregnancy and at term, **01:** 327
  threonine; free acid in • in early pregnancy and at term, **01:** 327
  tryptophan; free acid in • in early pregnancy and at term, **01:** 327
  tyrosine; free acid in • in early pregnancy and at term, **01:** 327
  valine; free acid in • in early pregnancy and at term, **01:** 327
AMP
  heat of proton ionization, pK, and related thermodynamic quantities, **06:** 160
  pK'_a values, **06:** 330
D-AMP-3, *see also* Thiamphenicol
  thiamphenicol (•); origin, structure, and characteristic as protein biosynthesis inhibitor, **04:** 609
Amphotericin B
  UV spectra, formula, molecular weight, **08:** 184
Amylase
  average hydrophobicity values, **01:** 213
  enzymatic activity, subcellular fractions, **02:** 698, 714
  molar absorptivity, and-or absorbance values, **02:** 393
  table of cofactors, molecular weights, stoichiometry and sources, **02:** 278
α-Amylase
  amino acid composition, complete data, **07:** 505
  average hydrophobicity values, **01:** 213
  carbohydrate content, **02:** 274
  circular dichroism
    in UV and near UV region, **07:** 84, 143

molar absorptivity and-or absorbance values, **02:** 393
optical rotatory dispersion
  UV region, **07:** 46
  visible and near UV regions, **07:** 17
refractive index increments, **02:** 374
subunit, constitution of, **02:** 332
β-Amylase
  circular dichroism in the UV region, **07:** 84
  luminescence of, table, **01:** 205
  molar absorptivity and-or absorbance values, **02:** 394
  optical rotatory dispersion
    UV region, **07:** 47
    visible and near UV regions, **07:** 17
  subunit, constitution of, **02:** 340
α-Amylase-I, II
  average hydrophobicity values, **01:** 213
Amylase PI, PII, PIII
  average hydrophobicity values, **01:** 213
Analgesics
  ligands binding to plasma albumin, **02:** 570
Analogs
  amino acids, *see also* Aromatic amino acids, *also* specific acids; α-Keto acids • of, properties, **01:** 181-182
  formula, molecular; prostaglandin •, **08:** 397-421
  molecular weight; prostaglandin •, **08:** 397-421
  prostaglandins; •
    names and structures, **08:** 396-421
    properties, physical and biological, **08:** 396-421
    synthesis and importance, general information, **08:** 394-395
  structure; prostaglandin •, **08:** 396-421
  trivial names; prostaglandin •, **08:** 396-421
C3a anaphyla
  toxin
    circular dichroism in the UV region, **07:** 84
C5a anaphyla
  toxin
    circular dichroism in the UV region, **07:** 84
Androgens
  structures and properties, **05:** 531-533
Angiotensin amide
  luminescence of, **01:** 204
Angiotensin I
  amino acid sequence, **07:** 375
Angiotensin II
  amino acid sequence, **07:** 375
Angiotensinogen
  amino acid sequence, **07:** 375
Angolamycin
  origin, structure, and characteristic as protein biosynthesis inhibitor, **04:** 559
Angusticeps-type toxins, *see* Toxins, angusticeps-type
Angustmycin A
  physicochemical constants, spectral, chemotherapeutic and biological properties, **03:** 282
Angustmycin C
  physicochemical constants, spectral, chemotherapeutic and biological properties, **03:** 284
Anhydrase
  pK; histidine in; carbonic •, values for residues, **02:** 691
Anhydrase B and C
  carbonic •, average hydrophobicity values, **01:** 216

Anhydrase C
  carbonic •, human erythrocyte structure, schematic il-
    lustrating, **02:** 765
Anhydrides
  monosaccharides; •, nomenclature rules, **05:** 130-132
Aniline
  derivatives
    heat of proton ionization, pK, and related thermody-
      namic quantities, **06:** 168-169
Anilines
  pK'_a values, **06:** 327-330
Anion
  N-acetyl-L-tyrosine ethyl ester •, UV spectra, **01:** 195
  riboflavin •
    UV spectra, formula, molecular weight, **08:** 161
Anions, *see also* Inorganic anions, Ions,
  albumin, plasma, *see also* Human plasma albumin;
    Plasma albumin; ligand binding; inorganic •, list of
    references, **02:** 563
Anisomycin
  origin, structure, and characteristics as protein biosyn-
    thesis inhibitor, **04:** 559
Anomers
  in carbohydrate nomenclature, **05:** 114-115
Antamanide
  proton NMR and suggested conformations, **07:** 570
Anthelmycin
  structure, **03:** 285
Anthracene 2-isocyanate
  covalent protein conjugates, data, **01:** 208
Anthranilate-PP-ribose-P phosphoribosyl-transferase
  Neurospora crassa mutant, **04:** 749
Anthranilate synthetase
  Neurospora crassa mutant, **04:** 754
Anthranylate
  synthetase, component I, II
    average hydrophobicity value, **01:** 213
Antibiotic 9-27, *see* Toyocamycin
Antibiotic 9-48, *see* Toyocamycin
Antibiotic 1037, C, D, D-13, E-212, R-285, T-3018
  physicochemical constants, spectral, chemotherapeutic
    and biological properties, **03:** 286-292
Antibiotic A-14, *see* Angustmycin A
Antibiotic A-128-OP
  Telomycin® (•); origin, structure, and characteristic as
    protein biosynthesis inhibitor, **04:** 607
Antibiotic T
  crotocin (•); origin, structure, and characteristic as
    protein biosynthesis inhibitor, **04:** 568
Antibiotic U-18496, *see* 5-Azacytidine
Antibiotic U-9586, *see* Angustmycin C
Antibiotics
  ligands binding to plasma albumin, **02:** 568-569
  pK'_a values, **06:** 348
Antibiotics, nucleoside, *see also* Nucleoside antibiotics
  chemotherapeutic properties; •, **03:** 271-393
  chromatography; •, **03:** 271-393
  formula, molecular; •, **03:** 271-393
  IR spectra; •, **03:** 271-393
  melting point; •, **03:** 271-393
  molecular weight; •, **03:** 271-393
  optical rotation; •, **03:** 271-393

physicochemical constants, spectral, chemotherapeutic
    and biological properties, **03:** 271-393
  pK; •, **03:** 271-393
  pMR spectra; •, **03:** 271-393
  solubility; •, **03:** 271-393
  structure; •, **03:** 271-393
  toxicity; •, **03:** 271-393
  UV spectra; •, **03:** 271-393
Antibodies
  serum •
    methods for detection, **07:** 543-544
Antibody
  -producing cells
    methods for detection, **07:** 542
Anticapsin
  physical and chemical properties, **01:** 136
Anticoagulants
  ligands binding to plasma albumin, **02:** 571
Antigen
  Australia •
    circular dichroism in the UV region, **07:** 86
  immobilizing •
  graft rejection; hisocompatibility •, presence of,
    04: 884
  human red cell. list, **04:** 880
    amino acid composition, complete data, **07:** 508
    molar absorptivity and-or absorbance values, **02:** 395
  serotypic • 51A
    amino acid composition, incomplete data, **07:** 514
Antigen K
  allergen (•)
    amino acid composition, complete data, **07:** 505
Antigen NN
  amino acid composition, incomplete data, **07:** 512
Antihemophilic factor
  physical data and characteristics, **02:** 254-255
Antihemorrhagic
  vitamins, properties of, **08:** 290
Antithrombin III
  animal sources, amino acid composition, **02:** 653
  carbohydrate composition, **02:** 666-667
  mammalian and chicken blood specificity and proper-
    ties, **02:** 636-637
  molecular parameters, **02:** 243
α^1-Antitrypsin
  animal sources, amino acid composition, **02:** 653
  carbohydrate composition, **02:** 666-667
  mammalian and chicken blood specificity and proper-
    ties, **02:** 636-637
  molecular parameters, **02:** 242
Apo-high density
  lipoprotein
    average hydrophobicity value, **01:** 214
Apocytocuprein
  cytocuprein; •, human
    molar absorptivity and-or absorbance values, **02:** 417
Apoferritin
  amino acid composition, complete data, **07:** 505
Apolipoprotein-
  valine
    average hydrophobicity value, **01:** 214

Apolipoprotein--alanine-I, II
average hydrophobicity value, 01: 214
Apolipoprotein--glutamine-I, II
average hydrophobicity value, 01: 214
Apolipoprotein Glu-II
molar absorptivity and-or absorbance values, 02: 395
ApoLP-Val
lipoprotein very low density, human •
molar absorptivity and-or absorbance values, 02: 467
Apomyoglobin
sperm whale
luminescence of, table, 01: 206
Apovitellinin-I
average hydrophobicity value, 01: 214
Aqueous
density; guanidine hydrochloride, • solutions with
added reagents, at 25°, 06: 406
Aqueous solution, see also Aqueous solutions
amino acids, see also Aromatic amino acids, also
specific acids; free energy of formation in • at 25°C,
06: 118
amino acids, see also Aromatic amino acids, also
specific acids; free energy of solution in • at 25°C,
06: 118
amino acids, see also Aromatic amino acids, also
specific acids; heats of solution in • at 25°C, 06:
116-117
arginine; far ultraviolet absorption spectra; • at pH5,
01: 184
cysteine; far ultraviolet absorption spectra; • at pH 5,
01: 184
½cystine; far ultraviolet absorption spectra; • at pH 5,
01: 184
free energy of formation; amino acids in • at 25°C, 06:
118
free energy of solution; amino acids in • at 25°C, 06:
118
heat of solution; amino acids in • at 25°C, 06: 116-117
histidine; far ultraviolet absorption spectra; • at pH 5,
01: 184
leucine; far ultraviolet absorption spectra; • at pH 5,
01: 184
lysine; far ultraviolet absorption spectra; • at pH 5, 01:
184
methionine; far ultraviolet absorption spectra, 01: 185;
• at pH 5, 01: 184
Aqueous solutions, see also Aqueous solution
density; urea, • with added reagents, at 25°, 06: 406
guanidine hydrochloride; densities of • with added reagents, at 25°, 06: 406
guanidine hydrochloride; viscosities of • with added
reagents, at 25°, 06: 407
guanidine hydrochloride; viscosity of • at 25°, 06: 405
urea; densities of • with added reagents, at 25°, 06: 406
urea; viscosities of • with added reagents, at 25°, 06:
407
urea; viscosity of • at 25°, 06: 405
viscosity; guanidine hydrochloride, • at 25°, 06: 405
viscosity; guanidine hydrochloride, • with added reagents, at 25°, 06: 407
viscosity; urea, • at 25°, 06: 405

α-L-Arabinofuranosidase
average hydrophobicity value, 01: 214
molar absorptivity and-or absorbance values, 02: 395
9-β-D-Arabinofuranosyladenine (Ara-A)
physicochemical constants, spectral, chemotherapeutic
and biological properties, 03: 293
1-β-D-Arabinofuranosylthymine
physical constants and spectral properties, 03: 135
1-β-D-Arabinofuranosyluracil
physical constants and spectral properties, 03: 135
Arabinose
heat of proton ionization, pK, and related thermodynamic quantities, 06: 169
pK'$_a$ values, 06: 317
L-Arabinose-binding protein
average hydrophobicity value, 01: 214
Arachidonic acid
biological and physical properties, 08: 322-328
isolation and synthesis of, 08: 326-327
liberation phosphatidyl inositol, 08: 320
occurrence, 08: 325
precursor in prostaglandin biosynthesis, 08: 334-338
Arachin
molar absorptivity and-or absorbance values, 02: 395
refractive index increments, 02: 374
subunit, constitution of, 02: 346
Arginase
amino acid composition, incomplete data, 07: 512
bovine liver
luminescence of, table, 01: 205
enzymatic activity, subcellular fractions, 02: 698
molar absorptivity and-or absorbance values, 02: 395
optical rotatory dispersion
UV region, 07: 47
visible and near UV regions, 07: 17
subunit, constitution of, 02: 335
Arginine
antagonism to lysine, 01: 178
antagonists of, 01: 177
bond distances and angles for side chain, 08: 222
decarboxylase
amino acid composition, complete data, 07: 505
average hydrophobicity value, 01: 214
molar absorptivity and-or absorbance values, 02: 395
subunit, constitution of, 02: 345, 350
far ultraviolet absorption spectra
aqueous solution at pH5, 01: 184
neutral water, table, 01: 185
0.1 M sodium dodecyl sulfate, table, 01: 185
free acid in amniotic fluid in early pregnancy and at
term, 01: 327
free acid in blood plasma of newborn infants and
adults, 01: 328
heat of proton ionization, pK, and related thermodynamic quantities, 06: 169
kinase
amino acid composition, complete data, 07: 505
circular dichroism
in UV and near UV region, 07: 85, 143
molar absorptivity and-or absorbance values, 02: 395
optical rotatory dispersion
UV region, 07: 47

Aspartate *(continued)*

pyrimidine-specific carbamyl phosphate synthetase; •
transcarbamylase
Neurospora crassa mutant, **04**: 748

transcarbamoylase
molar absorptivity and-or absorbance values, **02**: 397

transcarbamylase, average hydrophobicity values, **01**:
215

L-Aspartate

β-decarboxylase
amino acid composition, complete data, **07**: 505

Aspartate-8-semialdehyde
dehydrogenase, *Neurospora crassa* mutant, **04**: 743

Aspartate transaminase, *see* Aspartate aminotransferase

Aspartate transcarbamylase, *see* Aspartate carbamoyltransferase

Aspartic α-methylamide
structure and symbols for those incorporated into synthetic polypeptides, **01**: 99

Aspartic β-methylamide
structure and symbols for those incorporated into synthetic polypeptides, **01**: 99

Aspartic acid
active site peptides, **07**: 188

antagonists of, **01**: 177

free acid in amniotic fluid in early pregnancy and at
term, **01**: 327

free acid in blood plasma of newborn infants and
adults, **01**: 328

heat of proton ionization, pK, and related thermodynamic quantities, **06**: 170

neucleotide sequences of, **04**: 442-443

nucleoside composition, tables of values, **04**: 429

pK'_a values, **06**: 318

physical and chemical properties, **01**: 117

requirements of, for growth of various microorganisms,
table, **04**: 630-643

specific rotatory dispersion constants, 0.1 *M* solution,
01: 244

spectra, far UV, **01**: 184

symbols for atoms and bonds in side chains, **01**: 69, **02**:
73

thumbprint, content in, **08**: 121

β-Aspartic acid hydrazide
antagonism to aspartic acid, **01**: 177

Aspartokinase

lysine sensitive
average hydrophobicity value, **01**: 215

molar absorptivity and-or absorbance values, **02**: 398,
450

subunit, constitution of, **02**: 335, 336

Aspartokinase I--homoserine

dehydrogenase I
amino acid composition, complete data, **07**: 505

circular dichroism
in UV and near UV region, **07**: 86, 144

optical rotatory dispersion in the visible and near UV
regions, **07**: 18

Aspartophenone
antagonism to aspartic acid, **01**: 177

Aspartyl residues

active center
homology in sequences adjoining tryptophanyl and, in
pepsin, **07**: 359

tryptophanyl residues; homology in sequences adjoining
active center • and, in pepsin, **07**: 359

Aspergillopeptidase A, *see Aspergillus* acid proteinase

Aspergillopeptidase A, B
molar absorptivity and-or absorbance values,
02: 398

Aspergillopeptidase B, *see Aspergillus* alkaline proteinase
average hydrophobicity value, **01**: 215

Aspergillus

alkaline proteinase
optical rotatory dispersion
UV region, **07**: 48
UV region, **07**: 48
visible and near UV regions, **07**: 18

Aspiculamycin
physicochemical constants, spectral, chemotherapeutic
and biological properties, **03**: 296

Aspirin
prostaglandin biosynthesis by platelets, inhibition, **08**:
332

prostaglandins; biosynthesis inhibition by •,
08: 332

Astaxanthin
UV spectra, formula, molecular weight,
08: 195

Asteromycin
physicochemical constants, spectral, chemotherapeutic
and biological properties, **03**: 297

Atoms

alanine; symbols for • and bonds in side chains, **01**: 69,
02: 73

arginine; symbols for • and bonds in side chains, **01**:
70, **02**: 74

asparagine; symbols for • and bonds in side chains, **01**:
69, **02**: 73

aspartic acid; symbols for • and bonds in side chains,
01: 69, **02**: 73

cysteine; symbols for • and bonds in side chains, **01**:
69, **02**: 73

cystine; symbols for • and bonds in side chains, **01**: 69,
02: 73

glutamic acid; symbols for • and bonds in side chains,
01: 70, **02**: 74

glutamine; symbols for • and bonds in side chains, **01**:
70, **02**: 74

histidine; symbols for • and bonds in side chains, **01**:
70, **02**: 74

hydroxyproline; symbols for • and bonds in side chains,
01: 70, **02**: 74

isoleucine; symbols for • and bonds in side chains, **01**:
69, **02**: 73

leucine; symbols for • and bonds in side chains, **01**: 69,
02: 73

lysine; symbols for • and bonds in side chains, **01**: 69,
02: 73

methionine; symbols for • and bonds in side chains, **01**:
69, **02**: 73

Atoms *(continued)*

phenylalanine; symbols for • and bonds in side chains, **01:** 70, **02:** 74

proline; symbols for • and bonds in side chains, **01:** 70, **02:** 74

serine; symbols for • and bonds in side chains, **01:** 69, **02:** 73

threonine; symbols for • and bonds in side chains, **01:** 69, **02:** 73

tryptophan; symbols for • and bonds in side chains, **01:** 71, **02:** 75

tyrosine; symbols for • and bonds in side chains, **01:** 71, **02:** 75

valine; symbols for • and bonds in side chains, **01:** 69, **02:** 73

ATP

pK'_a values, **06:** 330

ATP phosphoribopyrophosphate

pyrophosphorylase, *Neurospora crassa* mutant, **04:** 741

ATPase, *see* Adenosinetriphosphatase

activity

enzymatic, subcellular fractions, **02:** 713

myosins, nonmuscle, table of values, **02:** 319

Atropine

pK'_a values, **06:** 326

Aureomycin

pK'_a values, **06:** 332

Aureomycin®

origin, structure, and characteristic as protein biosynthesis inhibitor, **04:** 560

Aurintricarboxylic acid

origin, structure, and characteristic as protein biosynthesis inhibitor, **04:** 560

Australia

antigen

circular dichroism in the UV region, **07:** 86

Avidin

average hydrophobicity value, **01:** 215

carbohydrate content, **02:** 268

circular dichroism

UV and near-UV region, **07:** 86, 144

luminescence of, table, **01:** 205

molar absorptivity and-or absorbance values, **02:** 398

optical rotatory dispersion

UV region, **07:** 48

visible and near UV regions, **07:** 18

subunit, constitution of, **02:** 329

Avilamycin

origin, structure, and characteristic as protein biosynthesis inhibitor, **04:** 561

5-Azacytidine

physicochemical constants, spectral, chemotherapeutic and biological properties, **03:** 298

4-Azaleucine

antagonism to leucine, 01: 178

4-Azalysine

antagonism to lysine, 01: 178

Azaserine

antagonism to glutamine, 01: 177

physical and chemical properties, 01: 134

7-Azatryptophan

antagonism to tryptophan, 01: 179

Azetidine-2-carboxylic acid

antagonism to proline, **01:** 179

physical and chemical properties, **01:** 137

structure and symbols for those incorporated into synthetic polypeptides, **01:** 99

Aziridinecarboxylic acid

structure and symbols for those incorporated into synthetic polypeptides, **01:** 99

Aziridinonecarboxylic acid

structure and symbols for those incorporated into synthetic polypeptides, **01:** 100

Azirinomycin

physical and chemical properties, **01:** 137

Azurin

amino acid composition, complete data, **07:** 505

amino acid sequence, **07:** 498

average hydrophobicity value, **01:** 215

circular dichroism in near-UV region, at room temperature, **07:** 144

cyanogen bromide cleavage, **02:** 199

luminescence of, table, **01:** 205

molar absorptivity and-or absorbance values, **02:** 399

molecular weights, stoichiometry and sources, **02:** 282

B

β

melanotropin; amino acid sequence; •, **07:** 386

B$_2$

plasma, *see also* Blood plasma; Human plasma; human, basic •

molar absorptivity and-or absorbance values, **02:** 498

BA-90912

physicochemical constants, spectral, chemotherapeutic and biological properties, **03:** 299

Bacterial protease, *see* Microbial metalloenzyme

Bacteriochlorophyll

-protein complex

amino acid composition, complete data, **07:** 505

UV spectra, formula, molecular weight, **08:** 159

Bacteriocin DF$_{13}$

origin, structure, and characteristic as protein biosynthesis inhibitor, **04:** 561

Bacteriophage

protein

amino acid sequence of coat proteins, **07:** 261-262

circular dichroism in the UV region, **07:** 86

optical rotatory dispersion

UV region, **07:** 48

visible and near UV regions, **07:** 18

Baikiain

physical and chemical properties, **01:** 137

Bamicetin

origin, structure, and characteristic as protein biosynthesis inhibitor, **04:** 561

physicochemical constants, spectral, chemotherapeutic and biological properties, **03:** 301

α Bands

heme-base complexes, positions and extinctions of •, **08:** 280

Barbitol
  buffer, preparation of, **06**: 375
Barbiturates
  ligands binding to plasma albumin, **02**: 569
Barbituric acid
  chemical structures and approved numbering schemes, **08**: 224
  derivatives
    heat of proton ionization, pK, and related thermodynamic quantities, **06**: 171-172
  pK'_a values, **06**: 330
Base
  DNA, *see also* Deoxyribonucleic acid; • compositions of eucaryotic protists, tables, **04**: 236-239
  RNA, *see* Nucleic acids, Transfer RNA, TRNA (TRNA); ribosomal; chloroplast, • composition, **04**: 361-362
  RNA, *see* Nucleic acids, Transfer RNA, TRNA (TRNA); ribosomal; cytoplasmic, • composition, **04**: 361-362
  Watson-Crick pairs; • stacking in standard models, diagrams, **04**: 414
Bases
  alkyl, UV spectral characteristics and pK_a values, **03**: 409-416
  commercial strength, table of concentration data, **06**: 384
  ionization constants; acids and •, tables of values, **06**: 307-348
  molecular weights; •, commercial strength, **06**: 384
  osmometry coefficients, vapor phase, **03**: 528-529
  pK'_a values, **06**: 307-348
  specific gravity; •, commercial strength, **06**: 384
  symbols for, use of, **03**: 8, **04**: 8
  UV spectra; unmodified • and some of their alkyl derivatives, **03**: 420-447
  UV spectra of unmodified, **03**: 420-447
Basic
  amino acid permease
    Neurospora crassa mutant, **04**: 755
Basic brain
  protein
    amino acid composition, incomplete data, **07**: 512
Beeswax
  fractions, composition of acids of, **05**: 504
Bence-Jones
  protein
    circular dichroism in the UV region, **07**: 86
    optical rotatory dispersion
      UV region, **07**: 49
      visible and near UV regions, **07**: 18
Benzaldehyde
  derivatives, heat of proton ionization, pK, and related thermodynamic quantities, **06**: 172
Benzene
  derivatives, heat of proton ionization, pK, and related thermodynamic quantities, **06**: 172
Benzoic acid
  derivatives
    heat of proton ionization, pK, and related thermodynamic quantities, **06**: 176-181
  pK'_a values, **06**: 313

β-(2-Benzothienyl)alanine
  antagonism to tryptophan, **01**: 179
S-Benzyl-β-mercaptopyruvic acid
  properties of, **01**: 182
N-Benzylglutamine
  antagonism to glutamine, **01**: 177
(α-Benzyl)phenylalanine
  structure and symbols for those incorporated into synthetic polypeptides, **01**: 100
3-Benzyltyrosine
  structure and symbols for those incorporated into synthetic polypeptides, **01**: 100
Berninamycin
  origin, structure, and characteristic as protein biosynthesis inhibitor, **04**: 562
Betaine of thiol histidine, *see* Ergothionine
Betonicine
  physical and chemical properties, **01**: 161
Bile
  pigments
    pK'_a values, **06**: 348
  pigments, UV spectra and formulas, **08**: 169
Bile acids
  structures and properties, **05**: 534-535
Bilirubin
  UV spectra, formula, molecular weight, **08**: 179
Bio-Gel A®
  filtration media, table of properties, **08**: 130
Bio-Gel P®
  filtration media, table of properties, **08**: 131-132
Biochemical nomenclature, *see* Nomenclature, biochemical
Biochemical pathways, chart of, **04**: insert
Biologically interesting
  structure; • compounds, **08**: 144-195
Biotin
  biological characteristics, **08**: 302
  properties of, **08**: 293
Biotin carboxyl carrier
  protein
    average hydrophobicity value, **01**: 215
2,2'-Bis(3-hydroxymethylbut-2-enyl)ϵ-carotene
  UV spectra, formula, molecular weight, **08**: 188
Bispyridine ferroprotoporphyrin IX, *see* Pyridine hemochromogen
  UV spectra, formula, molecular weight, **08**: 173
β,β-Bis(trifluoromethyl)alanine, *see* γ_6-Hexafluorovaline
Blasticidin S
  origin, structure, and characteristic as protein biosynthesis inhibitor, **04**: 562
  physicochemical constants, spectral, chemotherapeutic and biological properties, **03**: 303
Blastokinin
  average hydrophobicity value, **01**: 215
Blood
  α^1-antitrypsin; mammalian and chicken • specificity and properties, **02**: 636-637
  proteins, human, demonstrating quantitative abnormality, **04**: 881

Blood clotting
  factors
    amino acid sequences, **07:** 350-354
    serine proteases, trypsin-related; amino acid sequence
      data, index to; • factors, **07:** 350-354
Blood coagulation
  inheritance, mode of; • proteins, **02:** 255
  protein
    table of data and characteristics, **02:** 254-255
Blood coagulation factors
  nomenclature, **02:** 195
Blood coagulation proteins
  molecular weight; •, table of values, **02:** 255
Blood plasma, *see also* Human plasma; Plasma
  fibrin stabilizing factor system of, **02:** 670
  free amino acid content, newborn infants and adults,
    table, **01:** 328
Bluensomycin
  origin, structure, and characteristic as protein biosynthe-
    sis inhibitor, **04:** 563
Boat conformation
  in stereochemistry, **01:** 42-43, **02:** 42-43, **04:** 34-35, **06:**
    41, **08:** 41-42
Body fluids
  carbohydrate content; glycoproteins; •, **02:** 267
Bonds
  alanine; symbols for atoms and • in side chains, **01:** 69,
    02: 73
  arginine; symbols for atoms and • in side chains, **01:**
    70, **02:** 74
  asparagine; symbols for atoms and • in side chains, **01:**
    69, **02:** 73
  aspartic acid; symbols for atoms and • in side chains,
    01: 69, **02:** 73
  cysteine; symbols for atoms and • in side chains, **01:**
    69, **02:** 73
  glutamic acid; symbols for atoms and • in side chains,
    01: 70, **02:** 74
  glutamine; symbols for atoms and • in side chains, **01:**
    70, **02:** 74
  histidine; symbols for atoms and • in side chains, **01:**
    70, **02:** 74
  hydroxyproline; symbols for atoms and • in side chains,
    01: 70, **02:** 74
  isoleucine; symbols for atoms and • in side chains, **01:**
    69, **02:** 73
  leucine; symbols for atoms and • in side chains, **01:** 69,
    02: 73
  lysine; symbols for atoms and • in side chains, **01:** 69,
    02: 73
  methionine; symbols for atoms and • in side chains, **01:**
    69, **02:** 73
  peptide •
    hydrolysis, specificity of chymotrypsin, **02:** 212
    hydrolysis, specificity of papain, **02:** 218
    hydrolysis, specificity of pepsin, **02:** 215
    hydrolysis, specificity of subtilisin, **02:** 221
  phenylalanine; symbols for atoms and • in side chains,
    01: 70, **02:** 74
  proline; symbols for atoms and • in side chains, **01:** 70,
    02: 74

serine; symbols for atoms and • in side chains, **01:** 69,
  02: 73
threonine; symbols for atoms and • in side chains, **01:**
  69, **02:** 73
tryptophan; symbols for atoms and • in side chains, **01:**
  71, **02:** 75
tyrosine; symbols for atoms and • in side chains, **01:**
  71, **02:** 75
valine; symbols for atoms and • in side chains, **01:** 69,
  02: 73
Borax
  boric acid-• buffer, preparation of, **06:** 376
  -NaOH buffer, preparation of, **06:** 376
Boric acid
  -borax buffer, preparation of, **06:** 376
  heat of proton ionization, pK, related thermodynamic
    quantities, **06:** 182
Borrelidin
  origin, structure, and characteristic as protein biosynthe-
    sis inhibitor, **04:** 563
Bottromycin A$_2$
  origin, structure, and characteristic as protein biosynthe-
    sis inhibitor, **04:** 563
Bovine
  α thrombin A chain
    alignment of amino acid sequences homologous to,
      07: 342-343
Bowman-Birk inhibitor
  legume sources, specificity and properties, **02:** 588-589
  plant sources, amino acid composition, **02:** 606
Bradykinin
  group
    amino acid sequence, physical and biological proper-
      ties, **07:** 222-235
Bradykininogen
  amino acid composition, incomplete data, **07:** 512
  average hydrophobicity value, **01:** 215
Bredinin
  physicochemical constants, spectral, chemotherapeutic
    and biological properties, **03:** 305
Brij 35
  chromatography; • detergent, properties of, **08:** 216
Bromelain
  amino acid sequence, **07:** 356-357
  carbohydrate content, **02:** 274
  circular dichroism
    UV and near-UV region, **07:** 86, 144
  molar absorptivity and-or absorbance values, **02:** 399
  optical rotatory dispersion
    UV region, **07:** 49
    visible and near UV regions, **07:** 19
Bromophenylalanines
  antagonism to phenylalanine, **01:** 179
5-Bromouridine
  molal activity coefficients, **03:** 529
  molal osmotic coefficients, **03:** 528
Bryamycin
  origin, structure, and characteristic as protein biosynthe-
    sis inhibitor, **04:** 564
Bufanolide
  steroid nomenclature, use of term in, **05:** 65-66

Buffer
  acetate •
    preparation of, **06**: 372
    protonic activity tables, **06**: 529-539
  aconitate •, preparation of, **06**: 371
  2-amino-2-methyl-1,3-propanediol(ammediol) •,
    preparation of, **06**: 376
  barbitol •, preparation of, **06**: 375
  borax-NaOH •, preparation of, **06**: 376
  boric acid-borax •, preparation of, **06**: 376
  solutions
    amine types, table of structures and pK_a values, **06**:
      368-369
    enzyme studies, preparation of buffers for, **06**: 370-377
    equilibrium data measurement, recommendations, **06**:
      95
    histochemical studies, preparation of buffers for, **06**:
      370-377
    pH values at varying temperatures for several, **06**:
      360-361
    preparation data for several, **06**: 358-359
    preparation instructions for several, **06**: 362-363
    protonic activity for several, **06**: 529-539
    standard primary, pH values and preparation, **06**:
      354-355
Buffers
  amine •, structures and pK_a values, **06**: 368-369
  buffer solutions; enzyme studies, preparation of • for,
    06: 370-377
  buffer solutions; histochemical studies, preparation of •
    for, **06**: 370-377
  enzyme studies, preparation of • for, **06**: 370-377
  histochemical studies, preparation of •, **06**: 370-377
  protonic activity of some usual •, tables, **06**: 529-539
α-Bungarotoxin
  average hydrophobicity value, **01**: 215
  circular dichroism in near-UV region, at room tempera-
    ture, **07**: 145
β-Bungarotoxin
  circular dichroism in near-UV region, at room tempera-
    ture, **07**: 145
Butane
  derivatives
    heat of proton ionization, pK, and related thermody-
      namic quantities, **06**: 183
Butanoic acid
  derivatives
    heat of proton ionization, pK, and related thermody-
      namic quantities, **06**: 184-185
O-Butylhomoserine
  physical and chemical properties, **01**: 124
Butyric acid
  amino acid requirements for growth, table, **04**: 632

γ-Butyrobetaine
  physical and chemical properties, **01**: 161
By-products
  biosynthesis; prostaglandins, properties of intermediates,
    thromboxanes and •, **08**: 332-341
  formula, molecular; prostaglandin biosynthesis inter-
    mediates, thromboxanes and •, **08**: 334-340
  molecular weight; prostaglandin biosynthesis intermedi-
    ates, thromboxanes and •, **08**: 334-340
  nomenclature; prostaglandin biosynthesis intermediates,
    thromboxanes and •, **08**: 334-340
  prostaglandins; biosynthesis, intermediates, thrombox-
    anes and •
    isolation, biological effects, stability, **08**: 335-341
    occurrence, structure, molecular weight, **08**: 334-340
  structure; prostaglandin biosynthesis intermediates,
    thromboxanes and •, **08**: 334-340
  trivial names; prostaglandin biosynthesis intermediates,
    thromboxanes and •, **08**: 334-340

C

C_8
  density; fatty acids from • to C_{12}, **05**: 492
  specific volume; fatty acids from C_8 to •, **05**: 492
  temperature coefficient; fatty acids from C_8 to •, **05**:
    492
C_{12}
  density; fatty acids from C_8 to •, **05**: 492
  specific volume; fatty acids from • to C_{12}, **05**: 492
  temperature coefficient; fatty acids from • to C_{12}, **05**:
    492
C_{553}
  desulfovibrio •
    amino acid sequence, **07**: 302
Cacodylate buffer
  preparation of, **06**: 373
  protonic activity tables, **06**: 529-539
Caffeine
  ligands binding to plasma albumin, **02**: 573
  pK'_a values, **06**: 333
Calciferol, *see also* Vitamin D
  properties, **08**: 286
  UV spectra, formula, molecular weight, **08**: 152
Calcitonin
  average hydrophobicity value, **01**: 215
  molar absorptivity and-or absorbance values, **02**: 399
Calcitonins
  amino acid sequence, **07**: 383
Calcium
  -binding protein
    average hydrophobicity value, **01**: 215

Calcium *(continued)*
circular dichroism
in UV and near-UV regions, **07**: 86, 145
-binding protein (high affinity)
amino acid composition, incomplete data, **07**: 512
circular dichroism in the UV region, **07**: 87
precipitable protein
circular dichroism in the UV region, **07**: 87
Calsequestrin
circular dichroism in the UV region, **07**: 87
Canaline
antagonism to ornithine, **01**: 178
physical and chemical properties, **01**: 120
Canavanine
antagonism to arginine, **01**: 177
physical and chemical properties, **01**: 132
Canavanosuccinic acid
physical and chemical properties, **01**: 132
Canthaxanthin
UV spectra, formula, molecular weight, **08**: 190
Carbamate
kinase
amino acid composition, complete data, **07**: 505
N-Carbamoyl-2-(*p*-hydroxyphenyl)
glycine
physical and chemical properties, **01**: 137
Carbamoylglycine, *see* Hydantoic acid
Carbamoyltransferase
aspartate •
amino acid composition, complete data
catalytic subunit, **07**: 505
regulatory subunit, **07**: 505
amino acid sequences, **07**: 308
circular dichroism
near UV and UV region, **07**: 85, 143
optical rotatory dispersion
UV region, **07**: 47
visible and near UV regions, **07**: 18
O-Carbamyl-D-serine
antagonism to *D*-Alanine, **01**: 177
physical and chemical properties, **01**: 165
Carbamyl phosphate
synthetase
average hydrophobicity value, **01**: 215
S-Carbamylcysteine
antagonism to glutamine, **01**: 177
O-Carbamylserine
antagonism to glutamine, **01**: 177
Carbamyltaurine
physical and chemical properties, **01**: 152
O-Carbazylserine
antagonism to glutamine, **01**: 177
Carbohydrate
acyclic forms in • nomenclature, **05**: 113
agglutinin; • content, **02**: 270
alkaline phosphatase; • content, **02**: 274
α-Amylase; • content, **02**: 274
anomeric prefix in • nomenclature, **05**: 101, 114
anomers, in • nomenclature, **05**: 114-115
antithrombin III; • composition, **02**: 666-667
α¹-Antitrypsin; • composition, **02**: 666-667
avidin; • content, **02**: 268

bromelain; • content, **02**: 274
carboxylesterase; • content, **02**: 274
casein; • content, **02**: 268, 269
ceruloplasmin; plasma, human; • content, molecular
weights, sedimentation coefficients, **02**: 258
chloroperoxidase; • content, **02**: 273
cholinesterase; • content, **02**: 273
coagulation factors; plasma, nonhuman; • content, **02**:
260
composition
proteinase inhibitors, table of selected, **02**: 666-667
Tamm-Horsfall glycoprotein, **02**: 303
conalbumin, *see also* Ovotransferrin; • content, **02**: 268
content
glycoproteins
blood group substances, table, **02**: 262-263
body fluids, **02**: 267
cell membrane, **02**: 266
eggs, table of values, **02**: 268-269
enzymes, table of values, **02**: 273-274
hormones, table of values, **02**: 271-272
milk, table of values, **02**: 268-269
mucins, table, **02**: 262-263
plants, table of values, **02**: 270
plasma, human, table of values, **02**: 258
plasma, nonhuman, table of values, **02**: 259-260
tissues, table of values, **02**: 264-265
viruses, enveloped, **02**: 267
lectins, purified, table of values, **02**: 546-551
proteinase inhibitors
animal sources, **02**: 618-641
cereal grains, **02**: 598-599
deoxyribonuclease; • content, **02**: 273
desoxyribonuclease; • content, **02**: 274
DPNase; • content, **02**: 273
DPNase inhibitor; • content, **02**: 274
erythropoietin; • content, **02**: 272-273
fetuin; plasma, nonhuman; • content, **02**: 259
fibrinogen; plasma, human; • content, molecular
weights, sedimentation coefficients, **02**: 258
Fischer projection in • nomenclature, **05**: 100, 100-101
frictional coefficients; proteins; •, index to studies containing, **02**: 232
α-L-fucosidase; • content, **02**: 274
α-galactosidase; • content, **02**: 274
globulin, *see also* Macroglobulin; • content, **02**: 270
glucose oxidase; • content, **02**: 273
β-glucuronidase; • content, **02**: 274
γ-glutamyl transferase; • content, **02**: 274
gonadotrophin-transporting protein; plasma, nonhuman; • content, **02**: 259
Hageman factor; plasma, nonhuman; • content, **02**: 260
haptoglobin; plasma, human; • content, molecular
weights, sedimentation coefficients, **02**: 258
Haworth representation in • nomenclature, **05**: 100-101
hemagglutinin; • content, **02**: 270
hemopexin; plasma, human; • content, molecular
weight, sedimentation coefficient, **02**: 258
hormone, *see also* Luteinizing hormone; chorionic
gonadotropin, human; • content, **02**: 271
hormone, *see also* Luteinizing hormone; follicle-
stimulating, human; • content, **02**: 271

Carbohydrate (continued)

hormone, see also Luteinizing hormone; interstitial cell stimulating; • content, **02:** 271

hormone, see also Luteinizing hormone; luteinizing; • content, **02:** 272-273

immunoglobulin; plasma, human; • content, molecular weights, sedimentation coefficients, **02:** 258

immunoglobulin; plasma, nonhuman; • content, **02:** 259

cl-inactivator; • composition, 02: 666-667

invertase; • content, **02:** 274

lactoperoxidase; • content, **02:** 274

lactotransferrin; • content, **02:** 269

lectin; • content, **02:** 270

lipase, see Triacylglycerol, lipase; • content, **02:** 274

luteinizing hormone, see also Interstitial cell-stimulating hormone, **07:** 30, 66; • content, **02:** 272-273

macroglobulin, see also Ovomacroglobulin; plasma, nonhuman; • content, **02:** 259

α_2-macroglobulin; • composition, **02:** 666-667

mitogen; • content, **02:** 270

molecular weight; proteins; •, index to studies containing, **02:** 232

monoamine oxidase; • content, **02:** 273, 274

nomenclature, IUPAC tentative rules for, **05:** 100-136

nomenclature, journal references, **02:** 87

ovalbumin; • content, **02:** 268

ovoglycoprotein; • content, **02:** 268

ovoinhibitor; • composition, **02:** 666-667

ovomucin; • content, **02:** 268

ovomucoid; • composition, **02:** 666-667

ovomucoid; • content, **02:** 268

pepsinogen; • content, **02:** 274

peroxidase; • content, **02:** 273

plasminogen; plasma, human; • content, molecular weights, sedimentation coefficients, **02:** 258

progesterone; plasma, nonhuman; • content, **02:** 260

proteinase inhibitors; animal sources; • content, **02:** 618-628

proteins, see also Bacteriophage Flavoproteins, Matrix protein, also Protein, individual proteins, Molybdoproteins; • linkages, types of, **02:** 257

prothrombin; plasma, human; • content, molecular weights, sedimentation coefficients, **02:** 258

prothrombin; plasma, nonhuman; • content, **02:** 260

racemic forms, in • nomenclature, **05:** 103

reference carbon atom in • nomenclature, **05:** 101

ribonuclease; • content, **02:** 273, 274

stellacyanin; • content, **02:** 270

stem names in • nomenclature, **05:** 103

Tamm-Horsfall glycoprotein, see also Glycoproteins Tamm-Horsfall; • content, **02:** 267

thyroglobulin; • content, **02:** 271-272

thyrotrophin; • content, **02:** 271-272

transcortin; plasma, human; • content, molecular weight, sedimentation coefficients, **02:** 258

transferrin, see also Ovotransferrin; • content, **02:** 268

transferrin, see also Ovotransferrin; plasma, human; • content, molecular weights, sedimentation coefficients, **02:** 258

transferrin, see also Ovotransferrin; plasma, nonhuman; • content, **02:** 260

trivial names; • nomenclature, **05:** 102-103

trypsin inhibitors, see also Trypsin inhibitor; • composition, **02:** 666-667

Carbohydrate-amino acid linkages

found in mammalian glycoproteins, **05:** 281

Carbohydrate-protein linkages

types, **02:** 257

Carbohydrate content

coagulation factors; plasma, human; •, molecular weight, sedimentation coefficients, **02:** 258

corticosteroid-transporting protein; plasma, nonhuman, •, **02:** 259

α_2-macroglobulin; human; •, molecular weight, sedimentation coefficients, **02:** 258

Carbohydrate phosphate

esters

hydrolysis constant, **05:** 262-273

melting point, **05:** 253-258, 262-273

specific rotation, **05:** 253-258, 262-273

Carbohydrates, see also specific types

acids, natural, derived from

chemical formula, **05:** 153-176

chromatography, **05:** 153-176

melting point, **05:** 153-176

specific rotation, **05:** 153-176

amino sugar, naturally occurring

physical constants, structure, sources, electrophoretic mobility, **05:** 359-370

complex, of mammalian origin

disaccharide units isolated from, structure, **05:** 278-280

dimensions, average, of a sugar unit, **05:** 472

glycosaminoglycans, occurrence and physical data, **05:** 356-357

mucopolysaccharides, occurrence and physical data, **05:** 356-357

structures; •, IUPAC rules for nomenclature, **05:** 100-136

systematic nomenclature; •, **05:** 102

Carbohydrates, protein

physical-chemical data for, index to ultracentrifuge studies, **02:** 232

Carbomycin

origin, structure, and characteristic as protein biosynthesis inhibitor, **04:** 564

Carbon acids

pK'_a; •, **06:** 347

Carbon atom

reference • in carbohydrate nomenclature, **05:** 101

Carbon tetrachloride

fatty acids, see also Lipids, Wax fatty acids; methyl linoleate in • solution, NMR spectrum, **05:** 511

Carbon tetrachloride solution

methyl linoleate; NMR spectrum in •, **05:** 511

NMR spectra; methyl linoleate in •, **05:** 511

Carbonate-bicarbonate buffer

preparation of, **06:** 377

Carbonate buffers

protonic activity tables, **06:** 532-535

Carbonic

anhydrase B and C, average hydrophobicity values, **01:** 216

anhydrase C, human erythrocyte structure, schematic illustrating, **02:** 765

Carbonic *(continued)*

pK; histidine in; • anhydrase, values for residues, **02:** 691

Carbonic acid

heat of proton ionization, pK, and related thermodynamic quantities, **06:** 187-188

Carbonic anhydrase, *see* Carbonic dehydratase

average hydrophobicity value, **01:** 215

luminescence of, table, **01:** 205

molar absorptivity and-or absorbance values, **02:** 400-401

molecular weights, stoichiometry and sources, **02:** 283

subunit, constitution of, **02:** 339

Carbonic dehydratase

A or B

circular dichroism in the UV region, **07:** 87

optical rotatory dispersion in the UV region, **07:** 49

B

amino acid composition, complete data, **07:** 505

circular dichroism

in UV and near-UV region, **07:** 87, 145

optical rotatory dispersion

UV region, **07:** 49

visible and near UV regions, **07:** 19

C

circular dichroism

UV and near-UV region, **07:** 87, 145

optical rotatory dispersion

UV region, **07:** 50

visible and near UV regions, **07:** 19

2[S-(β-Carboxy-β-aminoethyl-tryptophan)]

physical and chemical properties, **01:** 152

2-Carboxy-3-carboxymethyl-4-1-methyl-2-carboxy-1,3-hexadienyl-pyrrolidine, *see* Domoic acid

3-Carboxy-6,7-dihydroxy-l,2,3,4-tetrahydroisoquinoline

physical and chemical proproperties, **01:** 137

D-(3-Carboxy-4-hydroxyphenyl)

glycine

physical and chemical properties, **01:** 165

3-Carboxy-4-hydroxyphenylalanine

physical and chemical properties, **01:** 129

β-(6-Carboxy-α-pyran-3-yl) alanine, *see* Stizolobinic acid

α-(Carboxyamino)-4,9-dihydro-4,6-dimethyl-9-oxo-1*H*-imidazo [1,2-α] purine-7-butyric acid

dimethyl ester

physical constants and spectral properties, **03:** 94

α-(Carboxyamino)-4,9-dihydro-4,6-dimethyl-9-oxo-3-β-D-ribofuranosyl-1*H*-imidazo [1,2-α] purine-7-butyric acid

dimethyl ester

physical constants and spectral properties, **03:** 139

α(Carboxyamino)-4,9-dihydro-β-hydroperoxy-4,6-dimethyl-9-oxo-l*H*-imidazo [1,2-α] purine-7-butyric acid

dimethyl ester

physical constants and spectral properties, **03:** 95

cis-α-(Carboxycyclopropyl)

glycine

physical and chemical properties, **01:** 115

N-α-(1-Carboxyethyl-arginine), *see* D-Octopine

S-(β-Carboxyethyl)-cysteine

physical and chemical properties, **01:** 152

N²-(D-1-Carboxyethyl)-lysine, *see* Lysopine

N-(1-Carboxyethyl)-taurine

physical and chemical properties, **01:** 152

Carboxyferrohemoglobin, HbCO

UV and visible absorption spectrum, **07:** 178

2-(1-Carboxyhydrazino)propane, *see* 2-Isopropyl-carbazic acid

S-(2-Carboxyisopropyl)-cysteine

physical and chemical properties, **01:** 152

Carboxykinase

phosphoenol pyruvate •

average hydrophobicity value, **01:** 229

phosphoenolpyruvate •

amino acid composition, complete data, **07:** 509

phospho*enol*pyruvate •

molar absorptivity and-or absorbance values, **02:** 494

Carboxyl

pK; • side chain, values estimated in lysozyme, **02:** 696

Carboxylase

β-methylcrotonylcoenzyme A •

average hydrophobicity value, **01:** 227

phosphoenolpyruvate •

phospho*enol*pyruvate •

molar absorptivity and-or absorbance values, **02:** 494

propionyl coenzyme A •

amino acid composition, incomplete data, **07:** 514

pyruvate •

Neurospora crassa mutant, **04:** 740

subunit, constitution of, **02:** 341, 348, 349

pyruvate • deficiency

characteristics of, **01:** 326

ribulose 1,5-diphosphate •

amino acid composition, complete data, **07:** 510

ribulose diphosphate •

average hydrophobicity value, **01:** 231

Carboxylesterase

carbohydrate content, **02:** 274

molar absorptivity and-or absorbance values, **02:** 402

subunit, constitution of, **02:** 339

Carboxylic acid

alkyl monoesters, refractive index, **05:** 494

Carboxylic acids

p*K'*$_a$ values, **06:** 309-313

5-Carboxymethoxyuridine

composition in various tRNA's, **04:** 428-441

isolation and detection of, in RNA, general remarks, **03:** 241

RNA, various, natural occurrence in, **03:** 230

S-(Carboxymethyl)-homocysteine

physical and chemical properties, **01:** 152

3-Carboxymethyl-4-isopropenyl proline, *see Allo*kainic acid

S-Carboxymethylboxymethylkerateine 2

refractive index increments, **02:** 374

trans-α-(2-Carboxymethylcyclopropyl)

glycine

physical and chemical properties, **01:** 115

5-Carboxymethyluridine

isolation and detection of, in RNA, general remarks, **03:** 241-242

RNA, various, natural occurrence in, **03:** 230

CDP, *see* Cytidylic acid

Celesticetin
origin, structure, and characteristic as protein biosynthesis inhibitor, **04:** 564

Cell constituents
cell and •, range of weights, **08:** 424

Cell membrane
carbohydrate content; glycoproteins; •, **02:** 266

Cellulase
amino acid composition, complete data, **07:** 506
circular dichroism in the UV region, **07:** 88
molar absorptivity and-or absorbance values, **02:** 404

Cellulose phosphate Whatman® P 11
Escherichia coli, see also E. coli; MRE 600 30 S ribosomal proteins, separation on •, **04:** 475
proteins, ribosomal; *Escherichia coli* MRE 600 30 S, separation on •, **04:** 475

Cellulosic
ion exchanges, properties, **08:** 136-138

Cenuloplasmin
molecular parameters, **02:** 245

Cephalosporin Pl
origin, structure, and characteristic as protein biosynthesis inhibitor, **04:** 565

Cephalosporinase
circular dichroism, **07:** 88
UV and near-UV region, **07:** 88, 155

Ceramide
generic term usage, **05:** 9

Cerebrocuprein
molar absorptivity and-or absorbance values, **02:** 404

Cerebroside
generic term usage, **05:** 10

Ceruloplasmin
amino acid composition, complete data, **07:** 506
circular dichroism in the UV region, **07:** 88
human
molar absorptivity and-or absorbance values, **02:** 404
molecular weight, stoichiometry and sources, **02:** 281
optical rotatory dispersion
UV region, **07:** 50
visible and near UV regions, **07:** 20
pig
molar absorptivity and-or absorbance values, **02:** 405
plasma, human
carbohydrate content, molecular weights, sedimentation coefficients, **02:** 258
rabbit
molar absorptivity and-or absorbance values, **02:** 405
rat
molar absorptivity and-or absorbance values, **02:** 405
serum, human
subunit, constitution of, **02:** 336

Cesium chloride
refractive index; density of • solution as function, table of values, **06:** 419-423
solution, density values as a function of refractive index, **06:** 419-423

Chain, *see also* Chains
amino acids among 60 species, frequency of occurrence, at different positions along •
table, **07:** 288-291

bovine α thrombin A •
alignment of amino acid sequences homologous to, **07:** 342-343
conformation angles in polynucleotide double helices, **04:** 416
γG immunoglobulin kappa •
amino acid composition, complete data, **07:** 508
glu(Asp)-plasminogen, amino-terminus of single •
alignment of amino-terminal amino acid sequences homologous to, **07:** 341
helical segments, nomenclature rules in polypeptides •, **01:** 72, **02:** 76
hemoglobin; α-• variants, **07:** 461-468
hemoglobin; β-• variants, **07:** 461-468
immunoglobulin; • structure, table, **07:** 530-531
constant regions, **07:** 408, 411, 414-419
variable region, **07:** 403-407, 409-410, 412-413
immunoglobulin; rabbit allotypes, • structures, **07:** 534
immunoglobulin, Eu heavy •
average hydrophobicity value, **01:** 224
immunoglobulin, newλ- •
average hydrophobicity value, **01:** 224
insulin B •
luminescence of, **01:** 204
length composition, herring oils and pilchard oil, **05:** 525
luciferase • α
amino acid composition, complete data, **07:** 508
myosin, light •
circular dichroism in the UV region, **07:** 115
nucleoside phosphotransferase-A-•
average hydrophobicity value, **01:** 228
nucleoside phosphotransferase-B-•
average hydrophobicity value, **01:** 228
polypeptide •
nomenclature rules, **01:** 59-73
primary structure of a segment, definition, **01:** 73
secondary structure of a segment, definition, **01:** 73

Chain termini
RNA, *see* Nucleic acids, Transfer RNA, TRNA (TRNA); • in partially hydrolyzed, discussion of, **03:** 403

Chains, *see also* Chain, Side chains
abbreviations; polypeptide •, conformation, journal reference, **02:** 87
amino acids, *see also* Aromatic amino acids, *also* specific acids; peptic hydrolysis in human α- and β-•, **02:** 216
chymotryptic hydrolysis; human globin, α-• of, **02:** 213
collagen •
amino acid sequences, **07:** 474-488
α-crystallin; composite sequence, α •, **07:** 503
α-crystallin; variable positions, α •, **07:** 502
globins, metazoan, aligned •
amino acid sequence, **07:** 456-458
hemoglobin, vertebrate tetrameric; amino acid sequence; α type •, **07:** 441-447
hemoglobin, vertebrate tetrameric; amino acid sequence; β type •, **07:** 448-455
human globin; chymotryptic hydrolysis of α-• of, **02:** 213

Chains *(continued)*

hydrolysis, *see also* Peptic hydrolysis; chymotryptic, of α-● of human globin, **02:** 213

hydrolysis, *see also* Peptic hydrolysis; peptic, aromatic amino acids in human α- and β-●, **02:** 216

hydrolysis, *see also* Peptic hydrolysis; peptic, leucine in human α- and β-●, **02:** 217

hydrolysis, *see also* Peptic hydrolysis; peptides from α- and β-● of human hemoglobin by papain, **02:** 219

insulin A ●
  amino acid sequence, **07:** 378

insulin B ●
  amino acid sequence, **07:** 379-380

leghemoglobin, soybean, aligned ●
  amino acid sequence, **07:** 456-458

leucine; peptic hydrolysis in human α- and β-●, **02:** 217

leucine; symbols for atoms and bonds in side ●, **01:** 69, **02:** 73

methionine; symbols for atoms and bonds in side ●, **01:** 69, **02:** 73

nomenclature; polypeptide ●, rules for abbreviations and symbols,, **01:** 59-73, **02:** 63-77

papain; hydrolysis peptides from α- and β-● of human hemoglobin, **02:** 219

peptic hydrolysis, *see also* Hydrolysis; aromatic amino acids in human α- and β-●, **02:** 216

peptides; hydrolysis from α- and β-● of human hemoglobin, **02:** 219

polypeptide ●
  blood coagulation proteins, table of values, **02:** 255
  immunoglobulin molecules, notation for, **02:** 180
  nomenclature rules, **02:** 63-77
  primary structure of a segment, definition, **02:** 77
  secondary structure of a segment, definition, **02:** 77

proline; symbols for atoms and bonds in side ●, **01:** 70, **02:** 74

serine proteases active, bearing the active site serine; alignments of the ● of, **07:** 344-349

symbols; polypeptide ●, nomenclature rules, **01:** 59-73, **02:** 63-77

symbols; side ● of, L-amino acids, **01:** 69

Chair conformation
  in stereochemistry, **01:** 42, **02:** 42, **04:** 34, **06:** 41, **08:** 41

Chalcomycin
  origin, structure, and characteristic as protein biosynthesis inhibitor, **04:** 565

Chartreusin
  origin, structure, and characteristic as protein biosynthesis inhibitor, **04:** 566

Chemical induced mutants
  tobacco mosaic virus; location of some amino acid replacements in naturally occurring and● of, **07:** 266-267

Chloramphenicol
  origin, structure, and characteristic as protein biosynthesis inhibitor, **04:** 566
  UV spectra, formula, molecular weight, **08:** 181

Chlorinated hydrocarbon
  lipids; solubility of selected, in ● solvents, **05:** 514

Chlorinated hydrocarbon mixtures
  lipids; solubility of selected, in ● with 33% methanol, **05:** 514

solubility; lipids in ● with 33% methanol, **05:** 514

Chlorinated hydrocarbon solvents
  solubility; lipids in ●, **05:** 514

Chloroacetate buffer
  protonic activity tables, **06:** 529-539

Chlorobium, C_{555}
  amino acid sequence, **07:** 303

Chlorocruorin
  refractive index increments, **02:** 374

2-Chloroethanol
  Lorentz correction factors; concentration dependence; ● at several wavelengths, **06:** 400-401

δ-Chloroleucine
  antagonism to leucine, **01:** 178

Chloroperoxidase
  amino acid composition, incomplete data, **07:** 512
  carbohydrate content, **02:** 273

(4-Chloro)phenylalanine
  structure and symbols for those incorporated into synthetic polypeptides, **01:** 100

Chlorophenylalanines
  antagonism to phenylalanine, **01:** 179

Chlorophyll
  UV spectra, formula, molecular weight, **08:** 170-171

5-Chloropiperidazine-3-carboxylic acid
  physical and chemical properties, **01:** 159

Chloroplast
  buoyant density; DNA; ●, table of values, **04:** 356-358
  chromosome, circular
    length and molecular weight, table of values, **04:** 359-360
  ribosomal RNA, base composition, table, **04:** 361-362

Chloroplast nucleic acids, *see* Nucleic acid, chloroplast

Chlortetracycline
  origin, structure, and characteristic as protein biosynthesis inhibitor, **04:** 567

Cholchisine-binding
  protein
    average hydrophobicity value, **01:** 216

Cholecalciferol
  properties of, **08:** 287

Cholecystokinin
  -pancreozymin
    cyanogen bromide cleavage, **02:** 199

Cholesteryl
  esters, content in various animal tissues, **05:** 519-520

Choline
  biological characteristics, **08:** 302
  properties of, **08:** 294
  sulfatase
    Neurospora crassa mutant, **04:** 744

Choline esterase, *see* Cholinesterase

Cholinesterase
  carbohydrate content, **02:** 273
  circular dichroism in the UV region, **07:** 88
  molar absorptivity and-or absorbance values, **02:** 405
  molecular parameters, **02:** 245
  optical rotatory dispersion in the visible and near UV regions, **07:** 20
  pseudoacetyl ●
    human
      luminescence of, table, **01:** 206

Citrate *(continued)*
  optical rotatory dispersion in the UV region, **07:** 51
Citrate buffer
  preparation of, **06:** 371
Citrate synthase, *see* Citrate *(si)*-synthase
  molar absorptivity and-or absorbance values, **02:** 407
  subunit, constitution of, **02:** 333, 343
Citric acid
  heat of proton ionization, pK, and related thermodynamic quantities, **06:** 188-189
  pK'_a values, **06:** 309
Citrinin
  UV spectra, formula, molecular weight, **08:** 164
Citrulline
  citrullinemia, effect of, **01:** 318
  free acid in amniotic fluid in early pregnancy and at term, **01:** 327
  free acid in blood plasma of newborn infants and adults, **01:** 328
  physical and chemical properties, **01:** 133
  structure and symbols for those incorporated into synthetic polypeptides, **01:** 100
  thumbprint, content in, **08:** 121
Clavicipitic acid
  physical and chemical properties, **01:** 137
Clindamycin
  origin, structure, and characteristic as protein biosynthesis inhibitor, **04:** 567
Clostridiopeptidase B, *see Clostridium histolyticum* proteinase B
Clostridium histolyticum
  proteinase B
    optical rotatory dispersion
      UV region, **07:** 52
      visible and near UV regions, **07:** 21
Clostripain, *see Clostridium histolyticum* proteinase B
Clotting
  genetic variations in man, tables of enzymes and variations in proteins and • factors, **04:** 879-883
  human; plasma; • factors, quantitative variation in, **04:** 881
Clotting factors
  plasma, human, quantitative variation in •, **04:** 881
Clupeine
  Pacific herring
    amino acid sequences, **07:** 498
CMP
  pK'_a values, **06:** 330
Coagulation
  factors
    plasma, human
      carbohydrate content, molecular weight, sedimentation coefficients, **02:** 258
    plasma, nonhuman
      carbohydrate content, **02:** 260
  vitamins, properties of, **08:** 290
Coat
  bacteriophage protein; amino acid sequence of • proteins, **07:** 261-262
  proteins
    amino acid sequences, **07:** 261

Cobramine B
  amino acid composition, complete data, **07:** 506
Cobro
  toxin
    circular dichroism
      UV and near-UV region, **07:** 89, 147
    optical rotatory dispersion in the UV region, **07:** 52
Cocaine
  pK'_a values, **06:** 326
Cocoonase
  average hydrophobicity value, **01:** 217
  molar absorptivity and-or absorbance values, **02:** 408
Codeine
  pK'_a values, **06:** 326
Codons
  found in the MS_2 coat protein gene, **04:** 340
  genetic code, table, **04:** 896
Coenzyme A
  3-hydroxyacyl • dehydrogenase
    average hydrophobicity value, **01:** 224
  β-methylcrotonyl• carboxylase
    average hydrophobicity value, **01:** 227
  propionyl • carboxylase
    amino acid composition, incomplete data, **07:** 514
  succinyl • synthetase
    average hydrophobicity value, **01:** 231
Coenzyme Q
  nomenclature recommendations, **08:** 9-11
Coenzymes
  abbreviations, use of, **08:** 6
  abbreviations for, use of, **01:** 6, **02:** 6, **03:** 6, **06:** 6
  nomenclature; •, trivial names and preferred usages, **08:** 8-19
  nomenclature, journal references for, **02:** 87
  trivial names; •, **08:** 8-19
  use of abbreviations, **05:** 6
  use of abbreviations for, **04:** 6
Cofactors
  aldolase, *see also* Fructose-bisphosphate aldolase; •, molecular weights, stoichiometry, sources **02:** 284
  enzyme •
    fluorescence of, **07:** 601-602
  metalloenzyme; •, molecular weights, stoichiometry and sources, **02:** 278-286
  metapyrocatechase, *see also* Catechol 2,3,-dioxygenase; table of •, molecular weights, stoichiometry and sources, **02:** 280
  monoamine oxidase; table of •, molecular weights, stoichiometry, and sources, **02:** 282
  nitrate reductase; •, molecular weights, stoichiometry and sources, **02:** 285
  protease; •, molecular weights, stoichiometry, sources, **02:** 284
  pyrocatechase, *see also* Catechol 1,2 -dioxygenase (pyrocatechase); table of •, molecular weights, stoichiometry and sources, **02:** 278
  thermolysin, *see also* Microbial metalloenzyme; •, molecular weights, stoichiometry, sources, **02:** 284
  xanthine oxidase; table of •, molecular weights, stoichiometry, and sources, **02:** 278
Coffearin, *see* Trigonelline

Coformycin
  physicochemical constants, spectral, chemotherapeutic
    and biological properties, **03:** 306
Colchicine
  pK'_a values, **06:** 326
Colicin E3
  origin, structure, and characteristic as protein biosynthe-
    sis inhibitor, **04:** 567
Colicin E$_1$
  circular dichroism in the UV region, **07:** 89
Colicin E$_2$
  circular dichroism in the UV region, **07:** 89
Colicin E$_3$
  circular dichroism in the UV region, **07:** 89
Colicin I$_a$-CA53
  average hydrophobicity value, **01:** 217
Colicin I$_b$-P9
  average hydrophobicity value, **01:** 217
Collagen
  amino acid composition, complete data, **07:** 506
  average hydrophobicity values, **01:** 217
  chains
    amino acid sequences, **07:** 474-488
  circular dichroism
    UV and spectra, **07:** 9, 89
  cross-linkage, **07:** 523
  cyanogen bromide cleavage, **02:** 199, 202
  heat capacity and entropy values, **06:** 110
  optical rotatory dispersion
    spectra, **07:** 9
    UV region, **07:** 52
  post-translational enzymes in, **07:** 524
  refractive index increments, **02:** 374
  selected amino acid analysis, **07:** 520-521
  subunit, constitution of, **02:** 342
Collagenase
  average hydrophobicity values, **01:** 217
  circular dichroism in the UV region, **07:** 90
  enzymatic hydrolysis of proteins, **02:** 209
  molar absorptivity and-or absorbance values, **02:** 408
  optical rotatory dispersion
    UV region, **07:** 52
    visible and near UV regions, **07:** 21
Complex, *see also* Complexes
  bacteriochlorophyll-protein •
    amino acid composition, complete data, **07:** 505
  ferrimyoglobin •
    heat of proton ionization, pK, and related thermody-
      namic quantities, **06:** 200
  major histocompatibility •
    definition, **04:** 885
    designation for a variety of mammalian species, **04:**
      885
    man, table of values, **04:** 886
    mouse, table of values, **04:** 886-887
    properties associated with differences at the MHC, **04:**
      885
  multienzyme • in tryptophan pathway
    amino acid composition, complete data, **07:** 509
  pyruvate dehydrogenase •
    subunit, constitution of, **02:** 351

trypsin-trypsin inhibitor •
  molar absorptivity and-or absorbance values, **02:** 511
Complexes, *see also* Complex
  amino acids, *see also* Aromatic amino acids, *also*
    specific acids; circular dichroism spectra of metal •
    of, **01:** 245-315
  extinction coefficients; heme-base •, α bands, **08:** 280
  heme-base •, positions and extinctions of α bands, **08:**
    280
  melting temperature; deoxyribohomopolymers and •,
    03: 581-582
  melting temperature; ribohomopolymers and •, **03:**
    575-580
  metal • of amino acids and peptides, circular dichroism
    spectra, **01:** 245-315
Component I, II
  anthranylate synthetase, •
    average hydrophobicity value, **01:** 213
Compounds
  absorbance bands; • used in biochemical studies, **06:**
    123-129
  aliphatic acids, long-chain, and related •, molecular di-
    mensions, **05:** 498
  amino acids, *see also* Aromatic amino acids, *also*
    specific acids; chromatography, ion exchange; nin-
    hydrin positive •, elution behavior, **08:** 122
  chiral •, cyclitol nomenclature, **05:** 98
  chromatography; ion exchange, amino acids; ninhydrin
    positive •, elution behavior, **08:** 122
  concentration dependence; Lorentz correction factors,
    values for several •, **06:** 396-403
  concentration dependence; refractive index, values for
    several •, **06:** 395
  concentration dependence; Sellmeier constants, values
    for several •, **06:** 395
  decarboxylation; free energy values for several •, **06:**
    303
  elution behavior, ninhydrin-positive •, **08:** 122
  entropy; chemical •, table of values, **06:** 153-262
  fluorescence; vitamin B$_6$ •, properties, **08:** 215
  fluorescent parameters, folic acid • of biological in-
    terest, **08:** 214
  folic acid •, fluorescent parameters, **08:** 214
  formula, structural, *see* Structure, *also* Structures;
    chemical •, table, **06:** 153-262
  free energy; decarboxylation, values for several •, **06:**
    303
  free energy; hydrolysis; acetic acid esters and related •,
    06: 300
  heat of proton ionization; chemical •, table of values,
    06: 153-262
  hydrolysis, *see also* Peptic hydrolysis; free energy values
    for •, tables, **06:** 300-303
  immunogenic properties; some low molecular weight •,
    table, **07:** 541
  infrared spectra, *see* IR spectra; characteristic frequen-
    cies between ~ 700-300 cm^{-1}, organic and inorganic
    •, **08:** 237-246
  molar absorbance; • used in biochemical studies, **06:**
    123-129
  molecular dimensions, long-chain aliphatic acids and
    related •, **05:** 498

Compounds *(continued)*

molecular weight; • of biological interest, **08:** 144-195

ninhydrin positive •, elution behavior, **08:** 122

nomenclature; isotopically labeled •, CEBJ rules for, **01:** 16, **02:** 16, **03:** 58, **04:** 58, **06:** 62, **08:** 62

oxidation-reduction potentials; • used in biochemical studies, **06:** 123-129

phenylalanyl model •

near-UV circular dichroism intensities, **07:** 168

phosphorylated •

symbols for, use of, **01:** 8, **02:** 8, **04:** 8

phosphorylated •, use of symbols for, **03:** 8, **05:** 8

pK; chemical •, table of values, **06:** 153-262

refractive index; concentration dependence; Lorentz correction factors, values for several •, **06:** 396-403

refractive index; concentration dependence; Sellmeier constants, values for several •, **06:** 395

Sellmeier constants, concentration dependence values for several •, **06:** 395

structure; biologically interesting •, **08:** 144-195

thermodynamic quantities, chemical •, table of values, **06:** 153-262

tryptophanyl model •

near-UV circular dichroism intensities, **07:** 169

tyrosyl model •

near-UV circular dichroism intensities, **07:** 170

UV spectra; • of biological interest, **08:** 144-195

vitamin B$_6$; fluorescence properties of •, **08:** 215

Conalbumin, *see also* Ovotransferrin

average hydrophobicity value, **01:** 217

carbohydrate content, **02:** 268

molar absorptivity and-or absorbance values, **02:** 408

molecular weight, stoichiometry, source, function, **02:** 276

refractive index increments, **02:** 374

α-Conarachin

optical rotatory dispersion in the visible and near UV regions, **07:** 21

Concanavalin A

amino acid composition, complete data, **07:** 506

circular dichroism

UV and near-UV region, **07:** 90, 147

optical rotatory dispersion

UV region, **07:** 52

visible and near UV regions, **07:** 21

γ-Conglycinin

circular dichroism in the UV region, **07:** 90

optical rotatory dispersion

UV region, **07:** 52

visible and near UV regions, **07:** 21

Conjugated proteins

chymotrypsin; enzymatic hydrolysis, •, **02:** 211

enzymatic hydrolysis; •, table, **02:** 211

fetuin; enzymatic hydrolysis, •, **02:** 211

hydrolysis, *see also* Peptic hydrolysis; enzymatic, •, table, **02:** 211

ovalbumin; enzymatic hydrolysis, •, **02:** 211

pancreatin; enzymatic hydrolysis, •, **02:** 211

papain; enzymatic hydrolysis, •, **02:** 211

pepsin, *see also* Pepsin A; enzymatic hydrolysis, •, **02:** 211

phosphorylase; enzymatic hydrolysis, •, **02:** 211

pronase; enzymatic hydrolysis, •, **02:** 211

trypsin; enzymatic hydrolysis, •, **02:** 211

Conjugates, covalent protein

table of data, **01:** 208

Constituents

chromatography; ion exchange, amino acids; urine, resolution of ninhydrin positive •, **08:** 114-119

ninhydrin positive •

urine, resolution of, by ion exchange chromatography, **08:** 114-119

urine; chromatography of, resolution of ninhydrin positive •, **08:** 114-119

Contractile

protein

molecular parameters, table, **02:** 306

Copolymers

of repeating sequence, melting temperatures, **03:** 583-585

Copper

blue • proteins

resonance raman spectra, **07:** 589

Copper phathalocyanine

UV spectra, formula, molecular weight, **08:** 178

Cordycepin

physicochemical constants, spectral, chemotherapeutic and biological properties, **03:** 308

Corrinoid protein

average hydrophobicity value, **01:** 217

Corrinoids, *see also* Cyanocobalamin, Vitamin B$_{12}$

abbreviations; • derivatives and vitamin B$_{12}$, **08:** 16-17

nomenclature, journal references for, **02:** 87

nomenclature and structures, **08:** 12-17

Corticoids

structures and properties, **05:** 536-538

Corticosteroid

-binding globulin

amino acid composition, complete data, **07:** 506

Corticosteroid-transporting

protein

plasma, nonhuman, carbohydrate content, **02:** 259

Corticotropin

amino acid sequence, **07:** 385

luminescence of, table, **01:** 205

Cortisol

metabolites binding large protein

amino acid composition, incomplete data, **07:** 512

Covalent protein conjugates, *see also* Conjugated proteins; Proteins, covalent conjugates

fluorescamine; •, data, **01:** 208

fluorescein isothiocyanate; •, data, **01:** 208

Creatine

enthalpy and free energy of formation, **06:** 112

heat capacity and entropy values, **06:** 110

heat of combustion, **06:** 112

kinase

average hydrophobicity value, **01:** 217

Creatine *(continued)*
circular dichroism
UV and near-UV region, **07**: 90, 148
molar absorptivity and-or absorbance values, **02**: 409
optical rotatory dispersion
UV region, **07**: 52
visible and near UV regions, **07**: 21
subunit, constitution of, **02**: 330
pK'_a values, **06**: 318
Creatine phosphokinase, *see* Creatine, kinase
Creatinine
enthalpy and free energy of formation, **06**: 112
heat capacity and entropy values, **06**: 110
heat of combustion, **06**: 112
all-trans-Crocetin
dimethyl ester
UV spectra, formula, molecular weight, **08**: 194
Crotocin
(Antibiotic T); origin, structure, and characteristic as
protein biosynthesis inhibitor, **04**: 568
Crotocol
origin, structure, and characteristic as protein biosynthesis inhibitor, **04**: 568
Crotonase
amino acid composition, complete data, **07**: 506
average hydrophobicity value, **01**: 217
molar absorptivity and-or absorbance values, **02**: 409
subunit, constitution of, **02**: 338, 339
Crotonoside
physical constants and spectral properties, **03**: 99
Crotoxin
average hydrophobicity value, **01**: 217
molar absorptivity and-or absorbance values, **02**: 409
Crotylalanine, *see* 2-Amino-5-heptenoic acid
Crotylglycine, *see* 2-Amino-4-hexenoic acid
β-Crustacyanin
amino acid composition, complete data, **07**: 506
Cryoglobulin
molar absorptivity and-or absorbance values, **02**: 409
refractive index increments, **02**: 374
Cryptopleurine
origin, structure, and characteristic as protein biosynthesis inhibitor, **04**: 569
Crystallin
molar absorptivity and-or absorbance values, **02**: 410,
411
α-Crystallin
circular dichroism in the UV region, **07**: 90
composite sequence, α chains, **07**: 503
optical rotatory dispersion
UV region, **07**: 52
visible and near UV regions, **07**: 21
variable positions, α chains, **07**: 502
γ-Crystallin
circular dichroism in the UV region, **07**: 90
optical rotatory dispersion in the UV region,
07: 52
β-Crystallin
amino acid composition, complete data, **07**: 506
Cs_2SO_4
RNA, *see also* Nucleic acids, Transfer RNA, TRNA
(TRNA); viral, buoyant density values, • gradient,
03: 569

Cs_2SO_4
buoyant density; RNA, viral, in the • gradient, **03**: 569
Cucurbitine
physical and chemical properties, **01**: 138
Cuproproteins
nomenclature rules, **02**: 121
γ-Cyano-α-aminobutyric acid
physical and chemical properties, **01**: 135
β-Cyanoalanine
physical and chemical properties, **01**: 134
structure and symbols for those incorporated into synthetic polypeptides, **01**: 100
Cyanocobalamin, *see also* Vitamin B_{12}
biological characteristics, **08**: 302
nomenclature and structure, **08**: 12-17
properties of, **08**: 294
UV spectra, formula, molecular weight, **08**: 144
N-(2-Cyanoethyl)
glycine
structure and symbols for those incorporated into synthetic polypeptides, **01**: 100
Cyanogen bromide
aldolase, *see also* Fructose-bisphosphate aldolase; •
cleavage, **02**: 199
azurin; • cleavage, **02**: 199
carboxypeptidase A; • cleavage, **02**: 199
cholecystokinin-pancreozymin; • cleavage, **02**: 199
chymotrypsin; • cleavage, **02**: 199
collagen; • cleavage, **02**: 199, 202
cytochrome *c*, *see also* Eukaryotic cytochromes *c*; •
cleavage, **02**: 199
cytochrome c_2; • cleavage, **02**: 199
cytochrome c_{551}; • cleavage, **02**: 199
ferredoxin; • cleavage, **02**: 199
β-galactosidase; • cleavage, **02**: 199
gastrin; • cleavage, **02**: 199
growth hormone; • cleavage, **02**: 199
histones; calf thymus, • cleavage, **02**: 199
hormone, *see also* Luteinizing hormone; parathyroid; •
cleavage, **02**: 199
immunoglobulin IgG; human; • cleavage, **02**: 199
immunoglobulin IgG; rabbit; • cleavage, **02**: 199
kininogen; • cleavage, **02**: 199
α-lactalbumin; • cleavage, **02**: 199
lysozyme; • cleavage, **02**: 199
myoglobin; • cleavage, **02**: 199
myosin A; • cleavage, **02**: 199
nuclease; • cleavage, **02**: 199
peptides; • cleavage of, table, **02**: 199-202
ribonuclease; bovine; • cleavage, **02**: 199
ribonuclease; bovine pancreatic; • cleavage, **02**: 199
ribonuclease; cross-linked bovine pancreatic; • cleavage,
02: 199
ribonuclease A, *see also* Ribonuclease I; • cleavage,
02: 199
streptokinase; • cleavage, **02**: 199
S-sulfopepsin; • cleavage, **02**: 199
thioredoxin; • cleavage, **02**: 199
thyrocalcitonin; • cleavage, **02**: 199
thyroglobulin; • cleavage, **02**: 199
trypsinogen; bovine pancreatic; • cleavage, **02**: 199
tryptophan synthetase; • cleavage, **02**: 199

Cysteine *(continued)*
  requirements of, for growth of various microorganisms,
    table, **04:** 630-643
  symbols for atoms and bonds in side chains, **01:** 69, **02:**
    73
  synthase
    molar absorptivity and-or absorbance values, **02:** 412
  synthetase
    subunit, constitution of, **02:** 345
    UV spectra of, **01:** 197
Cysteine β 93 SH
  pK values in human hemoglobin, **02:** 696
Cysteine β93 SH
  pK; • in human hemoglobin, **02:** 696
Cysteine sulfinic acid
  physical and chemical properties, **01:** 153
Cystine
  antagonism to α,ϵ-diaminopimelic acid, **01:** 177
  cystinosis, nephropathic, effect of, **01:** 318
  derivatives
    heat of proton ionization, pK, and related thermody-
      namic quantities, **06:** 191
  destruction of, during acid hydrolysis, **02:** 206
  N,N'-diacetyl-L-cystine dimethyl ester, UV spectra of,
    01: 199
  free acid in amniotic fluid in early pregnancy and at
    term, **01:** 327
  free acid in blood plasma of newborn infants and
    adults, **01:** 328
  molar extinctions: N-acetyl methyl esters of aromatic
    amino acids, • and N-acetylcysteine, **01:** 186
  pK'_a values, **06:** 318
  physical and chemical properties, **01:** 153
  requirements of, for growth of various microorganisms,
    table, **04:** 630-643
  spectra, far UV, **01:** 184
  symbols for atoms and bonds in side chains, **01:** 69, **02:**
    73
  thumbprint, content in, **08:** 121
  UV absorption characteristics, **01:** 186
  UV spectra of, **01:** 198
½Cystine
  far ultraviolet absorption spectra
    aqueous solution at pH 5, **01:** 184
    neutral water, table, **01:** 185
    0.1 M sodium dodecyl sulfate, table, **01:** 185
  molar extinctions, **01:** 185
Cystine disulfoxide
  physical and chemical properties, **01:** 153
Cystinyl
  compounds
    longest wavelength disulfide circular dichroism band,
      07: 173
Cytidine
  and derivatives
    UV spectra, **03:** 440-443
    UV spectral characteristics and acid dissociation con-
      stants, **03:** 414-415
  and nucleoside derivatives
    physical constants and spectral properties, index to,
      03: 70
  bond angles and distances, **08:** 224

  chemical structures and approved numbering schemes,
    08: 224
  composition in various tRNA's, **04:** 428-441
  derivatives
    heat of proton ionization, pK, and related thermody-
      namic quantities, **06:** 191
  molal activity coefficients, **03:** 529
  molal osmotic coefficients, **03:** 528
  pK'_a values, **06:** 330, 339
  raman frequencies, table of values, **03:** 540-541
Cytidine nucleotide derivatives
  physical constants and spectral properties, index to, **03:**
    73
Cytidylic acid
  derivatives, UV spectral characteristics and acid disso-
    ciation constants, **03:** 416
Cytisine
  pK'_a values, **06:** 326
Cytochrome, *see also* Cytochromes
  average hydrophobicity values, **01:** 217-218
Cytochrome *b*
  amino acid composition, complete data, **07:** 506
  molar absorptivity and-or absorbance values, **02:** 412
Cytochrome b_2, *see also* Lactate dehydrogenase (cyto-
    chrome b_2)
  enzymatic activity, subcellular fractions, **02:** 707
  subunit, constitution of, **02:** 343
Cytochrome b_5
  circular dichroism
    UV and near-UV region, **07:** 91, 148
  optical rotatory dispersion
    UV region, **07:** 53
    visible and near UV regions, **07:** 22
Cytochrome b_{563}
  circular dichroism
    UV and near-UV region, **07:** 91, 148
Cytochrome *c*, *see also* Eukaryotic cytochromes *c*
  amino acid composition, complete data, **07:** 506
  amino acid sequence, **07:** 304-306
  circular dichroism
    UV and near-UV region, **07:** 91, 148
  cyanogen bromide cleavage, **02:** 199
  enzymatic activity, subcellular fractions, **02:** 702
  molar absorptivity and-or absorbance values, **02:** 413
  optical rotatory dispersion in the UV region, **07:** 53
  oxidase
    circular dichroism in the UV region, **07:** 93
    optical rotatory dispersion in the UV region, **07:** 54
  peroxidase
    molar absorptivity and-or absorbance values, **02:** 417
  pK; histidine in; • specific values, **02:** 691
Cytochrome c_A
  circular dichroism in the UV region, **07:** 92
  optical rotatory dispersion in the UV region, **07:** 53
Cytochrome c_1
  circular dichroism
    UV and near-UV region, **07:** 93, 150
  molar absorptivity and-or absorbance values, **02:** 414
Cytochrome c_2
  amino acid sequence, **07:** 294-298
  cyanogen bromide cleavage, **02:** 199
  molar absorptivity and-or absorbance values, **02:** 414

D

Decarboxylase *(continued)*
  acetoacetic acid •
    average hydrophobicity value, **01:** 210
  amino acid •, aromatic
    average hydrophobicity value, **01:** 213
  arginine •
    amino acid composition, complete data, **07:** 505
    average hydrophobicity value, **01:** 214
    molar absorptivity and-or absorbance values, **02:** 395
    subunit, constitution of, **02:** 345, 350
  decarboxylation of α-keto acids; yeast •, by, **01:** 181
  glutamate •
    average hydrophobicity value, **01:** 221
    molar absorptivity and-or absorbance values, **02:** 432
    subunit, constitution of, **02:** 331, 345
  histidine •
    amino acid composition, complete data, **07:** 507
    average hydrophobicity value, **01:** 224
    molar absorptivity and-or absorbance values, **02:** 448
    subunit, constitution of, **02:** 334, 340
  α-keto acids; decarboxylation by yeast •, **01:** 69-70
  lysine •
    average hydrophobicity value, **01:** 226
    molar absorptivity and-or absorbance values, **02:** 468
    subunit, constitution of, **02:** 349
  oxaloglycolate reductive •
    amino acid composition, incomplete data, **07:** 513
  phosphatidyl serine •
    average hydrophobicity value, **01:** 229
  prohistidine •
    average hydrophobicity value, **01:** 230
  pyruvate •
    circular dichroism intensities at maxima in near-UV
      region, at room temperature, **07:** 160
  pyruvate • (cytoplasmic)
    optical rotatory dispersion
      UV region, **07:** 73
      visible and near UV regions, **07:** 34
β-Decarboxylase
  1-aspartate •
    amino acid composition, complete data, **07:** 505
  aspartate-•, average hydrophobicity values, **01:** 215
Decoylnine
  physicochemical constants, spectral, chemotherapeutic
    and biological properties, **03:** 312
Deferrichrysin
  proton NMR and suggested conformations, **07:** 567-568
Dehydrase
  dihydroxy-acid •
    Neurospora crassa mutant, **04:** 751
  β-hydroxydecanoyl thioester •
    amino acid composition, complete data, **07:** 507
  imidazole glycerol phosphate •
    Neurospora crassa mutant, **04:** 751
  oxyglutarate •
    Neurospora crassa mutant, **04:** 749
Dehydratase
  chorismate mutase-prephenate •
    average hydrophobicity value, **01:** 216
  prephenic •
    Neurospora crassa mutant, **04:** 747

serine •
  molar absorptivity and-or absorbance values, **02:** 507
  subunit, constitution of, **02:** 328
d-serine •
  average hydrophobicity value, **01:** 231
  molar absorptivity and-or absorbance values, **02:** 507
Dehydroalanine
  structure and properties, **01:** 175
ω-Dehydroalloisoleucine
  antagonism to valine, **01:** 180
Dehydrocysteine
  structure and properties, **01:** 175
Dehydrogenase, *see also* dehydrogenases
  alcohol •
    amino acid sequence, **07:** 314-315
    average hydrophobicity value, **01:** 212
    molar absorptivity and-or absorbance values, **02:** 388
    optical rotatory dispersion
      UV region, **07:** 45
      visible and near UV regions, **07:** 16
    subunit, constitution of, **02:** 328, 330, 337, 338
    table of cofactors, molecular weights, stoichiometry
      and sources, **02:** 284
  aldehyde •
    amino acid composition, complete data, **07:** 505
    molar absorptivity and-or absorbance values, **02:** 388
    subunit, constitution of, **02:** 343
  aldehyde •, protein A
    average hydrophobicity value, **01:** 212
  aspartate-8-semialdehyde •, *Neurospora crassa* mutant,
    04: 743
  dihydro orotate •
    Neurospora crassa mutant, **04:** 748
  estradiol •
    average hydrophobicity value, **01:** 220
    Neurospora crassa mutant, **04:** 755
    optical rotatory dispersion
      UV region, **07:** 56
      visible and near UV regions, **07:** 23
  glucose 6-phosphate •, **02:** 336
  glutamate •
    amino acid sequence, **07:** 316-318
    average hydrophobicity value, **01:** 221
    luminescence of, table, **01:** 205
    molar absorptivity and-or absorbance values, **02:** 432
    subunit, constitution of, **02:** 344, 345
  glutamic •
    cofactors, molecular weights, stoichiometry and
      sources, **02:** 284
    molar absorptivity and-or absorbance values, **02:** 432
    refractive index increments, **02:** 376
  glyceraldehyde-phosphate •
    circular dichroism in the UV region, **07:** 99
    optical rotatory dispersion
      UV region, **07:** 57
      visible and near UV regions, **07:** 24
  d-glyceraldehyde-3-phosphate •
    refractive index increments, **02:** 376
  glyceraldehyde-3-phosphate •
    amino acid sequence, **07:** 327-329
    circular dichroism in near-UV region, at room temper-
      ature, **07:** 151

Dehydrogenase *(continued)*
    molar absorptivity and-or absorbance values, **02:** 434
    subunit, constitution of, **02:** 349
    viscosity, intrinsic, **02:** 721
1-glycerol 3-phosphate •
    amino acid composition, complete data, **07:** 507
glycerol-3-phosphate •
    average hydrophobicity value, **01:** 222
    molar absorptivity and-or absorbance values, **02:** 434
α-glycerophosphate •
    optical rotatory dispersion
        UV region, **07:** 58
        visible and near UV regions, **07:** 25
gylceraldehyde-3-phosphate •
    average hydrophobicity value, **01:** 222
    luminescence of, table, **01:** 206
histidinol •
    amino acid composition, complete data, **07:** 507
    molar absorptivity and-or absorbance values, **02:** 449
    Neurospora crassa mutant, **04:** 741
    subunit, constitution of, **02:** 331
β-hydroxbutyrate •
    average hydrophobicity value, **01:** 224
3-hydroxyacyl coenzyme A •
    average hydrophobicity value, **01:** 224
α^1-hydroxysteroid •
    average hydrophobicity value, **01:** 224
17-β-hydroxysteroid •
    average hydrophobicity value, **01:** 224
20-β-hydroxysteroid •
    optical rotatory dispersion
        UV region, **07:** 61
        visible and near UV regions, **07:** 26
β-IPM •
    Neurospora crassa mutant, **04:** 740, 746
isocitrate •
    amino acid composition, complete data, **07:** 508
    average hydrophobicity value, **01:** 225
    circular dichroism in the UV region, **07:** 106
    molar absorptivity and-or absorbance values, **02:** 458
    optical rotatory dispersion
        UV region, **07:** 64
        visible and near UV regions, **07:** 28
β-isopropylmalate •
    amino acid composition, complete data, **07:** 508
α-keto acids; reduction by lactic •, **01:** 181-182
lactate •
    amino acid sequence, **07:** 320-321, 336-337
    circular dichroism
        UV and near UV-region, **07:** 107-108, 155
    luminescence of, table, **01:** 206
    molar absorptivity and-or absorbance values, **02:** 461-462
    optical rotatory dispersion
        UV region, **07:** 64
        visible and near UV regions, **07:** 28-29
    subunit, constitution of, **02:** 337
d-lactate •
    amino acid composition, complete data, **07:** 508
lactate •, dogfish
    structure, illustration, **02:** 766

lactic •
    reduction of α-keto acid, **01:** 181-182
    refractive index increments, **02:** 377
lipoamide • (NADH)
    amino acid composition, complete data, **07:** 508
    circular dichroism in the UV region, **07:** 108
    optical rotatory dispersion
        UV region, **07:** 65
        visible and near UV regions, **07:** 29
liver alcohol •
    amino acid sequence, **07:** 330-332
malate •
    average hydrophobicity value, **01:** 226
    molar absorptivity and-or absorbance values, **02:** 470
    optical rotatory dispersion
        UV region, **07:** 66
        visible and near UV regions, **07:** 30
    subunit, constitution of, **02:** 328, 329, 330, 338
malate •, porcine
    structure, illustration, **02:** 766
malic • (mitochondrial)
    amino acid composition, complete data, **07:** 508
methylmalonatesemialdehyde•
    average hydrophobicity value, **01:** 227
NADP-glutamate •
    Neurospora crassa mutant, **04:** 751
octopine •
    circular dichroism in the UV region, **07:** 116
    optical rotatory dispersion
        UV region, **07:** 69
        visible and near UV regions, **07:** 32
oxoglutarate •
    circular dichroism in the UV region, **07:** 117
    optical rotatory dispersion in the UV region, **07:** 69
2-oxoglutarate •
    average hydrophobicity value, **01:** 228
phosphogluconate • (decarboxylating)
    amino acid composition, complete data, **07:** 509
    optical rotatory dispersion in the UV region, **07:** 71
phosphoglycerate •
    amino acid composition, complete data, **07:** 509
polyol •
    amino acid composition, incomplete data, **07:** 514
pyruvate •
    molar absorptivity and-or absorbance values, **02:** 504
    subunit, constitution of, **02:** 332, 338
pyruvate • complex
    subunit, constitution of, **02:** 351
pyruvate • deficiency
    characteristics of, **01:** 326
pyruvate • multiple-enzyme complex
    circular dichroism in the UV region, **07:** 121
ribitol •
    molar absorptivity and-or absorbance values, **02:** 505
    subunit, constitution of, **02:** 334
subunit structures; dogfish lactate •, illustration, **02:** 766
subunit structures; porcine malate •, illustration, **02:** 766
tartrate •
    amino acid composition, complete data, **07:** 510
tetrahydrofolate •
    circular dichroism in the UV region, **07:** 124

Dehydrogenase *(continued)*
thermolabile prephenic •
Neurospora crassa mutant, **04:** 742
triosephosphate •
average hydrophobicity value, **01:** 233
UDPglucose •, **07:** 128
Dehydrogenase[3]
glutamate • neurospora (NADP)
amino acid sequence, **07:** 318-320
Dehydrogenase (cytochrome b_2)
lactate •
circular dichroism in near-UV region, at room temperature, **07:** 148-155
Dehydrogenase I
aspartokinase I--homoserine •
amino acid composition, complete data, **07:** 505
circular dichroism
in UV and near UV region, **07:** 86, 144
optical rotatory dispersion in the visible and near UV regions, **07:** 18
Dehydrogenase (NADP$^+$)
glutamate •
circular dichroism in the UV region, **07:** 98
optical rotatory dispersion
UV region, **07:** 57
visible and near UV regions, **07:** 24
Dehydrogenases, *see also* Dehydrogenase
dependent •
amino acid sequence, **07:** 314
ω-Dehydroisoleucine
antagonism to isoleucine, **01:** 178
Dehydroleucine
structure and properties, **01:** 175
trans-4-Dehydrolysine
antagonism to lysine, **01:** 178
Dehydrophenylalanine
structure and properties, **01:** 175
Dehydroproline
structure and properties, **01:** 175
3,4-Dehydroproline
antagonism to proline, **01:** 179
Dehydroquinase
synthetic •
Neurospora crassa mutant, **04:** 745
Dehydroquinic acid
synthetase
Neurospora crassa mutant, **04:** 745
Dehydroretinol
properties of, **08:** 284
Dehydroserine
structure and properties, **01:** 175
Dehydroshikimic acid
reductase
Neurospora crassa mutant, **04:** 745
Dehydrotryptophan
structure and properties, **01:** 175
Dehydrovaline
structure and properties, **01:** 175
3-Deoxy-D-arabinoheptulosonate 7-phosphate
synthetase-chroismate mutase
average hydrophobicity value, **01:** 218

(R)-3-(2-Deoxy-β-D-erythro-pentofuranosyl)3,6,7,8-tetrahydroimidazo-[4,5-d] [1,3]diazepin-8-ol
physicochemical constants, spectral, chemotherapeutic and biological properties, **03:** 314
Deoxyadenosine
nucleotide derivatives
physical constants and spectral properties, index to, **03:** 73
physical constants and spectral properties, **03:** 141
3'-Deoxyadenosine, *see* Cordycepin
Deoxyadenosine, N^6-Methyl-
physical constants and spectral properties, **03:** 141
2'-Deoxycoformycin
Parke Davis[7551] X41A, •, **03:** 314
Deoxycycline
origin, structure, and characteristic as protein biosynthesis inhibitor, **04:** 570
Deoxycytidine
and nucleoside derivatives
physical constants and spectral properties, index to, **03:** 70
Deoxycytidine nucleotide derivatives
physical constants and spectral properties, index to, **03:** 73
Deoxycytidylate
deaminase
average hydrophobicity value, **01:** 218
subunit, constitution of, **02:** 328
deaminase (T-2 bacteriophage induced)
subunit, constitution of, **02:** 336
Deoxyguanosine
and nucleoside derivatives
physical constants and spectral properties, index to, **03:** 70
nucleotide derivatives
physical constants and spectral properties, index to, **03:** 73
Deoxyhemoglobin, HB
UV and visible absorption spectrum, **07:** 176
Deoxynucleotide polymerizing enzymes
ape, properties of • from, **04:** 539-544
Bacillus subtilis; • from, enzymatic functions of, **04:** 545
Bacillus subtilis; • from, template specificity properties, **04:** 538
cat; • from, properties of, **04:** 539-544
chicken; • from, properties of, **04:** 539-544
cow; • from, properties of, **04:** 539-544
Escherichia coli, see also E. coli; • from, enzymatic functions of, **04:** 545
Escherichia coli, see also E. coli; • from, template specificity properties, **04:** 538
hamster; • from, properties of, **04:** 539-544
human; • from, properties of, **04:** 539-544
molecular weight; •, tables of values, **04:** 538-540
monkey; • from, properties of, **04:** 539-544
mouse; • from, properties of, **04:** 539-544
properties, template specificities of, and reactions, **04:** 536-545
rabbit; • from, properties of, **04:** 539-544
rat; • from, properties of , **04:** 539-544
turnover number; •, tables of values, **04:** 538-540

1-β-2'-Deoxyribofuranosyl-4-methylamino-2-pyrimidinone
physical constants and spectral properties, **03**: 142
Deoxyribohomopolymer complexes (purine·pyrimidine)
melting temperatures, **03**: 581-582
Deoxyribohomopolymers
melting temperatures, **03**: 581
Deoxyribonuclease
amino acid composition, complete data, **07**: 506
average hydrophobicity value, **01**: 218
carbohydrate content, **02**: 273
inhibitor
amino acid composition, complete data, **07**: 506
molar absorptivity and-or absorbance values, **02**: 418
pancreatic
refractive index increments, **02**: 374
Deoxyribonuclease A, B, C, II
average hydrophobicity values, **01**: 219
Deoxyribonuclease I
circular dichroism in the UV region, **07**: 93
molar absorptivity and-or absorbance values, **02**: 417
optical rotatory dispersion
UV region, **07**: 54
visible and near UV regions, **07**: 22
Deoxyribonuclease II-B
circular dichroism in near-UV region, at room temperature, **07**: 150
Deoxyribonucleases
characteristics, functional, **04**: 495-507
Escherichia coli, *see also E. coli*; • from, functional
characteristics, **04**: 497-502
Deoxyribonucleic acid, *see also* DNA, DNA
ligase
average hydrophobicity value, **01**: 218
Deoxyribonucleic acids, *see also* DNA; DNAs
annelida; • from, purine and pyrimidine distribution in,
04: 265
arthropoda; • from, purine and pyrimidine distribution
in, **04**: 266
aschelminthes; • from, purine and pyrimidine distribution in, **04**: 264
bacterial phages; • from, purine and pyrimidine distribution in, **04**: 276-278
chordata; • from, purine and pyrimidine distribution in,
04: 268-273
coelenterata; • from, purine and pyrimidine distribution
in, **04**: 264
corn (Zea mays), *see also* Maize; • from, purine and
pyrimidine distribution in, **04**: 259
echinodermata; • from, purine and pyrimidine distribution in, **04**: 267
Escherichia coli, *see also E. coli*; • from, purine and
pyrimidine distribution in, **04**: 247-248, 276
mollusca; • from, purine and pyrimidine distribution in,
04: 265
mouse; • from, purine and pyrimidine distribution in,
04: 270
nearest neighbor frequencies; • from diverse sources,
04: 312-318
Neurospora crassa; • from, purine and pyrimidine distribution in, **04**: 242
porifera; • from, purine and pyrimidine distribution in,
04: 264

protozoa; • from, purine and pyrimidine distribution in,
04: 263
purines; distribution of, in • from diverse sources, **04**:
241-281
pyrimidines; distribution of, in • from diverse sources,
04: 241-281
Salmonella typhimurium; • from, purine and pyrimidine
distribution in, **04**: 247
thallophyta; algae; • from, purine and pyrimidine distributionin, **04**: 256-257
thallophyta; fungi; • from, purine and pyrimidine distribution in, **04**: 242-253
tracheophyta; • from, purine and pyrimidine distribution in, **04**: 258-261
viruses; chordate; • from, purine and pyrimidine distribution in, **04**: 281
viruses; insect; • from, purine and pyrimidine distribution in, **04**: 280
viruses; plant DNA; • from purine and pyrimidine distribution in, **04**: 280
Deoxyribonucleosidase
pyrimidine •
Neurospora crassa mutant, **04**: 744
Deoxyribonucleoside, 6-methylaminopurine-
physical constants, and spectral properties, **03**: 141
Deoxyribonucleotidase
inhibitor II
average hydrophobicity value, **01**: 218
Deoxyribose 5-phosphate
aldolase
amino acid composition, incomplete data, **07**: 512
Deoxyuridine
and nucleoside derivatives
physical constants and spectral properties, index to,
03: 70
nucleotide derivatives
physical constants and spectral properties, index to,
03: 73
Dephosphorylase
phosphoribosyl-ATP-•
Neurospora crassa mutant, **04**: 741
Depolymerase
polysaccharide •
molar absorptivity and-or absorbance values, **02**: 500
subunit, constitution of, **02**: 347
Derivatives
abbreviations; amino acid •, journal reference to rules,
02: 87
abbreviations; corrinoid • and vitamin B$_{12}$, **08**: 16-17
absorption data; UV, pyridoxine, pyridoxal and
pyridoxamine •, **08**: 252-266
adenine and •
physical constants and spectral properties, index to,
03: 67
UV spectra, **03**: 420-423
UV spectral characteristics and acid dissociation constants, **03**: 409-410
adenosine; •, heat of proton ionization, pK, and related
thermodynamic quantities, **06**: 158-160
adenosine and •
molal osmotic coefficients, **03**: 528
UV spectra, **03**: 432-435

Derivatives *(continued)*

UV spectral characteristics and acid dissociation constants, 03: 413-414

adenylic acid; •, UV spectral characteristics and acid dissociation constants, 03: 416

alkaloids and •, pK'_a, 06: 326-327

amine •
heat of proton ionization, pK, and related thermodynamics quantities, 06: 162-164

amino acids, *see also* Aromatic amino acids, *also* specific acids; UV spectra of • of cysteine, cystine, histidine, phenylalanine, tyrosine, and tryptophan, 01: 192-199

aniline •
heat of proton ionization, pK, and related thermodynamic quantities, 06: 168-169

barbituric acid •
heat of proton ionization, pK, and related thermodynamic quantities, 06: 171-172

benzaldehyde •, heat of proton ionization, pK, and related thermodynamic quantities, 06: 172

benzene •, heat of proton ionization, pK, and related thermodynamic quantities, 06: 172

benzoic acid •
heat of proton ionization, pK, and related thermodynamic quantities, 06: 176-181

butane •
heat of proton ionization, pK, and related thermodynamic quantities, 06: 183

butanoic acid •
heat of proton ionization, pK, and related thermodynamic quantities, 06: 184-185

cyclohexane •
heat of proton ionization, pK, and related thermodynamic quantities, 06: 190

cystine •
heat of proton ionization, pK, and related thermodynamic quantities, 06: 191

cytidine and •
UV spectra, 03: 440-443
UV spectral characteristics and acid dissociation constants, 03: 414-415

cytidine •
heat of proton ionization, pK, and related thermodynamic quantities, 06: 191

cytidylic acid; •, UV spectral characteristics and acid dissociation constants, 03: 416

cytosine and •
physical constants and spectral properties, index to, 03: 67
UV spectra, 03: 427-428
UV spectral characteristics and acid dissociation constants, 03: 412

electronic charge distribution; monosaccharides and some of their •, 05: 474-477

formula, empirical; pyridoxine, pyridoxal and pyridoxamine •, 08: 252-266

guanine and •
physical constants and spectral properties, index to, 03: 67
UV spectra, 03: 423-427

UV spectral characteristics and acid dissociation constants, 03: 411-412

guanosine and •
UV spectra, 03: 436-440
UV spectral characteristics and acid dissociation constants, 03: 414

hemoglobin •
UV and visible absorption spectra from human normal adult, 07: 174-185

hypoxanthine and •
physical constants and spectral properties, index to, 03: 67
UV spectral characteristics and acid dissociation constants, 03: 413

imidazole • excreted in human urine, mg-day, 03: 252-269

inosine and •
molal osmotic coefficients, 03: 528
UV spectra, 03: 446-447
UV spectral characteristics and acid dissociation constants, 03: 415-416

molecular weight; pyridoxine, pyridoxal and pyridoxamine •, 08: 252-266

pK'_a; alkaloids and •, 06: 326-327

peptides and their •, immunogenic, 07: 549-550

purine • excreted in human urine, mg-day, 03: 252-269

pyridine • excreted in human urine, mg-day, 03: 252-269

pyridoxal •
structure, melting point, UV absorption data, 08: 256-261

pyridoxamine •
structure, melting point, UV absorption data, 08: 261-263

pyridoxine •
structure, melting point, UV absorption data, 08: 252-256

pyrimidine • excreted in human urine, mg-day, 03: 252-269

9-β-D-ribofuranosylpurine-6-one 3'(2')-phosphate •
physical constants and spectral properties, index to, 03: 74

9-β-D-ribofuranosylpurine 5'-phosphate •
physical constants and spectral properties, index to, 03: 74

6-ribosylaminoisocytosine 3'(2')-phosphate •
physical constants and spectral properties, index to, 03: 74

steroid •, nomenclature rules, 05: 71-73

structure; pyridoxine, pyridoxal and pyridoxamine •, 08: 252-266

sugar and sugar •, use of symbols for, 05: 8-9

2-thiouracil and •
physical constants and spectral properties, index to, 03: 68

thymidine and •
UV spectra, 03: 445-446
UV spectral characteristics and acid dissociation constants, 03: 415

thymine and •
homodimers, structure, 03: 52

Derivatives *(continued)*
    physical constants and spectral properties, index to, **03:** 68
    UV spectra, **03:** 431
    UV spectral characteristics and acid dissociation constants, **03:** 413
    trivial names vs. systematic names, steroid ●, **05:** 73
    tyrosine ●
        heat of proton ionization, pK, and related thermodynamic quantities, **06:** 258
    uracil and ●
        physical constants and spectral properties, index to, **03:** 68-69
        UV spectra, **03:** 430
        UV spectral characteristics and acid dissociation constants, **03:** 413
    uridine and ●
        molal activity coefficients, **03:** 529
        molal osmotic coefficients, **03:** 528
        UV spectra, **03:** 444-445
        UV spectral characteristics and acid dissociation constants, **03:** 415
    wye and ●
        physical constants and spectral properties, index to, **03:** 69
    xanthine and ●
        UV spectra, **03:** 428-429
        UV spectral characteristics and acid dissociation constants, **03:** 412
    xanthosine; ●, UV spectral characteristics and acid dissociation constants, **03:** 416
    zeatosine and ●
        physical constants and spectral properties, index to, **03:** 72
Desaminocanavanine
    physical and chemical properties, **01:** 133
Desmosine
    physical and chemical properties, **01:** 161
Desoxyribonuclease
    carbohydrate content, **02:** 274
Desulfovibrio
    C_{553}
        amino acid sequence, **07:** 302
Desulfyhydrase
    cysteine ●
        molar absorptivity and-or absorbance values, **02:** 412
        subunit, constitution of, **02:** 342
Detergent
    chromatography; Brij 35 ●, properties of, **08:** 216
    solubilizers, table of ● properties, **08:** 216
    table of properties, **08:** 216-217
Deuterium oxide
    heat of proton ionization, pK, and related thermodynamic quantities, **06:** 261
2-*N*,6-*N*-di-(2,3-dihydroxybenzoyl)lysine
    physical and chemical properties, **01:** 138
N,*N*′-diacetyl-L-cystine
    cystine; ● dimethyl ester, UV spectra of, **01:** 199
    dimethyl ester
        UV spectra of, **01:** 199
Dialdoses
    nomenclature rules, **05:** 109

α-Dialkylamino
    transamidase
        average hydrophobicity value, **01:** 218
L-Diamino, dicarboxylic acids
    physical and chemical properties, **01:** 121
2,6-Diamino-4-hexynoic acid
    structure and symbols for those incorporated into synthetic polypeptides, **01:** 101
2,6-Diamino-7-hydroxyazelaic acid
    physical and chemical properties, **01:** 120
α,ϵ-Diamino-α-hydroxycaproic acid, *see* α-Hydroxylysine
α,ϵ-Diamino-δ-hydroxycaproic acid, *see* δ-Hydroxylysine
α,ϵ-Diamino-β-hydroxypimelic acid, *see* Tabtoxinine
α,γ-Diaminobutyric acid
    physical and chemical properties, **01:** 120
2,4-Diaminobutyric acid
    structure and symbols for those incorporated into synthetic polypeptides, **01:** 101
α,ϵ-Diaminocaproic acid, *see* Lysine
β,ϵ-Diaminocaproic acid, *see* β-Lysine
2,6-Diaminoheptanoic acid
    antagonism to lysine, **01:** 178
3,5-Diaminohexanoic acid
    physical and chemical properties, **01:** 120
3,6-Diaminohexanoic acid
    physical and chemical properties, **01:** 121
    structure and symbols for those incorporated into synthetic polypeptides, **01:** 101
α,ϵ-Diaminopimelic acid
    antagonists of, **01:** 177
    γ-methyl-α,ϵ-diaminopimelic acid; antagonism to ●, **01:** 177
    physical and chemical properties, **01:** 122
2,2′-Diaminopimelic acid
    structure and symbols for those incorporated into synthetic polypeptides, **01:** 101
α,β-Diaminopropionic acid
    physical and chemical properties, **01:** 120
2,3-Diaminopropionic acid
    structure and symbols for those incorporated into synthetic polypeptides, **01:** 101
α,α-Diaminosebacic acid
    antagonism to α,ϵ-diaminopimelic acid, **01:** 177
α,α-Diaminosuberic acid
    antagonism to α,ϵ-diaminopimelic acid, **01:** 177
Diaminosuccinic acid
    antagonism to aspartic acid, **01:** 177
2,3-Diaminosuccinic acid
    physical and chemical properties, **01:** 122
α,δ-Diaminovaleric acid, *see* Ornithine
Diaphorase, *see* Lipoamide dehydrogenase (NADH)
ϵ-Diazo
    physical and chemical properties, **01:** 135
6-Diazo-5-oxonorleucine
    antagonism to Glutamine, **01:** 177
O-Diazoacetylserine, *see* Azaserine
3,5-Dibromotyrosine
    physical and chemical properties, **01:** 159
S-(1,2-Dicarboxy-ethyl)-cysteine
    physical and chemical properties, **01:** 154
Dicarboxylic acid
    alkyl, diesters, refractive index, **05:** 494

Diphosphatase
fructose •
subunit, constitution of, 02: 336
Diphosphokinase
nucleoside •
average hydrophobicity value, 01: 228
subunit, constitution of, 02: 333, 336
Dipyrimidines
singly bonded, proposal for abbreviations, 03: 53-55
singly bonded, proposals for abbreviations, 04: 53-55
Disaccharide units
isolated from complex carbohydrates of mammalian origin, structure of, 05: 278-280
Disaccharides
chemical formula, 05: 283-297, 327-334
derivatives, 05: 283-297, 327-334
melting point, 05: 283-297, 327-334
nomenclature rules, 05: 133-134
specific rotation, 05: 283-297, 327-334
synonyms, 05: 283-297, 327-334
Dismutase
superoxide •
amino acid composition, complete data, 07: 506
average hydrophobicity value, 01: 231
circular dichroism in the UV region: extrema between 185 and 250 NM^3, 07: 124
UV and near-UV region, 07: 94, 124, 161
optical rotatory dispersion in the UV region, 07: 55
subunit, constitution of, 02: 326, 327
Disodium salt
NADH$_2$ •
UV spectra, formula, molecular weight, 08: 168
Dispersoids
gas, chart of diameters for various, 08: 425
Disulfide
cystinyl compounds; longest wavelength • circular dichroism band, 07: 173
Disulfide-exchange
enzyme
amino acid composition, incomplete data, 07: 512
$\beta\beta'$-Dithiodi-(α-aminopropionic acid), *see* Cystine
Diuretics
ligands binding to plasma albumin, 02: 571
Djenkolic acid
physical and chemical properties, 01: 154
DNA, *see also* Deoxyribonucleic acid; DNAs
Absidia; G + C composition of • of, table arranged by specie, 04: 185
Acanthamoeba; G + C composition of • of, table arranged by specie, 04: 228
Acetobacter; G + C composition of • of, table arranged by specie, 04: 152-153
Achlya; G + C composition of • of, table arranged by specie, 04: 185
Achromobacter; G + C composition of • of, table arranged by specie, 04: 69-71
achromobacteriaceae; G + C composition of • of, table arranged by genera and specie, 04: 69-74
Aciddminococcus; G + C composition of • of, table arranged by specie, 04: 147
Acinetobacter; G + C composition of • of, table arranged by specie, 04: 89-90

Acrasis; G + C composition of • of, table arranged by specie, 04: 185
Acrothecium; G + C composition of • of, table arranged by specie, 04: 185
Actinobacillus; G + C composition of • of, table arranged by specie, 04: 90-91
Actinomucor; G + C composition of • of, table arranged by specie, 04: 185
Actinomyces; G + C composition of • of, table arranged by specie, 04: 75
actinoplanaceae; G+C composition of • of, table arranged by genera and specie, 04: 76-78
Actinoplanes; G + C composition of • of, table arranged by specie, 04: 76
Actinosporangium; G + C composition of • of, table arranged by specie, 04: 77
Acytostelium; G + C composition of • of, table arranged by specie, 04: 185
Aerobacter (Enterobacter); G + C composition of • of, table arranged by specie, 04: 104-105
Aerococcus; G + C composition of • of, table arranged by specie, 04: 127
Aeromonas; G + C composition of • of, table arranged by specie, 04: 153
Agaricus; G + C composition of • of, table arranged by specie, 04: 186
agnatha, • content per cell, 04: 293
Agrobacterium; G + C composition of • of, table arranged by specie, 04: 162-164
Alcaligenes; G + C composition of • of, table arranged by specie, 04: 71-73
algae; • base compositions for, 04: 236-237
algae; G + C composition of • of, table arranged by genera and specie, 04: 224-227
Amanita; G + C composition of • of, table arranged by specie, 04: 186
Amauroascus; G + C composition of • of, table arranged by specie, 04: 186
Amoeba; G + C composition of • of, table arranged by specie, 04: 228
Amorphosporangium; G + C composition of • of, table arranged by specie, 04: 77
amphibia, satellite •'s; buoyant density and G + C content of, table, 04: 389-390
amphibians; • content per cell for various, table, 04: 298-299
Ampullariella; G + C composition of • of, table arranged by specie, 04: 77
Anaplasma; G + C composition of • of, table arranged by specie, 04: 78
Anaplasmataceae; G + C composition of • of, table arranged by genera and specie, 04: 78
angiosperms; buoyant density and G + C content of satellite •s for several species, table, 04: 400-401
Anixiopsis; G + C composition of • of, table arranged by specie, 04: 186
Ankistrodesmus; G + C composition of • of, table arranged by specie, 04: 224
annelida; • content per cell, 04: 291
Arachniotus; G + C composition of • of, table arranged by specie, 04: 186

DNA *(continued)*

Archangiaceae; G + C composition of • of, table arranged by genera and specie, **04:** 78

Archangium; G + C composition of • of, table arranged by specie, **04:** 78

Arthrobacter; G + C composition of • of, table arranged by specie, **04:** 97-99

Arthrobotrys; G + C composition of • of, table arranged by specie, **04:** 186

arthropoda; • content per cell for various, table, **04:** 291-293

ascomycetes, • content per cell for various, table, **04:** 284

Aspergillus; G + C composition of • of, table arranged by specie, **04:** 186-188

Aspergillus nidulans; • content per cell, **04:** 284

Astasia; G + C composition of • of, table arranged by specie, **04:** 228

Athiohodaceae; G + C composition of • of, table arranged by genera and specie, **04:** 78-80

Aureobasidium; G + C compositon of • of, table arranged by specie, **04:** 188

Auxarthon; G + C composition of • of, table arranged by specie, **04:** 189

Azotobacter; G + C composition of • of, table arranged by specie, **04:** 80-81

Azotobacteriaceae; G + C composition of • of, table arranged by genera and specie, **04:** 80-81

Azotomonas; G + C composition of • of, table arranged by specie, **04:** 153

bacillaceae; G + C composition of • of, table arranged by genera and specie, **04:** 81-89

Bacillus; G + C composition of • of, table arranged by specie, **04:** 81-85

Bacillus subtilis; • content per cell for various, table, **04:** 284

G + C composition of, **04:** 84

Backusia; G + C composition of • of, table arranged by specie, **04:** 189

bacteria; G + C composition of • of, table, arranged by family, genera, specie, **04:** 69-183

bacteria; nearest neighbor frequencies, in • from various, **04:** 314-315

bacteriophage types; viral •
nucleotide sequences, **04:** 350-351

Bacterium; G + C composition of • of, table arranged by specie, **04:** 105

bacteroidaceae; G + C composition of • of, table arranged by genera and specie, **04:** 86-87

Bacteroides; G + C composition of • of, table arranged by specie, **04:** 86-87

base compositions of eucaryotic protists, tables, **04:** 236-239

Basidiobolus; G + C composition of • of, table arranged by specie, **04:** 189

Bdellovibrio; G + C composition of • of, table arranged by specie, **04:** 166

Beauveria; G + C composition of • of, table arranged by specie, **04:** 189

Beijerinckia; G + C composition of • of, table arranged by specie, **04:** 81

Bifidobacterium; G + C composition of • of, table arranged by specie, **04:** 75, 115

Bispora; G + C composition of • of, table arranged by specie, **04:** 189

Bjerkandera; G + C composition of • of, table arranged by specie, **04:** 189

Blakesleea; G + C composition of • of, table arranged by specie, **04:** 189

Blastocladiella; G + C composition of • of, table arranged by specie, **04:** 189

Blastocrithidia; G + C composition of • of, table arranged by specie, **04:** 228

Bordetella; G + C composition of • of, table arranged by specie, **04:** 91

Borrelia; G + C composition of • of, table arranged by specie, **04:** 180

Botrytis; G + C composition of • of, table arranged by specie, **04:** 190

Bovista; G + C composition of • of, table arranged by specie, **04:** 190

Brettanomyces; G + C composition of • of, table arranged by specie, **04:** 190

brevibacteriaceae; G + C composition of • of, table arranged by genera and specie, **04:** 87-89

Brevibacterium; G + C composition of • of, table arranged by specie, **04:** 87-89

Brucella; G + C composition of • of, table arranged by specie, **04:** 91

brucellaceae; G + C composition of • of, table arranged by genera and specie, **04:** 89-93

buoyant density; satellite •s
amphibia, **04:** 389-390
birds, **04:** 390-391
crustaceae, **04:** 384-387
insects, **04:** 380-384
mammals, **04:** 391-399
molluscs, **04:** 387
plants, **04:** 399-402
tunicates, **04:** 388

Byssochlamys; G + C composition of • of, table arranged by specie, **04:** 190

Candida; G + C composition of • of, table arranged by specie, **04:** 190-191

Catenabacterium; G + C composition of • of, table arranged by specie, **04:** 115

Caulobacter; G + C composition of • of, table arranged by specie, **04:** 95

caulobacteriaceae; G + C composition of • of, table arranged by genera and specie, **04:** 95

cellular, buoyant density values for several, **03:** 565-566

Cellulomonas; G + C composition of • of, table arranged by specie, **04:** 99

Ceratocystis; G + C composition of • of, table arranged by specie, **04:** 192

Cercospora; G + C composition of • of, table arranged by specie, **04:** 192

Ceriporiopsis; G + C composition of • of, table arranged by specie, **04:** 192

Chaetoceras; G + C composition of • of, table arranged by specie, **04:** 224

Chaetocladium; G + C composition of • of, table arranged by specie, **04:** 192

DNA *(continued)*

Chaetomium; G + C composition of • of, table arranged by specie, **04**: 192-193

Chara; G + C composition of • of, table arranged by specie, **04**: 224

Chlamydia; G + C composition of • of, table arranged by specie, **04**: 95

chlamydiaceae; G + C composition of • of, table arranged by genera and specie, **04**: 95

chlamydobacteriaceae; G + C composition of • of, table arranged by genera and specie, **04**: 95

Chlamydomonas; G + C composition of • of, table arranged by specie, **04**: 224-225

Chlorella; G + C composition of • of, table arranged by specie, **04**: 225

Chloridium; G + C composition of • of, table arranged by specie, **04**: 193

chlorobacteriaceae; G + C composition of • of, table arranged by genera and specie, **04**: 96-97

Chlorobium; G + C composition of • of, table arranged by specie, **04**: 96

Chlorogonium; G + C composition of • of, table arranged by specie, **04**: 225

chloroplast
   buoyant density, table of values, **04**: 356-358
   GC mol %, table of values, **04**: 356-358

Chloropseudomonas; G + C composition of • of, table arranged by specie, **04**: 97

Choanephora; G + C composition of • of, table arranged by specie, **04**: 193

Chondrococcus; G + C composition of • of, table arranged by specie, **04**: 145

Chondromyces; G + C composition of • of, table arranged by specie, **04**: 150-151

chondrostei, • content per cell, **04**: 293

Chromatium; G + C composition of • of, table arranged by specie, **04**: 178-179

Chromobacterium; G + C composition of • of, table arranged by specie, **04**: 164

Circinella; G + C composition of • of, table arranged by specie, **04**: 193

circular dichroism parameters; oligonucleotides of •, **03**: 465-468

Citeromyces; G + C composition of • of, table arranged by specie, **04**: 193

Citrobacter; G + C composition of • of, table arranged by specie, **04**: 105

Cladosporium; G + C composition of • of, table arranged by specie, **04**: 193

Claviceps; G + C composition of • of, table arranged by specie, **04**: 193

Clostridium; G + C composition of • of, table arranged by specie, **04**: 85-86

Coccolithus; G + C composition of • of, table arranged by specie, **04**: 225

Coemansia; G + C composition of • of, table arranged by specie, **04**: 194

Cokeromyces; G + C composition of • of, table arranged by specie, **04**: 194

Colletotrichum; G + C composition of • of, table arranged by specie, **04**: 194

Colpidium; G + C composition of • of, table arranged by specie, **04**: 228

Comamonas; G + C composition of • of, table arranged by specie, **04**: 166

content per cell
   algae from various sources, table, **04**: 286
   amphibians from various sources, table, **04**: 298-299
   animal viruses from various sources, table, **04**: 310
   annelida from various sources, table, **04**: 291
   arthropoda from various sources, table, **04**: 291-293
   bacteriophages from various sources, table, **04**: 307-308
   birds from various sources, table, **04**: 300-301
   chordata from various sources, table, **04**: 293-305
   coelenterata from various sources, table, **04**: 290
   echinodermata from various sources, table, **04**: 290
   fish from various sources, table, **04**: 293-297
   fungi from various sources, table, **04**: 284-285, 289
   mammals from various sources, table, **04**: 302-305
   mollusca from various sources, table, **04**: 291
   nematoda from various sources, table, **04**: 291
   porifera from various sources, table, **04**: 290
   pteropsida from various sources, table, **04**: 287-288
   reptiles from various sources, table, **04**: 298-299

Coprinus; G + C composition of • of, table arranged by specie, **04**: 194

corynebacteriaceae; G + C composition of • of, table arranged by genera and specie, **04**: 97-103

Corynebacterium; G + C composition of • of, table arranged by specie, **04**: 99-103

Cricosphaera; G + C composition of • of, table arranged by specie, **04**: 225

Crithidia; G + C composition of • of, table arranged by specie, **04**: 228

Cryptococcus; G + C composition of • of, table arranged by specie, **04**: 194-195

Ctenomyces; G + C composition of • of, table arranged by specie, **04**: 195

Cunninghamella; G + C composition of • of, table arranged by specie, **04**: 195

Curvularia; G + C composition of • of, table arranged by specie, **04**: 196

Cyclotella; G + C composition of • of, table arranged by specie, **04**: 225

Cylindrocephalum; G + C composition of • of, table arranged by specie, **04**: 196

Cylindrotheca; G + C composition of • of, table arranged by specie, **04**: 225

Cystoseira; G + C composition of • of, table arranged by specie, **04**: 225

Cytophaga; G + C composition of • of, table arranged by specie, **04**: 103-104

cytophagaceae; G + C composition of • of, table arranged by genera and specie, **04**: 103-104

Dactylium; G + C composition of • of, table arranged by specie, **04**: 196

Dactylosporangium; G + C composition of • of, table arranged by specie, **04**: 77

Daedalea; G + C composition of • of, table arranged by specie, **04**: 196

Debaryomyces; G + C composition of • of, table arranged by specie, **04**: 196

DNA *(continued)*

density; kinetoplast •, table, **04:** 375-377

Derxia; G + C composition of • of, table arranged by specie, **04:** 81

Desulfotomaculum; G + C composition of • of, table arranged by specie, **04:** 167

Desulfovibrio; G + C composition of • of, table arranged by specie, **04:** 167

Dictyostelium; G + C composition of • of, table arranged by specie, **04:** 196

Dictyuchus; G + C composition of • of, table arranged by specie, **04:** 197

Diplococcus; G + C composition of • of, table arranged by specie, **04:** 116

dipnoans, • content per cell, **04:** 293

Dipodascus; G + C composition of • of, table arranged by specie, **04:** 197

Dipsacomyces; G + C composition of • of, table arranged by specie, **04:** 197

dog; mitochondrial • from, properties, **04:** 371

drosophila, buoyant density and G + C content of satellite •s for several strains, table, **04:** 380-382

Drosophila melanogaster; mitochondrial •, properties of, **04:** 369

Dunaliella; G + C composition of • of, table arranged by specie, **04:** 225

echinodermata; • content per cell for various, table, **04:** 290

Eidamella; G + C composition of • of, table arranged by specie, **04:** 197

elasmobranchii, • content per cell, **04:** 293

Elfvingia; G + C composition of • of, table arranged by specie, **04:** 197

Emericella; G + C composition of • of, table arranged by specie, **04:** 197

Emericellopsis; G + C composition of • of, table arranged by specie, **04:** 197

Endomyces; G + C composition of • of, table arranged by specie, **04:** 197

Endomycopsis; G + C composition of • of, table arranged by specie, **04:** 198

Entamoeba; G + C composition of • of, table arranged by specie, **04:** 228

enterobacteriaceae; G + C composition of • of, table arranged by genera and specie, **04:** 104-114

Epicoccum; G + C composition of • of, table arranged by specie, **04:** 198

Eremascus; G + C composition of • of, table arranged by specie, **04:** 198

Erwinia; G + C composition of • of, table arranged by specie, **04:** 105-109

Escherichia coli, see also E. coli; • content per cell for various, table, **04:** 285

Escherichia coli, see also E. coli; G + C composition of • of, table arranged by specie, **04:** 110

Escherichia coli, see also E. coli; nearest neighbor frequencies in • from various, **04:** 314

Euglena; G + C composition of • of, table arranged by specie, **04:** 228

eukaryotes, multicellular; nearest neighbor frequencies

in • from various, **04:** 316-318

eukaryotes, unicellular; nearest neighbor frequencies in • from various, **04:** 315-316

eukaryotic satellite •s, properties of selected, **04:** 379-402

Eupenicillium; G + C composition of • of, table arranged by specie, **04:** 198

T-even coliphage, buoyant density values, **03:** 568

extinction coefficient; •, double-strand, as a function of A + T content, graph, **03:** 590

extinction coefficient; •, single-strand, **03:** 589

extinction coefficients for double-strand types as a function of A + T content, graph, **03:** 590

extinction coefficients for single-strand types, **03:** 589

Flavobacterium; G + C composition of • of, table arranged by specie, **04:** 74

Flexibacter; G + C composition of • of, table arranged by specie, **04:** 104

Flexibacteria; G + C composition of • of, table arranged by specie, **04:** 181

Flexothrix; G + C composition of • of, table arranged by specie, **04:** 182

fluorescent dyes bound to, data tables, **04:** 470

Fomes; G + C composition of • of, table arranged by specie, **04:** 199

Fomitopsis (Fomes); G + C composition of • of, table arranged by specie, **04:** 199

Fulgio; G + C composition of • of, table arranged by specie, **04:** 199

fungi; G + C composition of • of, table arranged by specie, **04:** 185-224

Fusarium; G + C composition of • of, table arranged by specie, **04:** 199

Fusobacterium; G + C composition of • of, table arranged by specie, **04:** 87

G + C composition; algae •, arranged by genera and specie, **04:** 224-227

G + C composition; bacteria •, arranged by family, genera, specie, **04:** 69-183

G + C composition; fungi •, arranged by genera and specie, **04:** 185-224

G + C composition; protozoa •, arranged by genera and specie, **04:** 228-229

G + C composition of • of, table arranged by specie, **04:** 192

G + C content; mitochondrial •s, table, **04:** 363-372

G + C content; satellite •s

amphibia, **04:** 389-390

birds, **04:** 390-391

crustaceae, **04:** 384-387

insects, **04:** 380-384

mammals, **04:** 391-399

molluscs, **04:** 387

plants, **04:** 399-402

tunicates, **04:** 388

G + C content; viral •, **03:** 560-562

Gaffkya; G + C composition of • of, table arranged by specie, **04:** 127

Ganoderma; G + C composition of • of, table arranged by specie, **04:** 127

DNA *(continued)*

Gelasinospora; G + C composition of • of, table arranged by specie, **04:** 199-200

Geotrichum; G + C composition of • of, table arranged by specie, **04:** 200

Gilbertella; G + C composition of, • of, table arranged by specie, **04:** 200

Glaucoma; G + C composition of • of, table arranged by specie, **04:** 228

Gliocladium; G + C composition of • of, table arranged by specie, **04:** 200

Gloeophyllum (Lenzites); G + C composition of • of, table arranged by specie, **04:** 200

Gluconobacter; G + C composition of • of, table arranged by specie, **04:** 153

guinea pig; mitochondrial • from, properties, **04:** 371

guinea pig; satellite •s buoyant density and G + C content of, table, **04:** 394

Gymnoascus; G + C composition of • of, table arranged by specie, **04:** 200

Haemophilus; G + C composition of • of, table arranged by specie, **04:** 91

Halobacterium; G + C composition of • of, table arranged by specie, **04:** 154

hamster; mitochondrial • from, properties, **04:** 371

Hanseniaspora; G + C composition of • of, table arranged by specie, **04:** 200

Hansenula; G + C composition of • of, table arranged by specie, **04:** 200-203

Haplosporangium; G + C composition of • of, table arranged by specie, **04:** 203

Helicoma; G + C composition of • of, table arranged by specie, **04:** 203

Helicostylium; G + C composition of • of, table arranged by specie, **04:** 203

Helminthosporium; G + C composition of • of, table arranged by specie, **04:** 203

Helvella; G + C composition of • of, table arranged by specie, **04:** 203

Herellea; G + C composition of • of, table arranged by specie, **04:** 91-92

Herpetosiphon; G + C composition of • of, table arranged by specie, **04:** 182

Histoplasma; G + C composition of • of, table arranged by specie, **04:** 203

holostei, • content per cell, **04:** 293

human; • content per cell, **04:** 305

human; mitochondrial • from, properties, **04:** 372

human; satellite •s; buoyant density and G + C content of, table, **04:** 397-398

Humicola; G + C composition of • of, table arranged by specie, **04:** 204

Hydrodictyon; G + C composition of • of, table arranged by specie, **04:** 225

Hypocrea; G + C composition of • of, table arranged by specie, **04:** 204

Inonotus; G + C composition of • of, table arranged by specie, **04:** 204

insects, satellite •s; buoyant density and G + C content of, table, **04:** 380-384

intrasporangium; G + C composition of • of, table arranged by specie, **04:** 172

Irpex; G + C composition of • of, table arranged by specie, **04:** 204

Isoachyla; G + C composition of • of, table arranged by specie, **04:** 204

kinetoplast, properties of, table, **04:** 375-377

Klebsiella; G + C composition of • of, table arranged by specie, **04:** 111

Kloeckera; G + C composition of • of, table arranged by specie, **04:** 204

Kluyveromyces; G + C composition of • of, table arranged by specie, **04:** 204-205

Labyrinthula; G + C composition of • of, table arranged by specie, **04:** 205

lactobacillaceae; G + C composition of • of, table arranged by genera and specie, **04:** 115-126

Lactobacillus; G + C composition of • of, table arranged by specie, **04:** 116-122

Laetiporus; G + C composition of • of, table arranged by specie, **04:** 205

Lagerheimia; G + C composition of • of, table arranged by specie, **04:** 225

lambda molecule of *Escherichia coli*, genetic and molecular map, **04:** 678

Laricifomes (Fomes); G + C composition of • of, table arranged by specie, **04:** 206

Leishmania; G + C composition of • of, table arranged by specie, **04:** 228

Lenzites; G + C composition of • of, table arranged by specie, **04:** 206

Leptosphaeria; G + C composition of • of, table arranged by specie, **04:** 206

Leptospira; G + C composition of • of, table arranged by specie, **04:** 180

Leptotrichia; G + C composition of • of, table arranged by specie, **04:** 95

Leuconostoc; G + C composition of • of, table arranged by specie, **04:** 122

Leucothrix; G + C composition of • of, table arranged by specie, **04:** 126

leucotrichaceae; G + C composition of • of, table arranged by genera and specie, **04:** 126-127

Lichtheimia (Absidia); G + C composition of • of, table arranged by specie, **04:** 206

Linderina; G + C composition of • of, table arranged by specie, **04:** 206

Lipomyces; G + C composition of • of, table arranged by specie, **04:** 206

Listeria; G + C composition of • of, table arranged by specie, **04:** 103

Lodderomyces; G + C composition of • of, table arranged by specie, **04:** 206

Lophomonas; G + C composition of • of, table arranged by specie, **04:** 154

Lycogala; G + C composition of • of, table arranged by specie, **04:** 206

Lyngbya; G + C composition of • of, table arranged by specie, **04:** 226

mammals; satellite •s buoyant density and G + C content of, table, **04:** 391-399

melting temperature; viral •, **03:** 560-562

DNA *(continued)*

Meruliopsis (Poria); G + C composition of • of, table
arranged by specie, **04**: 206

Methanobacterium; G + C composition of • of, table
arranged by specie, **04**: 168

6-methylaminopurine, content of, **04**: 282-283

5-methylcytosine; content in •s, discussion of hypothesis, **04**: 358

5-methylcytosine, content of, **04**: 282-283

Metschnikowia; G + C composition of • of, table arranged by specie, **04**: 206

Microbacterium; G + C composition of • of, table arranged by specie, **04**: 103

Microbispora (Waksmania); G + C composition of • of,
table arranged by specie, **04**: 149

micrococcaceae; G + C composition of • of, table arranged by genera and specie, **04**: 127-138

Micrococcus (Staphylococcus); G + C composition of •
of, table arranged by specie, **04**: 128-134

Microcoleus; G + C composition of • of, table arranged
by specie, **04**: 226

Microcyclus; G + C composition of • of, table arranged
by specie, **04**: 168

Microellobosporia; G + C composition of • of, table arranged by specie, **04**: 77

Micromonospora; G + C composition of • of, table arranged by specie, **04**: 138

micromonosporaceae; G + C composition of • of, table
arranged by genera and specie, **04**: 138

Micropolyspora; G + C composition of • of, table arranged by specie, **04**: 149

Mima; G + C composition of • of; table arranged by
specie, **04**: 92

mitochondrial, properties of, table,
04: 363-372

monkey; mitochondrial • from, properties, **04**: 371

Monodus; G + C composition of • of, table arranged
by specie, **04**: 226

Monosporium; G + C composition of • of, table arranged by specie, **04**: 206

Moraxella; G + C composition of • of, table arranged
by specie, **04**: 92

Mortierella; G + C composition of • of, table arranged
by specie, **04**: 207

mouse; buoyant density and G + C content of satellite
•s for several varieties, table, **04**: 391-393

mouse; • content per cell, **04**: 302

mouse; mitochondrial • from, properties, **04**: 371

mouse; nearest neighbor frequencies in • from various
parts of, **04**: 317

Mucor; G + C composition of • of, table arranged by
specie, **04**: 207

mycobacteriaceae; G + C composition of • of, table
arranged by genera and specie, **04**: 139-141

Mycobacterium; G + C composition of • of, table arranged by specie, **04**: 139-141

Mycoplasma; G + C composition of • of, table arranged by specie, **04**: 141-145

Mycoplasmataceae; G + C composition of • of, table
arranged by genera and specie, **04**: 141

Mycotypha; G + C composition of • of, table arranged
by specie, **04**: 208

Myrothecium; G + C composition of • of, table arranged by specie, **04**: 208

Myxobacterium; G + C composition of • of, table arranged by species, **04**: 146

myxococcaceae; G + C composition of • of, table arranged by genera and specie, **04**: 145

Myxococcus (Myxobacterium); G + C composition of •
of, table arranged by specie, **04**: 146

Myxotrichum; G + C composition of • of, table arranged by specie, **04**: 208

Naegleria; G + C composition of • of, table arranged
by specie, **04**: 229

Naganishia; G + C composition of • of, table arranged
by specie, **04**: 208

Navicula; G + C composition of • of, table arranged
by specie, **04**: 226

nearest neighbor frequencies in acids from diverse
sources, **04**: 312-318

Neisseria; G + C composition of • of, table arranged
by specie, **04**: 147-148

neisseriaceae; G + C composition of • of, table arranged by genera and specie, **04**: 147-148

Neurospora; G + C composition of • of, table arranged
by specie, **04**: 208

Neurospora crassa; mitochondrial •, properties of, **04**:
368

Nigrospora; G + C composition of • of, table arranged
by specie, **04**: 209

Nitella; G + C composition of • of, table arranged by
specie, **04**: 226

Nitrobacter; G + C composition of • of, table arranged
by specie, **04**: 148

nitrobacteraceae; G + C composition of • of, table arranged by genera and specie, **04**: 148

Nitrosomonas; G + C composition of • of, table arranged by specie, **04**: 148

Nitzschia; G + C composition of • of, table arranged
by specie, **04**: 226

Nocardia; G + C composition of • of, table arranged
by specie, **04**: 149-150

nocardiaceae; G + C composition of • of, table arranged by genera and specie, **04**: 149-150

Nodularia; G + C composition of • of, table arranged
by specie, **04**: 226

non-human primates; satellite •s
buoyant density and G + C content of, table, **04**:
398-399

Nostoc; G + C composition of • of, table arranged by
specie, **04**: 226

nuclear
buoyant density, table of values, **04**: 356-358
GC mol %, table of values, **04**: 356-358

nucleotide; sequences and models for several RNAs and
•s, **04**: 324-353

Ochromonas; G + C composition of • of, table arranged by specie, **04**: 226

Oerskovia; G + C composition of • of, table arranged
by specie, **04**: 75-76

oligonucleotides, circular dichroism parameters, **03**:
465-468

oligonucleotides, optical dispersion parameters, **03**:
459-460

DNA *(continued)*

optical rotatory dispersion parameters; oligonucleotides of•, **03**: 459-460

Pachysolen; G + C composition of • of, table arranged by specie, **04**: 209

Paecilomyces; G + C composition of • of, table arranged by specie, **04**: 209

Paracolobactrum; G + C composition of • of, table arranged by specie, **04**: 112

Paramecium; G + C composition of • of, table arranged by specie, **04**: 229

Pasteurella; G + C composition of • of, table arranged by specie, **04**: 94

Pectobacterium; G + C composition of • of, table arranged by specie, **04**: 112

Pediococcus; G + C composition of • of, table arranged by specie, **04**: 123

Penicillium; G + C composition of • of, table arranged by specie, **04**: 209-212

Pestalotiopsis; G + C composition of • of, table arranged by species, **04**: 212

Petalosporus; G + C composition of • of, table arranged by specie, **04**: 212

Phaeocoriolellus (Lenzites); G + C composition of • of, table arranged by specie, **04**: 212

Phaeolus (Polyporus); G + C composition of • of, table arranged by specie, **04**: 212

Phellinus; G + C composition of • of, table arranged by specie, **04**: 212

Phialophora; G + C composition of • of, table arranged by specie, **04**: 213

Phoma; G + C composition of • of, table arranged by specie, **04**: 213

Phycomyces; G + C composition of • of, table arranged by specie, **04**: 213

Physarum; G + C composition of • of, table arranged by specie, **04**: 213

Phytophthora; G + C composition of • of, table arranged by specie, **04**: 213

Pichia; G + C composition of • of, table arranged by specie, **04**: 214

Pilaira; G + C composition of • of, table arranged by specie, **04**: 214

Piptoporus (Polyporus); G + C composition of • of, table arranged by specie, **04**: 214

Planobispora; G + C composition of • of, table arranged by specie, **04**: 77

plants, satellite •s; buoyant density and G + C content of, table, **04**: 399-402

Plasmodium; G + C composition of • of, table arranged by specie, **04**: 229

Plectonema; G + C composition of • of, table arranged by specie, **04**: 226

Pleurotus; G + C composition of • of, table arranged by specie, **04**: 214

polyangiaceae; G + C composition of • of, table arranged by genera and specie, **04**: 150-151

Polyangium; G + C composition of • of, table arranged by specie, **04**: 151

Polyides; G + C composition of • of, table arranged by specie, **04**: 226

polymerase
amino acid composition, complete data, **07**: 506
enzymatic activity, subcellular fractions, **02**: 699, 718
properties, template specificities, tables of, **04**: 538-540
reactions catalyzed by, **04**: 536
sources of, **04**: 536

polynucleotide double helices with Watson-Crick base pairs
atomic coordinates and molecular conformations for, **04**: 411-412

Polypaecilum; G + C composition of • of, table arranged by specie, **04**: 214

Polysphondylium; G + C composition of • of, table arranged by specie, **04**: 214

Polytoma; G + C composition of • of, table arranged by specie, **04**: 227

Polytomella; G + C composition of • of, table arranged by specie, **04**: 227

Poria; G + C composition of • of, table arranged by specie, **04**: 215

porifera; • content per cell for various, table, **04**: 290

primates, satellite •s; buoyant density and G + C content of, table, **04**: 397-399

Promicromonospora; G + C composition of • of, table arranged by specie, **04**: 76

propionibacteriaceae; G + C composition of • of, table arranged by genera and specie, **04**: 151-152

Propionibacterium; G + C composition of • of, table arranged by specie, **04**: 151-152

Prosthecomicrobium; G + C composition of • of, table arranged by specie, **04**: 182

Proteus; G + C composition of • of, table arranged by specie, **04**: 112-113

Protoachlya; G + C composition of • of, table arranged by specie, **04**: 215

Protostelium; G + C composition of • of, table arranged by specie, **04**: 215

protozoa; • content per cell for various, table, **04**: 289

protozoa; G + C composition of • of, table arranged by genera and specie, **04**: 228-229

Providencia; G + C composition of • of, table arranged by specie, **04**: 113

Prymnesium; G + C composition of • of, table arranged by specie, **04**: 227

Psalliota; G + C composition of • of, table arranged by specie, **04**: 215

Pseudeurotium; G + C composition of • of, table arranged by specie, **04**: 215

Pseudoarachniotus; G + C composition of • of, table arranged by specie, **04**: 215

Pseudogymnoascus; G + C composition of • of, table arranged by specie, **04**: 215

pseudomonadaceae; G + C composition of • of, table arranged by genera and species, **04**: 152-162

Pseudomonas; G + C composition of • of, table arranged by specie, **04**: 154-160

Pseudonocardia; G + C composition of • of, table arranged by specie, **04**: 150

pteropsida; • content per cell for various, table, **04**: 287-288

DNA *(continued)*

purine and pyrimidine, distribution of, in acids from diverse sources, **04:** 241-281

Pycnidiophora; G + C composition of ● of, table arranged by specie, **04:** 215

Pycnoporus; G + C composition of ● of, table arranged by specie, **04:** 215

Pythium; G + C composition of ● of, table arranged by specie, **04:** 215

rabbit; mitochondrial ● from, properties, **04:** 371

Radiomyces; G + C composition of ● of, table arranged by specie, **04:** 216

raman spectral changes, melting calf thymus DNA, **03:** 544

Ramibacterium; G + C composition of ● of, table arranged by specie, **04:** 123

range of weights, **08:** 424

rat; ● content per cell, **04:** 302

Rhabdonema; G + C composition of ● of, table arranged by specie, **04:** 227

rhizobiaceae; G + C composition of ● of, table arranged by genera and specie, **04:** 162-165

Rhizobium; G + C composition of ● of, table arranged by specie, **04:** 164-165

Rhizoclonium; G + C composition of ● of, table arranged by specie, **04:** 227

Rhizophlyctis; G + C composition of ● of, table arranged by specie, **04:** 216

Rhizophydium; G + C composition of ● of, table arranged by specie, **04:** 216

Rhizopus; G + C composition of ● of, table arranged by specie, **04:** 216

Rhodopseudomonas; G + C composition of ● of, table arranged by specie, **04:** 78-79

Rhodospirillum; G + C composition of ● of, table arranged by specie, **04:** 80

Rhodotorula; G + C composition of ● of, table arranged by specie, **04:** 216-217

Rhodymenia; G + C composition of ● of, table arranged by specie, **04:** 227

Rickettsia (Coxiella); G + C composition of ● of, table arranged by specie, **04:** 165

rickettsiaceae; G + C composition of ● of, table arranged by genera and specie, **04:** 165

Rothia; G + C composition of ● of, table arranged by specie, **04:** 76

Saccharomyces; G + C composition of ● of, table arranged by specie, **04:** 217-218

Saccharomyces cerevisiae; ● content per cell for various, table, **04:** 284

Saccharomyces cerevisiae; mitochondrial ●, properties, **04:** 367

salmonella; G + C composition of ● of, table arranged by specie, **04:** 113

Salmonella typhimurium; ● content per cell, **04:** 285

Saprolegnia; G + C composition of ● of, table arranged by specie, **04:** 219

Sapromyces; G + C composition of ● of, table arranged by specie, **04:** 219

Saprospira; G + C composition of ● of, table arranged by specie, **04:** 171

Sarcina; G + C composition of ● of, table arranged by specie, **04:** 134-135

Sartorya; G + C composition of ● of, table arranged by specie, **04:** 219

Scenedesmus; G + C composition of ● of, table arranged by specie, **04:** 227

schizomycetes; ● content per cell for various, table, **04:** 284

Schizophyllum; G + C composition for ● of, table arranged by specie, **04:** 219

Schizosaccharomyces; G + C composition of ● of, table arranged by specie, **04:** 219

Schwanniomyces; G + C composition of ● of, table arranged by specie, **04:** 219

Sclerotinia; G + C composition of ● of, table arranged by specie, **04:** 219

Scopulariopsis; G + C composition of ● of, table arranged by specie, **04:** 219-220

sequences in eukaryotes, **04:** 319-322

Serratia; G + C composition of ● of, table arranged by specie, **04:** 114

sheep; mitochondrial ● from, properties, **04:** 371

Shigella; G + C composition of ● of, table arranged by specie, **04:** 114

sorangiaceae; G + C composition of ● of, table arranged by specie, **04:** 166

Sorangium; G + C composition of ● of, table arranged by specie, **04:** 166

Sordaria; G + C composition of ● of, table arranged by specie, **04:** 220

Spadicoides; G + C composition of ● of, table arranged by specie, **04:** 220

Sphaerophorus; G + C composition of ● of, table arranged by specie, **04:** 87

Sphaerotilus; G + C composition of ● of, table arranged by specie, **04:** 95

spirillaceae; G + C composition of ● of, table arranged by genera and specie, **04:** 166-171

Spirillospora; G + C composition of ● of, table arranged by specie, **04:** 77

Spirillum; G + C composition of ● of, table arranged by specie, **04:** 168-169

Spirochaeta; G + C composition of ● of, table arranged by specie, **04:** 172

spirochaetaceae; G + C composition of ● of, table arranged by genera and specie, **04:** 171-172

Spirogyra; G + C composition of ● of, table arranged by specie, **04:** 227

Spirosoma; G + C composition of ● of, table arranged by specie, **04:** 182

Spondylocladium; G + C composition of ● of, table arranged by specie, **04:** 220

Spongipellis (Polyporus); G + C composition of ● of, table arranged by specie, **04:** 220

Sporobolomyces; G + C composition of ● of, table arranged by specie, **04:** 220-221

Sporocytophaga; G + C composition of ● of, table arranged by specie, **04:** 146

Sporomia; G + C composition of ● of, table arranged by specie, **04:** 221

DNA *(continued)*

Sporotrichum; G + C composition of ● of, table arranged by specie, **04:** 221

Stachybotrys; G + C composition of ● of, table arranged by specie, **04:** 221

Staphylococcus; G + C composition of ● of, table arranged by specie, **04:** 128-134

Stemphylium; G + C composition of ● of, table arranged by specie, **04:** 221

strand separation; mitochondrial ●s, table, **04:** 363-372

Streptobacillus; G + C composition of ● of, table arranged by specie, **04:** 87

Streptococcus; G + C composition of ● of, table arranged by specie, **04:** 123-126

Streptomyces; G + C composition of ● of, table arranged by specie, **04:** 172-177

streptomycetaceae; G + C composition of ● of, table arranged by genera and specie, **04:** 172-177

Streptosporangium; G + C composition of ● of, table arranged by specie, **04:** 78

Streptoverticillium; G + C composition of ● of, table arranged by specie, **04:** 177

Syncephalastrum; G + C composition of ● of, table arranged by specie, **04:** 221

synthesis; pathways chart, **04:** insert

Talaromyces; G + C composition of ● of, table arranged by specie, **04:** 221-222

telostei; ● content per cell for various, table, **04:** 293-297

temperature midpoint; kinetoplast ●s, table, **04:** 375-377

temperature midpoint; mitochondrial ●s, table, **04:** 363-372

Tetrahymena; G + C composition of ● of, table arranged by specie, **04:** 229

Thalassiosira; G + C composition of ● of, table arranged by specie, **04:** 227

Thamnidium; G + C composition of ● of, table arranged by specie, **04:** 222

Thermoactinomyces; G + C composition of ● of, table arranged by specie, **04:** 150

Thermoactinopolyspora; G + C composition of ● of, table arranged by specie, **04:** 150

Thermomonospora; G + C composition of ● of, table arranged by specie, **04:** 150

Thermoplasma; G + C composition of ● of, table arranged by specie, **04:** 145

Thermus; G + C composition of ● of, table arranged by specie, **04:** 182

Thielavia; G + C composition of ● of, table arranged by specie, **04:** 222

Thiobacillus; G + C composition of ● of, table arranged by specie, **04:** 177

thiobacteriaceae; G + C composition of ● of, table arranged by genera and specie, **04:** 177

thiorhodaceae; G + C composition of ● of, table arranged by genera and specie, **04:** 178-180

Thraustotheca; G + C composition of ● of, table arranged by specie, **04:** 222

Torula; G + C composition of ● of, table arranged by specie, **04:** 222

Torulopsis; G + C composition of ● of, table arranged by specie, **04:** 223

Toxoplasma; G + C composition of ● of, table arranged by specie, **04:** 229

Toxotrichum; G + C composition of ● of, table arranged by specie, **04:** 223

Tremella; G + C composition of ● of, table arranged by specie, **04:** 223

Treponema; G + C composition of ● of, table arranged by specie, **04:** 181

treponemataceae; G + C composition of ● of, table arranged by genera and specie, **04:** 180-181

Trichithecium; G + C composition of ● of, table arranged by specie, **04:** 223

Trichoderma; G + C composition of ● of, table arranged by specie, **04:** 223

Trichomonas; G + C composition of ● of, table arranged by specie, **04:** 229

Trichosporon; G + C composition of ● of, table arranged by specie, **04:** 223

Trigonopsis; G + C composition of ● of, table arranged by specie, **04:** 223

Trypanosoma; G + C composition of ● of, table arranged by specie, **04:** 229

Tuberculosis; G + C composition of ● of, table arranged by specie, **04:** 94

tunicates; ● content per cell, **04:** 293

Ulothrix; G + C composition of ● of, table arranged by specie, **04:** 227

Veillonella; G + C composition of ● of, table arranged by specie, **04:** 148

Verticillium; G + C composition of ● of, table arranged by specie, **04:** 224

Vibrio; G + C composition of ● of, table arranged by specie, **04:** 169-171

viral
   nucleotide sequences, **04:** 350-353

viral, buoyant densities, melting temperature and GC content, **03:** 560-562

viral, buoyant density values for several, **03:** 566-567

viral ●, buoyant densities, melting temperatures and GC content, **03:** 560-562

viral DNA molecules, content per virion, **03:** 551-556

viral molecules, composition and physical properties, **03:** 552-556

viruses; nearest neighbor frequencies in ● from various, **04:** 313-314

viruses; plant ●
   deoxyribonucleic acids from purine and pyrimidine distribution in, **04:** 280

Vitreoscilla; G + C composition of ● of, table arranged by specie, **04:** 181

vitreoscillaceae; G + C composition of ● of, table arranged by genera and specie, **04:** 181

Wickerhamia; G + C composition of ● of, table arranged by specie, **04:** 224

Wolbachia; G + C composition of ● of, table arranged by specie, **04:** 165

Xanthomonas; G + C composition of ● of, table arranged by specie, **04:** 161-162

Zygorhynchus; G + C composition of ● of, table arranged by specie, **04:** 224

DNA base
   fungi; ● compositions for, **04:** 237-239

DNA base *(continued)*

Neurospora crassa; • composition, **04:** 239
protozoa; • compositions for, **04:** 236
Saccharomyces cerevisiae; • composition, **04:** 239

DNA molecules

DNA, *see also* Deoxyribonucleic acid; viral •, content
per virion, **03:** 551-556
G + C content; viral •, **03:** 551-556
mapping, physical; viral •, **03:** 551-556
molecular weight; viral •, **03:** 551-556
strand separation in viral •, **03:** 551-556
sucrose; viral •, relative content in, **03:** 551-556
viral •, composition and physical properties, **03:** 551-556
Watson-Crick duplexes, viral •, 03: 549

DNAs, *see also* Deoxyribonucleic acid; DNA

birds; satellite •
buoyant density and G + C content of, table, **04:** 390-391
crabs; buoyant density and G + C content of satellite •
for several varieties, **04:** 384-387
crustaceae, satellite •; buoyant density and G + C content of,table, **04:** 384-387
density; mitochondrial •, table, **04:** 363-372
gymnosperms; buoyant density and G + C content of satellite • for several varieties, table, **04:** 399-400
molluscs, satellite •; buoyant density and G + C content of, table, **04:** 387
monocotyledons; buoyant density and G + C content of satellite • for several species, table, **04:** 402
tunicates; satellite •
buoyant density and G + C content of, table, **04:** 388

DNase, *see* Deoxyribonuclease I

D₂O

mononucleotides; ultraviolet absorbance in 97% •, **03:** 408
UV absorbance; mononucleotides in 97% •, **03:** 408

Domoic acid

physical and chemical properties, **01:** 139

DOPA, *see* 3,4-Dihydroxyphenylalanine

Dopamine-

β-hydroxylase
average hydrophobicity value, **01:** 219

Double helical complexes

molar residue ellipticity; nucleotides, •, and double stranded RNA, **03:** 601
molar residue rotation; nucleotides, • and double-stranded RNA, table of values, **03:** 599

Double helices

RNA, *see* Nucleic acids, Transfer RNA, TRNA
(TRNA); • at atomic resolution, geometry of, **04:** 463-469

Double stranded RNA

molar residue ellipticity; nucleotides, double helical complexes, and •, **03:** 601
molar residue rotation; nucleotides, double helical complexes and •, table of values, **03:** 599

DPNase

carbohydrate content, **02:** 273
inhibitor
carbohydrate content, **02:** 274

molar absorptivity and-or absorbance values, **02:** 419

Drugs

ligands binding to plasma albumin, **02:** 568-574

Duomycin, *see* Aureomycin, Chlortetracycline

Dyes

fluorescent, bound to nucleic acids, data tables, **04:** 470
pK'_a values, **06:** 348
visible, ligands binding to plasma albumin, **02:** 564-568

γ₁

immunoglobulin, specific; •, guinea pig
molar absorptivity and-or absorbance values, **02:** 456

γ₂

immunoglobulin, specific; •, guinea pig
molar absorptivity and-or absorbance values, **02:** 456

E

Echinine

physical and chemical properties, **01:** 140

Edeine

origin, structure, and characteristic as protein biosynthesis inhibitor, **04:** 571

Edestin

optical rotatory dispersion in the visible and near UV regions, **07:** 22
refractive index increments, **02:** 374
subunit, constitution of, **02:** 345

EDTA

heat of proton ionization, pK, and related thermodynamic quantities, **06:** 197
inhibition of transamitase activity, **02:** 669-673

Egg white

cross-reacting protein
amino acid composition, complete data, **07:** 506
lysozyme; •
luminescence of, table, **01:** 206

Egg whites

birds
proteinase inhibitors from, specificities and properties, **02:** 624-629
ovoinhibitor; bird •, specificities and properties, **02:** 628-629
ovomucoid; bird •, specificities and properties, **02:** 624-629

Eicosapentaenoic acid

biological and physical properties, **08:** 322-328
isolation and synthesis of, **08:** 326-327
occurrence, **08:** 325

Eicosatetraenoic acid

biological and physical properties, **08:** 322-328
isolation and synthesis of, **08:** 326-327
occurrence, **08:** 325

Eicosatrienoic acid

biological and physical properties, **08:** 322-328
isolation and synthesis of, **08:** 326-327
occurrence, **08:** 325

Elastase

circular dichroism
UV and near-UV region, **07:** 93, 150

Elastase *(continued)*
  luminescence of, table, **01**: 205
  molar absorptivity and-or absorbance values, **02**: 419
  optical rotatory dispersion
    UV region, **07**: 54
    visible and near UV regions, **07**: 22
Elastase-like
  enzyme
    molar absorptivity and-or absorbance values, **02**: 419
Elastase inhibitor
  legume sources, specificity and properties, **02**: 588-589
  mammalian organs and secretions, specificities and
    properties, **02**: 632-641
Elastin
  average hydrophobicity value, **01**: 219
α-Elastin
  circular dichroism in the UV region, **07**: 93
Electron-transfer proteins
  nomenclature; •, **02**: 114-121
Eledoisin
  group, natural and related synthetic oligopeptide
    amino acid sequence, physical and biological proper-
      ties, **07**: 236-257
Elements
  bond angles and distances; • having biochemical impor-
    tance, values for, **08**: 221
  covalent radii of common •, **08**: 221
  radii; covalent and van der Waals, of common •, **08**:
    221
  van der Waals' radii of common •, **08**: 221
EMB
  microorganisms; sugar fermentation, preparation of •
    medium for detecting, **04**: 650
EMB medium
  for detecting sugar fermentation, preparation of, **04**: 650
Emetine
  origin, structure, and characteristic as protein biosynthe-
    sis inhibitor, **04**: 572
Enamel
  proteins
    optical rotatory dispersion in the visible and near UV
      regions, **07**: 22
Enantiomers
  definition and nomenclature, **01**: 36-58, **02**: 36-58, **03**:
    28-50, **04**: 28-50, **05**: 33-55, **06**: 35, **08**: 35-40
Encephalitogenic
  protein
    amino acid composition, complete data, **07**: 506
    circular dichroism in the UV region, **07**: 94
    optical rotatory dispersion
      UV region, **07**: 54
      visible and near UV regions, **07**: 22
Encephalitogenic A-1
  protein
    average hydrophobicity value, **01**: 219
Endo-β-*N*-acetylglucosaminidase
  circular dichroism in the UV region, **07**: 94
Endonucleases
  Escherichia coli, *see also E. coli*; restriction • from, func-

tional characteristics, **04**: 493-494
    luminescence of, table, **01**: 205
  restriction
    characteristics, functional, **04**: 493-494
    cleavage sites, number of, for several, **04**: 532-534
    definition and discussion, **04**: 491-492
    recognition sequences for several, **04**: 532-534
Endopolygalacturonase
  average hydrophobicity value, **01**: 219
  molar absorptivity and-or absorbance values, **02**: 420
Endotoxin-receptor, *see* Lipopolysaccharide-receptor
Enduracididine
  physical and chemical properties, **01**: 140
Enniatin B
  proton NMR and suggested conformations, **07**: 561
Enolase
  amino acid composition, complete data, **07**: 506
  average hydrophobicity value, **01**: 219
  circular dichroism in the UV region, **07**: 94
  enzymatic activity, subcellular fractions, **02**: 698, 715
  molar absorptivity and-or absorbance values, **02**: 420
  optical rotatory dispersion
    UV region, **07**: 54
    visible and near UV regions, **07**: 22
  subunit, constitution of, **02**: 331, 332, 346
3-Enolpyruvylshikimic acid-5PO₄
  synthetase
    Neurospora crassa mutant, **04**: 745
Enomycin
  origin, structure, and chracteristic as protein biosynthe-
    sis inhibitor, **04**: 572
Enterotoxin A
  average hydrophobicity value, **01**: 220
Enterotoxin A, B, C, E
  molar absorptivity and-or absorbance values, **02**:
    420-421
Enterotoxin C
  amino acid composition, complete data, **07**: 506
  average hydrophobicity value, **01**: 220
Enterotoxin E
  average hydrophobicity value, **01**: 220
Envelope protein, *see* Matrix protein
Enzyme, *see also* Enzymes, Isoenzymes, Isozymes
  buffer solutions; • studies, preparation of buffers for,
    06: 370-377
  cis,cis-muconate lactonizing •
    average hydrophobicity value, **01**: 227
  citrate condensing •, *see* Citrate (*si*)-synthase
  cofactors
    fluorescence of, **07**: 601-602
  condensing •
    Neurospora crassa mutant, **04**: 749
  cysteamine to hypotaurine •
    amino acid composition, complete data, **07**: 506
  disulfide-exchange •
    amino acid composition, incomplete data, **07**: 512
  Drosophila melanogaster; biochemical mutants; • and
    structural protein, **04**: 848-849
  elastase-like •
    molar absorptivity and-or absorbance values, **02**: 419
  inhibition constant; • kinetics, definition, **02**: 112

Enzyme *(continued)*
  kinetics
    Michaelis constant, equation and symbols, **02:** 111
    rate constants, definition, **02:** 112
    symbols used in, **02:** 111-114
  malic •
    molar absorptivity and-or absorbance values, **02:** 470-471
    subunit, constitution of, **02:** 343, 344
  1-malic •
    average hydrophobicity value, **01:** 226
  old yellow •
    amino acid composition, incomplete data, **07:** 513
  pyruvate dehydrogenase multiple-• complex
    circular dichroism in the UV region, **07:** 121
  studies, preparation of buffers for, **06:** 370-377
  substrate concentration; • kinetics, definition, **02:** 112
  substrate constant; • kinetics, definition, **02:** 112
  thrombin-like
    molar absorptivity and-or absorbance values, **02:** 421
Enzyme cofactors
  fluorescent probes; •, **07:** 601-602
Enzyme inhibitors
  fluorescent probes; •, **07:** 598-599
  fluorescent properties, table, **07:** 598-599
Enzymes, *see also* Coenzyme, Metalloenzyme, Multienzyme
  amino acid sequences of proteins, **07:** 308-313
  classification of, **02:** 93-109
  cleavage sites, number of, for restriction and modification types, **04:** 532-534
  collagen; post-translational • in, **07:** 524
  defects in amino acid metabolism errors, **01:** 317-322
  defects in organic acid metabolism errors, **01:** 326
  deoxynucleotide polymerizing
    enzymatic functions of several, **04:** 545
    eucaryotes sources, template specificities and properties for some, **04:** 539-544
    procaryotes sources, template specificity properties, molecular weights, **04:** 538
  dissociation constants; prostaglandin metabolizing •, **08:** 364-367
  dissociation constants, glycohydrolases, table of, **05:** 426-445
  DNA polymerase, sources of and reactions, **04:** 536
  electron-transfer proteins, nomenclature, **02:** 114-121
  enzymes, *see also* Coenzyme, Metalloenzyme, Multienzyme; restriction and modification • in several strains, recognition sequences for, **04:** 532-534
  Escherichia coli, see also E. coli; restriction and modification • present in several strains, recognition sequences for, **04:** 532
  genetic variations in man, tables of • and variations in proteins and clotting factors, **04:** 879-883
  genetically variant, nomenclature, **02:** 86
  glycolytic •
    amino acid sequences, **07:** 324, 337
  glycoproteins, carbohydrate content, **02:** 273-274
  human disorders demonstrating deficient activity of specific enzymes, list, **04:** 882-883
  immobilization of
    absorption method, table of supports, **02:** 723

    covalent bond method, table of polymeric supports, **02:** 725-734
    entrapment method, table of supports, **02:** 724
    fixation on solid supports, multifunctional reagents for, **02:** 735
    methods used, description, **02:** 722
  immobilized, uses of, **02:** 722
  inhibitors; prostaglandin metabolizing •, **08:** 364-367
  isoenzymes, definition and nomenclature of, **02:** 84-86
  isozymes, definition and nomenclature of, **02:** 84-86
  list of recommended and systematic names, **02:** 121-172
  metalloenzymes, table of cofactors, molecular weights, stoichiometry and sources, **02:** 278-286
  Michaelis constants, glycohydrolases, table of, **05:** 426-445
  molar activity; •, defined, **02:** 109
  molecular turnover in animal tissue, table, **07:** 552-556
  molecular weight; • found in normal human urine, table, **02:** 301
  molecular weight; prostaglandin metabolizing •, **08:** 364-367
  multiple forms, list of groups, **02:** 85
  names, list of recommended and systematic, **02:** 121-172
  nomenclature; •, recommendations, **02:** 91-172
  nomenclature, multiple forms of, **02:** 84-86
  nomenclature, recommendations, **02:** 91-172
  pH values (optimum and stable) in glycohydrolase reactions, **05:** 426-445
  prostaglandin metabolizing
    properties and activity, **08:** 364-367
    target sites, diagram, **08:** 320
  prostaglandins; •, metabolizing, table of properties and activity, **08:** 364-367
  prostaglandins; metabolizing •, target sites, **08:** 320
  proteolytic, digestion cross-linked proteins, **02:** 669
  reaction rates, parameters for glycohydrolases, **05:** 426-445
  restriction and modification enzymes in several strains, recognition sequences for, **04:** 532-534
  reverse transcriptase, sources of and reactions, **04:** 536
  ribonucleotide polymerizing, subunits, molecular weights, **04:** 549-553
  specific activity; •, defined, **02:** 109
  specificity, for glycohydrolases, **05:** 426-445
  substrates used in glycohydrolase reactions, **05:** 426-445
  supports, tables of, used in immobilization of •, **02:** 723-734
  susceptibility of poly(α-amino acids) to, **01:** 393-396
  terminal transferase, sources of and reactions, **04:** 536
  transamidase activity, detection and sources, **02:** 670, 671
  urine, normal human, molecules weight of those found in, **02:** 301
  velocity of reaction, maximum for glycohydrolases, **05:** 426-445
Eosin-methylene blue medium
  for detecting sugar fermentation, preparation of, **04:** 650
Epidermal
  growth factor
    circular dichroism in the UV region, **07:** 94

Epimerase, *see* UDPglucose 4-epimerase
  aldose l-●
    molar absorptivity and-or absorbance values, **02:** 390
4-Epimerase
  1-ribulose 5-phosphate ●
    amino acid composition, complete data, **07:** 510
  UDPglucose ●
    circular dichroism in the UV region, **07:** 128
  uridine diphosphate galactose ●
    amino acid composition, complete data, **07:** 511
Epimerases
  definition and nomenclature, **02:** 98
  numbering and classification of, **02:** 108
Epon®
  chemical resistance and other properties, **08:** 429
Epoxidase
  tartrate ●
    amino acid composition, complete data,
      07: 510
Epoxy
  fatty acids, *see also* Lipids, Wax fatty acids; ●
    chemical characteristics, **05:** 488-489
    chemical formula, **05:** 488-489
    common name, **05:** 488-489
    physical characteristics, **05:** 488-489
  used as prefix in nomenclature, **06:** 68,
    08: 68
Erabutoxin
  amino acid composition, incomplete data, **07:** 512
Erabutoxin a
  molar absorptivity and-or absorbance values, **02:** 421
Ergocalciferol
  properties of, **08:** 286
Ergothionine
  physical and chemical properties, **01:** 161
Erythrocruorin
  molar absorptivity and-or absorbance values, **02:** 421
  subunit, constitution of, **02:** 351
Erythrocuprein, *see* Superoxide dismutase
  average hydrophobicity value, **01:** 220
  molar absorptivity and-or absorbance values, **02:** 421,
    422
  subunit, constitution of, **02:** 328
Erythrocyte
  fatty acids, *see also* Lipids, Wax fatty acids; composi-
    tion in plasma and ● lipids, effect of dietary fat, **05:**
    522
Erythromycin
  cation
    UV spectra, formula, molecular weight, **08:** 182
Erythromycin A
  origin, structure, and characteristic as protein biosynthe-
    sis inhibitor, **04:** 573
Erythropoietin
  carbohydrate content, **02:** 272-273
  molar absorptivity and-or absorbance values, **02:** 422
Ester
  leucine; methyl and ethyl ● of, as protein biosynthesis
    inhibitor, **04:** 584
  phenylalanine; *N*-acetyl-DL- -phenylalanine methyl ●,
    UV spectra of, **01:** 193

Esterase
  average hydrophobicity value, **01:** 220
  enzymatic activity, subcellular fractions, **02:** 698, 706
  molar absorptivity and-or absorbance values, **02:** 422
  subunit, constitution of, **02:** 337
Esterases
  nucleophosphodi ●, functional characterization of, **04:**
    491
Esters
  acid value; polyol ● table, **05:** 515
  carbohydrate phosphate ●
    hydrolysis constant, **05:** 262-273
    melting point, **05:** 253-258, 262-273
    specific rotation, **05:** 253-258, 262-273
  carboxylic acid, alkyl mono●, refractive index, **05:** 494
  cholesteryl ●, content in various animal tissues, **05:**
    519-520
  dielectric constants of some fats, fatty acids, and fatty
    acid ●, **05:** 494
  fatty acids, *see also* Lipids, Wax fatty acids; alkyl ● re-
    fractive index and equations for some, **05:** 493
  fatty acids, *see also* Lipids, Wax fatty acids; dielectric
    constants of some fats, fatty acids and ●, **05:** 494
  fatty acids, *see also* Lipids, Wax fatty acids; linseed oil
    acids and ●, force-area data, **05:** 497
  fatty acids, *see also* Lipids, Wax fatty acids; wax ● and
    sterol esters from vernix caseosa and from human
    skin surface lipid, **05:** 509
  force-area data, linseed oil acids and ●, **05:** 497
  free energy; hydrolysis; acetic acid ● and related com-
    pounds, **06:** 300
  free energy; hydrolysis; thiol ●, **06:** 301
  glycosyl ● of polyisoprenol phosphate and pyrophos-
    phate, structures and organisms, **05:** 391-393
  human skin surface; carbohydrate phosphate ●, **05:**
    253-258, 262-273
  human skin surface; lipid, fatty acids from wax ● and
    sterol esters, **05:** 509-510
  hydroxyl value; polyol ●, table, **05:** 515
  linseed oil acids and ●, force-area data, **05:** 497
  lipids; animal tissues, content of total, of cholesteryl ●
    and of phospholipids, **05:** 519-520
  lipids; human skin surface, fatty acids of wax esters and
    sterol ●, **05:** 509
  melting point; carbohydrate phosphate ●, **05:** 253-258,
    262-273
  molar extinctions; *N*-Acetyl methyl ● of aromatic
    amino acids, cystine and *N*-acetylcysteine, **01:** 186
  molecular weight; linseed oil acids and ●, **05:** 497
  monomolecular film measurements; linseed oil acids
    and ●, force-area data, **05:** 497
  refractive index; linseed oil acids and ●, **05:** 497
  specific rotation; carbohydrate phosphate ●, **05:**
    253-258, 262-273
  thiol ●
    hydrolysis, kinetic constants, **02:** 682
  vernix caseosa; lipid, fatty acids from wax esters and
    sterol ●, **05:** 509-510
Estradiol
  dehydrogenase
    average hydrophobicity value, **01:** 220

Estrogens
structures and properties, **05**: 539-540
Etamycin®, *see* Viridogrisein
Ethane derivatives
heat of proton ionization, pK, and related thermodynamic quantities, **06**: 195-197
Ethanolamine
deaminase
amino acid composition, complete data, **07**: 506
free acid in blood plasma of newborn infants and adults, **01**: 328
Ether
absorption data; hemin and hematin spectra in •, **08**: 279
hematin; absorption maxima in •, **08**: 279
hemin; absorption maxima in •, **08**: 279
intramolecular •, nomenclature rules, **05**: 130-132
soret band data; hemin and hematin spectra in •, **08**: 279
thio • protein group, chemical modification of reagents used, table of specificities, **02**: 203-204
Ethers
of 3,5-diiodotyrosine
antagonism to thyroxine, **01**: 179
Ethionine
antagonism to methionine, **01**: 178
physical and chemical properties, **01**: 154
structure and symbols for those incorporated into synthetic polypeptides, **01**: 102
Ethyl
refractive index; • alcohol, equation for change with temperature, **06**: 540
P-Ethyl-γ-phosphonoglutamic acid
antagonism to Glutamic acid, **01**: 177
Ethyl ester
N-acetyl-L-tyrosine •, UV spectra, **01**: 194
N-acetyl-L-tyrosine • anion, UV spectra, **01**: 195
γ-Ethyl ester
α-ketoglutaric • acid
properties of, **01**: 181
Ethylasparagine
physical and chemical properties, **01**: 118
Ethylene glycol
mononucleotides; ultraviolet absorbance in 90% v-v •, **03**: 408
UV absorbance; mononucleotides in 90% v-v •, **03**: 408
-water mixtures, dielectric constants and freezing points, **06**: 522
Ethylene glycol-methanol
-water mixtures
dielectric constants and freezing points, **06**: 528
viscosity table, **06**: 521
*tele*Ethylhistidine
structure and symbols for those incorporated into synthetic polypeptides, **01**: 102
1-Ethylhistidine, *see tele*Ethylhistidine
O-Ethylhomoserine
physical and chemical properties, **01**: 124
γ-Ethylidene glutamic acid
physical and chemical properties, **01**: 118

Eucaryotic
DNA, *see also* Deoxyribonucleic acid; base compositions of • protists, tables, **04**: 236-239
Eukaryotic
protists, DNA base compositions of, table, **04**: 236-239
Eukaryotic cytochromes *c*
amino acid sequences of protein, tables, **07**: 268-285
animals, **07**: 268-272, 282-283
plants, **07**: 273-277, 284-285
T-even coliphage
DNA, *see also* Deoxyribonucleic acid; •, buoyant density values, **03**: 568
Evolidine
proton NMR and suggested conformations, **07**: 566
Excelsin
molar absorptivity and-or absorbance values, **02**: 422
subunit, constitution of, **02**: 345
Excretion
porphyrins; • in humans, normal values, **08**: 279
porphyrins; • in laboratory animals, average normal values, **08**: 279
Exo-β-D-(1→3)
-glucanase
amino acid composition, complete data, **07**: 506
Exo-3,4-methanoproline
physical and chemical properties, **01**: 143
Exonucleases
definitions, discussion of, **04**: 491
Ezomycin A_1, A_2, B_1, B_2
physicochemical constants, spectral, chemotherapeutic and biological properties, **03**: 316-319

F

Factor
epidermal growth •
circular dichroism in the UV region, **07**: 94
fibrin stabilizing •
disc gel electrophoresis, **02**: 678
measurement of, graph, **02**: 677
molar absorptivity and-or absorbance values, **02**: 425
physical data and characteristics, **02**: 254-255
system in blood plasma, description, **02**: 670
Hageman •
amino acid composition, incomplete data, **07**: 513
physical data and characteristics, **02**: 254-255
plasma, nonhuman
carbohydrate content, **02**: 260
intrinsic •
amino acid composition, incomplete data, **07**: 513
lathyrus •
physical and chemical properties, **01**: 121
nerve growth •
molar absorptivity and-or absorbance values, **02**: 482
subunit, constitution of, **02**: 326
nerve growth • fraction A
amino acid composition, incomplete data, **07**: 513
rheumatoid •
plasma, human
carbohydrate content, molecular weights, sedimentation coefficients, **02**: 258

Fetuin *(continued)*
  animal sources, amino acid composition, **02**: 653
  circular dichroism, **07**: 95
    UV and near-UV region, **07**: 95, 150
  enzymatic hydrolysis, conjugated proteins, **02**: 211
  mammalian and chicken blood, specificity and proper-
    ties, **02**: 638-639
  molar absorptivity and-or absorbance values, **02**: 425
  optical rotatory dispersion
    UV region, **07**: 55
    visible and near UV regions, **07**: 22
  plasma, nonhuman
    carbohydrate content, **02**: 259
Fiber
  protein
    circular dichroism in the UV region, **07**: 95
Fibers
  cilia protein, outer •
    amino acid composition, complete data, **07**: 506
    optical rotatory dispersion in the visible and near UV
      regions, **07**: 21
Fibrin
  calorimetric ΔH values accompanying conformational
    changes, **06**: 270
  molar absorptivity and-or absorbance values, **02**: 425
Fibrin stabilizing
  factor
    disc gel electrophoresis, **02**: 678
    measurement of, graph, **02**: 677
    molar absorptivity and-or absorbance values, **02**: 425
    physical data and characteristics, **02**: 254-255
    system in blood plasma, description, **02**: 670
Fibrinogen
  calorimetric Δ values accompanying conformational
    changes, **06**: 270
  circular dichroism in the UV region, **07**: 95
  iodinated
    refractive index increments, **02**: 375
  molar absorptivity and-or absorbance values, **02**:
    425-426
  molecular parameters, **02**: 248
  optical rotatory dispersion
    UV region, **07**: 55
    visible and near UV regions, **07**: 23
  physical data and characteristics, **02**: 254-255
  plasma, human
    carbohydrate content, molecular weights, sedimenta-
      tion coefficients, **02**: 258
  refractive index increments, **02**: 375
Fibrinogen B
  average hydrophobicity value, **01**: 220
Fibrinoligase
  transamidase activity, **02**: 671-681
Fibrinopeptides A
  amino acid sequences, **07**: 431-433
Fibrinopeptides B
  amino acid sequences, **07**: 433-435
Fibroin
  average hydrophobicity value, **01**: 220
  molar absorptivity and-or absorbance values, **02**: 426
  silk •
    circular dichroism in the UV region, **07**: 123

optical rotatory dispersion
    UV region, **07**: 75
    visible and near UV regions, **07**: 35
Ficin
  amino acid sequence, **07**: 356-357
  molar absorptivity and-or absorbance values, **02**: 426
Ficin II
  average hydrophobicity value, **01**: 221
Ficin III
  average hydrophobicity value, **01**: 221
Film
  monomolecular • measurements
    linseed oil acids and esters, force-area data, **05**: 497
Flagellin
  amino acid composition, complete data, **07**: 506
  average hydrophobicity value, **01**: 221
  circular dichroism in the UV region, **07**: 95
  optical rotatory dispersion
    UV region, **07**: 55
    visible and near UV regions, **07**: 23
Flavins
  luminescence data table, **08**: 154-158
Flaviolin
  UV spectra, formula, molecular weight, **08**: 163
Flavodoxin
  amino acid composition, complete data, **07**: 506
  amino acid sequence, **07**: 430
  average hydrophobicity value, **01**: 221
  circular dichroism in the UV region, **07**: 95
  molar absorptivity and-or absorbance values, **02**:
    426-427
Flavoprotein
  riboflavin •
    circular dichroism in the UV region: extrema between
      185 and 250 NM^3, **07**: 122
    optical rotatory dispersion in the visible and near UV
      regions, **07**: 35
    optical rotatory dispersion in the UV region: extrema
      between 185 and 250 NM^3, **07**: 74
  shethna •
    circular dichroism at maxima in near UV region, at
      room temperature, **07**: 161
Flavoprotein containing FMN, *see* Flavodoxin
Flavoprotein containing riboflavin, *see* Riboflavin flavo-
    protein
Fluids
  glycoproteins; body •
    carbohydrate content, **02**: 267
Fluorescamine
  covalent protein conjugates, data, **01**: 208
Fluorescein isothiocyanate
  covalent protein conjugates, data, **01**: 208
Fluorescent probes
  commonly used for membrane studies, properties, **07**:
    608-610
  enzyme cofactors, **07**: 601-602
  enzyme inhibitors, **07**: 598-599
  naphthalene sulfonates, protein structure, **07**: 604-606
γ-Fluoroglutamic acid
  antagonism to glutamic acid, **01**: 177
Fluorophenylalanines
  antagonism to phenylalanine, **01**: 179

5-Fluorotryptophan
  antagonism to tryptophan, 01: 179
Fluorotyrosines
  antagonism to tyrosine, 01: 180
6-Flurotryptophan
  antagonism to tryptophan, 01: 179
Folacin
  nomenclature and structures, 08: 17-18
  properties of, 08: 295
Folic acid
  biological characteristics, 08: 303
  compounds, fluorescent parameters, 08: 214
  nomenclature, journal references for, 02: 87
  nomenclature and structure, 08: 17-18
  properties of, 08: 295
Folic acid reductase, see Tetrahydrofolate dehydrogenase
Folinic acid
  properties of, 08: 295
Formic acid
  heat of proton ionization, pK, and related thermody-
      namic quantities, 06: 200
N-Formimino-L-glutamate
  iminohydrolase
    average hydrophobicity value, 01: 221
Formycin
  physicochemical constants, spectral, chemotherapeutic
      and biological properties, 03: 320
Formycin B
  physicochemical constants, spectral, chemotherapeutic
      and biological properties, 03: 322
N-Formyl-N-hydroxyaminoacetic acid, see Hadacidin
γ-Formyl-N-methylnorvaline
  physical and chemical properties, 01: 148
N-Formyl methionine
  physical and chemical properties, 01: 154
Forocidin
  origin, structure, and characteristic as protein biosynthe-
      sis inhibitor, 04: 574
Fraction 1
  protein
    amino acid composition, complete data, 07: 507
Fraction A
  nerve growth factor •
    amino acid composition, incomplete data, 07: 513
Fraction II
  phosvitin •
    amino acid composition, complete data, 07: 509
Free acid
  penicillin V •
    UV spectra, formula, molecular weight, 08: 158
Frequencies
  calculated characteristic polypeptide table, 07: 596
  from, physical properties
    Escherichia coli, see also E. coli; RNA molecules•, 04:
      406,409
Fructosan-specific
  protein
    circular dichroism in the UV region, 07: 96
Fructose
  heat of proton ionization, pK, and related thermody-
      namic quantities, 06: 201
  pK'$_a$ values, 06: 317

Fructose-bisphosphate
  aldolase
    amino acid composition, complete date, 07: 507
    amino acid sequence, 07: 333-335
    circular dichroism in the UV region, 07: 96
    optical rotatory dispersion
      UV region, 07: 56
      visible and near UV regions, 07: 23
Fructose-1,6-diphosphatase, see Hexosediphosphatase
  average hydrophobicity value, 01: 221
Fructose 1,6-diphosphate
  adolase A
    amino acid composition, complete data, 07: 507
Fructose-1,6-diphosphate aldolase, see Fructose-
      bisphosphate aldolase
Fucose
  content of, in glycoproteins, 02: 258-267, 271-274
α-L-Fucosidase
  carbohydrate content, 02: 274
  subunit, constitution of, 02: 341
Fumarase
  amino acid composition, complete data, 07: 507
  circular dichroism in near-UV region, at room tempera-
      ture, 07: 150
  enzymatic activity, subcellular fractions, 02: 702
  molar absorptivity and-or absorbance values, 02: 429
  subunit, constitution of, 02: 340
Fumarate
  hydratase
    circular dichroism in the UV region, 07: 97
    optical rotatory dispersion
      UV region, 07: 56
      visible and near UV regions, 07: 23
N-Fumarylalanine
  physical and chemical properties, 01: 118
Furanomycin
  origin, structure, and characteristic as protein biosynthe-
      sis inhibitor, 04: 574
  physical and chemical properties, 01: 140
Furosine
  physical and chemical properties, 01: 140
Furostans
  names, new standard vs. old, 05: 69-70
  steroid nomenclature, use of term, 05: 68-69
  structures, 05: 69-70
ε-N-(2-Furoyl-methyl)-lypine, see Furosine
β-2-Furylalanine
  antagonism to Phenylalanine, 01: 179
β-3-Furylalanine
  antagonism to Phenylalanine, 01: 179
Fusarenone X
  origin, structure, and characteristic as protein biosynthe-
      sis inhibitor, 04: 574
Fusarinine
  physical and chemical properties, 01: 149
Fusidic acid
  origin, structure, and characteristic as protein biosynthe-
      sis inhibitor, 04: 575
Fusidin
  inhibitor of protein biosynthesis, 04: 575

G

γG
immunoglobulin, specific; •, horse
  molar absorptivity and-or absorbance values, 02: 456
immunoglobulin, specific; •, human
  molar absorptivity and-or absorbance values, 02: 456
immunoglobulin, specific; •, lemon shark
  molar absorptivity and-or absorbance values, 02: 456
immunoglobulin, specific; •, rabbit
  molar absorptivity and-or absorbance values, 02: 456
γG Immunoglobulin
kappa chain
  amino acid composition, complete data, 07: 508
G + C
Absidia; • composition of DNA of, table arranged by
  specie, 04: 185
Acanthamoeba; • composition of DNA of, table arranged by specie, 04: 228
Acetobacter; • composition of DNA of, table arranged
  by specie, 04: 152-153
Achlya; • composition of DNA of, table arranged by
  specie, 04: 185
Achromobacter; • composition of DNA of, table arranged by specie, 04: 69-71
achromobacteriaceae; • composition of DNA of, table
  arranged by genera and specie, 04: 69-74
Aciddminococcus; • composition of DNA of, table arranged by specie, 04: 147
Acinetobacter; • composition of DNA of, table arranged
  by specie, 04: 89-90
Acrasis; • composition of DNA of, table arranged by
  specie, 04: 185
Acrothecium; • composition of DNA of, table arranged
  by specie, 04: 185
Actinobacillus; • composition of DNA of, table arranged
  by specie, 04: 90-91
Actinomucor; • composition of DNA of, table arranged
  by specie, 04: 185
Actinomyces; • composition of DNA of, table arranged
  by specie, 04: 75
actinoplanaceae; • composition of DNA of, table arranged by genera and specie, 04: 76-78
Actinoplanes; • composition of DNA of, table arranged
  by specie, 04: 76
Actinosporangium; • composition of DNA of, table arranged by specie, 04: 77
Acytostelium; • composition of DNA of, table arranged
  by specie, 04: 185
Aerobacter (Enterobacter); • composition of DNA of,
  table arranged by specie, 04: 104-105
Aerococcus; • composition of DNA of, table arranged
  by specie, 04: 127
Aeromonas; • composition of DNA of, table arranged
  by specie, 04: 153
Agaricus; • composition of DNA of, table arranged by
  specie, 04: 186
Agrobacterium; • composition of DNA of, table arranged by specie, 04: 162-164
Alcaligenes; • composition of DNA of, table arranged
  by specie, 04: 71-73

Amanita; • composition of DNA of, table arranged by
  specie, 04: 186
Amauroascus; • composition of DNA of, table arranged
  by specie, 04: 186
Amoeba; • composition of DNA of, table arranged by
  specie, 04: 228
Amorphosporangium; • composition of DNA of, table
  arranged by specie, 04: 77
amphibia, satellite DNA's; buoyant density and • content of, table, 04: 389-390
Ampullariella; • composition of DNA of, table arranged
  by specie, 04: 77
Anaplasma; • composition of DNA of, table arranged
  by specie, 04: 78
Anaplasmataceae; • composition of DNA of, table arranged by genera and specie, 04: 78
angiosperms; buoyant density and • content of satellite
  DNAs for several species, table, 04: 400-401
Anixiopsis; • composition of DNA of, table arranged by
  specie, 04: 186
Ankistrodesmus; • composition of DNA of, table arranged by specie, 04: 224
Arachniotus; • composition of DNA of, table arranged
  by specie, 04: 186
Archangiaceae; • composition of DNA of, table ar-
  ranged by genera and specie, 04: 78
Archangium; • composition of DNA of, table arranged
  by specie, 04: 78
Arthrobacter; • composition of DNA of, table arranged
  by specie, 04: 97-99
Arthrobotrys; • composition of DNA of, table arranged
  by specie, 04: 186
Aspergillus; • composition of DNA of, table arranged
  by specie, 04: 186-188
Aspergillus nidulans; • composition of, 04: 187
Astasia; • composition of DNA of, table arranged by
  specie, 04: 228
Athiohodaceae; • composition of DNA of, table arranged by genera and specie, 04: 78-80
Aureobasidium; • compositon of DNA of, table arranged by specie, 04: 188
Auxarthon; • composition of DNA of, table arranged
  by specie, 04: 189
Azotobacter; • composition of DNA of, table arranged
  by specie, 04: 80-81
Azotobacteriaceae; • composition of DNA of, table arranged by genera and specie, 04: 80-81
Azotomonas; • composition of DNA of, table arranged
  by specie, 04: 153
bacillaceae; • composition of DNA of, table arranged
  by genera and specie, 04: 81-89
Bacillus; • composition of DNA of, table arranged by
  specie, 04: 81-85
Bacillus subtilis; DNA content per cell for various,
  table, 04: 284; • composition of, 04: 84
Backusia; • composition of DNA of, table arranged by
  specie, 04: 189
Bacterium; • composition of DNA of, table arranged by
  specie, 04: 105
bacteroidaceae; • composition of DNA of, table ar-

G + C *(continued)*

ranged by genera and specie, **04:** 86-87

Bacteroides; • composition of DNA of, table arranged by specie, **04:** 86-87

Basidiobolus; • composition of DNA of, table arranged by specie, **04:** 189

Bdellovibrio; • composition of DNA of, table arranged by specie, **04:** 166

Beauveria; • composition of DNA of, table arranged by specie, **04:** 189

Beijerinckia; • composition of DNA of, table arranged by specie, **04:** 81

Bifidobacterium; • composition of DNA of, table arranged by specie, **04:** 75, 115

Bispora; • composition of DNA of, table arranged by specie, **04:** 189

Bjerkandera; • composition of DNA of, table arranged by specie, **04:** 189

Blakesleea; • composition of DNA of, table arranged by specie, **04:** 189

Blastocladiella; • composition of DNA of, table arranged by specie, **04:** 189

Blastocrithidia; • composition of DNA of, table arranged by specie, **04:** 228

Bordetella; • composition of DNA of, table arranged by specie, **04:** 91

Borrelia; • composition of DNA of, table arranged by specie, **04:** 180

Botrytis; • composition of DNA of, table arranged by specie, **04:** 190

Bovista; • composition of DNA of, table arranged by specie, **04:** 190

Brettanomyces; • composition of DNA of, table arranged by specie, **04:** 190

brevibacteriaceae; • composition of DNA of, table arranged by genera and specie, **04:** 87-89

Brevibacterium; • composition of DNA of, table arranged by specie, **04:** 87-89

Brucella; • composition of DNA of, table arranged by specie, **04:** 91

brucellaceae; • composition of DNA of, table arranged by genera and specie, **04:** 89-93

Byssochlamys; • composition of DNA of, table arranged by specie, **04:** 190

Candida; • composition of DNA of, table arranged by specie, **04:** 190-191

Catenabacterium; • composition of DNA of, table arranged by specie, **04:** 115

Caulobacter; • composition of DNA of, table arranged by specie, **04:** 95

caulobacteriaceae; • composition of DNA of, table arranged by genera and specie, **04:** 95

Cellulomonas; • composition of DNA of, table arranged by specie, **04:** 99

Ceratocystis; • composition of DNA of, table arranged by specie, **04:** 192

Cercospora; • composition of DNA of, table arranged by specie, **04:** 192

Ceriporiopsis; • composition of DNA of, table arranged by specie, **04:** 192

Chaetoceras; • composition of DNA of, table arranged

by specie, **04:** 224

Chaetocladium; • composition of DNA of, table arranged by specie, **04:** 192

Chaetomium; • composition of DNA of, table arranged by specie, **04:** 192-193

Chara; • composition of DNA of, table arranged by specie, **04:** 224

Chlamydia; • composition of DNA of, table arranged by specie, **04:** 95

chlamydiaceae; • composition of DNA of, table arranged by genera and specie, **04:** 95

chlamydobacteriaceae; • composition of DNA of, table arranged by genera and specie, **04:** 95

Chlamydomonas; • composition of DNA of, table arranged by specie, **04:** 224-225

Chlorella; • composition of DNA of, table arranged by specie, **04:** 225

Chloridium; • composition of DNA of, table arranged by specie, **04:** 193

chlorobacteriaceae; • composition of DNA of, table arranged by genera and specie, **04:** 96-97

Chlorobium; • composition of DNA of, table arranged by specie, **04:** 96

Chlorogonium; • composition of DNA of, table arranged by specie, **04:** 225

Chloropseudomonas; • composition of DNA of, table arranged by specie, **04:** 97

Choanephora; • composition of DNA of, table arranged by specie, **04:** 193

Chondrococcus; • composition of DNA of, table arranged by specie, **04:** 145

Chondromyces; • composition of DNA of, table arranged by specie, **04:** 150-151

Chromatium; • composition of DNA of, table arranged by specie, **04:** 178-179

Chromobacterium; • composition of DNA of, table arranged by specie, **04:** 164

Circinella; • composition of DNA of, table arranged by specie, **04:** 193

Citeromyces; • composition of DNA of, table arranged by specie, **04:** 193

Citrobacter; • composition of DNA of, table arranged by specie, **04:** 105

Cladosporium; • composition of DNA of, table arranged by specie, **04:** 193

Claviceps; • composition of DNA of, table arranged by specie, **04:** 193

Clostridium; • composition of DNA of, table arranged by specie, **04:** 85-86

Coccolithus; • composition of DNA of, table arranged by specie, **04:** 225

Coemansia; • composition of DNA of, table arranged by specie, **04:** 194

Cokeromyces; • composition of DNA of, table arranged by specie, **04:** 194

Colletotrichum; • composition of DNA of, table arranged by specie, **04:** 194

Colpidium; • composition of DNA of, table arranged by specie, **04:** 228

Comamonas; • composition of DNA of, table arranged by specie, **04:** 166

G + C *(continued)*

composition

algae DNA, arranged by genera and specie, **04:** 224-227

bacteria DNA, arranged by family, genera, specie, **04:** 69-183

calculation of, from buoyant density, **04:** 356

DNA

chloroplast, table of values, **04:** 356-358

nuclear, table of values, **04:** 356-358

DNA, *see also* Deoxyribonucleic acid; chloroplast; • mol %, table of values, **04:** 356-358

DNA, *see also* Deoxyribonucleic acid; nuclear; • mol %, table of values, **04:** 356-358

DNA, *see also* Deoxyribonucleic acid; viral, buoyant densities, melting temperature and • content, **03:** 560-562

viral DNA, buoyant densities, melting temperatures and • content, **03:** 560-562

DNA base composition of eucaryotic protists, table, **04:** 236-239

fungi DNA, arranged by genera and specie, **04:** 185-224

protozoa DNA, arranged by genera and specie, **04:** 228-229

composition of DNA of, table arranged by specie, **04:** 192

content

mitochondrial DNAs, table, **04:** 363-372

satellite DNAs

amphibia, **04:** 389-390

birds, **04:** 390-391

crustaceae, **04:** 384-387

insects, **04:** 380-384

mammals, **04:** 391-399

molluscs, **04:** 387

plants, **04:** 399-402

tunicates, **04:** 388

viral DNA, **03:** 560-562

viral DNA molecules, **03:** 551-556

Coprinus; • composition of DNA of, table arranged by specie, **04:** 194

corynebacteriaceae; • composition of DNA of, table arranged by genera and specie, **04:** 97-103

Corynebacterium; • composition of DNA of, table arranged by specie, **04:** 99-103

crabs; buoyant density and • content of satellite DNAs for several varieties, **04:** 384-387

Cricosphaera; • composition of DNA of, table arranged by specie, **04:** 225

Crithidia; • composition of DNA of, table arranged by specie, **04:** 228

Cryptococcus; • composition of DNA of, table arranged by specie, **04:** 194-195

Ctenomyces; • composition of DNA of, table arranged by specie, **04:** 195

Cunninghamella; • composition of DNA of, table arranged by specie, **04:** 195

Curvularia; • composition of DNA of, table arranged by specie, **04:** 196

Cyclotella; • composition of DNA of, table arranged by specie, **04:** 225

Cylindrocephalum; • composition of DNA of, table arranged by specie, **04:** 196

Cylindrotheca; • composition of DNA of, table arranged by specie, **04:** 225

Cystoseira; • composition of DNA of, table arranged by specie, **04:** 225

Cytophaga; • composition of DNA of, table arranged by specie, **04:** 103-104

cytophagaceae; • composition of DNA of, table arranged by genera and specie, **04:** 103-104

Dactylium; • composition of DNA of, table arranged by specie, **04:** 196

Dactylosporangium; • composition of DNA of, table arranged by specie, **04:** 77

Daedalea; • composition of DNA of, table arranged by specie, **04:** 196

Debaryomyces; • composition of DNA of, table arranged by specie, **04:** 196

Derxia; • composition of DNA of, table arranged by specie, **04:** 81

Desulfotomaculum; • composition of DNA of, table arranged by specie, **04:** 167

Desulfovibrio; • composition of DNA of, table arranged by specie, **04:** 167

Dictyostelium; • composition of DNA of, table arranged by specie, **04:** 196

Dictyuchus; • composition of DNA of, table arranged by specie, **04:** 197

Diplococcus; • composition of DNA of, table arranged by specie, **04:** 116

Dipodascus; • composition of DNA of, table arranged by specie, **04:** 197

Dipsacomyces; • composition of DNA of, table arranged by specie, **04:** 197

drosophila, buoyant density and • content of satellite DNAs for several strains, table, **04:** 380-382

Dunaliella; • composition of DNA of, table arranged by specie, **04:** 225

Eidamella; • composition of DNA of, table arranged by specie, **04:** 197

Elfvingia; • composition of DNA of, table arranged by specie, **04:** 197

Emericella; • composition of DNA of, table arranged by specie, **04:** 197

Emericellopsis; • composition of DNA of, table arranged by specie, **04:** 197

Endomyces; • composition of DNA of, table arranged by specie, **04:** 197

Endomycopsis; • composition of DNA of, table arranged by specie, **04:** 198

Entamoeba; • composition of DNA of, table arranged by specie, **04:** 228

enterobacteriaceae; • composition of DNA of, table arranged by genera and specie, **04:** 104-114

Epicoccum; • composition of DNA of, table arranged by specie, **04:** 198

Eremascus; • composition of DNA of, table arranged by specie, **04:** 198

Erwinia; • composition of DNA of, table arranged by specie, **04:** 105-109

Escherichia coli, *see also* E. coli; • composition of DNA of, table arranged by specie, **04:** 110

G + C *(continued)*

Euglena; • composition of DNA of, table arranged by specie, **04:** 228

Eupenicillium; • composition of DNA of, table arranged by specie, **04:** 198

Eurotium; • composition of, table arranged by specie, **04:** 198

Flavobacterium; • composition of DNA of, table arranged by specie, **04:** 74

Flexibacter; • composition of DNA of, table arranged by specie, **04:** 104

Flexibacteria; • composition of DNA of, table arranged by specie, **04:** 181

Flexothrix; • composition of DNA of, table arranged by specie, **04:** 182

Fomes; • composition of DNA of, table arranged by specie, **04:** 199

Fomitopsis (Fomes); • composition of DNA of, table arranged by specie, **04:** 199

Fulgio; • composition of DNA of, table arranged by specie, **04:** 199

Fusarium; • composition of DNA of, table arranged by specie, **04:** 199

Fusobacterium; • composition of DNA of, table arranged by specie, **04:** 87

Gaffkya; • composition of DNA of, table arranged by specie, **04:** 127

Ganoderma; • composition of DNA of, table arranged by specie, **04:** 127

Gelasinospora; • composition of DNA of, table arranged by specie, **04:** 199-200

Geotrichum; • composition of DNA of, table arranged by specie, **04:** 200

Gilbertella; • composition of, DNA of, table arranged by specie, **04:** 200

Glaucoma; • composition of DNA of, table arranged by specie, **04:** 228

Gliocladium; • composition of DNA of, table arranged by specie, **04:** 200

Gloeophyllum (Lenzites); • composition of DNA of, table arranged by specie, **04:** 200

Gluconobacter; • composition of DNA of, table arranged by specie, **04:** 153

guinea pig; satellite DNAs; buoyant density and • content of, table, **04:** 394

Gymnoascus; • composition of DNA of, table arranged by specie, **04:** 200

gymnosperms; buoyant density and • content of satellite DNAs for several varieties, table, **04:** 399-400

Haemophilus; • composition of DNA of, table arranged by specie, **04:** 91

Halobacterium; • composition of DNA of, table arranged by specie, **04:** 154

Hanseniaspora; • composition of DNA of, table arranged by specie, **04:** 200

Hansenula; • composition of DNA of, table arranged by specie, **04:** 200-203

Haplosporangium; • composition of DNA of, table arranged by specie, **04:** 203

Helicoma; • composition of DNA of, table arranged by specie, **04:** 203

Helicostylium; • composition of DNA of, table arranged by specie, **04:** 203

Helminthosporium; • composition of DNA of, table arranged by specie, **04:** 203

Helvella; • composition of DNA of, table arranged by specie, **04:** 203

Herellea; • composition of DNA of, table arranged by specie, **04:** 91-92

Herpetosiphon; • composition of DNA of, table arranged by specie, **04:** 182

Histoplasma; • composition of DNA of, table arranged by specie, **04:** 203

human; satellite DNAs; buoyant density and • content of, table, **04:** 397-398

Humicola; • composition of DNA of, table arranged by specie, **04:** 204

Hydrodictyon; • composition of DNA of, table arranged by specie, **04:** 225

Hypocrea; • composition of DNA of, table arranged by specie, **04:** 204

Inonotus; • composition of DNA of, table arranged by specie, **04:** 204

intrasporangium; • composition of DNA of, table arranged by specie, **04:** 172

Irpex; • composition of DNA of, table arranged by specie, **04:** 204

Isoachyla; • composition of DNA of, table arranged by specie, **04:** 204

Klebsiella; • composition of DNA of, table arranged by specie, **04:** 111

Kloeckera; • composition of DNA of, table arranged by specie, **04:** 204

Kluyveromyces; • composition of DNA of, table arranged by specie, **04:** 204-205

Labyrinthula; • composition of DNA of, table arranged by specie, **04:** 205

lactobacillaceae; • composition of DNA of, table arranged by genera and specie, **04:** 115-126

Lactobacillus; • composition of DNA of, table arranged by specie, **04:** 116-122

Laetiporus; • composition of DNA of, table arranged by specie, **04:** 205

Lagerheimia; • composition of DNA of, table arranged by specie, **04:** 225

Laricifomes (Fomes); • composition of DNA of, table arranged by specie, **04:** 206

Leishmania; • composition of DNA of, table arranged by specie, **04:** 228

Lenzites; • composition of DNA of, table arranged by specie, **04:** 206

Leptosphaeria; • composition of DNA of, table arranged by specie, **04:** 206

Leptospira; • composition of DNA of, table arranged by specie, **04:** 180

Leptotrichia; • composition of DNA of, table arranged by specie, **04:** 95

Leuconostoc; • composition of DNA of, table arranged by specie, **04:** 122

Leucothrix; • composition of DNA of, table arranged by specie, **04:** 126

leucotrichaceae; • composition of DNA of, table arranged by genera and specie, **04:** 126-127

Lichtheimia (Absidia); • composition of DNA of, table

G + C *(continued)*

    arranged by specie, **04:** 206

Linderina; • composition of DNA of, table arranged by specie, **04:** 206

Lipomyces; • composition of DNA of, table arranged by specie, **04:** 206

Listeria; • composition of DNA of, table arranged by specie, **04:** 103

Lodderomyces; • composition of DNA of, table arranged by specie, **04:** 206

Lophomonas; • composition of DNA of, table arranged by specie, **04:** 154

Lycogala; • composition of DNA of, table arranged by specie, **04:** 206

Lyngbya; • composition of DNA of, table arranged by specie, **04:** 226

mammals; satellite DNAs; buoyant density and • content of, table, **04:** 391-399

Meruliopsis (Poria); • composition of DNA of, table arranged by specie, **04:** 206

Methanobacterium; • composition of DNA of, table arranged by specie, **04:** 168

Metschnikowia; • composition of DNA of, table arranged by specie, **04:** 206

Microbacterium; • composition of DNA of, table arranged by specie, **04:** 103

Microbispora (Waksmania); • composition of DNA of, table arranged by specie, **04:** 149

micrococcaceae; • composition of DNA of, table arranged by genera and specie, **04:** 127-138

Micrococcus (Staphylococcus); • composition of DNA of, table arranged by specie, **04:** 128-134

Microcoleus; • composition of DNA of, table arranged by specie, **04:** 226

Microcyclus; • composition of DNA of, table arranged by specie, **04:** 168

Microellobosporia; • composition of DNA of, table arranged by specie, **04:** 77

Micromonospora; • composition of DNA of, table arranged by specie, **04:** 138

micromonosporaceae; • composition of DNA of, table arranged by genera and specie, **04:** 138

Micropolyspora; • composition of DNA of, table arranged by specie, **04:** 149

Mima; • composition of DNA of, table arranged by specie, **04:** 92

molluscs, satellite DNAs; buoyant density and • content of, table, **04:** 387

monocotyledons; buoyant density and • content of satellite DNAs for several species, table, **04:** 402

Monodus; • composition of DNA of, table arranged by specie, **04:** 226

Monosporium; • composition of DNA of, table arranged by specie, **04:** 206

Moraxella; • composition of DNA of, table arranged by specie, **04:** 92

Mortierella; • composition of DNA of, table arranged by specie, **04:** 207

mouse; buoyant density and • content of satellite DNAs for several varieties, table, **04:** 391-393

Mucor; • composition of DNA of, table arranged by specie, **04:** 207

mycobacteriaceae; • composition of DNA of, table arranged by genera and specie, **04:** 139-141

Mycobacterium; • composition of DNA of, table arranged by specie, **04:** 139-141

Mycoplasma; • composition of DNA of, table arranged by specie, **04:** 141-145

Mycoplasmataceae; • composition of DNA of, table arranged by genera and specie, **04:** 141

Mycotypha; • composition of DNA of, table arranged by specie, **04:** 208

Myrothecium; • composition of DNA of, table arranged by specie, **04:** 208

Myxobacterium; • composition of DNA of, table arranged by species, **04:** 146

myxococcaceae; • composition of DNA of, table arranged by genera and specie, **04:** 145

Myxococcus (Myxobacterium); • composition of DNA of, table arranged by specie, **04:** 146

Myxotrichum; • composition of DNA of, table arranged by specie, **04:** 208

Naegleria; • composition of DNA of, table arranged by specie, **04:** 229

Naganishia; • composition of DNA of, table arranged by specie, **04:** 208

Navicula; • composition of DNA of, table arranged by specie, **04:** 226

Neisseria; • composition of DNA of, table arranged by specie, **04:** 147-148

neisseriaceae; • composition of DNA of, table arranged by genera and specie, **04:** 147-148

Neurospora; • composition of DNA of, table arranged by specie, **04:** 208

Neurospora crassa; • composition, **04:** 208

Nigrospora; • composition of DNA of, table arranged by specie, **04:** 209

Nitella; • composition of DNA of, table arranged by specie, **04:** 226

Nitrobacter; • composition of DNA of, table arranged by specie, **04:** 148

nitrobacteraceae; • composition of DNA of, table arranged by genera and specie, **04:** 148

Nitrosomonas; • composition of DNA of, table arranged by specie, **04:** 148

Nitzschia; • composition of DNA of, table arranged by specie, **04:** 226

Nocardia; • composition of DNA of, table arranged by specie, **04:** 149-150

nocardiaceae; • composition of DNA of, table arranged by genera and specie, **04:** 149-150

Nodularia; • composition of DNA of, table arranged by specie, **04:** 226

non-human primates; satellite DNAs; buoyant density and • content of, table, **04:** 398-399

Nostoc; • composition of DNA of, table arranged by specie, **04:** 226

Ochromonas; • composition of DNA of, table arranged by specie, **04:** 226

Oerskovia; • composition of DNA of, table arranged by specie, **04:** 75-76

Pachysolen; • composition of DNA of, table arranged by specie, **04:** 209

Paecilomyces; • composition of DNA of, table arranged

G + C *(continued)*
by specie, **04**: 209

Paracolobactrum; ● composition of DNA of, table arranged by specie, **04**: 112

Paramecium; ● composition of DNA of, table arranged by specie, **04**: 229

Pasteurella; ● composition of DNA of, table arranged by specie, **04**: 94

Pectobacterium; ● composition of DNA of, table arranged by specie, **04**: 112

Pediococcus; ● composition of DNA of, table arranged by specie, **04**: 123

Penicillium; ● composition of DNA of, table arranged by specie, **04**: 209-212

Pestalotiopsis; ● composition of DNA of, table arranged by species, **04**: 212

Petalosporus; ● composition of DNA of, table arranged by specie, **04**: 212

Phaeocoriolellus (Lenzites); ● composition of DNA of, table arranged by specie, **04**: 212

Phaeolus (Polyporus); ● composition of DNA of, table arranged by specie, **04**: 212

Phellinus; ● composition of DNA of, table arranged by specie, **04**: 212

Phialophora; ● composition of DNA of, table arranged by specie, **04**: 213

Phoma; ● composition of DNA of, table arranged by specie, **04**: 213

Phycomyces; ● composition of DNA of, table arranged by specie, **04**: 213

Physarum; ● composition of DNA of, table arranged by specie, **04**: 213

Phytophthora; ● composition of DNA of, table arranged by specie, **04**: 213

Pichia; ● composition of DNA of, table arranged by specie, **04**: 214

Pilaira; ● composition of DNA of, table arranged by specie, **04**: 214

Piptoporus (Polyporus); ● composition of DNA of, table arranged by specie, **04**: 214

Planobispora; ● composition of DNA of, table arranged by specie, **04**: 77

plants, satellite DNAs; buoyant density and ● content of, table, **04**: 399-402

Plasmodium; ● composition of DNA of, table arranged by specie, **04**: 229

Plectonema; ● composition of DNA of, table arranged by specie, **04**: 226

Pleurotus; ● composition of DNA of, table arranged by specie, **04**: 214

polyangiaceae; ● composition of DNA of, table arranged by genera and specie, **04**: 150-151

Polyangium; ● composition of DNA of, table arranged by specie, **04**: 151

Polyides; ● composition of DNA of, table arranged by specie, **04**: 226

Polypaecilum; ● composition of DNA of, table arranged by specie, **04**: 214

Polysphondylium; ● composition of DNA of, table arranged by specie, **04**: 214

Polytoma; ● composition of DNA of, table arranged by

specie, **04**: 227

Polytomella; ● composition of DNA of, table arranged by specie, **04**: 227

Poria; ● composition of DNA of, table arranged by specie, **04**: 215

primates, satellite DNAs; buoyant density and ● content of, table, **04**: 397-399

Promicromonospora; ● composition of DNA of, table arranged by specie, **04**: 76

propionibacteriaceae; ● composition of DNA of, table arranged by genera and specie, **04**: 151-152

Propionibacterium; ● composition of DNA of, table arranged by specie, **04**: 151-152

Prosthecomicrobium; ● composition of DNA of, table arranged by specie, **04**: 182

Proteus; ● composition of DNA of, table arranged by specie, **04**: 112-113

Protoachlya; ● composition of DNA of, table arranged by specie, **04**: 215

Protostelium; ● composition of DNA of, table arranged by specie, **04**: 215

protozoa, ● composition of DNA of, table arranged by genera and specie, **04**: 228-229

Providencia; ● composition of DNA of, table arranged by specie, **04**: 113

Prymnesium; ● composition of DNA of, table arranged by specie, **04**: 227

Psalliota; ● composition of DNA of, table arranged by specie, **04**: 215

Pseudeurotium; ● composition of DNA of, table arranged by specie, **04**: 215

Pseudoarachniotus; ● composition of DNA of, table arranged by specie, **04**: 215

Pseudogymnoascus; ● composition of DNA of, table arranged by specie, **04**: 215

pseudomonadaceae; ● composition of DNA of, table arranged by genera and species, **04**: 152-162

Pseudomonas; ● composition of DNA of, table arranged by specie, **04**: 154-160

Pseudonocardia; ● composition of DNA of, table arranged by specie, **04**: 150

Pycnidiophora; ● composition of DNA of, table arranged by specie, **04**: 215

Pycnoporus; ● composition of DNA of, table arranged by specie, **04**: 215

Pythium; ● composition of DNA of, table arranged by specie, **04**: 215

Radiomyces; ● composition of DNA of, table arranged by specie, **04**: 216

Ramibacterium; ● composition of DNA of, table arranged by specie, **04**: 123

Rhabdonema; ● composition of DNA of, table arranged by specie, **04**: 227

rhizobiaceae; ● composition of DNA of, table arranged by genera and specie, **04**: 162-165

Rhizobium; ● composition of DNA of, table arranged by specie, **04**: 164-165

Rhizoclonium; ● composition of DNA of, table arranged by specie, **04**: 227

Rhizophlyctis; ● composition of DNA of, table arranged by specie, **04**: 216

G + C *(continued)*

Rhizophydium; • composition of DNA of, table arranged by specie, **04:** 216

Rhizopus; • composition of DNA of, table arranged by specie, **04:** 216

Rhodopseudomonas; • composition of DNA of, table arranged by specie, **04:** 78-79

Rhodospirillum; • composition of DNA of, table arranged by specie, **04:** 80

Rhodotorula; • composition of DNA of, table arranged by specie, **04:** 216-217

Rhodymenia; • composition of DNA of, table arranged by specie, **04:** 227

Rickettsia (Coxiella); • composition of DNA of, table arranged by specie, **04:** 165

rickettsiaceae; • composition of DNA of, table arranged by genera and specie, **04:** 165

Rothia; • composition of DNA of, table arranged by specie, **04:** 76

Saccharomyces; • composition of DNA of, table arranged by specie, **04:** 217-218

Saccharomyces cerevisiae; • composition of, **04:** 217

salmonella; • composition of DNA of, table arranged by specie, **04:** 113

Salmonella typhimurium; • composition of, **04:** 113

Saprolegnia; • composition of DNA of, table arranged by specie, **04:** 219

Sapromyces; • composition of DNA of, table arranged by specie, **04:** 219

Saprospira; • composition of DNA of, table arranged by specie, **04:** 171

Sarcina; • composition of DNA of, table arranged by specie, **04:** 134-135

Sartorya; • composition of DNA of, table arranged by specie, **04:** 219

Scenedesmus; • composition of DNA of, table arranged by specie, **04:** 227

Schizophyllum; • composition for DNA of, table arranged by specie, **04:** 219

Schizosaccharomyces; • composition of DNA of, table arranged by specie, **04:** 219

Schwanniomyces; • composition of DNA of, table arranged by specie, **04:** 219

Sclerotinia; • composition of DNA of, table arranged by specie, **04:** 219

Scopulariopsis; • composition of DNA of, table arranged by specie, **04:** 219-220

Serratia; • composition of DNA of, table arranged by specie, **04:** 114

Shigella; • composition of DNA of, table arranged by specie, **04:** 114

sorangiaceae; • composition of DNA of, table arranged by specie, **04:** 166

Sorangium; • composition of DNA of, table arranged by specie, **04:** 166

Sordaria; • composition of DNA of, table arranged by specie, **04:** 220

Spadicoides; • composition of DNA of, table arranged by specie, **04:** 220

Sphaerophorus; • composition of DNA of, table arranged by specie, **04:** 87

Sphaerotilus; • composition of DNA of, table arranged by specie, **04:** 95

spirillaceae; • composition of DNA of, table arranged by genera and specie, **04:** 166-171

Spirillospora; • composition of DNA of, table arranged by specie, **04:** 77

Spirillum; • composition of DNA of, table arranged by specie, **04:** 168-169

Spirochaeta; • composition of DNA of, table arranged by specie, **04:** 172

spirochaetaceae; • composition of DNA of, table arranged by genera and specie, **04:** 171-172

Spirogyra; • composition of DNA of, table arranged by specie, **04:** 227

Spirosoma; • composition of DNA of, table arranged by specie, **04:** 182

Spondylocladium; • composition of DNA of, table arranged by specie, **04:** 220

Spongipellis (Polyporus); • composition of DNA of, table arranged by specie, **04:** 220

Sporobolomyces; • composition of DNA of, table arranged by specie, **04:** 220-221

Sporocytophaga; • composition of DNA of, table arranged by specie, **04:** 146

Sporomia; • composition of DNA of, table arranged by specie, **04:** 221

Sporotrichum; • composition of DNA of, table arranged by specie, **04:** 221

Stachybotrys; • composition of DNA of, table arranged by specie, **04:** 221

Staphylococcus; • composition of DNA of, table arranged by specie, **04:** 128-134

Stemphylium; • composition of DNA of, table arranged by specie, **04:** 221

Streptobacillus; • composition of DNA of, table arranged by specie, **04:** 87

Streptococcus; • composition of DNA of, table arranged by specie, **04:** 123-126

Streptomyces; • composition of DNA of, table arranged by specie, **04:** 172-177

Streptomyces coelicolor; • composition coelicolor, **04:** 173

streptomycetaceae; • composition of DNA of, table arranged by genera and specie, **04:** 172-177

Streptosporangium; • composition of DNA of, table arranged by specie, **04:** 78

Streptoverticillium; • composition of DNA of, table arranged by specie, **04:** 177

Syncephalastrum; • composition of DNA of, table arranged by specie, **04:** 221

Talaromyces; • composition of DNA of, table arranged by specie, **04:** 221-222

Tetrahymena; • composition of DNA of, table arranged by specie, **04:** 229

Thalassiosira; • composition of DNA of, table arranged by specie, **04:** 227

Thamnidium; • composition of DNA of, table arranged by specie, **04:** 222

Thermoactinomyces; • composition of DNA of, table arranged by specie, **04:** 150

Thermoactinopolyspora; • composition of DNA of, table

G + C *(continued)*
arranged by specie, **04**: 150
Thermomonospora; • composition of DNA of, table arranged by specie, **04**: 150
Thermoplasma; • composition of DNA of, table arranged by specie, **04**: 145
Thermus; • composition of DNA of, table arranged by specie, **04**: 182
Thielavia; • composition of DNA of, table arranged by specie, **04**: 222
Thiobacillus; • composition of DNA of, table arranged by specie, **04**: 177
thiobacteriaceae; • composition of DNA of, table arranged by genera and specie, **04**: 177
thiorhodaceae; • composition of DNA of, table arranged by genera and specie, **04**: 178-180
Thraustotheca; • composition of DNA of, table arranged by specie, **04**: 222
Torula; • composition of DNA of, table arranged by specie, **04**: 222
Torulopsis; • composition of DNA of, table arranged by specie, **04**: 223
Toxoplasma; • composition of DNA of, table arranged by specie, **04**: 229
Toxotrichum; • composition of DNA of, table arranged by specie, **04**: 223
Tremella; • composition of DNA of, table arranged by specie, **04**: 223
Treponema; • composition of DNA of, table arranged by specie, **04**: 181
treponemataceae; • composition of DNA of, table arranged by genera and specie, **04**: 180-181
Trichithecium; • composition of DNA of, table arranged by specie, **04**: 223
Trichoderma; • composition of DNA of, table arranged by specie, **04**: 223
Trichomonas; • composition of DNA of, table arranged by specie, **04**: 229
Trichosporon; • composition of DNA of, table arranged by specie, **04**: 223
Trigonopsis; • composition of DNA of, table arranged by specie, **04**: 223
Trypanosoma; • composition of DNA of, table arranged by specie, **04**: 229
Tuberculosis; • composition of DNA of, table arranged by specie, **04**: 94
Ulothrix; • composition of DNA of, table arranged by specie, **04**: 227
Veillonella; • composition of DNA of, table arranged by specie, **04**: 148
Verticillium; • composition of DNA of, table arranged by specie, **04**: 224
Vibrio; • composition of DNA of, table arranged by specie, **04**: 169-171
Vitreoscilla; • composition of DNA of, table arranged by specie, **04**: 181
vitreoscillaceae; • composition of DNA of, table arranged by genera and specie, **04**: 181
Wickerhamia; • composition of DNA of, table arranged by specie, **04**: 224
Wolbachia; • composition of DNA of, table arranged by specie, **04**: 165

Xanthomonas; • composition of DNA of, table arranged by specie, **04**: 161-162
Zygorhynchus; • composition of DNA of, table arranged by specie, **04**: 224
Galactokinase
amino acid composition, complete data, **07**: 507
Galactose
heat of proton ionization, pK, and related thermodynamic quantities, **06**: 201
oxidase
amino acid composition, incomplete data, **07**: 512
circular dichroism in the UV region, **07**: 97
UV and near-UV region, **07**: 97, 151
pK'_a values, **06**: 317
uridine diphosphate • 4-epimerase
amino acid composition, complete data, **07**: 511
uridine diphosphate •: lipopolysaccharide α-3-galactosyl transferase
amino acid composition, incomplete data, **07**: 514
Galactose 1-phosphate
uridylyltransferase
amino acid composition, incomplete data, **07**: 512
α-Galactosidase
carbohydrate content, **02**: 274
molar absorptivity and-or absorbance values, **02**: 429
β-Galactosidase
amino acid composition, complete data, **07**: 507
average hydrophobicity value, **01**: 221
cyanogen bromide cleavage, **02**: 199
molar absorptivity and-or absorbance values, **02**: 429
subunit, constitution of, **02**: 348
α-D-Galactoside galactohydrolase
enzymatic reactions, velocity and parameters, table, **05**: 440-441
β-D-Galactoside galactohydrolase
enzymatic reactions, velocity and parameters, table, **05**: 435-438
Gas
dispersoids, •, chart of diameters for various, **08**: 425
Gastricin
average hydrophobicity value, **01**: 221
Gastrin
cyanogen bromide cleavage, **02**: 199
molar absorptivity and-or absorbance values, **02**: 429
Gastrin I
amino acid composition, incomplete data, **07**: 512
circular dichroism in the UV region, **07**: 97
Gastrins
amino acid sequence, **07**: 323
Gaugliodise
generic term usage, **05**: 10
GDP, *see* Guanylic acid
pK'_a values, **06**: 331
Gel
filtration media
Bio-Gel A®, properties, **08**: 130
Bio-Gel P®, properties, **08**: 131-132
Sephadex®, properties, **08**: 133-134
Sepharose®, properties, **08**: 135

Gelatin
   refractive index increments, **02:** 375
Gene product
   bacteriophage T4; genes; •, **04:** 665-673
Genetic
   factors
      immunoglobulins, human, notation for, **02:** 186
Genetic code, codons
   table, **04:** 896
Genetic markers, *see also* Morphogenetic markers
   designation of, for *Bacillus subtilis*, **04:** 686-698
   Escherichia coli, **04:** 654-659
   Streptomyces coelicolor, list, **04:** 724-727
   maize (*Zea mays* L.), annotated list, **04:** 835-844
   mouse (*Mus musculus*), **04:** 857-870
   Saccharomyces cerevisiae, **04:** 767-826
   Salmonella typhimurium, **04:** 705-717
Gentamycin (C$_1$ and C$_2$)
   origin, structure, and characteristic as protein biosynthe-
      sis inhibitor, **04:** 575
Gigartinine
   physical and chemical properties, **01:** 133
Gliadin
   circular dichroism in the UV region, **07:** 97
   optical rotatory dispersion
      UV region, **07:** 56
      visible and near UV regions, **07:** 23
α-Gliadin
   amino acid composition, incomplete data, **07:** 512
   circular dichroism in the UV region, **07:** 97
   optical rotatory dispersion
      UV region, **07:** 56
      visible and near UV regions, **07:** 23
Gliadin SP 2-2, SP 2-1
   average hydrophobicity values, **01:** 221
Globin, *see also* Haptoglobin, Hemoglobin listings
   chymotryptic hydrolysis; human •, α-chains of, **02:** 213
   ferriprotoporphyrin IX-•
      UV spectra, molecular weight, **08:** 172
   human •
      chymotryptic hydrolysis of α-chains of, **02:** 213
   hydrolysis, *see also* Peptic hydrolysis; chymotryptic, of
      α-chains of human •, **02:** 213
   metazoan, aligned chains
      amino acid sequence, **07:** 456-458
   molar absorptivity and-or absorbance values, **02:** 430
   refractive index increments, **02:** 375, 376
   stereo drawings of several,
      02: 761
Globulin, *see also* Macroglobulin
   carbohydrate content, **02:** 270
   corticosteroid-binding •
      amino acid composition, complete data, **07:** 506
   molar absorptivity and-or absorbance values, **02:** 430
   plasma, human
      carbohydrate content, molecular weights, sedimenta-
         tion coefficients, **02:** 258
   progesterone-binding •
      molar absorptivity and-or absorbance values, **02:** 501
   subunit, constitution of, **02:** 349
   thyroxine-binding •
      amino acid composition, incomplete data, **07:** 514

α$_2$-Globulin
   refractive index increments, **02:** 376
γ-Globulin, *see* Immunoglobulin
   immunoglobulin, specific; • fraction, chicken
      molar absorptivity and-or absorbance values, **02:** 456
   refractive index increments, **02:** 376
γI-Globulin
   luminescence of, table, **01:** 205
γ$_1$-globulin
   immunoglobulin, specific; •, human
      molar absorptivity and-or absorbance values, **02:** 456
β$_1$-Globulin
   refractive index increments, **02:** 376
Globulin, 0.6 S γ$_2$
   average hydrophobicity value, **01:** 221
Glu(Asp)-plasminogen
   amino-terminus of single chain
      alignment of amino-terminal amino acid sequences
         homologous to, **07:** 341
Glucagon
   amino acid sequence, **07:** 376
   average hydrophobicity value, **01:** 221
   circular dichroism in the UV region, **07:** 97
   luminescence of, table, **01:** 205
   molar absorptivity and-or absorbance values, **02:** 431
   optical rotatory dispersion in the UV region, **07:** 56
Glucanase
   exo-β-D-(1→3)-•
      amino acid composition, complete data, **07:** 506
S-β-1-(Gluco-pyranosyl)-3-indolylacetothiohydroximyl-
      O-sulfate, *see* Glucobrassicin
Glucobrassicin
   physical and chemical properties, **01:** 154
Glucose
   oxidase
      carbohydrate content, **02:** 273
      circular dichroism in the UV region, **07:** 97
      molar absorptivity and-or absorbance values, **02:** 431
      optical rotatory dispersion
         UV region, **07:** 56
         visible and near UV region, **07:** 23
   pK$_a$ values, **06:** 317
Glucose-6-phosphate isomerase, *see* Glucosephosphate,
      isomerase
Glucose derivatives
Glucosephosphate
   isomerase
      circular dichroism in the UV region, **07:** 97
      optical rotatory dispersion
         UV region, **07:** 56
         visible and near UV regions, **07:** 23
υ-Glucuronidase
   amino acid composition, incomplete data, **07:** 512
β-Glucuronidase
   carbohydrate content, **02:** 274
   molar absorptivity and-or absorbance values, **02:** 432
Glutamase
   formimino•
      molar absorptivity and-or absorbance values, **02:** 428
Glutamate
   decarboxylase
      average hydrophobicity value, **01:** 221

Glyceraldehyde-3-phosphate *(continued)*
circular dichroism in near-UV region, at room temperature, **07**: 151
molar absorptivity and-or absorbance values, **02**: 434
subunit, constitution of, **02**: 349
viscosity, intrinsic, **02**: 721
Glyceroglycolipids
nomenclature and classification, **05**: 416, 421-423
Glycerokinase
optical rotatory dispersion
UV region, **07**: 58
visible and near UV regions, **07**: 25
Glycerol
Beckman rotors, construction data for isokinetic sucrose and ● gradients, **06**: 432-464
centrifugation, density gradient; isokinetic gradients, sucrose and ●, data for construction
Beckman rotors, **06**: 432-464
Christ rotors, **06**: 465-479
geometrical parameters used in calculations, **06**: 428
International rotors, **06**: 480-488
MSE rotors, **06**: 489-518
Christ rotors, construction data for isokinetic sucrose and ● gradients, **06**: 465-479
International rotors, construction data for isokinetic sucrose and ● gradients, **06**: 480-488
MSE rotors, construction data for isokinetic sucrose and ● gradients, **06**: 489-518
L-Glycerol 3-phosphate
dehydrogenase
amino acid composition, complete data, **07**: 507
Glycerol-water
mixtures, dielectric constants and freezing points, **06**: 526
Glycerol derivatives
heat of proton ionization, pK, and related thermodynamic quantities, **06**: 202
stereospecific nomenclature, **05**: 10
α-Glycerophosphate
dehydrogenase
optical rotatory dispersion
UV region, **07**: 58
visible and near UV regions, **07**: 25
Glycine
3-aminomethylcyclohexane ●
antagonism to lysine, **01**: 178
antagonism to α alanine, **01**: 177
antagonists of, **01**: 177
N-carbamoyl-2-(*p*-hydroxyphenyl) ●
physical and chemical properties, **01**: 137
d-(3-carboxy-4-hydroxyphenyl) ●
physical and chemical properties, **01**: 165
cis-α-(carboxycyclopropyl) ●
physical and chemical properties, **01**: 115
trans-α-(2-carboxymethylcyclopropyl) ●
physical and chemical properties, **01**: 115
m-carboxyphenyl-●
physical and chemical properties, **01**: 165
N-(2-cyanoethyl)●
structure and symbols for those incorporated into synthetic polypeptides, **01**: 100

α-(Cyclopentyl)●
structure and symbols for those incorporated into synthetic polypeptides, **01**: 101
free acid in amniotic fluid in early pregnancy and at term, **01**: 327
free acid in blood plasma of newborn infants and adults, **01**: 328
hyperglycinemia ketotic (severe infantile), effect of, **01**: 318
α-(methylene-cyclopropyl) ●
physical and chemical properties, **01**: 116
ninhydrin reaction, absorption ratio, **08**: 123
nucleoside composition, tables of values, **04**: 430-432
nucleotide sequences of, **04**: 444-445
pK'_a values, **06**: 318
physical and chemical properties, **01**: 116
requirements of, for growth of various microorganisms, table, **04**: 630-643
thumbprint, content in, **08**: 121
(*trans*)-α-(carboxycyclorpopyl) ●
physical and chemical properties, **01**: 115
Glycine-HCl buffer
preparation of, **06**: 370
Glycine-NaOH buffer
preparation of, **06**: 376
Glycine betaine, *see* Lycin
Glycine buffers
protonic activity tables, **06**: 537-539
Glycine derivatives
heat of proton ionization, pK, and related thermodynamic quantities, **06**: 203-205
Glycinin
circular dichroism in the UV region, **07**: 99
optical rotatory dispersion
UV region, **07**: 58
visible and near UV regions, **07**: 25
N^6-Glycinocarbonyladenosine
isolation and detection of, in RNA, general remarks, **03**: 234
RNA, various, natural occurrence in, **03**: 218
Glyco-proteins
acetyl hexosamine, content of, in ●, **02**: 258-274
Glycocyamine, *see* Guanidinoacetyl
Glycocyamine kinase, *see* Guanidinoacetate, kinase
average hydrophobicity value, **01**: 222
Glycocyaminekinase
molar absorptivity and-or absorbance values, **02**: 435
Glycogen
phosphorylase
amino acid composition, incomplete data, **07**: 507
average hydrophobicity value, **01**: 222
Glycohydrolase
enzymes, *see also* Coenzyme, Metalloenzyme, Multienzyme; pH values (optimum and stable) in ● reactions, **05**: 426-445
enzymes, *see also* Coenzyme, Metalloenzyme, Multienzyme; substrates used in ● reactions, **05**: 426-445
Escherichia coli, *see also* E. coli; ● from, enzymatic reaction parameters, **05**: 435-436
Neurospora crassa; ● from, enzymatic reaction, parameters, **05**: 437
specificity, for ● reactions, table, **05**: 426-445

Glycohydrolase *(continued)*
  substrates used in • reactions, **05:** 426-445
Glycohydrolases
  dissociation constants; • table, **05:** 426-445
  enzymatic reactions, velocity and parameters, tables, **05:** 426-445
  enzymes, *see also* Coenzyme, Metalloenzyme, Multienzyme; dissociation constants, •, table of, **05:** 426-445
  enzymes, *see also* Coenzyme, Metalloenzyme, Multienzyme; Michaelis constants, •, table of, **05:** 426-445
  enzymes, *see also* Coenzyme, Metalloenzyme, Multienzyme; reaction rates, parameters for •, **05:** 426-445
  enzymes, *see also* Coenzyme, Metalloenzyme, Multienzyme; specificity, for •, **05:** 426-445
  enzymes, *see also* Coenzyme, Metalloenzyme, Multienzyme; velocity of reaction, maximum for •, **05:** 426-445
  Michaelis constants for •, table of, 05: 426-445
  pH values for • reactions, **05:** 426-445
Glycolipids
  classification and nomenclature of, **05:** 416-423
  lipids; •
    classification and nomenclature of, **05:** 416-423
    of bacteria, structures and organisms, **05:** 373-393
  of bacteria, structures and organisms, **05:** 373-393
  structures; • of bacteria, **05:** 373-393
Glycolytic
  enzymes
    amino acid sequences, **07:** 324, 337
Glycoprotein, *see also* Glycoproteins
  α,-acid •
    amino acid composition, incomplete data, **07:** 512
    optical rotatory dispersion
      UV region, **07:** 44
      visible and near UV regions, **07:** 15
  α₁-acid •
    average hydrophobicity value, **01:** 210
  acidic •
    circular dichroism in the UV region, **07:** 82
    amino acid composition; Tamm-Horsfall •, **02:** 303
    amino acid composition, complete data, **07:** 507
    amino acid composition, incomplete data, **07:** 512
    carbohydrate composition; Tamm-Horsfall •, **02:** 303
    circular dichroism in the UV region, **07:** 99
    hormones
      amino acid sequences of α subunit, **07:** 393-394
    Tamm-Horsfall
      circular dichroism in the UV region, **07:** 98
  γ-Glycoprotein
    average hydrophobicity value, **01:** 222
Glycoprotein M-1
  amino acid composition, incomplete data, **07:** 513
Glycoproteins, *see also* Glycoprotein
  blood group substances
    carbohydrate content, **02:** 262-263
  body fluids
    carbohydrate content, **02:** 267
  carbohydrate content; •
    blood group substances, table, **02:** 262-263
    body fluids, **02:** 267
    cell membrane, **02:** 266
    eggs, table of values, **02:** 268-269

enzymes, table of values, **02:** 273-274
hormones, table of values, **02:** 271-272
milk, table of values, **02:** 268-269
mucins, table, **02:** 262-263
plants, table of values, **02:** 270
plasma, human, table of values, **02:** 258
plasma, nonhuman, table of values, **02:** 259-260
tissues, table of values, **02:** 264-265
viruses, enveloped, **02:** 267
cell membrane
  carbohydrate content, **02:** 266
definition of, **02:** 257
eggs
  carbohydrate content, **02:** 268-269
enzymes
  carbohydrate content, **02:** 273-274
enzymes, *see also* Coenzyme, Metalloenzyme, Multienzyme; •, carbohydrate content, **02:** 273-274
fucose, content of, in •, **02:** 258-267, 271-274
hexose, content of, in •, **02:** 258
hormones
  carbohydrate content, **02:** 271-272
lectins, purified, table of properties, **02:** 546-551
mammalian, carbohydrate-amino acid linkages found in, **05:** 281
milk
  carbohydrate content, **02:** 268-269
molar absorptivity and-or absorbance values, **02:** 435-436
molecular parameters, **02:** 242
molecular weight; •
  plasma, human, table of values, **02:** 258
mouse plasma, tumor
  molar absorptivity and-or absorbance values, **02:** 435
mucins
  carbohydrate content, **02:** 262-263
plants
  carbohydrate content, **02:** 270
plasma, human
  carbohydrate content, molecular weights, sedimentation coefficients, **02:** 258
plasma, nonhuman
  carbohydrate content, **02:** 259-260
proteins, *see also* Bacteriophage Flavoproteins, Matrix protein, *also* Protein, individual proteins, Molybdoproteins; carbohydrate content tables for • from various sources, **02:** 257-274
sialic acid, content of, in •, **02:** 258-269, 271-274
sugar, neutral, content of in •, **02:** 259-274
Tamm-Horsfall, *see also* Tamm-Horsfall glycoprotein; Tamm-Horsfall mucoprotein
  molar absorptivity and-or absorbance values, **02:** 435
Tamm-Horsfall, rabbit urine
  molar absorptivity and-or absorbance values, **02:** 435
Tamm-Horsfall, rat intestinal mucosa
  molar absorptivity and-or absorbance values, **02:** 435
tissues
  carbohydrate content, **02:** 264-265
viruses, enveloped
  carbohydrate content, **02:** 267

Glycosaminoglycans, *see* Mucopolysaccharides
　table of data and characteristics, 02: 686-687
Glycoses, acyl
　structures and organisms, 05: 373-375
Glycoside derivatives
　of phospholipids, structures and organisms, 05: 385-387
Glycosides
　cardiac •, ligands binding to plasma albumin, 02: 572
　free energy; hydrolysis; •, 06: 303
　free energy values of hydrolysis, 06: 303
　nomenclature rules, 05: 116-117
Glycosidic lipids
　miscellaneous, structures and organisms, 05: 388-390
Glycosphingolipid
　generic term usage, 05: 9
Glycosyl
　diglycerides, structures and organisms, 05: 376-385
　esters of polyisoprenol phosphate and pyrophosphate,
　　structures and organisms, 05: 391-393
Glycosyl radicals
　and glycosylamines, nomenclature rules, 05: 117-118
Glycosylamines
　glycosyl radicals and •, nomenclature rules, 05: 117-118
Glycosyloxy radicals
　nomenclature rules, 05: 119
Glycylglycine
　heat capacity and entropy values, 06: 110
Glyoxalase
　optical rotatory dispersion
　　UV region, 07: 58
　　visible and near UV region, 07: 25
Glyoxylate
　cycle; pathways chart, 04: insert
　reductase
　　optical rotatory dispersion
　　　UV region, 07: 58
　　　visible and near UV regions, 07: 25
Glyoxylic acid
　properties of, 01: 181
Golgi material
　enzymatic activity, table, 02: 714
Gonadotropin
　-transporting protein
　　plasma, nonhuman
　　　carbohydrate content, 02: 259
Gonadotropin
　hormone, *see also* Luteinizing hormone; chorionic •,
　　human
　　carbohydrate content, 02: 271
　　molar absorptivity and-or absorbance values, 02: 450
Gonadotropin-α
　chorionic •
　　average hydrophobicity value, 01: 216
Gonadotropin-β
　chorionic •
　　average hydrophobicity value, 01: 216
Gonadotropin, chorionic, *see* Chorionic gonadotropin
Gougerotin
　origin, structure, and characteristic as protein biosynthe-
　　sis inhibitor, 04: 576
　physicochemical constants, spectral, chemotherapeutic
　　and biological properties, 03: 324

Gramicidin S-A
　proton NMR and suggested conformations, 07: 563
Granules
　zymogen •
　　enzymatic activity, table, 02: 714
Griseoviridine
　origin, structure, and characteristic as protein biosynthe-
　　sis inhibitor, 04: 576
O-group
　salmonella; lipopolysaccharides of; sugar composition
　　for •, 05: 396-399
Growth
　epidermal • factor
　　circular dichroism in the UV region, 07: 94
　hormone
　　amino acid composition, complete data, 07: 507
　　amino acid sequence, 07: 376, 388-389, 392-393
　　average hydrophobicity value, 01: 222
　　bovine
　　　pituitary gland, constitution of subunit, 02: 327
　　circular dichroism
　　　UV and near UV region, 07: 98, 151
　　cyanogen bromide cleavage, 02: 199
　　luminescence of, table, 01: 206
　　molar absorptivity and-or absorbance values, 02: 437
　　optical rotatory dispersion
　　　UV regions, 07: 58
　　　visible and near UV regions, 07: 25
Guanidine
　pK'_a values, 06: 344
Guanidine-1-pyrroline-5-carboxylic acid, *see* Viomycidine
Guanidine hydrochloride
　densities of aqueous solutions with added reagents, at
　　25°, 06: 406
　density, summary of data, 06: 404
　index of refraction, summary of data, 06: 404
　viscosities of aqueous solutions with added reagents, at
　　25°, 06: 407
　viscosity of aqueous solutions at 25°, 06: 405
Guanidinoacetate
　kinase
　　optical rotatory dispersion in the visible and near UV
　　　regions, 07: 25
Guanidinoacetyl
　structure and symbols for those incorporated into syn-
　　thetic polypeptides, 01: 102
β-Guanidinoalanine
　structure and symbols for those incorporated into syn-
　　thetic polypeptides, 01: 102
Guanidinomethylarginine, *see* ω-N-Methylarginine
5-Guanidinovaleric acid
　structure and symbols for those incorporated into syn-
　　thetic polypeptides, 01: 102
β-Guanido-γ-hydroxyvaline
　physical and chemical properties, 01: 124
Guanido amino acids
　physical and chemical properties, 01: 132-134
Guanidotaurine
　physical and chemical properties, 01: 154

Guanine
 and derivatives
  physical constants and spectral properties, index to, **03:** 67
  UV spectra, **03:** 423-427
  UV spectral characteristics and acid dissociation constants, **03:** 411-412
 pK'_a values, **06:** 331
Guanosine
 and derivatives
  UV spectra, **03:** 436-440
  UV spectral characteristics and acid dissociation constants, **03:** 414
 and nucleoside derivatives
  physical constants and spectral properties, index to, **03:** 70
 bond angles and distances, **08:** 225
 chemical structures and approved numbering schemes, **08:** 224
 composition in various tRNA's, **04:** 428-441
 pK'_a values, **06:** 331
 raman frequencies, table of values, **03:** 538-539
Guanosine derivatives
 heat of proton ionization, pK, and related thermodynamic quantities, **06:** 206
Guanosine nucleotide derivatives
 physical constants and spectral properties, index to, **03:** 73-74
Guanylic acid
 derivatives, UV spectral characteristics and acid dissociation constants, **03:** 416
Guanyloribonuclease
 amino acid composition, complete data, **07:** 510
 amino acid sequences, **07:** 311
 circular dichroism
  UV and near UV region, **07:** 99, 161
 optical rotatory dispersion
  UV region, **07:** 58
  visible and near UV regions, **07:** 25
5'-Guanylylmethylene diphosphate
 origin, structure, and characteristic as protein biosynthesis inhibitor, **04:** 577
Guvacine
 physical and chemical properties, **01:** 140
Gylceraldehyde-3-phosphate
 dehydrogenase
  average hydrophobicity value, **01:** 222
  luminescence of, table, **01:** 206

H

H1' and H2' protons
 coupling constants; dinucleoside monophosphates, of the •, **03:** 531-532
 coupling constants; dinucleotides, of the •, **03:** 531-532
 coupling constants; mononucleotides, of the •, **03:** 530
 coupling constants; oligonucleotides, of the •, **03:** 531-532
 coupling constants; polynucleotides, of the •, **03:** 533

Hadacidin
 antagonism to aspartic acid, **01:** 177
 physical and chemical properties, **01:** 135
Hageman
 factor
  amino acid composition, incomplete data, **07:** 513
  physical data and characteristics, **02:** 254-255
  plasma, nonhuman
   carbohydrate content, **02:** 260
L-Halogen-containing amino acids
 physical and chemical properties, **01:** 159-160
Haploid chromosome
 numbers in fungi, table of values, **04:** 874-877
Haptoglobin
 amino acid composition, complete data, **07:** 507
 circular dichroism in the UV region, **07:** 99
 molar absorptivity and-or absorbance values, **02:** 437
 optical rotatory dispersion in the visible and near UV regions, **07:** 25
 plasma, human
  carbohydrate content, molecular weights, sedimentation coefficients, **02:** 258
Haptoglobin 1-1
 human
  molar absorptivity and-or absorbance values, **02:** 437
  subunit, constitution of, **02:** 331
Haptoglobin, $\alpha_{1 s}$-chain
 average hydrophobicity value, **01:** 222
Haptoglobin, α_2-chain
 average hydrophobicity value, **01:** 222
Haptoglobin, β-chain
 average hydrophobicity value, **01:** 222
Haptoglobulin
 human
  molar absorptivity and-or absorbance values, **02:** 437
Harringtonine
 origin, structure, and characteristic as protein biosynthesis inhibitor, **04:** 577
Hb
 hemoglobin; human •, subunits
  molar absorptivity and-or absorbance values, **02:** 447
HbO_2
 oxyferrohemoglobin,•
  UV and visible absorption spectrum, **07:** 177
HCl
 absorption data; porphyrin dications in aqueous •, **08:** 269-271
 numbers, porphyrins, **08:** 275
 porphyrins; absorption maxima; dications in aqueous •, **08:** 269-271
 porphyrins; • numbers, table, **08:** 275
 soret band data; porphyrin dications in aqueous •, **08:** 269-271
Heavy merromyosin (HMM), *see* Myosin, HMM
Helical complexes, double
 molar residue ellipticity, table of values, **03:** 601
 molar residue rotation, **03:** 599
Helical segments
 nomenclature rules in polypeptides chain, **01:** 72, **02:** 76
Helicorubin
 definition and nomenclature, **02:** 118

α-Helix content
  tropomyosin from nonmuscle values, **02:** 321
Hemagglutin
  average hydrophobicity value, **01:** 222-223
Hemagglutin I and II
  average hydrophobicity values, **01:** 222
Hemagglutinin
  amino acid composition, complete data, **07:** 507
  amino acid composition, incomplete data, **07:** 513
  carbohydrate content, **02:** 270
  molar absorptivity and-or absorbance values, **02:** 437
  subunit, constitution of, **02:** 327
Hematin
  absorption data; hemin and ● spectra in ether, **08:** 279
  absorption maxima in ether, **08:** 279
Heme
  proteins
    resonance raman spectra, **07:** 589
Heme-base
  complexes, positions and extinctions of α bands, **08:** 280
  extinction coefficients; ● complexes, α bands, **08:** 280
Hemerythrin
  amino acid composition, complete data, **07:** 507
  amino acid sequences, **07:** 498
  average hydrophobicity value, **01:** 223
  circular dichroism
    UV and near UV region, **07:** 99, 151
  molar absorptivity and-or absorbance values, **02:** 437
  molecular weight, stoichiometry, source, function, **02:** 276
  optical rotatory dispersion in the UV region, **07:** 58
  refractive index increments, **02:** 376
  subunit, constitution of, **02:** 327, 334
Hemin
  absorption maxima in ether, **08:** 279
  R_F value in 2,6-lutidine-water system, **08:** 276
Hemin chloride
  dimethyl ester
    UV and visible absorption spectrum, **07:** 183
    UV spectra, formula, molecular weight, **08:** 174
Hemochrome
  spectra, pyridine, **08:** 280
Hemochromogen
  pyridine ●
    UV and visible absorption spectrum, **07:** 182
    UV spectra, formula, molecular weight, **08:** 173
Hemocuprein, *see* Superoxide dismutase
Hemocyanin
  amino acid composition, complete data, **07:** 507
  average hydrophobicity value, **01:** 223
  circular dichroism
    UV and near UV region, **07:** 99, 152
  molar absorptivity and-or absorbance values, **02:** 438
  molecular weight, stoichiometry, source, function, **02:** 277
  subunit, constitution of, **02:** 350
Hemoglobin
  amino acid composition, complete data, **07:** 507
  average hydrophobicity value, **01:** 223
  beef
    molar absorptivity and-or absorbance values, **02:** 443

bovine
  refractive index increments, **02:** 376
canine
  refractive index increments, **02:** 376
α-chain variants, **07:** 461-468
β-chain variants, **07:** 461-468
circular dichroism
  UV and near UV region, **07:** 152
  UV and near UV region, **07:** 152
cysteine β 93 SH; pK values in human ●, **02:** 696
derivatives
  UV and visible absorption spectra from human normal adult, **07:** 174-185
helical number, **07:** 461-468
horse
  molar absorptivity and-or absorbance values, **02:** 443
human, *see also* Human hemoglobin
  heat of proton ionization, pK, and related thermodynamic quantities, **06:** 206
  molar absorptivity and-or absorbance values, **02:** 444
  pK values, α-amino groups, table, **02:** 693
  pK values, cysteine β 93 SH, **02:** 696
  pK values, histidine, **02:** 690
  pK values, histidine 146 β, **02:** 690
  pK values, tyrosine, **02:** 695
  refractive index increments, **02:** 376
human Hb, subunits
  molar absorptivity and-or absorbance values, **02:** 447
human ●, *see also* Hemoglobin, human
  hydrolysis peptides by leucine, **02:** 217
  hydrolysis peptides by papain, **02:** 219
hydrolysis, *see also* Peptic hydrolysis; peptides from α- and β-chains of human ● by papain, **02:** 219
known substitutions deletions, index to, **07:** 461-468
luminescence of, table, **01:** 206
molar absorptivity and-or absorbance values, **02:** 439-445
mouse
  molar absorptivity and-or absorbance values, **02:** 444
optical rotatory dispersion
  UV region, **07:** 58
  visible and near UV regions, **07:** 25
oxidation-reduction potentials of, **06:** 137-139
papain; hydrolysis peptides from α- and β-chains of human ●, **02:** 219
peptides; hydrolysis from α- and β-chains of human ●, **02:** 219
pK; histidine in; ● human, values for His 146β, **02:** 690
pK; tyrosine in; ●, table of values, **02:** 695
sheep
  molar absorptivity and-or absorbance values, **02:** 443
subunit, constitution of, **02:** 328, 351
viscosity, intrinsic, **02:** 721
Hemoglobin, deoxy(ferro)-
  optical rotatory dispersion in the UV region, **07:** 59
Hemoglobin, met (ferri)-
  circular dichroism in the UV region, **07:** 100
  optical rotatory dispersion in the UV region, **07:** 59
Hemoglobin, oxy (ferro)-
  optical rotatory dispersion in the UV region, **07:** 60

Hormone *(continued)*
  thyroid stimulating •β-chain
    average hydrophobicity value, **01:** 232
Hormone-binding
  polypeptide
    amino acid composition, complete data, **07:** 507
Hormones, *see also* Hormone
  amino acid sequence, **07:** 375-376, 378-381
  anterior pituitary
    amino acid sequence, **07:** 385-397
  follicle-stimulating •
    amino acid composition, complete data, **07:** 506
    amino acid sequence of α subunit, **07:** 393-394
    circular dichroism in the UV region, **07:** 96
  glycoprotein •
    amino acid sequences of α subunit, **07:** 393-394
  neurohypophysial
    distribution in vertebrates, table, **07:** 400-401
  parathyroid
    amino acid sequence, **07:** 399
  pituitary •, nomenclature, **02:** 176-178
  placenta
    amino acid sequence, **07:** 385-397
Human
  carbohydrate content; glycoproteins; plasma, •, table of
    values, **02:** 258
Human urine, *see* Urine, human
Hyaluronic acid
  table of data and characteristics, **02:** 686
Hyaluronidase
  amino acid composition, complete data, **07:** 507
  average hydrophobicity value, **01:** 224
  bovine testicle
    luminescence of, table, **01:** 206
  circular dichroism in the UV region, **07:** 103
  optical rotatory dispersion in the visible and near UV
    regions, **07:** 26
Hyaluronoglucosidase, *see* Hyaluronidase
Hydantoic acid
  structure and symbols for those incorporated into syn-
    thetic polypeptides, **01:** 102
5-Hydantoinacetyl
  structure and symbols for those incorporated into syn-
    thetic polypeptides, **01:** 103
Hydratase
  fumarate •
    circular dichroism in the UV region, **07:** 97
    optical rotatory dispersion
      UV region, **07:** 56
      visible and near UV regions, **07:** 23
Hydrazines
  pK'_a values, **06:** 344
Hydrochloric acid
  -potassium chloride buffer, preparation of, **06:** 370
Hydrogen
  equivalents, oxidation and reduction reagents, **06:** 352
  NMR spectra; • in organic structures, characteristic po-
    sitions, **08:** 247
  NMR spectral positions, in organic structures, **08:** 247
  Watson-Crick pairs; standard polynucleotide double he-
    lices, values for constrained • bonds, **04:** 413

Hydrogenase
  average hydrophobicity value, **01:** 224
  ferredoxin •
    circular dichroism in the UV region, **07:** 95
  molar absorptivity and-or absorbance values, **02:** 451
  subunit, constitution of, **02:** 328
  table of cofactors, molecular weights, stoichiometry and
    sources, **02:** 280
Hydrogenase (*C. pasteurianum* W5), *see* Ferredoxin, hy-
    drogenase
Hydrolases
  definition and nomenclature, **02:** 97
  numbering and classification of, **02:** 107
7-[(2-Hydroperoxy)-3-(methoxycarbonyl)-3-
    (methoxyformamido)propyl] wyosine
  isolation and detection of, in RNA, general remarks, **03:**
    246
  RNA, various, natural occurrence in, **03:** 233
Hydroquinine
  pK'_a values, **06:** 326
β-Hydroxbutyrate
  dehydrogenase
    average hydrophobicity value, **01:** 224
α-Hydroxy-ε-amino caproic acid
  physical and chemical properties, **01:** 125
1-Hydroxy-2-amino ethylphosphonic acid
  physical and chemical properties, **01:** 161
Hydroxy-β-aminobutyramide
  structure and mode of action as protein biosynthesis in-
    hibitor, **04:** 578
α-Hydroxy-γ-aminobutyric acid
  physical and chemical properties, **01:** 125
β-Hydroxy-γ-aminobutyric acid
  physical and chemical properties, **01:** 125
S-(3-Hydroxy-3-carboxy-*n*-propyl)
  cysteine
    physical and chemical properties, **01:** 156
S-(3-Hydroxy-3-carboxy-*n*-propyl-thio)-homocysteine
    physical and chemical properties, **01:** 156
S-(3-Hydroxy-3-carboxy-*n*-propyl thio)-cysteine
    physical and chemical properties, **01:** 156
S-(β-Hydroxy-β-carboxyethane-sulfonyl methyl) cysteine,
    see Dichrostachinic acid
S-(2-Hydroxy-2-carboxyethyl)-homocysteine
    physical and chemical properties, **01:** 155
S(2-Hydroxy-2-carboxyethylthio)-homocysteine
    physical and chemical properties, **01:** 155
β-Hydroxy-α,ε-diaminopimelic acid
    antagonism to α,ε-diaminopimelic acid, **01:** 177
4-Hydroxy-3-hydroxymethylphenylalanine
    physical and chemical properties, **01:** 130
δ-Hydroxy-γ-ketonorvaline
    physical and chemical properties, **01:** 126
δ-*N*-(*cis*-5-Hydroxy-3-methylpent-2-enoyl)-f-*N*-
    hydroxy-ornithine, *see* Fusarinine
4-Hydroxy-*N*-methylproline
    physical and chemical properties, **01:** 149
4-Hydroxy-4-methylproline
    physical and chemical properties, **01:** 141
5-Hydroxy-piperidazine-3-carboxylic acid
    physical and chemical properties, **01:** 141

I

Immunoglobulin *(continued)*
γM, human
molar absorptivity and-or absorbance values, **02:** 456
γM, human, subunit
molar absorptivity and-or absorbance values, **02:** 456
γG, lemon shark
molar absorptivity and-or absorbance values, **02:** 456
γA, rabbit
molar absorptivity and-or absorbance values, **02:** 456
γG, rabbit
molar absorptivity and-or absorbance values, **02:** 456
Immunoglobulin, Eu heavy
chain
average hydrophobicity value, **01:** 224
Immunoglobulin, newλ-
chain
average hydrophobicity value, **01:** 224
Immunoglobulin IgG
human
cyanogen bromide cleavage, **02:** 199
rabbit
cyanogen bromide cleavage, **02:** 199
Immunoglobulins
nomenclature; •, genetic factors, **02:** 186
Inactivator
cl-•
carbohydrate composition, **02:** 666-667
molar absorptivity and-or absorbance values, **02:** 399
molecular parameters, **02:** 244
kallikrein •
molar absorptivity and-or absorbance values, **02:** 459
trypsin inhibitor, basic (kallikrein •)
amino acid composition, complete data, **07:** 510
circular dichroism at maxima in near-UV region, **07:** 163
C_1-Inactivator
average hydrophobicity value, **01:** 215
Inacton
origin and structure, **04:** 580
Indicators
acid-base types, pH range and color change table, **06:** 357
adsorption, applications of several, **06:** 383
mixed, transition pH and color change, **06:** 382
oxidation-reduction, transition potential and color change, **06:** 383
oxidation-reduction •, transition potential and color change, **06:** 383
pK'_a values, **06:** 330, 348
pH; determination, • for, **06:** 380-383
pH determination, table of color change, pH range and preparation data, **06:** 380-382
pH ranges for various, **06:** 378-379
reduction-oxidation •, transition potential and color change, **06:** 383
universal, for approximate pH determination, **06:** 383
use in pH measurement, **06:** 357
volumetric work, • for, **06:** 380-382
volumetric work, table of color change, pH range and preparation data, **06:** 380-382
Indole
antagonism to tryptophan, **01:** 179

Indole-3-acetly-ε-lysine
physical and chemical properties, **01:** 143
N-(Indole-3-acetyl)-aspartic acid
physical and chemical properties, **01:** 142
Indole-3-glycerol phosphate
synthetase
amino acid composition, complete data, **07:** 508
Indoleacrylic acid
antagonism to tryptophan, **01:** 179
β-Indolypyruvic acid
properties of, **01:** 182
Indospicine
physical and chemical properties, **01:** 134
Inhibitor, *see also* Inhibitors, Repressor
deoxyribonuclease •
amino acid composition, complete data, **07:** 506
molar absorptivity and-or absorbance values, **02:** 418
dPNase •
carbohydrate content, **02:** 274
kallikrein •
mammalian and chicken blood, specificity and properties, **02:** 638-639
mammalian organs and secretions, specificity and properties, **02:** 630-631
plant sources, amino acid composition, **02:** 606
potato tuber sources, specificity and properties, **02:** 586-587
Kunitz •
legume sources, specificity and properties, **02:** 588-589
mammalian organs and secretions, specificity and properties, **02:** 630-631
plant sources, amino acid composition, **02:** 606
myxovirus hemagglutination •
amino acid composition, incomplete data, **07:** 513
soybean trypsin •
refractive index increments, **02:** 380
soybean trypsin • F_3
amino acid composition, complete data, **07:** 510
troponin • (Tn-I), rabbit skeletal
amino acid sequence, **07:** 494
trypsin-trypsin • complex
molar absorptivity and-or absorbance values, **02:** 511
urokinase •
mammalian organs and secretions, specificities and properties, **02:** 632-641
Inhibitor, protease, *see also* Protease inhibitor
Inhibitor I, II
trypsin •
average hydrophobicity value, **01:** 234
Inhibitor II
deoxyribonucleotidase •
average hydrophobicity value, **01:** 218
Inhibitors, *see also* Inhibitor
human serum, *see also* Serum, human; proteinase •
from, specificity and properties, **02:** 636-641
pepsin •
animal sources, amino acid composition, **02:** 649
lower animal sources, specificity and properties, **02:** 618-619
prostaglandin metabolizing enzymes, **08:** 364-367
Inhibitors, proteinase, *see* Proteinase inhibitors

Iodine *(continued)*
　value
　　fats and oils, table of values, **05**: 502-503
　　fatty acids, **05**: 485-491
　　herring oils and Pacific pilchard oils, **05**: 523-524
　　vegetable oils, **05**: 512
Iodoacetamide
　inhibition of transamidase activity, **02**: 672
Iodogorgoic acid, *see* 3,5-Diiodotyrosine
Ion
　amino acids, *see also* Aromatic amino acids, *also*
　　　specific acids; chromatography, • exchange
　　ninhydrin positive compounds, elution behavior, **08**:
　　　122
　　thumbprint, constituents of, **08**: 121
　　urine, resolution of ninhydrin positive constituents, **08**:
　　　114-119
　　variables, mathematical relationships, **08**: 112-113
　chromatography; • exchange, amino acids
　　ninhydrin positive compounds, elution behavior, **08**:
　　　122
　　thumbprint, constituents of, **08**: 121
　　urine, resolution of ninhydrin positive constituents, **08**:
　　　114-119
　　variables, mathematical relationship, **08**: 112-113
Ion exchangers
　cellulosic, properties, **08**: 136-138
Ions, *see also* Anions
　absorbance; transmission limits of common •, **08**: 196
　albumin, plasma, *see also* Human plasma albumin;
　　　Plasma albumin; ligand binding; metal •, list of re-
　　　ferences, **02**: 563
　common, transmission limits, **08**: 196
　metal •, ligands binding to plasma albumin, **02**: 563
　spectra; transmission limits of common •, **08**: 196
IPM
　isomerase
　　Neurospora crassa mutant, **04**: 740
α-IPM
　synthetase
　　Neurospora crassa mutant, **04**: 740
β-IPM
　dehydrogenase
　　Neurospora crassa mutant, **04**: 740, 746
Iron
　adrenal •-sulfur protein
　　amino acid composition, complete data, **07**: 505
　high-potential •-sulfur protein
　　circular dichroism in near UV region, at room temper-
　　　ature, **07**: 154
　molybdenum-• protein
　　average hydrophobicity value, **01**: 227
　proteins, *see also* Bacteriophage Flavoproteins, Matrix
　　　protein, *also* Protein, individual proteins, Molybdo-
　　　proteins; •, classification of, **02**: 90
　proteins, •-sulfur primary structures
　　amino acid sequences, **07**: 425-427

-sulfur proteins
　resonance raman spectra, **07**: 589
Iron protein, *see* High potential iron protein
Iron-sulfur proteins, *see also* Iron; Proteins, iron-sulfur
　high potential • protein
　　average hydrophobicity value, **01**: 224
　nomenclature recommendations, **02**: 89-90
　table of cofactors, molecular weights, stoichiometry and
　　　sources, **02**: 278-280
Iron transport
　proteins
　　resonance raman spectra, **07**: 589
Isoamylase I, II
　average hydrophobicity value, **01**: 225
Isoasparagine
　structure and symbols for those incorporated into syn-
　　　thetic polypeptides, **01**: 104
Isocitrate
　dehydrogenase
　　amino acid composition, complete data, **07**: 508
　　average hydrophobicity value, **01**: 225
　　circular dichroism in the UV region, **07**: 106
　　molar absorptivity and-or absorbance values, **02**: 458
　　optical rotatory dispersion
　　　UV region, **07**: 64
　　　visible and near UV regions, **07**: 28
　lyase
　　amino acid composition, complete data, **07**: 508
　　Neurospora crassa mutant, **04**: 752
Isocytosine, 6-amino-5-*N*-methylformamido
　physical constants and spectral properties, **03**: 82
Isocytosine, 5-*N*-methylformamido-6-ribosylamino-
　physical constants and spectral properties, **03**: 116
Isodesmosine
　physical and chemical properties, **01**: 163
Isoenzymes
　definition of, **02**: 84
　nomenclature of, **02**: 84-86
Isoglutamine
　structure and symbols for those incorporated into syn-
　　　thetic polypeptides, **01**: 104
Isoguanine
　physical constants and spectral properties, **03**: 77
Isoguanosine
　physical constants and spectral properties, **03**: 99
Isolectin
　content, purified lectins, **02**: 547-551
Isoleucine
　antagonism to leucine, **01**: 178
　antagonism to valine, **01**: 180
　antagonists of, **01**: 178
　free acid in amniotic fluid in early pregnancy and at
　　　term, **01**: 327
　free acid in blood plasma of newborn infants and
　　　adults, **01**: 328
　maple syrup urine disease (intermittent form), effect of,
　　　01: 319

α-Ketophenylacetic acid
properties of, **01:** 181
4-Ketopipecolic acid
physical and chemical properties, **01:** 143
4-Ketoproline
physical and chemical properties, **01:** 143
Ketoses
natural
chemical formula, **05:** 226-239
chromatography, **05:** 226-239
melting point, **05:** 226-239
specific rotation, **05:** 226-239
nomenclature rules, **05:** 106-107
Δ^5-3-Ketosteroid
isomerase
amino acid composition, complete data, **07:** 508
average hydrophobicity value, **01:** 225
α-Ketosuccinamic acid
properties of, **01:** 181
α-Ketovaleric acid
properties of, **01:** 182
Kinase
adenylate •
amino acid composition, complete data, **07:** 505
optical rotatory dispersion
UV region, **07:** 45
visible and near UV regions, **07:** 16
arginine •
amino acid composition, complete data, **07:** 505
circular dichroism
in UV and near UV region, **07:** 85, 143
molar absorptivity and-or absorbance values, **02:** 395
optical rotatory dispersion
UV region, **07:** 47
visible and near UV regions, **07:** 17
arginine •, average hydrophobicity values, **01:** 214
carbamate •
amino acid composition, complete data, **07:** 505
creatine •
average hydrophobicity value, **01:** 217
circular dichroism
UV and near-UV region, **07:** 90, 148
molar absorptivity and-or absorbance values, **02:** 409
optical rotatory dispersion
UV region, **07:** 52
visible and near UV regions, **07:** 21
subunit, constitution of, **02:** 330
guanidinoacetate •
optical rotatory dispersion in the visible and near UV regions, **07:** 25
lombricine •
circular dichroism, **07:** 110
UV and near-UV region, **07:** 110, 156
molar absorptivity and-or absorbance values, **02:** 467
optical rotatory dispersion
UV region, **07:** 66
visible and near UV regions, **07:** 29
phosphocreatine •
phosphoglycerate •
average hydrophobicity value, **01:** 229
circular dichroism in the UV region, **07:** 118

3-phosphoglycerate •
optical rotatory dispersion in the UV region: extrema between 185 and 250 NM[3], **07:** 71
phosphorylase •
molar absorptivity and-or absorbance values, **02:** 497
subunit, constitution of, **02:** 350
protein •
subunit, constitution of, **02:** 344
pyruvate •
amino acid composition, complete data, **07:** 510
average hydrophobicity value, **01:** 230
circular dichroism
UV and near UV region, **07:** 121, 160
molar absorptivity and-or absorbance values, **02:** 504
optical rotatory dispersion
UV region, **07:** 73
visible and near UV regions, **07:** 34
rabbit
luminescence of, table, **01:** 206
subunit, constitution of, **02:** 340, 341, 342, 343
shikimic acid •
Neurospora crassa mutant, **04:** 745
taurocyamine •
circular dichroism, **07:** 124
UV and near-UV region, **07:** 161
molar absorptivity and-or absorbance values, **02:** 509
optical rotatory dispersion
UV region, **07:** 75
visible and near UV regions, **07:** 36
subunit, constitution of, **02:** 331
Kinase modulator
protein •
average hydrophobicity value, **01:** 230
Kininogen
cyanogen bromide cleavage, **02:** 199
molecular parameters, **02:** 245
Kininogenase, *see* Kininogenin
Kininogenin
circular dichroism in the UV region, **07:** 107
Kirromycin
(Mocimycin), origin, structure, and characteristic as protein biosynthesis inhibitor, **04:** 581
Kunitz
inhibitor
legume sources, specificity and properties, **02:** 588-589
mammalian organs and secretions, specificity and properties, **02:** 630-631
plant sources, amino acid composition, **02:** 606
Kynurenine
physical and chemical properties, **01:** 131

L

Labile aggregation stimulating
substances, *see* LASS
Lac
repressor
circular dichroism, **07:** 107
repressor
molar absorptivity and-or absorbance values, **02:** 460
subunit, constitution of, **02:** 338

Laccase B
circular dichroism
UV and near UV-region, **07**: 107, 155
α-Lactalbumin
amino acid sequence, **07**: 499
average hydrophobicity value, **01**: 225
circular dichroism
UV and near UV-region, **07**: 155
cyanogen bromide cleavage, **02**: 199
luminescence of, table, **01**: 206
molar absorptivity and-or absorbance values, **02**: 460
optical rotatory dispersion, **07**: 61
UV region, **07**: 64
visible and near UV regions, **07**: 28
refractive index increments, **02**: 377
β-Lactamase I, *see* Penicillinase
β-Lactamase I, II
molar absorptivity and-or absorbance values, **02**: 461
β-Lactamase II, *see* Cephalosporinase
Lactate
dehydrogenase
amino acid sequence, **07**: 320-321, 336-337
circular dichroism
UV and near UV-region, **07**: 107-108, 155
luminescence of, table, **01**: 206
molar absorptivity and-or absorbance values, **02**: 461-462
optical rotatory dispersion
UV region, **07**: 64
visible and near UV regions, **07**: 28-29
subunit, constitution of, **02**: 337
dehydrogenase, dogfish
structure, illustration, **02**: 766
dehydrogenase (cytochrome b_2)
circular dichroism in near-UV region, at room temperature, **07**: 148-155
malate-• transhydrogenase
molar absorptivity and-or absorbance values, **02**: 470
subunit structures; dogfish • dehydrogenase, illustration, **02**: 766
D-Lactate
dehydrogenase
amino acid composition, complete data, **07**: 508
Lactic
dehydrogenase
reduction of α-Keto acid, **01**: 181-182
refractive index increments, **02**: 377
Lactic acid
pK'_a values, **06**: 310
Lactic acid dehydrogenase, *see* Lactate, dehydrogenase
Lactoferrin
average hydrophobicity value, **01**: 225
circular dichroism in the UV region, **07**: 108
molar absorptivity and-or absorbance values, **02**: 462
molecular parameters, **02**: 250
optical rotatory dispersion in the visible and near UV regions, **07**: 29
Lactogen
placental •, human
amino acid sequence compared with human growth hormone and human prolactin, **07**: 392-393

Lactogen (MPL-2)
hormone, *see also* Luteinizing hormone; •
molar absorptivity and-or absorbance values, **02**: 450
Lactogenic
hormone
amino acid sequence, **07**: 390-392
circular dichroism
UV and near UV-region, **07**: 108, 156
β-Lactoglobulin
amino acid composition, complete data, **07**: 508
average hydrophobicity value, **01**: 225
circular dichroism
UV and near-UV region, **07**: 108, 156
molar absorptivity and-or absorbance values, **02**: 462-463
optical rotatory dispersion
UV region, **07**: 65
visible and near UV regions, **07**: 29
raman spectrum; •, native and denatured, **07**: 582
refractive index increments, **02**: 377
subunit, constitution of, **02**: 327
viscosity, intrinsic, **02**: 721
β-Lactoglobulin A
average hydrophobicity values, **01**: 225
luminescence of, table, **01**: 206
β-Lactoglobulin AB
bovine
luminescence of, table, **01**: 206
β-Lactoglobulin B and C
average hydrophobicity values, **01**: 225
Lactollin
amino acid composition, complete data, **07**: 508
Lactoperoxidase
amino acid composition, complete data, **07**: 508
average hydrophobicity value, **01**: 225
carbohydrate content, **02**: 274
molar absorptivity and-or absorbance values, **02**: 463
Lactose
synthetase, A protein
molar absorptivity and-or absorbance values, **02**: 463
synthetase (A protein)
circular dichroism in the UV region, **07**: 108
Lactosiderophilin
lactotransferrin, human milk
molar absorptivity and-or absorbance values, **02**: 463
Lactosomatotropin
circular dichroism in the UV region, **07**: 108
Lactotransferrin
carbohydrate content, **02**: 269
lactosiderophilin •, human milk
molar absorptivity and-or absorbance values, **02**: 463
molecular weight, stoichiometry, source, function, **02**: 276
Laminine
physical and chemical properties, **01**: 163
Lankamycin
origin, structure, and characteristic as protein biosynthesis inhibitor, **04**: 582
Lanthionine
physical and chemical properties, **01**: 156
LASS
biological activity of, **08**: 332

Ligands *(continued)*

barbiturates, • binding to plasma albumin, **02:** 569

binding to plasma albumin, table, **02:** 556-574

caffeine, • binding to plasma albumin, **02:** 573

cardiac glycosides, • binding to plasma albumin, **02:** 572

diuretics; • binding to plasma albumin, **02:** 571

drugs, • binding to plasma albumin, **02:** 568-574

dyes, visible, • binding to plasma albumin, **02:** 564-568

endogenous • binding to plasma albumin, **02:** 556-557

exogenous • binding to plasma albumin, **02:** 558-574

fatty acids, • binding to plasma albumin, **02:** 558-562

hypoglycemic agents, • binding to plasma albumin, **02:** 572

inorganic anions, • binding to plasma albumin, **02:** 563

metal ions, • binding to plasma albumin, **02:** 563

methadone, • binding to plasma albumin, **02:** 574

procaine, • binding to plasma albumin, **02:** 574

radio-opaque agents, • binding to plasma albumin, **02:** 572

saccharin, • binding to plasma albumin, **02:** 574

steroids; • binding to plasma albumin, **02:** 563

sulfonamides; • binding to plasma albumin, **02:** 568

tranquilizers; • binding to plasma albumin, **02:** 571

warfarin, • binding to plasma albumin, **02:** 572

Ligase

deoxyribonucleic acid •

average hydrophobicity value, **01:** 218

lysyl: tRNA •

average hydrophobicity value, **01:** 226

valine:tRNA •

average hydrophobicity value, **01:** 235

Ligases

definition and nomenclature, **02:** 98

numbering and classification of, **02:** 108

Light merromyosin (LMM), *see* Myosin, LMM

Lincomycin

origin, structure, and characteristic as protein biosynthesis inhibitor, **04:** 583

Linolenic acid

trivial names; • isomers, usage, **08:** 316

Linseed oil acids

molecular weight; • and esters, **05:** 497

monomolecular film measurements; • and esters, force-area data, **05:** 497

refractive index; • and esters, **05:** 497

Lipase, *see* Triacylglycerol, lipase

average hydrophobicity value, **01:** 225

carbohydrate content, **02:** 274

enzymatic activity, subcellular fractions, **02:** 698, 711, 714

molar absorptivity and-or absorbance values, **02:** 466

triacylglycerol •

circular dichroism in the UV region, **07:** 125

optical rotatory dispersion

UV region, **07:** 76

visible and near UV regions, **07:** 36

Lipid

fatty acids, *see also* Lipids, Wax fatty acids; wax esters and sterol esters from vernix caseosa and from human skin surface •, **05:** 509

human skin; • composition of various parts of adult, **05:** 507

metabolism; pathways chart, **04:** insert

vernix caseosa; •, fatty acids from wax esters and sterol esters, **05:** 509-510

Lipids

adult human skin, composition of various parts, **05:** 507

animal tissues, content of total, of cholesteryl esters and of phospholipids, **05:** 519-520

beeswax fractions, composition of acids of, **05:** 504

chain length composition, herring oils and pilchard oils, **05:** 525

fatty acids, *see also* Lipids, Wax fatty acids; composition in plasma and erythrocyte •, effect of dietary fat, **05:** 522

generic terms, for •, **05:** 9-10

glycolipids

classification and nomenclature of, **05:** 416-423

of bacteria, structures and organisms, **05:** 373-393

glycosidic, miscellaneous, structures and organisms, **05:** 388-390

herring oil, monethylenic isomer content in partially hydrogenated, **05:** 513

human skin surface, fatty acids of wax esters and sterol esters, **05:** 509

human skin surface, type and amount of fatty acid, **05:** 508

isomers, monoethylenic; content in rat cardiac •, **05:** 513

mass spectra of methyl esters of alkenyl branched chain acids, intensities of key fragments, **05:** 517

mass spectrum of α-toctrienol-TMS derivative, **05:** 520

methyl octadecadienoates and octadecatrienoates, equivalent chain lengths, **05:** 505

nomenclature; •

list of generic terms, **05:** 9-10

stereospecific, use of, **05:** 10

use of trivial names, **05:** 9-12

nomenclature, journal references for, **02:** 87

polyol esters, properties, **05:** 515

properties of interest, comparison of, for herring oils and pilchard oil, **05:** 526-527

rat cardiac, monoethylenic isomer content, **05:** 513

solubility of selected, in chlorinated hydrocarbon solvents, **05:** 514

solubility of selected, in chlorinated hydrocarbon mixtures with 33% methanol, **05:** 514

solubility of selected, in organic solvents, **05:** 512

stereospecific nomenclature, •, **05:** 10

surface areas for pure methyl esters and triglycerides, **05:** 515

trivial names, use of, **05:** 9-12

vegetable oils, % content unsaponifiables, **05:** 512

vegetable oils, individual tocopherol contents, **05:** 512

Lipoamide

dehydrogenase (NADH)

amino acid composition, complete data, **07:** 508

circular dichroism in the UV region, **07:** 108

optical rotatory dispersion

UV region, **07:** 65

visible and near UV regions, **07:** 29

Lipoate
  succinyltransferase
    circular dichroism in the UV region, **07:** 108
    optical rotatory dispersion in the UV region, **07:** 65
γ-Lipolytic
  hormone
    average hydrophobicity value, **01:** 225
β-Lipolytic
  hormone
    average hydrophobicity value, **01:** 225
Lipopolysaccharides
  Escherichia coli, see also E. coli; • of
    sugar composition for O-type, **05:** 396-399
    sugar sequences, general structures, **05:** 406, 409-411
  of gram-negative bacteria
    sugar composition, **05:** 396-402
    sugar sequences, general structure, **05:** 403-412
  receptor
    circular dichroism in the UV region, **07:** 109
  salmonella; • of
    sugar composition for O-group, **05:** 396-399
    sugar sequences, general structures, **05:** 403-406, 409, 412
Lipoprotein
  amino acid composition, complete data, **07:** 508
  amino acid composition, incomplete data, **07:** 513
  apo-high density •
    average hydrophobicity value, **01:** 214
  circular dichroism in the UV region, **07:** 109
  high density
    subunit, constitution of, **02:** 347
  optical rotatory dispersion
    UV region, **07:** 65
    visible and near UV regions, **07:** 29
  very low density, human ApoLP-Val
    molar absorptivity and-or absorbance values, **02:** 467
  very low density, rat serum
    molar absorptivity and-or absorbance values, **02:** 467
$α_1$-Lipoprotein
  molecular parameters, **02:** 242
  refractive index increments, **02:** 378
$α_2$-Lipoprotein
  molecular parameters, **02:** 245
β-Lipoprotein
  molecular parameters, **02:** 247
  refractive index increments, **02:** 378
$β_1$-Lipoprotein
  refractive index increments, **02:** 378
Lipoprotein B
  amino acid sequence, **07:** 387, 499
  circular dichroism in the UV region, **07:** 110
  optical rotatory dispersion
    UV region, **07:** 65
    visible and near UV regions, **07:** 29
Lipoprotein HDL_2
  human
    molar absorptivity and-or absorbance values, **02:** 467
Lipovitellin
  circular dichroism in the UV region, **07:** 110
  molar absorptivity and-or absorbance values, **02:** 467

optical rotatory dispersion in the UV region, **07:** 66
  refractive index increments, **02:** 379
  subunit, constitution of, **02:** 347
α-Lipovitellin
  average hydrophobicity value, **01:** 225
Lipoyl dehydrogenase, *see* Lipoamide, dehydrogenase (NADH)
Liquids
  refractive index; •, table of values, **06:** 408-410
  specific gravity; •, table of values, **06:** 411-414
Lithium bromide
  refractive index; • versus concentration, **06:** 387
Liver
  alcohol dehydrogenase
    amino acid sequence, **07:** 330-332
α-Livetin
  refractive index increments, **02:** 379
γ-Livetin
  refractive index increments, **02:** 379
β-Livetin
  refractive index increments, **02:** 379
Lividomycin
  origin, structure, and characteristic as protein biosynthesis inhibitor, **04:** 583
Lombricine
  kinase
    circular dichroism, **07:** 110
      UV and near-UV region, **07:** 110, 156
    molar absorptivity and-or absorbance values, **02:** 467
    optical rotatory dispersion
      UV region, **07:** 66
      visible and near UV regions, **07:** 29
  physical and chemical properties, **01:** 161
Long-chain aliphatic acids
  molecular dimensions, • and related compounds, **05:** 498
Long chain base
  generic term usage, **05:** 9
Long neurotoxins, *see* Neurotoxins, long
Luciferase
  average hydrophobicity values, **01:** 226
  chain α
    amino acid composition, complete data, **07:** 508
    subunit, constitution of, **02:** 330, 332
Luteinizing
  hormone-α chain
    average hydrophobicity value, **01:** 226
  hormone-β chain
    average hydrophobicity value, **01:** 226
Luteinizing hormone, **07:** 30, 66
  amino acid sequence
    α subunit, **07:** 393-394
    β subunit, **07:** 395-397
  carbohydrate content, **02:** 272-273
  circular dichroism
    UV and near-UV region, **07:** 106, 156
  molar absorptivity and-or absorbance values, **02:** 468
2,6-Lutidine-water system
  hemin; R_F value in •, **08:** 276

2,6-Lutidine-water systems
  chromatography; porphyrins R_F values in •, **08:** 276
  porphyrins; R_F values in •, **08:** 276
Lyase
  adenylosuccinate-AMP-•
    average hydrophobicity value, **01:** 212
  alliin •
    molar absorptivity and-or absorbance values, **02:** 391
  citrate oxaloacetate •
    amino acid composition, incomplete data, **07:** 512
  definition and nomenclature, **02:** 98
  histidine ammonia •
    average hydrophobicity value, **01:** 224
    molar absorptivity and-or absorbance values, **02:** 448
  isocitrate •
    amino acid composition, complete data, **07:** 508
    Neurospora crassa mutant, **04:** 752
  numbering and classification of, **02:** 108
  phenylalanine ammonia •
    average hydrophobicity value, **01:** 229
  1-phenylalanine ammonia •
    molar absorptivity and-or absorbance values, **02:** 492
Lycin
  physical and chemical properties, **01:** 163
Lycopene
  UV spectra, formula, molecular weight, **08:** 189
Lymphocytes
  immunological response, **07:** 536-537
  mitogenic activity on •, purified lectins, **02:** 547-551
Lys_n
  raman spectrum; •, **07:** 579
Lysergic acid
  pK'_a values, **06:** 313, 326
Lysin
  molar absorptivity and-or absorbance values, **02:** 468
Lysine
  active site peptides, **07:** 188
  antagonism to arginine, **01:** 177
  antagonists of, **01:** 178
  aspartokinase, • sensitive
    average hydrophobicity value, **01:** 215
  decarboxylase
    average hydrophobicity value, **01:** 226
    molar absorptivity and-or absorbance values, **02:** 468
    subunit, constitution of, **02:** 349
  endo-γ-glutamine: ε-• transferase
    transamilase activity, discussion and data, **02:** 669-683
  far ultraviolet absorption spectra
    aqueous solution at pH 5, **01:** 184
    neutral water, table, **01:** 185
    0.1 M sodium dodecyl sulfate, table, **01:** 185
  free acid in amniotic fluid in early pregnancy and at
    term, **01:** 327
  free acid in blood plasma in newborn infants and
    adults, **01:** 328
  heat of proton ionization, pK, and related thermody-
    namic quantities, **06:** 215
  hyperlysinemia, effect of, **01:** 320
  metabolism; pathways chart, **04:** insert
  nucleoside composition, tables of values, **04:** 434
  nucleotide sequences of, **04:** 446-447
  pK'_a values, **06:** 319

physical and chemical properties, **01:** 121
requirements of, for growth of various microorganisms,
  table, **04:** 630-643
specific rotatory dispersion constants, 0.1 M solution,
  01: 244
spectra, far UV, **01:** 184
symbols for atoms and bonds in side chains, **01:** 69, **02:**
  73
thumbprint, content in, **08:** 121
tRNA synthetase
  subunit, constitution of, **02:** 336
vasopressin, •
  average hydrophobicity value, **01:** 235
L-Lysine
  monooxygenase
    amino acid composition, complete data, **07:** 508
    average hydrophobicity value, **01:** 226
β-Lysine, *see also* 3,6-Diaminohexanoic acid
  mutase
    subunit, constitution of, **02:** 339
Lysine-vasopressin
  amino acid sequence, physical and biological properties,
    07: 197-198
Lysopine
  physical and chemical properties, **01:** 121
Lysosomes
  enzymatic activity, table, **02:** 711
  molecular parameters, **02:** 250
Lysostaphin
  amino acid composition, incomplete data, **07:** 513
  average hydrophobicity value, **01:** 226
Lysozyme
  amino acid composition, complete data, **07:** 508
  amino acid sequences of proteins, **07:** 309
  average hydrophobicity values, **01:** 226
  calorimetric ΔH values accompanying conformational
    changes, **06:** 273
  circular dichroism
    UV and near-UV region, **07:** 111, 157
  cyanogen bromide cleavage, **02:** 199
  egg white
    luminescence of, table, **01:** 206
  molar absorptivity and-or absorbance values, **02:** 468,
    469
  optical rotatory dispersion
    UV region, **07:** 66
    visible and near UV regions, **07:** 30
  pK; carboxyl side chain, values estimated in •, **02:** 696
  refractive index increments, **02:** 379
  viscosity, intrinsic, **02:** 721
Lysyl
  : tRNA ligase
    average hydrophobicity value, **01:** 226
  tRNA synthetase
    molar absorptivity and-or absorbance values, **02:** 469
Lysylaminoadenosine
  physicochemical constants, spectral, chemotherapeutic
    and biological properties, **03:** 328
α-Lytic
  protease
    average hydrophobicity value, **01:** 226

Me₂ SO-chymotrypsin
  calorimetric ΔH values accompanying conformational
    changes, **06:** 274
Media
  Bacillus; standard ● for growth of, **04:** 649
  Bacillus subtilis; standard ● for growth of, **04:** 649
  Bio-Gel A® filtration ●, table of properties, **08:** 130
  Bio-Gel P® filtration ●, table of properties, **08:** 131-132
  Escherichia; standard ● for growth, **04:** 649
  gel filtration ●
    Bio-Gel A®, properties, **08:** 130
    Bio-Gel P®, properties, **08:** 131-132
    Sephadex®, properties, **08:** 133-134
    Sepharose®, properties, **08:** 135
  microorganisms; growth of, standard ● for, **04:** 649
  salmonella; standard ● for growth of, **04:** 649
  Sephadex® filtration ●, table of properties, **08:** 133-134
  Sepharose® filtration ●, table of properties, **08:** 135
Medium
  Davis's minimal ●, preparation of, **04:** 649
  microorganisms; sugar fermentation, preparation of
    EMB ● for detecting, **04:** 650
  Vogel and Bonner minimal ●, preparation of, **04:** 649
β-Melanocyte stimulating
  hormone
    average hydrophobicity value, **01:** 226
Melanotropin
  amino acid sequence
    α, **07:** 385
    natural, **07:** 375
    β, **07:** 386
Membrane
  fluorescent probes; commonly used for ● studies,
    properties, **07:** 608-610
  glycoproteins; cell ●
    carbohydrate content, **02:** 266
  protein
    circular dichroism in the UV region, **07:** 112
  protein, mitochondria
    circular dichroism in the UV region, **07:** 112
    optical rotatory dispersion
      UV region, **07:** 66
      visible and near UV regions, **07:** 30
  protein, mycoplasma
    circular dichroism in the UV region, **07:** 112
  protein, purple
    circular dichroism in the UV region, **07:** 112
  protein, thylakoid
    circular dichroism in the UV region, **07:** 113
Menaquinone
  melting point; ●, properties of, **08:** 291
Mercaptalbumin
  calorimetric ΔH values accompanying conformational
    changes, **06:** 270
α-Mercaptoalanine
  structure and symbols for those incorporated into syn-
    thetic polypeptides, **01:** 104
β-Mercaptolactate-cysteine disulfide
  β-mercaptolactate cysteinuria, effect of, **01:** 317
  physical and chemical properties, **01:** 156
β-Mercaptolactate cysteinuria, effect of
  β-mercaptolactate-cysteine disulfide; ●, **01:** 317

β-Mercaptopyruvic acid
  properties of, **01:** 181
β-Mercaptovaline, *see* β,β-Dimethylcysteine
Merodesmosine
  physical and chemical properties, **01:** 149
Mesaconate
  pathway; pathways chart, **04:** insert
Mesotocin
  amino acid sequence, **07:** 195
Mesoxalic acid
  properties of, **01:** 181
Metabolites
  cortisol ● binding large protein
    amino acid composition, incomplete data, **07:** 512
  formula, molecular; prostaglandin ●, **08:** 368-391
  molecular weight; prostaglandin ●, **08:** 368-391
  prostaglandins; ●, table of physical and biological
    properties, **08:** 368-391
  structure; prostaglandin ●, **08:** 368-391
Metal
  amino acids, *see also* Aromatic amino acids, *also*
    specific acids; circular dichroism spectra of ● com-
    plexes of, **01:** 245-315
  complexes of amino acids and peptides, circular
    dichroism spectra, **01:** 245-315
  ions, ligands binding to plasma albumin, **02:** 563
  requirement, purified lectins, **02:** 547-551
Metalloenzyme
  cofactors, molecular weights, stoichiometry and sources,
    02: 278-286
  microbial ●
    amino acid sequence, **07:** 322
    optical rotatory dispersion
      UV region, **07:** 67
      visible and near UV regions, **07:** 30
Metalloporphyrins
  absorption data table, **08:** 279
  methyl esters
    absorption spectra, **08:** 278
    Soret band data using organic solvents, **08:** 278
  oxidation-reduction potentials, **06:** 139-144
Metalloprotein
  model systems
    resonance raman spectra, **07:** 590
  molecular weight, source, stoichiometry, function, **02:**
    276-277
  nomenclature rules, **02:** 121
Metallothionein (Cd, Zn-thionein)
  circular dichroism in the UV region, **07:** 113
Metapyrocatechase, *see* Catechol 2,3, -dioxygenase
  molar absorptivity and-or absorbance values, **02:** 472
  table of cofactors, molecular weights, stoichiometry and
    sources, **02:** 280
Metazoan globins, *see* Globins, metazoan, aligned chains
Methadone
  ligands binding to plasma albumin, **02:** 574
Methallylglycine
  antagonism to isoleucine, **01:** 178
  antagonism to leucine, **01:** 178
  antagonism to valine, **01:** 180

Mixtures *(continued)*
  N-N-dimethylformamide-water •, dielectric constants and freezing points, **06:** 528
  dimethylsulfoxide-water •, dielectric constants and freezing points, **06:** 527
Mo
  -Fe Protein
    subunit, constitution of, **02:** 340
Mocimycin, *see also* Kirromycin
  kirromycin (•), origin, structure, and characteristic as protein biosynthesis inhibitor, **04:** 581
Model compounds
  tyrosinate •
    near-UV circular dichroism intensities, **07:** 171-172
Molecular conformations,
  polynucleotide double helices, **04:** 411-418
Molecular map
  Escherichia coli bacteriophage lambda (λ), **04:** 678
Molecule
  achiral •, nomenclature for, **02:** 36-58, **03:** 28-33, **04:** 28-33, **05:** 33-38, **06:** 35, **08:** 35-40
  achiral • nomenclature for, **01:** 36-58
  conformer • in stereochemistry, **01:** 42-46, **02:** 42-46, **04:** 34-38, **06:** 41, **08:** 41-49
  DNA, *see also* Deoxyribonucleic acid; lambda • of *Escherichia coli*, genetic and molecular map, **04:** 678
  Moffitt equation; for estimate or content in protein •, **07:** 3-4
  protein, *see also* Bacteriophage protein, Conjugated proteins, Covalent protein conjugates, Covalent conjugates, Flavoproteins, Glycoprotein listings, Human plasma proteins, Iron proteins, Iron-sulfur proteins, Lipoprotein, Matrix protein, Metalloproteins, Molybdoproteins, Mucoprotein, Plasma proteins, human, Proteins, conjugated, Proteins, iron-sulfur, Serum proteins, Tamm-Horsfall, Tamm-Horsfall glycoproteins, Tamm-Horsfall mucoprotein, *also* Proteins; quaternary structure of a •, definition, **02:** 77
  protein, *see also* Bacteriophage protein, Conjugated proteins, Covalent protein conjugates, Covalent conjugates, Flavoproteins, Glycoprotein listings, Human plasma proteins, Iron proteins, Iron-sulfur proteins, Lipoprotein, Matrix protein, Metalloproteins, Molybdoproteins, Mucoprotein, Plasma proteins, human, Proteins, conjugated, Proteins, iron-sulfur, Serum proteins, Tamm-Horsfall, Tamm-Horsfall glycoproteins, Tamm-Horsfall mucoprotein, *also* Proteins; quaternary structure of a •, definition, **01:** 73
  protein, *see also* Bacteriophage protein, Conjugated proteins, Covalent protein conjugates, Covalent conjugates, Flavoproteins, Glycoprotein listings, Human plasma proteins, Iron proteins, Iron-sulfur proteins, Lipoprotein, Matrix protein, Metalloproteins, Molybdoproteins, Mucoprotein, Plasma proteins, human, Proteins, conjugated, Proteins, iron-sulfur, Serum proteins, Tamm-Horsfall, Tamm-Horsfall glycoproteins, Tamm-Horsfall mucoprotein, *also* Proteins; tertiary structure of a •, definition, **02:** 77

protein, *see also* Bacteriophage protein, Conjugated proteins, Covalent protein conjugates, Covalent conjugates, Flavoproteins, Glycoprotein listings, Human plasma proteins, Iron proteins, Iron-sulfur proteins, Lipoprotein, Matrix protein, Metalloproteins, Molybdoproteins, Mucoprotein, Plasma proteins, human, Proteins, conjugated, Proteins, iron-sulfur, Serum proteins, Tamm-Horsfall, Tamm-Horsfall glycoproteins, Tamm-Horsfall mucoprotein, *also* Proteins; tertiary structure of •, definition, **01:** 73
yeast phenylalanine transfer RNA; •, side views of, **04:** 459
Molecules
  DNA, *see also* Deoxyribonucleic acid; viral •, composition and physical properties, **03:** 552-556
Molybdenum
  -iron protein
    average hydrophobicity value, **01:** 227
Molybdoproteins
  nomenclature rules, **02:** 121
Monellin
  average hydrophobicity value, **01:** 227
  molar absorptivity and-or absorbance values, **02:** 472
Monethylenic isomer
  lipids; herring oil, • content in partially hydrogenated, **05:** 513
Monoamine
  oxidase
    amino acid composition, complete data, **07:** 509
    carbohydrate content, **02:** 273, 274
    molar absorptivity and-or absorbance values, **02:** 473
    subunit, constitution of, **02:** 335, 345, 350
    table of cofactors, molecular weights, stoichiometry, and sources, **02:** 282
L-Monoamino, dicarboxylic acids
  physical and chemical properties, **01:** 116-119
L-Monoamino, monocarboxylic acids
  physical and chemical properties, **01:** 112-115
3-Monobromo-5-monochlorotyrosine
  physical and chemical properties, **01:** 160
3-Monobromotyrosine
  physical and chemical properties, **01:** 160
Monochlorotyrosine
  physical and chemical properties, **01:** 160
Monoesters
  fatty acids, *see also* Lipids, Wax fatty acids; alkyl • of carboxylic acid, refractive index, **05:** 494
Monoethylenic isomer
  lipids; rat cardiac, • content, **05:** 513
2-Monoiodohistidine
  physical and chemical properties, **01:** 160
Monoiodotyrosine
  physical and chemical properties, **01:** 160
Monomer
  molecular weight; nonmuscle actin, of •, **02:** 314-315
Mononucleotides
  chemical shifts, **03:** 530
  coupling constants (Hz) of the H1' and H2' protons, **03:** 530
  ultraviolet absorbance, **03:** 405-406
  ultraviolet absorbance, in 7 M urea, **03:** 407

Mononucleotides *(continued)*
  ultraviolet absorbance in 97% D_2O, **03:** 408
  ultraviolet absorbance in 90% v-v ethylene glycol, **03:** 408
Monooxygenase
  l-lysine ●
    amino acid composition, complete data, **07:** 508
    average hydrophobicity value, **01:** 226
  monophenol ●
    amino acid composition, complete data, **07:** 511
    circular dichroism in the UV region, **07:** 113
3-Monooxygenase
  4-hydroxybenzoate ● (*p*-hydroxybenzoate hydroxylase)
    circular dichroism in near UV region, at room temperature, **07:** 154
    optical rotatory dispersion in the UV region, **07:** 61
Monophenol
  monooxygenase
    amino acid composition, complete data, **07:** 511
    circular dichroism in the UV region, **07:** 113
Monophosphate succinate synthetase
  adenosine; ●
    neurospora crassa mutant, **04:** 753
Monophosphates
  dinucleoside
    mean residue absorptivities, table of values, **03:** 597
    molar residue ellipticities, table of values, **03:** 600
    molar residue rotations, table of values, **03:** 598
2,3-Monophosphates, nucleoside
  molar absorptivity, table of values, **03:** 597
Monosaccharides
  anhydrides, nomenclature rules, **05:** 130-132
  circular dichroism, table, **05:** 465-468
  dimensions, average, of a unit, **05:** 472
  electronic charge distribution, **05:** 474-477
  nomenclature rules for some, **05:** 102-105, 109-112
  optical rotatory dispersion, table, **05:** 459-462
Monosaturated fatty acids
  spectra; pyrrolidides of ●, key fragments, **05:** 506
Moroyamycin
  structure, **03:** 331
Morphine
  pK'_a values, **06:** 327
Morphogenetic markers, *see also* Genetic markers
  Bacillus subtilis, **04:** 699-701
Motilin
  average hydrophobicity value, **01:** 227
MRE 600 30 S
  proteins, ribosomal; *Escherichia coli* ●, separation on cellulose phosphate Whatman® P11, **04:** 475
MSD-125 A, *see* Showdomycin
Mucin
  hypobranchial ●
    amino acid composition, incomplete data, **07:** 513 (major)
    amino acid composition, incomplete data, **07:** 513
Mucins
  carbohydrate content; glycoproteins; ●, table, **02:** 262-263
  glycoproteins; ●
    carbohydrate content, **02:** 262-263
Cis,cis-Muconate lactonizing

  enzyme
    average hydrophobicity value, **01:** 227
Muconolactone
  isomerase
    average hydrophobicity value, **01:** 227
Mucopolysaccharides
  carbohydrates, *see also* specific types; ●, occurrence and physical data, **05:** 356-357
  IR spectral data; ●, **05:** 356-357
  molecular weight; ●, **05:** 356-357
  occurrence, repeating unit and physical data, **05:** 356-357
  specific rotation; ●, **05:** 356-357
  table of data and characteristics, **02:** 686-687
  viscosity, intrinsic, ●, **05:** 356-357
Mucoprotein
  axial ratio; Tamm-Horsfall ●, **02:** 304
  diffusion coefficients; Tamm-Horsfall ●, **02:** 304
  frictional ratio; Tamm-Horsfall ●, **02:** 304
  Tamm-Horsfall, *see also* Tamm-Horsfall mucoprotein
    amino acid composition, complete data, **07:** 510
    properties of, **02:** 304
Multhiomycin
  origin, structure, and characteristic as protein biosynthesis inhibitor, **04:** 586
Multienzyme
  complex in tryptophan pathway
    amino acid composition, complete data, **07:** 509
Muramidase, *see* Lysozyme
Muscazone
  physical and chemical properties, **01:** 145
Muscle contractile
  proteins
    amino acid sequence, **07:** 490-496
Mutagens
  chemical
    alkylating, classes of, table, **04:** 891-892
    properties of selected, table, **04:** 888-889
Mutants, biochemical
  Coprinus radiatus
    loci, number of alleles, precursors, characteristics, **04:** 763-764
    map, **04:** 762
  Drosophila melanogaster, list, **04:** 848-855
Mutarotase
  average hydrophobicity value, **01:** 227
Mutase
  chorismate ●
    molar absorptivity and-or absorbance values, **02:** 406
  chorismate ●-prephenate dehydratase
    average hydrophobicity value, **01:** 216
  chorismic ●
    Neurospora crassa mutant, **04:** 748
  definition and nomenclature, **02:** 98
  3-deoxy-D-arabinoheptulosonate 7-phosphate synthetase-chroismate ●
    average hydrophobicity value, **01:** 218
  glutamate ● component
    amino acid composition, incomplete data, **07:** 512
  β-lysine ●
    subunit, constitution of, **02:** 339
Mycoplasma membrane, *see* Membrane, protein, mycoplasma

Myelin
  protein
    circular dichroism in the UV region, **07:** 113
    optical rotatory dispersion in the visible and near UV
      regions, **07:** 31
Myeloma
  protein, *see* Immunoglobulin
Myeloperoxidase
  amino acid composition, complete data, **07:** 509
  molar absorptivity and-or absorbance values, **02:** 473
Myoglobin
  amino acid sequence, **07:** 437-440
  average hydrophobicity value, **01:** 227
  calorimetric ΔH values accompanying conformational
    changes, **06:** 270
  circular dichroism
    UV and near-UV region, **07:** 113, 157
  conformation for sperm whale, **02:** 760
  cyanogen bromide cleavage, **02:** 199
  molar absorptivity and-or absorbance values, **02:**
    476-479
  optical rotatory dispersion
    UV region, **07:** 67
    visible and near UV regions, **07:** 31
  oxidation-reduction potentials of, **06:** 137-139
  pK; histidine in; •, values for residues, **02:** 690
  pK; tyrosine in; •, table of values, **02:** 695
  sperm whale
    heat of proton ionization, pK, and related thermody-
      namic quantities, **06:** 220
  vertebrate
    amino acid sequence, **07:** 437-440
  viscosity, intrinsic, **02:** 721
Myoglobin, met (ferri)-
  optical rotatory dispersion in the UV region: extrema
    between 185 and 250 NM³, **07:** 67
Myoglobin, metcyano-
  circular dichroism in the UV region: extrema between
    185 and 250 NM³, **07:** 114
Myohemerythrin
  average hydrophobicity value, **01:** 227
Myokinase, *see* Adenylate, kinase
Myosin
  amino acid composition, complete data, **07:** 509
  amino acid sequence, **07:** 493
  average hydrophobicity value, **01:** 227
  circular dichroism in the UV region, **07:** 115
  identification of, in nonmuscle cells, table, **02:** 307-313
  interaction of nonmuscle actin with, **02:** 316
  light chain
    circular dichroism in the UV region, **07:** 115
  molar absorptivity and-or absorbance values, **02:** 481
  molecular parameters, **02:** 306
  nonmuscle
    enzymatic activity of, **02:** 319
    filament data for several, **02:** 318
    interaction with action, **02:** 320
    physical properties for several, **02:** 317
  optical rotatory dispersion, **07:** 62
    UV region, **07:** 68
    visible and near UV regions, **07:** 31

rabbit
    luminescence of, table, **01:** 206
  refractive index increments, **02:** 379
  viscosity, intrinsic, **02:** 721
Myosin, HMM
  circular dichroism in the UV region, **07:** 115
  optical rotatory dispersion
    UV region, **07:** 68
    visible and near UV regions, **07:** 31
Myosin, HMM (S-1)
  circular dichroism in the UV region, **07:** 115
Myosin, LMM
  circular dichroism in the UV region, **07:** 115
  optical rotatory dispersion
    UV region, **07:** 68
    visible and near UV regions, **07:** 31
Myosin A
  cyanogen bromide cleavage, **02:** 199
Myosins
  activation energy; •, nonmuscle, table of values, **02:** 319
  ATPase activity; •, nonmuscle, table of values, 02: 319
  molecular weight; •, nonmuscle, table of values, **02:** 317
  sedimentation coefficient; •, nonmuscle, table of values,
    02: 317
  Stokes radius; •, nonmuscle, table of values, 02: 317
  substrate specificity; •, nonmuscle, table of values, **02:**
    319
  subunit composition; •, nonmuscle, table of values, **02:**
    317
Myosmine
  p*K'*$_a$ values, **06:** 327
Myxovirus hemagglutination
  inhibitor
    amino acid composition, incomplete data, **07:** 513

N

NAD
  UV spectra, formula, molecular weight, **08:** 167
NADH
  lipoamide dehydrogenase (•)
    amino acid composition, complete data, **07:** 508
    circular dichroism in the UV region, **07:** 108
    optical rotatory dispersion
      UV region, **07:** 65
      visible and near UV regions, **07:** 29
NADH$_2$
  disodium salt
    UV spectra, formula, molecular weight, **08:** 168
NAD(P)$^+$
  transhydrogenase
    circular dichroism in the UV region, **07:** 115
    optical rotatory dispersion in the UV region, **07:** 68
NADP-glutamate
  dehydrogenase
    Neurospora crassa mutant, **04:** 751
NAD(P)H
  glutathione reductase (•)
    amino acid composition, incomplete data, **07:** 512
    optical rotatory dispersion
      UV region, **07:** 57

NAD(P)H *(continued)*
   visible and near UV regions, **07:** 24
N-α-Nalonyl-D-alanine
   physical and chemical properties, **01:** 165
NaOH
   borax-• buffer, preparation of, **06:** 376
Naphthalene derivatives
   heat of proton ionization, pK, and related thermody-
      namic quantities, **06:** 221-223
Naphthalene sulfonates
   fluorescent probes of protein structure, **07:** 604-606
Naphthylacrylic acid
   antagonism to tryptophan, **01:** 179
β-(1-Naphthyl)alanine
   structure and symbols for those incorporated into syn-
      thetic polypeptides, **01:** 105
β-(2-Naphthyl)alanine
   structure and symbols for those incorporated into syn-
      thetic polypeptides, **01:** 105
Naphthylalanines
   antagonism to tryptophan, **01:** 179
Naramycin® B
   origin, structure, and characteristic as protein biosynthe-
      sis inhibitor, **04:** 586
Nariterashin
   physicochemical constants, spectral, chemotherapeutic
      and biological properties, **03:** 332
Naritheracin
   physicochemical constants, spectral, chemotherapeutic
      and biological properties , **03:** 332
Nebrancyin, *see* Tobramycin
N-(Nebularin-6-ylcarbamoyl)glycine
   physical constants and spectral properties, **03:** 103
N-(Nebularin-6-ylcarbamoyl)threonine
   physical constants and spectral properties, **03:** 103
Nebularine
   physical and spectral properties, **03:** 122
   physicochemical constants, spectral, chemotherapeutic
      and biological properties, **03:** 334
Neocarzinostatin
   average hydrophobicity value, **01:** 227
   circular dichroism in the UV region, **07:** 115
   optical rotatory dispersion in the UV region, **07:** 68
Neoglucobrassicin
   physical and chemical properties, **01:** 157
Neomycin A, B, and C
   origin, structure, and characteristic as protein biosynthe-
      sis inhibitor, **04:** 587
Neospiramycin
   origin, structure, and characteristic as protein biosynthe-
      sis inhibitor, **04:** 588
Nerve growth
   factor
      molar absorptivity and-or absorbance values, **02:** 482
      subunit, constitution of, **02:** 326
   factor fraction A
      amino acid composition, incomplete data, **07:** 513
Neucleotide
   aspartic acid; • sequences of, **04:** 442-443
Neuraminic acid
   generic term usage, **05:** 10

Neurohypophysial hormones, *see* Hormones, neurohypo-
      physial
Neurophysin
   circular dichroism in near-UV region, at room tempera-
      ture, **07:** 158
Neurophysin I, II, III
   average hydrophobicity values, **01:** 227
Neurotoxin, *see also* Neurotoxins, Toxin
   molar absorptivity and-or absorbance values, **02:** 482
Neurotoxin α
   amino acid composition, complete data, **07:** 509
   amino acid sequence, **07:** 499
Neurotoxin I
   optical rotatory dispersion in the UV region, **07:** 68
Neurotoxin I, II, III, IV, V
   average hydrophobicity values, **01:** 227,228
Neurotoxin II
   amino acid composition, complete data, **07:** 509
   circular dichroism in the UV region, **07:** 115
   optical rotatory dispersion in the UV region, **07:** 68
Neurotoxin III
   optical rotatory dispersion in the UV region, **07:** 68
Neurotoxins, *see also* Neurotoxin
   long
      amino acid sequences, **07:** 366-369
      from venom of various snakes, **07:** 366-369
   short
      amino acid sequence, **07:** 360-365
      from venom of various snakes, **07:** 360-365
Neutral proteinase, *see* Microbial metalloenzyme
α-NH₂-n-butyric acid
   free acid in blood plasma of newborn infants and
      adults, **01:** 328
Niacin
   nomenclature, preferred usage, **08:** 19
   properties of, **08:** 296
Nicotianamine
   physical and chemical properties, **01:** 145
Nicotianine
   physical and chemical properties, **01:** 163
Nicotinamide
   deamidase
      amino acid composition, complete data, **07:** 509
   properties of, **08:** 296
β-Nicotinamide adenine
   dinucleotide
      UV spectra, formula, molecular weight, **08:** 167
Nicotine
   pK'_a values, **06:** 327
Nicotinic acid
   biological characteristics, **08:** 303
   properties of, **08:** 296
Niddamycin
   origin, structure, and characteristic as protein biosynthe-
      sis inhibitor, **04:** 588
Ninhydrin
   amino acids, *see also* Aromatic amino acids, *also*
      specific acids; chromatography, ion exchange; urine,
      resolution of • positive constituents, **08:** 114-119
   glycine; • reaction, absorption ratio, **08:** 123
   positive compounds, elution behavior, **08:** 122

Nomenclature *(continued)*

quinones, references for rules, **02:** 87

RCS, suggested use of term in prostaglandin studies, **08:** 314

rules and recommendations affecting, list, **03:** 3, 4

sequence-rule procedure in fundamental stereochemistry, **02:** 50-58, **03:** 42-50, **04:** 42-50, **05:** 47-55, **06:** 49, **08:** 49-57

sequence-rule procedure in fundamental stereochemistry, **01:** 50-58

sequence rule, use of, **01:** 61-63, **02:** 65-67

stereochemistry, fundamental, IUPAC rules, **06:** 20, **08:** 20-57

stereochemistry, fundamental, IUPAC rules for, **05:** 18-55

stereochemistry, fundamental, IUPAC rules for nomenclature, **01:** 21-58, **02:** 21-58, **04:** 13-50

steroids, IUPAC definitive rules for, **05:** 56-88

steroids, references for rules, **02:** 87

symbols, use of, **03:** 7-12

abeo system, usage for steroids, **05:** 81-83

torsion angle, choice of, **01:** 62-63, **02:** 66-67

vitamins, references for rules, **02:** 87

vitamins, trivial names and preferred usages, **08:** 8-19

Nonhuman

carbohydrate content; glycoproteins; plasma, •, table of values, **02:** 259-260

Nonsaponifiables

herring oils and Pacific pilchard oil, **05:** 523-524

N-Nor-amicetin, *see* Bamicetin

Norleucine

antagonism to leucine, **01:** 178

antagonism to methionine, **01:** 178

structure and symbols for those incorporated into synthetic polypeptides, **01:** 105

Norvaline

antagonism to leucine, **01:** 178

antagonism to valine, **01:** 180

pK'_a values, **06:** 319

structure and symbols for those incorporated into synthetic polypeptides, **01:** 105

Noryl

chemical and physical properties, **08:** 427

Novobiocin

UV spectra, formula, molecular weight, **08:** 183

Nuclease

amino acid composition, complete data, **07:** 509

average hydrophobicity value, **01:** 227

cyanogen bromide cleavage, **02:** 199

(extracellular)

circular dichroism at maxima in near-UV region, at room temperature, **07:** 158

molar absorptivity and-or absorbance values, **02:** 485

Neurospora crassa; mitochondrial •, functional characteristics, **04:** 518

Neurospora crassa; •, functional characteristics, **04:** 518

optical rotatory dispersion

UV region, **07:** 69

visible and near UV regions, **07:** 32

pK; histidine in; •, table of values, **02:** 691

staphylococcus aureus •

luminescence of, table, **01:** 206

Nuclease-T

amino acid sequences of protein, **07:** 310

Nucleases

nonspecific for the sugar moiety, functional characteristics, **04:** 518-523

Nuclei

enzymatic activity, subcellular fraction, **02:** 698-700

Nucleic acid bases

activity coefficients, molal; • and nucleosides, vapor phase, **03:** 529

molal osmotic coefficients; nucleosides and •, **03:** 528

osmometry coefficients, vapor phase; • and nucleosides, **03:** 528-529

Nucleic acids, *see also* DNA, RNA

abbreviations; •, journal reference to, **02:** 87

abbreviations for, use of, **01:** 7, **02:** 7, **04:** 7, **05:** 7, **06:** 7 **08:** 7

buoyant density; •, **03:** 565-566

chloroplast, quantitative data tables, **04:** 356-362

circular dichroism; spectra of representative naturally occurring •, **03:** 591

fluorescent dyes bound to, data tables, **04:** 470

optical properties; absorption and circular dichroism spectra, •, **03:** 589-595

spectral data, *see also* IR spectra, PMR spectra, UV spectra, Circular dichroism; circular dichroism, of representative naturally occurring •, **03:** 591

symbols; •, journal reference to, **02:** 87

Nucleocidin

origin, structure, and characteristic as protein biosynthesis inhibitor, **04:** 589

physicochemical constants, spectral, chemotherapeutic and biological properties, **03:** 336

Nucleoli

enzymatic activity for several, table, **02:** 701

Nucleophosphodi

esterases, functional characterization of, **04:** 491

Nucleoproteins

circular dichroic spectra, graph, **06:** 393

Nucleosidase

adenosine monophosphate •

average hydrophobicity value, **01:** 211

diphosphopyridine •

amino acid composition, complete data, **07:** 506

Nucleoside

alanine; • composition, table of values, **04:** 428

arginine; • composition, table of values, **04:** 428

aspartic acid; • composition, tables of values, **04:** 429

cysteine; • composition, tables of values, **04:** 429

diphosphokinase

average hydrophobicity value, **01:** 228

subunit, constitution of, **02:** 333, 336

factor A •

physical constants and spectral properties, **03:** 111

glutamic acid; • composition, tables of values, **04:** 429

glutamine; • composition, tables of values, **04:** 430

glycine; • composition, tables of values, **04:** 430-432

histidine; • composition, tables of values, **04:** 432

isoleucine; • composition, tables of values, **04:** 432

leucine; • composition, tables of values, **04:** 433-434

lysine; • composition, tables of values, **04:** 434

Nucleoside *(continued)*

  methionine; • composition, tables of values, **04:** 434–436

  phenylalanine; • composition, tables of values, **04:** 437

  phosphorylase

    optical rotatory dispersion

      UV region, **07:** 69

      visible and near UV regions, **07:** 32

  phosphorylase, purine-•

    molar absorptivity and-or absorbance values, **02:** 497

  phosphotransferase-A-chain

    average hydrophobicity value, **01:** 228

  phosphotransferase-B-chain

    average hydrophobicity value, **01:** 228

  proline T4; • composition, tables of values, **04:** 437

  purine • phosphorylase

    amino acid composition, complete data, **07:** 509

  serine; • composition, tables of values, **04:** 438–439

  threonine; • composition, tables of values, **04:** 439

  tryptophan; • composition, tables of values, **04:** 439

  tyrosine; • composition, tables of values, **04:** 440

  valine; • composition, tables of values,
    04: 441

Nucleoside 2,3-monophosphates

  molar absorptivity, table of values, **03:** 597

Nucleoside antibiotics, *see also* Antibiotics, nucleoside

  octosyl acids A, B and C as •, **03:** 337

  physicochemical constants, spectral, chemotherapeutic
    and biological properties, **03:** 271–393

Nucleoside derivatives

  adenosine and •

    physical constants and spectral properties, index to,
      03: 69

  cytidine and •

    physical constants and spectral properties, index to,
      03: 70

  deoxycytidine and •

    physical constants and spectral properties, index to,
      03: 70

  deoxyguanosine and •

    physical constants and spectral properties, index to,
      03: 70

  deoxyuridine and •

    physical constants and spectral properties, index to,
      03: 70

  guanosine and •

    physical constants and spectral properties, index to,
      03: 70

  inosine and •

    physical constants and spectral properties, index to,
      03: 70

  9-β-D-ribofuranosylpurine, and •

    physical constants and spectral properties, index to,
      03: 71

  ribosylthymine and •

    physical constants and spectral properties, index to,
      03: 71

  2-thiouridine and •

    physical constants and spectral properties, index to,
      03: 71-72

  thymidine and •

    physical constants and spectral properties, index to,
      03: 72

  uridine and •

    physical constants and spectral properties, index to,
      03: 72

Nucleoside phosphorothioates

  symbols for, use of, **03:** 12, **04:** 12

Nucleosides

  activity coefficients, molal; nucleic acid bases and •,
    vapor phase, **03:** 529

  alkyl derivatives of unmodified bases and •, UV spectra
    of some, **03:** 420–447

  chemical shifts; •, **03:** 530-533

  dissociation constants, acidic, **03:** 409-416

  Escherichia coli, see also E. coli; RNA from, natural oc-
    currence of the modified • in, **03:** 217-232

  formula, molecular; •, index to table, **03:** 69-72

  melting point; •, index to table of values, **03:** 69-72

  modified

    isolation and detection of, in RNA, general remarks
      about several compounds, **03:** 233-246

    RNA, natural occurrence in, tables, **03:** 216-233

  molal activity coefficients; •, values for several, **03:** 529

  molal osmotic coefficients; • and nucleic acid bases, **03:**
    528

  molecular weight; •, index to table of values, **03:** 69-72

  mouse; RNA from, natural occurrence of the modified
    • in, **03:** 217-232

  Neurospora; RNA from, natural occurrence of the
    modified • in, **03:** 217-232

  one-letter symbols; purines, pyrimidines, •, and nucleo-
    tides index to table, **03:** 67-75

  osmometry coefficients, vapor phase, **03:** 528-529

  pK'_a values, **06:** 330-331

  physical constants and spectral properties, **03:** 69-72

  pK; •, index to table of values, **03:** 69-72

  pKa; •, table of values, **03:** 409-416

  proton chemical shifts, **03:** 530-533

  specific rotation; •, index to table of values, **03:** 69-72

  spectral data, *see also* IR spectra, PMR spectra, UV
    spectra, Circular dichroism; acidic; •, index to table
    of values, **03:** 69-72

  spectral data, *see also* IR spectra, PMR spectra, UV
    spectra, Circular dichroism; alkaline; •, index to
    table of values, **03:** 69-72

  spectral data, *see also* IR spectra, PMR spectra, UV
    spectra, Circular dichroism; neutral; •, index to
    table of values, **03:** 69-72

  structure; •, index to table of values, **03:** 69-72

  symbols; 1-letter; •, index to table of values, **03:** 67-69

  symbols; 3-letter; •, index to table, **03:** 69-72

  symbols for, use of, **03:** 8, **04:** 8

  three-letter symbols; purines, pyrimidines, •, and nu-
    cleotides, index to table, **03:** 67-65

  tRNA, content in, tables of values, **04:** 428-441

  tRNA secondary structure; identification, location, dis-
    tribution, **04:** 427

  UV spectra of some, including their alkyl derivatives,
    03: 420-447

  UV spectral characteristics, **03:** 409-416

5'-Nucleotidase

  amino acid composition, incomplete data, **07:** 513

  average hydrophobicity value, **01:** 228

Nucleotide, *see also* Nucleotides
  abbreviations for, use of, **04:** 6
  adenovirus 2--VA RNA, • sequence model, **04:** 349
  alanine; • sequences of, **04:** 442-443
  arginine; • sequences of, **04:** 442-443
  Bacillus subtilis; ribosomal RNA from, • composition, **04:** 409
  bacteriophage types; viral DNA; • sequences, **04:** 350-351
  bacteriophage types; viral RNA; • sequences and models, **04:** 337-344
  bacteriophage types; virus-induced RNA; • sequences and models, **04:** 346-348
  composition in high molecular weight ribosomal RNA, **04:** 409
  composition in viral RNA, **04:** 410
  cysteine; • sequences of, **04:** 442-443
  DNA, *see also* Deoxyribonucleic acid; viral; • sequences, **04:** 350-353
  Escherichia coli, see also E. coli; 5S-ribosomal RNA from, • sequences, **04:** 324-327
  Escherichia coli, see also E. coli; 4.5S RNA from, • sequence model, **04:** 331
  Escherichia coli, see also E. coli; 6S RNA from, • sequence model, **04:** 332
  glutamic acid; • sequences of, **04:** 442-443
  glutamine; • sequences of, **04:** 444-445
  glycine; • sequences of, **04:** 444-445
  histidine; • sequences of, **04:** 444-445
  isoleucine; • sequences of, **04:** 446-447
  leucine; • sequences of, **04:** 446-447
  lysine; • sequences of, **04:** 446-447
  methionine; • sequences of, **04:** 448-449
  phenylalanine; • sequences of, **04:** 448-449
  proline; • sequences of, **04:** 450-451
  pyridine •
    amino acid sequence, **07:** 314
  RNA, *see also* Nucleic acids, Transfer RNA, TRNA (TRNA); ribosomal; • sequence data 5 S RNA from *Escherichia coli*, **04:** 473
  RNA, *see also* Nucleic acids, Transfer RNA, TRNA (TRNA); ribosomal; 5S type, • sequences for several, **04:** 324-327
  RNA, *see also* Nucleic acids, Transfer RNA, TRNA (TRNA); ribosomal; 5.85 type from yeast, • sequence model, **04:** 330
  RNA, *see also* Nucleic acids, Transfer RNA, TRNA (TRNA); viral; bacteriophage types, • sequences and models, **04:** 337-344
  RNA, *see also* Nucleic acids, Transfer RNA, TRNA (TRNA); virus-induced; • sequences and models, **04:** 346-349
  sequence data
    phenylanine transfer RNA, **04:** 458
    ribosomal RNA, **04:** 473
    transfer RNA, tables, **04:** 442-453
  sequences and models for several RNAs and DNAs, **04:** 324-353
  serine; • sequences of, **04:** 450-451
  sugar •
    isolation and enzymatic synthesis of, **05:** 446-452
  threonine; • sequences of, **04:** 450-451

  tryptophan; • sequences of, **04:** 450-451
  tyrosine; • sequences of, **04:** 452-453
  valine; • sequences of, **04:** 452-453
  yeast phenylalanine transfer RNA; • sequence, **04:** 458
Nucleotide derivatives
  deoxyadenosine •
    physical constants and spectral properties, index to, **03:** 73
  deoxyguanosine •
    physical constants and spectral properties, index to, **03:** 73
  deoxyuridine •
    physical constants and spectral properties, index to, **03:** 73
Nucleotides
  abbreviations for, use of, **01:** 6, **02:** 6, **03:** 6, **05:** 6, **06:** 6, **08:** 6
  dissociation constants, acidic, **03:** 409-416
  formula, molecular; •, index to table, **03:** 72-75
  melting point; •, index to table of values, **03:** 72-75
  molar residue ellipticity, table of values, **03:** 601
  molar residue rotation, table of values, **03:** 599
  molecular weight; •, index to table of values, **03:** 72-75
  one-letter symbols; purines, pyrimidines, nucleosides, and • index to table, **03:** 67-75
  physical constants and spectral properties, index to, **03:** 72-75
  pK; •, index to table of values, **03:** 72-75
  pK'_a values, **06:** 330-331
  pKa; •, table of values, **03:** 409-416
  specific rotation; •, index to table of values, **03:** 72-75
  spectral data, *see also* IR spectra, PMR spectra, UV spectra, Circular dichroism; acidic; •, index to table of values, **03:** 72-75
  spectral data, *see also* IR spectra, PMR spectra, UV spectra, Circular dichroism; alkaline; •, index to table of values, **03:** 72-75
  spectral data, *see also* IR spectra, PMR spectra, UV spectra, Circular dichroism; neutral; •, index to table of values, **03:** 72-75
  structure; •, index to table of values, **03:** 72-75
  sugar, isolation and enzymatic synthesis of, **05:** 446-452
  symbols; 1-letter; •, index to table, **03:** 72-75
  symbols; 3-letter; •, index to table, **03:** 72-75
  three-letter symbols; purines, pyrimidines, nucleosides, and •, index to table, **03:** 67-65
  UV spectral characteristics, **03:** 409-416
Nucleotidyltransferase
  RNA •
    amino acid composition, complete data, **07:** 510
    circular dichroism in the UV region, **07:** 123
    optical rotatory dispersion
      UV region, **07:** 75
      visible and near UV regions, **07:** 35
Nystatin
  UV spectra, formula, molecular weight, **08:** 185

O

Octadecadienoates, methyl
  equivalent chain lengths, **05:** 505

Oxidase *(continued)*
  table of cofactors, molecular weights, stoichiometry
    and sources, **02:** 282
d-amino-acid •
  molar absorptivity and-or absorbance values, **02:** 392
  subunit, constitution of, **02:** 333
l-amino-acid •
  molar absorptivity and, **02:** or absorbance values, **02:**
    392
  subunit, constitution of, **02:** 336
d-amino acid •
  amino acid composition, complete data, **07:** 505
  average hydrophobicity value, **01:** 213
  circular dichroism in the UV region, **07:** 84
  optical rotatory dispersion
    UV region, **07:** 46
    visible and near UV regions, **07:** 17
l-amino acid •
  amino acid composition, complete data, **07:** 505
  optical rotatory dispersion in the UV region, **07:** 46
ascorbate •
  circular dichroism in the UV region, **07:** 85
ascorbic acid •
  amino acid composition, incomplete data, **07:** 512
cytochrome *c* •
  circular dichroism in the UV region, **07:** 93
  optical rotatory dispersion in the UV region, **07:** 54
diamine •
  molar absorptivity and-or absorbance values, **02:** 418
  table of cofactors, molecular weights, stoichiometry
    and sources, **02:** 282
galactose •
  amino acid composition, incomplete data, **07:** 512
  circular dichroism in the UV region, **07:** 97
  UV and near-UV region, **07:** 97, 151
glucose •
  carbohydrate content, **02:** 273
  circular dichroism in the UV region, **07:** 97
  molar absorptivity and-or absorbance values, **02:** 431
  optical rotatory dispersion
    UV region, **07:** 56
    visible and near UV region, **07:** 23
monoamine •
  amino acid composition, complete data, **07:** 509
  carbohydrate content, **02:** 273, 274
  molar absorptivity and-or absorbance values, **02:** 473
  subunit, constitution of, **02:** 335, 345, 350
  table of cofactors, molecular weights, stoichiometry,
    and sources, **02:** 282
putrescine •
  average hydrophobicity value, **01:** 230
  molar absorptivity and-or absorbance values, **02:** 504
sulfite • deficiency
  characteristics of, **01:** 322
xanthine •
  amino acid composition, complete data, **07:** 511
  circular dichroism
    UV and near-UV region, **07:** 128, 163
  molar absorptivity and-or absorbance values, **02:** 514
  optical rotatory dispersion
    UV region, **07:** 78
    visible and near UV regions, **07:** 38

  table of cofactors, molecular weights, stoichiometry,
    and sources, **02:** 278
Oxidoreductases
  definition and nomenclature of, **02:** 96
  intramolecular, numbering and classification, **02:** 108
  numbering and classification of, **02:** 104-106
β-3-Oxindolylalanine
  physical and chemical properties, **01:** 145
Oxoglutarate
  dehydrogenase
    circular dichroism in the UV region, **07:** 117
    optical rotatory dispersion in the UV region, **07:** 69
2-Oxoglutarate
  dehydrogenase
    average hydrophobicity value, **01:** 228
5-Oxoproline, *see* Pyrrolidone carboxylic acid
Δ5→4 3-Oxosteroid isomerase, *see* Steroid, Δ-isomerase
Oxyferrohemoglobin
  HbO$_2$
    UV and visible absorption spectrum, **07:** 177
Oxygen
  alcohols and other • acids, pK'_a values, **06:** 315-317
Oxygen acids
  pK'_a; alcohols and other •, **06:** 315-317
Oxygenase
  3,4-dihydroxyphenylacetate-2,3-•
    average hydrophobicity value, **01:** 218
  tryptophan •
    amino acid composition, complete data, **07:** 510
    molar absorptivity and-or absorbance values, **02:** 511
    subunit constitution of, **02:** 335, 339
Oxyglutarate
  dehydrase
    Neurospora crassa mutant, **04:** 749
Oxytetracycline, structure and characteristic as protein bi-
    osynthesis inhibitor, *see also* Terramycin and Tetra-
    cycline, **04:** 593
Oxytocin
  average hydrophobicity value, **01:** 228
  circular dichroism at maxima in near-UV region, at
    room temperature, **07:** 158
  luminescence of, **01:** 204
  proton NMR and suggested conformations, **07:** 570-572
  ser, Ile •
    amino acid sequence, **07:** 194-195
Oxytocins
  natural and related synthetic oligopeptides
    amino acid sequence, physical and biological proper-
    ties, **07:** 193-218
Oyamvcid
  physicochemical constants, spectral, chemotherapeutic
    and biological properties, **03:** 340

P

P11
  protein •
    subunit, constitution of, **02:** 329
PA114-A-1
  synergistin® A-1 (•); origin, structure, and characteris-
    tic as protein biosynthesis inhibitor, **04:** 605

PA 114-B
 origin, structure, and characteristic as protein biosynthesis inhibitor, **04**: 594
PA 114A, *see also* Osteogrycin A, Staphylomycin
  M₁,Virginiamycin M₁; origin and mode of action as
  protein biosynthesis inhibitor, **04**: 594
PABA
 properties of, **08**: 293
Pactamycin
 origin, structure, and characteristic as protein biosynthesis inhibitor, **04**: 593
Pancreatic DNase, *see* Deoxyribonuclease I
Pancreatin
 enzymatic hydrolysis, conjugated proteins, **02**: 211
Pancreozymin
 cholecystokinin-●
  cyanogen bromide cleavage, **02**: 199
Pantonine
 physical and chemical properties, **01**: 128
Pantothenic acid
 biological characteristics, **08**: 304
 properties of, **08**: 296-297
PAP
 phytolacca americana peptide (●); origin, structure, and
  characteristic as protein biosynthesis inhibitor, **04**:
  595
Papain
 amino acid sequence, **07**: 356-357
 average hydrophobicity value, **01**: 228
 circular dichroism in the UV region, **07**: 117
 enzymatic hydrolysis, conjugated proteins, **02**: 211
 enzymatic hydrolysis of proteins, **02**: 209
 fragments produced by digestion with, **02**: 182
 hydrolysis peptides from α- and β-chains of human
  hemoglobin, **02**: 219
 luminescence of, table, **01**: 206
 molar absorptivity and-or absorbance values, **02**: 487
 optical rotatory dispersion
  UV region, **07**: 69
  visible and near UV regions, **07**: 32
 specificity for hydrolysis of peptide bonds, **02**: 218
 viscosity, intrinsic, **02**: 721
Paracrystal
 period
  tropomyosin from nonmuscle cells, **02**: 321
Paramyosin
 circular dichroism in the UV region, **07**: 117
 molar absorptivity and-or absorbance values, **02**: 488
 molecular parameters, **02**: 306
 optical rotatory dispersion
  UV region, **07**: 70
  visible and near UV regions, **07**: 32
 subunit, constitution of, **02**: 342
 viscosity, intrinsic, **02**: 721
Parathyroid
 hormone
  amino acid composition, complete data, **07**: 509
  average hydrophobicity value, **01**: 228
  circular dichroism in the UV region, **07**: 117

molar absorptivity and-or absorbance values, **02**:
  450, 488
 optical rotatory dispersion in the UV region, **07**: 70
 cyanogen bromide cleavage, **02**: 199
polypeptide
 amino acid composition, complete data, **07**: 509
Parke Davis [7551 X41A]
 2'-deoxycoformycin, **03**: 314
Paromomycin
 origin, structure, and characteristic as protein biosynthesis inhibitor, **04**: 594
Particle
 size analysis, methods used, **08**: 425
Particles
 chart of diameters for various, **08**: 425
 frictional coefficients; proteins; ●, index to studies containing, **02**: 232
 partial specific volume; proteins; ●, index to studies
  containing, **02**: 232
Particles, protein
 physical-chemical data for, index to ultracentrifuge
  studies, **02**: 232
Parvalbumin
 average hydrophobicity value, **01**: 228
Parvalbumins
 amino acid sequence, **07**: 496
 circular dichroism
  UV and near-UV region, **07**: 117, 158
 optical rotatory dispersion
  UV region, **07**: 70
  visible and near UV regions, **07**: 32
Pathways, biochemical; chart of, **04**: insert
Patricin A
 proton NMR and suggested conformations, **07**: 565
Pectenoxanthin
 UV spectra, formula, molecular weight, **08**: 191
Pederin
 origin, structure, and characteristic as protein biosynthe-
  sis inhibitor, **04**: 595
Penicillamine, *see* β,β-Dimethylcysteine
D-Penicillamine
 physical and chemical properties, **01**: 166
Penicillin G
 UV spectra, formula, molecular weight, **08**: 157
Penicillin V
 free acid
  UV spectra, formula, molecular weight, **08**: 158
Penicillinase
 amino acid composition, complete data, **07**: 509
 amino acid composition, incomplete data, **07**: 513
 amino acid sequences of proteins, **07**: 310
 circular dichroism
  UV and near-UV region, **07**: 117, 155
Penicillo
 carboxypeptidase-S
  average hydrophobicity value, **01**: 228
  molar absorptivity and-or absorbance values, **02**: 488
(Pentafluorophenyl)alanine
 structure and symbols for those incorporated into synthetic polypeptides, **01**: 105

Peptides *(continued)*

hydrolysis, *see also* Peptic hydrolysis; acid, of •, relative rate table, **02:** 208

hydrolysis from α- and β-chains of human hemoglobin, **02:** 219

hydrolysis in acid solution, relative rates, **02:** 208

lysine; active site •, **07:** 188

molal activity coefficients, table of values, **06:** 120

natural

abbreviations, use of, for synthetic modification, **01:** 14, **02:** 14-15

rules for naming synthetic modifications of, **02:** 79-83

semitrivial names for variants, **02:** 79

nomenclature for those prepared by solid phase peptide synthesis, table, **01:** 374-375

pK'_a values, **06:** 321

prepared by solid phase peptide synthesis, table of characteristics, **01:** 374-390

proton NMR data, suggested conformations; biologically active cyclic •, **07:** 561-573

serine; active site •, **07:** 186

symbols for, rules, **01:** 88-90

symbols for, use of, **01:** 8-15, **02:** 8-15

torsion angle; • of L-amino acids, table of, **01:** 65, **02:** 69

tyrosine; active site •, **07:** 187

Permease

sulfate •

Neurospora crassa mutant, **04:** 744

Permease-I

sulfur •, conidial type

Neurospora crassa mutant, **04:** 741

Permease II

sulfur •

Neurospora crassa mutant, **04:** 750

Peroxidase

carbohydrate content, **02:** 273

circular dichroism

UV and near UV-region, **07:** 118, 159

cytochrome *c* •

molar absorptivity and-or absorbance values, **02:** 417

glutathione •

circular dichroism

UV and near-UV region, **07:** 98, 151

molar absorptivity and-or absorbance values, **02:** 433

molecular weight, stoichiometry and source, **02:** 285

molar absorptivity and-or absorbance values, **02:** 489, 492

optical rotatory dispersion

UV region, **07:** 70

visible and near UV regions, **07:** 33

subunit, constitution of, **02:** 340

Peroxidase B

amino acid composition, complete data, **07:** 509

Peroxisomes

enzymatic activity, table, **02:** 710

Peroxy Y base

physical constants and spectral properties, **03:** 95

Peroxywybutosine, *see* 7-[2-(Hydroperoxy)-3-(methoxycarbonyl)-3-(methoxyformamido)propyl] wyosine

composition in various tRNA's, **04:** 428-441

isolation and detection of, in RNA, general remarks, **03:** 240

PG, *see* Prostaglandins

PGF$_{1\beta}$

phospholipids; stereoconfiguration of •, **08:** 318

Phage protein, *see* Bacteriophage protein

Phalloidin

circular dichroism at maxima in near-UV region, at room temperature, **07:** 159

proton NMR and suggested conformations, **07:** 569

Phenanthrene derivatives

heat of proton ionization, pK, and related thermodynamic quantities, **06:** 228-229

Phenobarbital

heat of proton ionization, pK, and related thermodynamic quantities, **06:** 172

Phenol protein

group, chemical modification of

reagents used, table of specificities, **02:** 203-204

Phenols

heat of proton ionization, pK, and related thermodynamic quantities, **06:** 230-232

pK'_a values, **06:** 314

Phenomycin

origin, structure, and characteristic as protein biosynthesis inhibitor, **04:** 595

Phenoxymethylpenicillin

UV spectra, formula, molecular weight, **08:** 158

Phenylalanine

N-acetyl-DL- -phenylalanine methyl ester, UV spectra of, **01:** 193

acid vs. neutral difference spectra, **01:** 191

alkaline vs. neutral difference spectra, **01:** 190-191

antagonists of, **01:** 179

far ultraviolet absorption spectra

aqueous solution at pH 5, **01:** 184

neutral water, table, **01:** 185

0.1 *M* sodium dodecyl sulfate, table, **01:** 185

free acid in amniotic fluid in early pregnancy and at term, **01:** 327

free acid in blood plasma of newborn infants and adults, **01:** 328

hydrophobic stacking interactions, yeast • transfer RNA, **04:** 461

hydroxylase

average hydrophobicity value, **01:** 229

luminescence of, table, **01:** 200

luminescence of derivatives of, table, **01:** 203

molar extinctions, **01:** 185

molecular absorbances of, table, **01:** 189

nucleoside composition, tables of values, **04:** 437

nucleotide sequences of, **04:** 448-449

pK'_a values, **06:** 319

phenylketonuria

atypical, effect of, **01:** 320

classical, effect of, **01:** 320

physical and chemical properties, **01:** 131

β-(4-pyrazolyl)alanine; antagonism to •, **01:** 179

requirements of, for growth of various microorganisms, table, **04:** 630-643

Phenylalanine *(continued)*

RNA, *see also* Nucleic acids, Transfer RNA, TRNA (TRNA); transfer type, structure, three-dimensional, yeast
* transfer RNA, **04**: 457-461
spectra, far UV, **01**: 184
symbols for atoms and bonds in side chains, **01**: 70, **02**: 74
thumbprint, content in, **08**: 121
UV absorption characteristics, **01**: 186
Phenylalanine ammonia
lyase
average hydrophobicity value, **01**: 229
L-Phenylalanine ammonia
lyase
molar absorptivity and-or absorbance values, **02**: 492
Phenylalanyl model
compounds
near-UV circular dichrism intensities, **07**: 168
Phenylanine transfer RNA
nucleotide; sequence data; •, **04**: 458
Phenylglycine
pK'_a values, **06**: 319
structure and symbols for those incorporated into synthetic polypeptides, **01**: 106
Phenylpyruvate
tautomerase
amino acid composition, incomplete data, **07**: 513
Phenylpyruvic acid
properties of, **01**: 182
(α-Phenylsarcosine), *see* N-Methylphenylglycine
β-Phenylserine
antagonism to phenylalanine, **01**: 179
Threo-β-Phenylserine
physical and chemical properties, **01**: 128
Phosphatase
acid •
wheat bran
luminescence of, table, **01**: 206
acyl •
amino acid composition, incomplete data, **07**: 512
average hydrophobicity value, **01**: 211
molar absorptivity and-or absorbance values, **02**: 384
alkaline •
amino acid composition, complete data, **07**: 505
average hydrophobicity value, **01**: 213
carbohydrate content, **02**: 274
circular dichroism in the UV region, **07**: 83
molecular weights, stoichiometry and sources, **02**: 284
optical rotatory dispersion
UV region, **07**: 45
visible and near UV regions, **07**: 16
subunit, constitution of, **02**: 331, 335, 337
hexosedi•
amino acid composition, complete data, **07**: 507
circular dichroism in the UV region, **07**: 101
optical rotatory dispersion in the UV region, **07**: 60
histidinol phosphate •
Neurospora crassa mutant, **04**: 749

molar absorptivity and-or absorbance values, **02**: 493
subunit, constitution of, **02**: 334
Phosphate
acetyltransferase
optical rotatory dispersion
UV region, **07**: 70
visible and near UV regions, **07**: 33
and phosphonates, pK'_a values, **06**: 308
citrate-• buffer, preparation of, **06**: 372
Phosphate buffer
preparation of, **06**: 374
protonic activity tables, **06**: 529-539
Phosphatidic acid
generic term usage, **05**: 9
Phosphatidyl
arachidonic acid; liberation • inositol, **08**: 320
Phosphatidyl inositol
prostaglandins; liberation of precursor from •, **08**: 320
Phosphatidyl serine
decarboxylase
average hydrophobicity value, **01**: 229
3-*sn*-Phosphatidylcholine
generic term usage, **05**: 9
Phospho-2-keto-3-deoxygluconate
aldolase
optical rotatory dispersion
UV region, **07**: 71
visible and near UV regions, **07**: 33
Phosphoenol pyruvate
carboxykinase
average hydrophobicity value, **01**: 229
Phosphoenolpyruvate
carboxykinase
amino acid composition, complete data, **07**: 509
carboxylase
Phosphoethanolamine
hypophosphatasia, effect of, **01**: 321
Phosphofructokinase
amino acid composition, complete data, **07**: 509
average hydrophobicity value, **01**: 229
molar absorptivity and-or absorbance values, **02**: 494
subunit, constitution of, **02**: 349
Phosphoglucoisomerase
molar absorptivity and-or absorbance values, **02**: 494
Phosphoglucomutase
amino acid composition, complete data, **07**: 509
average hydrophobicity value, **01**: 229
molar absorptivity and-or absorbance values, **02**: 494
Neurospora crassa mutant, **04**: 741
optical rotatory dispersion
UV region, **07**: 70
visible and near UV regions, **07**: 33
Phosphogluconate
dehydrogenase (decarboxylating)
amino acid composition, complete data, **07**: 509
optical rotatory dispersion in the UV region, **07**: 71
6-Phosphogluconate dehydrogenase, *see also* Phosphogluconate, dehydrogenase (decarbosylating)
molar absorptivity and-or absorbance values, **02**: 494
Neurospora crassa mutant, **04**: 755
subunit, constitution of, **02**: 332, 333

Placental
lactogen, human
amino acid sequence compared with human growth
hormone and human prolactin, **07**: 392-393
Plasma, *see also* Blood plasma; Human plasma
albumin, •, *see also* Human plasma albumin; Plasma albumin
ligand binding
drugs, list of references, **02**: 568-574
endogenous ligands, list of references, **02**: 556-557
fatty acids, list of references, **02**: 558-562
inorganic anions, list of references, **02**: 563
measurement of, list of techniques, **02**: 555
metal ions, list of references, **02**: 563
steroids, list of references, **02**: 563-564
visible dyes, list of references, **02**: 564-568
amino acids, *see also* Aromatic amino acids, *also*
specific acids; •, normal or low, renal aminoacidurias, **01**: 323-324
basic • protein
amino acid composition, complete data, **07**: 505
carbohydrate content; glycoproteins; •, human, table of
values, **02**: 258
carbohydrate content; glycoproteins; •, nonhuman,
table of values, **02**: 259-260
ceruloplasmin; •, human
carbohydrate content, molecular weights, sedimentation coefficients, **02**: 258
coagulation factors; •, human
carbohydrate content, molecular weight, sedimentation
coefficients, **02**: 258
coagulation factors; •, nonhuman
carbohydrate content, **02**: 260
concentration
blood coagulation proteins, table of values, **02**: 255
corticosteroid-transporting protein; •, nonhuman, carbohydrate content, **02**: 259
diffusion coefficients; proteins; •, human, table of
values, **02**: 242-250
electrophoretic mobility; proteins; human •, table of
values, **02**: 242-250
fatty acids, *see also* Lipids, Wax fatty acids; composition in • and erythrocyte lipids, effect of dietary fat,
05: 522
fetuin; •, nonhuman
carbohydrate content, **02**: 259
fibrin stabilizing factor; system in blood •, description,
02: 670
fibrinogen; •, human
carbohydrate content, molecular weights, sedimentation coefficients, **02**: 258
frictional ratio; proteins; human •, table of values, **02**:
242-250
globulin, *see also* Macroglobulin; •, human
carbohydrate content, molecular weights, sedimentation coefficients, **02**: 258
glycoproteins; mouse •, tumor
molar absorptivity and-or absorbance values, **02**: 435
glycoproteins; •, human

carbohydrate content, molecular weights, sedimentation coefficients, **02**: 258
glycoproteins; •, nonhuman
carbohydrate content, **02**: 259-260
gonadotrophin-transporting protein; •, nonhuman
carbohydrate content, **02**: 259
Hageman factor; •, nonhuman
carbohydrate content, **02**: 260
haptoglobin; •, human
carbohydrate content, molecular weights, sedimentation coefficients, **02**: 258
hemopexin; •, human
carbohydrate content, molecular weight, sedimentation
coefficient, **02**: 258
human, basic B_2
molar absorptivity and-or absorbance values, **02**: 498
human, quantitative variation in clotting factors, **04**: 881
glycoproteins from, carbohydrate content, **02**: 258
ligand binding
drugs, list of references, **02**: 568-574
endogenous ligands, list of references, **02**: 556-557
fatty acids, list of references, **02**: 558-562
inorganic anions, list of references, **02**: 563
metal ions, list of references, **02**: 563-564
steroids, list of references, **02**: 563-564
visible dyes, list of references, **02**: 564-568
human • proteins
content in normal plasma, **02**: 242-250
molecular parameters, table, **02**: 242-250
immunoglobulin; •, human
carbohydrate content, molecular weights, sedimentation coefficients, **02**: 258
immunoglobulin; •, nonhuman
carbohydrate content, **02**: 259
isoelectric point; proteins, human •, **02**: 242-250
macroglobulin, *see also* Ovomacroglobulin; •, nonhuman
carbohydrate content, **02**: 259
membrane, *see* Membrane protein, plasma
enzymatic activity, table, **02**: 713
molecular weight; glycoproteins; •, human, table of
values, **02**: 258
molecular weight; proteins; human •, table of values,
02: 242-250
partial specific volume; proteins; •, human, table of
values, **02**: 242-250
plasminogen; •, human
carbohydrate content, molecular weights, sedimentation coefficients, **02**: 258
progesterone; •, nonhuman
carbohydrate content, **02**: 260
proteins
human, *see also* Human plasma proteins
refractive index increments, **02**: 380
proteins, *see also* Bacteriophage Flavoproteins, Matrix
protein, *also* Protein, individual proteins, Molybdoproteins; human •, molecular parameters, table, **02**:
242-250

Plasma (continued)
  prothrombin; •, human
    carbohydrate content, molecular weights, sedimentation coefficients, 02: 258
  prothrombin; •, nonhuman
    carbohydrate content, 02: 260
  rheumatoid factor; •, human
    carbohydrate content, molecular weights, sedimentation coefficients, 02: 258
  sedimentation coefficient; glycoproteins; •, human, table of values, 02: 258
  sedimentation coefficient; proteins; •, human, table of values, 02: 242-250
  thrombin; zymogen conversion during coagulation of •, 02: 670
  transcortin; •, human
    carbohydrate content, molecular weight, sedimentation coefficients, 02: 258
    molecular absorptivity and-or absorbance values, 02: 510
  transferrin, see also Ovotransferrin; •, human
    carbohydrate content, molecular weights, sedimentation coefficients, 02: 258
    molar absorptivity and-or absorbance values, 02: 510
  transferrin, see also Ovotransferrin; •, nonhuman
    carbohydrate content, 02: 260
  zymogen; conversion during coagulation of •, 02: 670
Plasma albumin, see also Albumin, plasma; Human plasma albumin
  analgesics, ligands binding to •, 02: 570
  antibiotics; ligands binding to •, 02: 568-569
  anticoagulants; ligands binding to •, 02: 571
  barbiturates, ligands binding to •, 02: 569
  caffeine, ligands binding to •, 02: 573
  cardiac glycosides, ligands binding to •, 02: 572
  diuretics; ligands binding to •, 02: 571
  drugs, ligands binding to •, 02: 568-574
  dyes, visible, ligands binding to •, 02: 564-568
  endogenous ligands binding to •, 02: 556-557
  exogenous ligands binding to •, 02: 558-574
  fatty acids, ligands binding to •, 02: 558-562
  hypoglycemic agents, ligands binding to •, 02: 572
  inorganic anions, ligands binding to •, 02: 563
  ligands binding to •, table, 02: 556-574
  metal ions, ligands binding to •, 02: 563
  methadone, ligands binding to •, 02: 574
  procaine, ligands binding to •, 02: 574
  radio-opaque agents, ligands binding to •, 02: 572
  saccharin, ligands binding to •, 02: 574
  steroids; ligands binding to •, 02: 563
  sulfonamides; ligands binding to •, 02: 568
  tranquilizers; ligands binding to •, 02: 571
  warfarin, ligands binding to •, 02: 572
Plasmin
  human
    molar absorptivity and-or absorbance values, 02: 498
  human, urokinase activated
    molar absorptivity and-or absorbance values, 02: 498
  molecular parameters, 02: 246
Plasminogen
  general building plan, 07: 353

human
  molar absorptivity and-or absorbance values, 02: 499
human, A
  molar absorptivity and-or absorbance values, 02: 499
human, B
  molar absorptivity and-or absorbance values, 02: 499
molecular parameters, 02: 245
physical data and characteristics, 02: 254-255
plasma, human
  carbohydrate content, molecular weights, sedimentation coefficients, 02: 258
sequence of the 69 residue amino-terminal peptide released from, upon activation with urokinase, 07: 354
Plastics
  commercial
    chemical and physical properties, 08: 427
    chemical compatibility of Millipore® filters, O-rings and filter holders, 08: 431-432
    chemical resistance of those used in ultracentrifuge, 08: 428-429
    ultracentrifuge tubes, chemical resistance, 08: 434
  specific gravity; •, commercial, 08: 427
  ultracentrifuge tubes, chemical resistance of • used, 08: 434
Plastocyanin
  average hydrophobicity value, 01: 230
  molar absorptivity and-or absorbance values, 02: 499
  molecular weights, stoichiometry and sources, 02: 282
Platelets
  aspirin; prostaglandin biosynthesis by •, inhibition, 08: 332
Plicacetin
  origin, structure, and characteristic as protein biosynthesis inhibitor, 04: 596
  physicochemical constants, spectral chemotherapeutic and biological properties, 03: 345
Poly(α-amino acids)
  amino acids, see also Aromatic amino acids, also specific acids; •
    enzymatic activities, susceptibility to, 01: 393-396
    solubility, table, 01: 393-396
  enzymes, see also Coenzyme, Metalloenzyme, Multienzyme; susceptibility of • to, 01: 393-396
  solubility; •, table, 01: 393-396
Poly (β-benzyl-L-aspartate)
  calorimetric ΔH values accompanying conformational changes, 06: 275-276
Poly (γ-benzyl-L-glutamate)
  calorimetric ΔH values accompanying conformational changes, 06: 276-280
Poly (N-γ-carbobenzoxy-L-α,γ-(diaminobutric acid)
  calorimetric ΔH values accompanying conformational changes, 06: 280
Poly(ε-carbobenzoxy-L-lysine)
  calorimetric ΔH values accompanying conformational changes, 06: 280
Poly(N-δ-carbobenzoxy-L-ornithine)
  calorimetric ΔH values accompanying conformational changes, 06: 280

Polypeptide *(continued)*

configuration; • chemistry, use of term, **01**: 73, **02**: 77

conformation; • chemistry, use of term, **01**: 73, **02**: 77

frequencies, calculated characteristic • table, **07**: 596

hormone-binding •

amino acid composition, complete data, **07**: 507

parathyroid •

amino acid composition, complete data, **07**: 509

symbols; • chains, conformation, journal reference, **02**: 87

Polypeptide chains

IUPAC-IUB Commission on Biochemical Nomenclature; •, abbreviations and symbols, tentative rules, **01**: 59-73, **02**: 63-77

Polypeptides, *see also* Polypeptide

abbreviations; •, synthetic, journal reference, **02**: 87

2-Acetamidoacrylic acid; structure and symbols for those incorporated into synthetic •, **01**: 97

N^α-Acetyl-2-fluorophenylalanine; structure and symbols for those incorporated into synthetic •, **01**: 97

N^α-Acetyllysine-N-methylamide; structure and symbols for those incorporated into synthetic •, **01**: 97

β-Alanine; structure and symbols for those incorporated into synthetic •, **01**: 97

alloisoleucine; structure and symbols for those incorporated into synthetic •, **01**: 97

3-Amino-2-benzylpropionic acid; structure and symbols for those incorporated into synthetic •, **01**: 97

3-Amino-3-benzylpropionic acid; structure and symbols for those incorporated into synthetic •, **01**: 97

2-Amino-6-dimethylamino-4-hexynoic acid; structure and symbols for those incorporated into synthetic •, **01**: 98

2-Amino-3-ethylvaleric acid; structure and symbols for those incorporated into synthetic •, **01**: 98

4-Amino-3-hydroxy-6-methylheptanoic acid; structure and symbols for those incorporated into synthetic •, **01**: 98

2-Amino-3-(2-imidazolyl)propionic acid; structure and symbols for those incorporated into synthetic •, **01**: 98

2-Amino-4-methyl-hexenoic acid; structure and symbols for those incorporated into synthetic •, **01**: 98

2-Amino-4-methyl-4-hexenoic acid; structure and symbols for those incorporated into synthetic •, **01**: 98

2-Amino-5-methyl-5-hexenoic acid; structure and symbols for those incorporated into synthetic •, **01**: 98

3-Amino-4-phenylbutyric acid; structure and symbols for those incorporated into synthetic •, **01**: 99

2-Amino-3-(2-pyridyl)propionic acid; structure and symbols for those incorporated into synthetic •, **01**: 99

2-Amino-3-(2-pyrimidyl)propionic acid; structure and symbols for those incorporated into synthetic •, **01**: 99

2-Amino-6-(trimethylammonio)hexanoic acid; structure and symbols for those incorporated into synthetic •, **01**: 99

amino acids, *see also* Aromatic amino acids, *also* specific acids; synthetic; structures and symbols for those incorporated into synthetic •, **01**: 96

2-Aminoadipic acid; structure and symbols for those incorporated into synthetic •, **01**: 97

3-Aminoadipic acid, **01**: 97; structure and symbols for those incorporated into synthetic •, **01**: 97

2-Aminobutyric acid; structure and symbols for those incorporated into synthetic •, **01**: 97

3-Aminobutyric acid; structure and symbols for those incorporated into synthetic •, **01**: 97

4-Aminobutyric acid; structure and symbols for those incorporated into synthetic •, **01**: 97

2-Aminocrotonic acid; structure and symbols for those incorporated into synthetic •, **01**: 97

1-Aminocyclohexane-1-carboxylic acid; structure and symbols for those incorporated into synthetic •, **01**: 97

1-Aminocyclopentane-1-carboxylic acid; structure and symbols for those incorporated into synthetic •, **01**: 97

6-Aminohexanoic acid; structure and symbols for those incorporated into synthetic •, **01**: 98

2-Aminoisobutyric acid; structure and symbols for those incorporated into synthetic •, **01**: 98

aminomethanesulfonic acid; structure and symbols for those incorporated into synthetic •, **01**: 98

4-Aminomethylbenzoic acid; structure and symbols for those incorporated into synthetic •, **01**: 98

8-Aminooctanoic acid; structure and symbols for those incorporated into synthetic •, **01**: 98

(4-Amino)phenylalanine; structure and symbols for those incorporated into synthetic •, **01**: 98

2-Aminopimelic acid; structure and symbols for those incorporated into synthetic •, **01**: 99

3-Aminotyrosine; structure and symbols for those incorporated into synthetic •, **01**: 99

aspartic α-methylamide; structure and symbols for those incorporated into synthetic •, **01**: 99

aspartic β-methylamide; structure and symbols for those incorporated into synthetic •, **01**: 99

azetidine-2-carboxylic acid; structure and symbols for those incorporated into synthetic •, **01**: 99

aziridinecarboxylic acid; structure and symbols for those incorporated into synthetic •, **01**: 99

aziridinonecarboxylic acid; structure and symbols for those incorporated into synthetic •, **01**: 100

(α-Benzyl)phenylalanine; structure and symbols for those incorporated into synthetic •, **01**: 100

3-Benzyltyrosine; structure and symbols for those incorporated into synthetic •, **01**: 100

(4-Chloro)phenylalanine; structure and symbols for those incorporated into synthetic •, **01**: 100

citrulline; structure and symbols for those incorporated into synthetic •, **01**: 100

β-Cyanoalanine; structure and symbols for those incorporated into synthetic •, **01**: 100

N-(2-Cyanoethyl)glycine; structure and symbols for those incorporated into synthetic •, **01**: 100

cyclic

symbols for, use of, **01**: 11, **02**: 11

β-(1,4-Cyclohexadienyl)alanine; structure and symbols for those incorporated into synthetic •, **01**: 100

β-(Cyclohexyl)alanine; structure and symbols for those incorporated into synthetic •, **01**: 100

α-(Cyclohexyl)glycine; structure and symbols for those incorporated into synthetic •, **01**: 100

Polypeptides *(continued)*

polymerization of product, determination for sequential
•, **01**: 332

β-(1-Pyrazolyl)alanine; structure and symbols for those
incorporated into synthetic •, **01**: 106

β-(3-Pyrazolyl)alanine; structure and symbols for those
incorporated into synthetic •, **01**: 106

β-(4-Pyrazolyl)alanine; structure and symbols for those
incorporated into synthetic •, **01**: 106

pyro-2-aminoadipic acid; structure and symbols for
those incorporated into synthetic •, **01**: 106

pyroglutamic acid; structure and symbols for those incorporated into synthetic •, **01**: 106

sarcosine; structure and symbols for those incorporated
into synthetic •, **01**: 107

sequential
abbreviations, **01**: 333
polymerization, determination of degree of, **01**: 332
preparation and product analysis, index to table, **01**:
334-339
racemization, determination of degree of, **01**: 332

succinamic acid; structure and symbols for those incorporated into synthetic •, **01**: 107

symbols for, rules, **01**: 88-90

symbols for, use of, **01**: 10-11, **02**: 10-11

synthetic
symbols for, use of, 01: 13, 02: 13-14

synthetic immunogenic, **07**: 546-547

taurine; structure and symbols for those incorporated
into synthetic •, **01**: 107

thiazolidine-4-carboxylic acid; structure and symbols for
those incorporated into synthetic •, **01**: 107

β-2-Thienylalanine; structure and symbols for those incorporated into synthetic •, **01**: 107

β-(2-Thienyl)serine; structure and symbols for those incorporated into synthetic •, **01**: 107

ε-(Trimethylammonio)hexanoic acid; structure and symbols for those incorporated into synthetic •, **01**: 107

m-Tyrosine; structure and symbols for those incorporated into synthetic •, **01**: 107

o-Tyrosine; structure and symbols for those incorporated into synthetic •, **01**: 107

Polypropylene
chemical and physical properties, **08**: 427

Polyribonucleotides
absorption, •, use of tables in calculation of, **03**: 596
circular dichroism; •, use of table in calculation of, **03**:
591
molar absorptivity; •, calculation of, **03**: 596
molar ellipticity; •, calculation of, **03**: 596
molar rotation; •, calculation of, **03**: 596
optical parameters; •, calculation of, **03**: 596
optical rotatory dispersion; •, use of tables in calculation of, **03**: 596

Polysaccharide
depolymerase

molar absorptivity and-or absorbance values, **02**: 500
subunit, constitution of, **02**: 347

Polysaccharides
circular dichroism; •, table, **05**: 468-470
connective tissues, table of data and characteristics, **02**:
686-687
electronic charge distribution, **05**: 478-481
IR spectra; •, fingerprint region, **02**: 686-687
molecular weight; •, table of values, **02**: 686-687
optical rotatory dispersion; •, table, **05**: 463-464
specific rotation; •, table of values, **02**: 686-687
viscosity; intrinsic; •, table of values, **02**: 686-687

Polystyrene
chemical and physical properties, **08**: 427

Polyvinyl chloride
chemical and physical properties, **08**: 427

Polyvinyl sulfate
mode of action as protein biosynthesis inhibitor, **04**: 596

Porcine pepsin, *see* Pepsin, porcine

Poricin
amino acid composition, incomplete data, **07**: 514

Porphyrins
absorption maxima
dications in aqueous HCl, **08**: 269-271
organic solvents, data table, **08**: 273-274
various solutions, data table, **08**: 272
excretion in humans, normal values, **08**: 279
excretion in laboratory animals, average normal values,
08: 279
fluorescence maxima in various solvents, **08**: 275
HCl numbers, table, **08**: 275
methylesters, melting points, **08**: 276
nomenclature and structure, **08**: 268-269
oxidation-reduction potentials of metalloporphyrins, **06**:
139-144
pK'_a values, **06**: 348
R_F values in 2,6-lutidine-water systems, **08**: 276
Soret band data; • dications in aqueous HCl, 08:
269-271
Soret band data; • in organic solvents, 08: 273-274
structure; •, **08**: 268-269
trivial names; •, **08**: 269

Postalbumin
4.6S
molar absorptivity and-or absorbance values, **02**: 500
molecular parameters, **02**: 242

Potassium chloride
hydrochloric acid-• buffer, preparation of, **06**: 370

Prealbumin
amino acid composition, complete data, **07**: 509
average hydrophobicity value, **01**: 230
circular dichroism in the UV region, **07**: 120
molar absorptivity and-or absorbance values, **02**: 500
molecular parameters, **02**: 242
optical rotatory dispersion in the UV region, **07**: 72
subunit, constitution of, **02**: 328

Prealbumin *(continued)*

(thyroxine-binding prealbumin)

circular dichroism intensities at maxima in near-UV region, at room temperature, **07:** 159

Precursors

chromatography; prostaglandin •, isolation and detection, **08:** 327

fatty acids, *see also* Lipids, Wax fatty acids; prostaglandin •

biological and physical properties, **08:** 322-328

isolation and synthesis of, **08:** 326-327

mammalian diet, metabolism reactions, **08:** 322-323

nomenclature, **08:** 315-316

occurrence, **08:** 323

formula, molecular; prostaglandin •, **08:** 325

molecular weight; prostaglandin •, **08:** 325

nomenclature; prostaglandins and •, **08:** 313-316

prostaglandins; liberation of • from phosphatidyl inositol, **08:** 320

prostaglandins; •

biological actions, **08:** 322-324, 328

isolation, detection and assay, methods for, **08:** 32

nomenclature of essential fatty acids, **08:** 315-316

occurrence of several, **08:** 325

structure and molecular weight, **08:** 325

synthesis, methods, **08:** 326

structure; prostaglandin •, **08:** 325

trivial names; prostaglandin •, **08:** 325

Prekallikrein

molecular parameters, **02:** 248

physical data and characteristics, **02:** 254-255

Prenylmenaquinone-6

properties of, **08:** 291

Prephenic

dehydratase

Neurospora crassa mutant, **04:** 747

thermolabile • dehydrogenase

Neurospora crassa mutant, **04:** 742

Prephospholipase A$_2$, *see* Prophospholipase A$_2$

Pristinamycin I, II

origin, structure, and characteristic as protein biosynthesis inhibitor, **04:** 596-597

Proaccelerin

physical data and characteristics, **02:** 254-255

Procaine

ligands binding to plasma albumin, **02:** 574

Procarboxypeptidase A

average hydrophobicity value, **01:** 230

molar absorptivity and-or absorbance values, **02:** 500

Procarboxypeptidase B

molar absorptivity and-or absorbance values, **02:** 501

Prococoonase

average hydrophobicity value, **01:** 217

Procollagen I

circular dichroism in the UV region, **07:** 120

Progestagens

structures and properties, **05:** 541-543

Progesterone

plasma, nonhuman

carbohydrate content, **02:** 260

Progesterone-binding

globulin

molar absorptivity and-or absorbance values, **02:** 501

protein

average hydrophobicity value, **01:** 230

Prohistidine

decarboxylase

average hydrophobicity value, **01:** 230

Proinsulin

amino acid composition, complete data, **07:** 509

amino acid sequence, **07:** 381

circular dichroism, **07:** 120

molar absorptivity and-or absorbance values, **02:** 501

optical rotatory dispersion in the UV region, **07:** 73

Prokaryotic

cytochromes *b*

amino acid sequence, **07:** 280-281

cytochromes *c*

amino acid sequence, **07:** 292-306

Prolactin

average hydrophobicity value, **01:** 230

hormone, *see also* Luteinizing hormone; •, sheep

molar absorptivity and-or absorbance values, **02:** 450

molar absorptivity and-or absorbance values, **02:** 501

Prolamin

circular dichroism in the UV region, **07:** 120

optical rotatory dispersion

UV region, **07:** 73

visible and near UV regions, **07:** 34

Proline

antagonists of, **01:** 179

3,4-dehydroproline; antagonism to •, **01:** 179

far ultraviolet absorption spectra

aqueous solution at pH 5, **01:** 184

neutral water, table, **01:** 185

0.1 *M* sodium dodecyl sulfate, table, **01:** 185

free acid in amniotic fluid in early pregnancy and at term, **01:** 327

free acid in blood plasma of newborn infants and adults, **01:** 328

heat of proton ionization, pK, and related thermodynamic quantities, **06:** 235

hyperprolinemia type I, effect of, **01:** 321

nucleotide sequences of, **04:** 450-451

pK'_a values, **06:** 319

physical and chemical properties, **01:** 146

requirements of, for growth of various microorganisms, table, **04:** 630-643

specific rotatory dispersion constants, 0.1 *M* solution, **01:** 244

spectra, far UV, **01:** 184

symbols for atoms and bonds in side chains, **01:** 70, **02:** 74

thumbprint, content in, **08:** 121

Proline betaine, *see* Stachydrine

Proline dation, seizures

hyperprolinemia type II, effect of, **01:** 321

Proline T4

nucleoside composition, tables of values, **04:** 437

Pronase

enzymatic hydrolysis, conjugated proteins, **02:** 211

S-(Prop-1-enyl)-cysteine
  physical and chemical properties, **01**: 157
S-(Prop-1-enyl)-cysteine sulfoxide
  physical and chemical properties, **01**: 157
Propane derivatives
  heat of proton ionization, pK, and related thermody-
    namic quantities, **06**: 235-236
1-2-Propanediol-water
  mixtures, dielectric constants and freezing points, **06**:
    525
Propanoic acid
  heat of proton ionization, pK, and related thermody-
    namic quantities, **06**: 237-239
Properdin
  molecular parameters, **02**: 250
Prophospholipase A$_2$
  circular dichroism in the UV region, **07**: 120
  optical rotatory dispersion in the UV region, **07**: 73
Propionic acid
  antagonism to β-Alanine, **01**: 177
Propionyl
  coenzyme A carboxylase
    amino acid composition, incomplete data, **07**: 514
S-n-Propylcysteine
  physical and chemical properties, **01**: 157
S-Propylcysteine sulfoxide, *see* Dihydroallin
S-n-Propylcysteine sulfoxide
  physical and chemical properties, **01**: 157
O-Propylhomoserine
  physical and chemical properties, **01**: 128
Prostaglandin, *see also* Prostaglandins
  arachidonic acid; precursor in • biosynthesis, **08**:
    334-338
  aspirin; • biosynthesis by platelets, inhibition, **08**: 332
  dissociation constants; • metabolizing enzymes, **08**:
    364-367
  fatty acids, *see also* Lipids, Wax fatty acids; • precur-
    sors
    biological and physical properties, **08**: 322-328
    isolation and synthesis of, **08**: 326-327
    mammalian diet, metabolism reactions, **08**: 322-323
    nomenclature, **08**: 315-316
    occurrence, **08**: 323
  formula, molecular; • analogs, **08**: 397-421
  formula, molecular; • biosynthesis intermediates, throm-
    boxanes and by-products, **08**: 334-340
  formula, molecular; • metabolites, **08**: 368-391
  formula, molecular; • precursors, **08**: 325
  inhibitors; • metabolizing enzymes, **08**: 364-367
  LASS; • nomenclature, suggested use of term, **08**: 314
  molecular weight; • analogs, **08**: 397-421
  molecular weight; • biosynthesis intermediates, throm-
    boxanes and by-products, **08**: 334-340
  molecular weight; • metabolites, **08**: 368-391
  molecular weight; • metabolizing enzymes, **08**: 364-367
  molecular weight; • precursors, **08**: 325
  nomenclature; LASS, suggested use of term in • studies,
    08: 314
  nomenclature; • biosynthesis intermediates, throwbox-
    anes and by-products, **08**: 334-340
  nomenclature; RCS, suggested use of term in • studies,
    08: 314

phospholipase A; • biosynthesis, importance, **08**: 320
prostanoic acid; • nomenclature system, **08**: 315
RCS; • nomenclature, suggested use of term, **08**: 314
structure; • analogs, **08**: 396-421
structure; • biosynthesis intermediates, thromboxanes
  and by-products, **08**: 334-340
structure; • metabolites, **08**: 368-391
trivial names; • analogs, **08**: 396-421
trivial names; • biosynthesis intermediates, thromboxanes and by-products, **08**: 334-340
trivial names; • precursors, **08**: 325
Prostaglandins, *see also* Prostaglandin
  analogs
    names and structures, **08**: 396-421
    properties, physical and biological, **08**: 396-421
    synthesis and importance, general information, **08**:
      394-395
  biological significance, **08**: 312-313
  biosynthesis; •, pathways diagram, **08**: 317
  biosynthesis; •, properties of intermediates, thrombox-
    anes and by-products, **08**: 332-341
  biosynthesis, intermediates, thromboxanes and by-
    products
    isolation, biological effects, stability, **08**: 335-341
    occurrence, structure, molecular weight, **08**: 334-340
  biosynthesis, pathways diagram, **08**: 317
  biosynthesis inhibition by aspirin, **08**: 332
  classification of, **08**: 313-315
  detection and assay of, general information, **08**: 344
  enzymes, metabolizing, table of properties and activity,
    08: 364-367
  formula, molecular; •, naturally occurring, **08**: 346-358
  isolation of, general information, **08**: 344
  liberation of precursor from phosphatidyl inositol, **08**:
    320
  metabolites, table of physical and biological properties,
    08: 368-391
  metabolizing enzymes, target sites, **08**: 320
  molecular weight; •, naturally occurring, **08**: 346-358
  naturally occurring, structures, sources, and biological
    actions, **08**: 346-359
  nomenclature; •, naturally occurring, **08**: 346-358
  nomenclature; • and precursors, **08**: 313-316
  nomenclature, series and classes, **08**: 313-315
  occurrence, general information, **08**: 312-313
  phospholipids; •, pathways diagram, **08**: 317
  precursors
    biological actions, **08**: 322-324, 328
    isolation, detection and assay, methods for, **08**: 327
    nomenclature of essential fatty acids, **08**: 315-316
    occurrence of several, **08**: 325
    structure and molecular weight, **08**: 325
    synthesis, methods, **08**: 326
  trivial names; •, naturally occurring, **08**: 346-358
Prostanoic acid
  prostaglandin nomenclature system, **08**: 315
  structure, **08**: 316
Protease, *see also* Proteases
  acid
    average hydrophobicity value, **01**: 230
    molar absorptivity and-or absorbance values, **02**: 502
  average hydrophobicity value, **01**: 230

Protease *(continued)*
circular dichroism in the UV region, **07**: 120
cofactors, molecular weights, stoichiometry, sources, **02**: 284
α-lytic •
average hydrophobicity value, **01**: 226
β-lytic •
average hydrophobicity value, **01**: 226
molar absorptivity and-or absorbance values, **02**: 501
optical rotatory dispersion in the visible and near UV regions, **07**: 34
Protease-A
average hydrophobicity value, **01**: 230
Protease A
optical rotatory dispersion
UV region, **07**: 73
visible and near UV regions, **07**: 34
Protease inhibitor
molar absorptivity and-or absorbance values, **02**: 457, 503
Proteases, *see also* Protease
serine •, trypsin-related
amino acid sequence data, index to
blood clotting factors, **07**: 350-354
explanation of tables, **07**: 340-341
sequence alignments, **07**: 341-349
serine • active, bearing the active site serine
alignments of the chains of, **07**: 344-349
Protein, *see also* Bacteriophage protein, Conjugated proteins, Covalent protein conjugates, Covalent conjugates, Flavoproteins, Glycoprotein listings, Human plasma proteins, Iron proteins, Iron-sulfur proteins, Lipoprotein, Matrix protein, Metalloproteins, Molybdoproteins, Mucoprotein, Plasma proteins, human, Proteins, conjugated, Proteins, iron-sulfur, Serum proteins, Tamm-Horsfall, Tamm-Horsfall glycoproteins, Tamm-Horsfall mucoprotein, *also* Proteins
acetylcholine receptor •
circular dichroism in the UV region, **07**: 82
acidic brain •
amino acid composition, incomplete data, **07**: 512
acyl carrier •
amino acid composition, complete data, **07**: 505
amino acid sequence, **07**: 498
average hydrophobicity value, **01**: 211
cyanogen bromide cleavage, **02**: 199
molar absorptivity and-or absorbance values, **02**: 384
optical rotatory dispersion
UV region, **07**: 44
visible and near UV regions, **07**: 15
adrenal iron-sulfur •
amino acid composition, complete data, **07**: 505
amino • group, chemical modification of
reagents used, table of specificities, **02**: 203-204
bacteriochlorophyll-• complex
amino acid composition, complete data, **07**: 505
bacteriophage •
amino acid sequence of coat proteins, **07**: 261-262
circular dichroism in the UV region, **07**: 86
optical rotatory dispersion
UV region, **07**: 48

visible and near UV regions, **07**: 18
basic brain •
amino acid composition, incomplete data, **07**: 512
basic plasma •
amino acid composition, complete data, **07**: 505
bee venom •
amino acid sequences, **07**: 498
Bence-Jones •
circular dichroism in the UV region, **07**: 86
optical rotatory dispersion
UV region, **07**: 49
visible and near UV regions, **07**: 18
biosynthesis, inhibitors of; characteristics, origin and structures, table, **04**: 555-618
biotin carboxyl carrier •
average hydrophobicity value, **01**: 215
blood coagulation •
table of data and characteristics, **02**: 254-255
S-100 brain-
amino acid composition, incomplete data, **07**: 514
brain acidic • (S-100--)
optical rotatory dispersion in the UV region, **07**: 49
brain proteolipid •
optical rotatory dispersion
UV region, **07**: 49
visible and near UV regions, **07**: 19
calcium-binding •
average hydrophobicity value, **01**: 215
circular dichroism
in UV and near-UV regions, **07**: 86, 145
calcium-binding • (high affinity)
amino acid composition, incomplete data, **07**: 512
circular dichroism in the UV region, **07**: 87
calcium precipitable •
circular dichroism in the UV region, **07**: 87
carboxyl • group, chemical modification of
reagents used, table of specificities, **02**: 203-204
carcinogen-binding •
amino acid composition, incomplete data, **07**: 512
chemical data on *Escherichia coli* ribosomes, **04**: 471-486
cholchisine-binding •
average hydrophobicity value, **01**: 216
cilia •, outer fibers
amino acid composition, complete data, **07**: 506
optical rotatory dispersion in the visible and near UV regions, **07**: 21
codons found in the MS$_2$ coat • gene, **04**: 340
composition
Tamm-Horsfall glycoprotein, **02**: 303
contractile •
molecular parameters, table, **02**: 306
corticosteroid-transporting •
plasma, nonhuman, carbohydrate content, **02**: 259
cortisol metabolites binding large •
amino acid composition, incomplete data, **07**: 512
cotton effect; in UV region, • conformation, spectra, **07**: 9
disulfide • group, chemical modification of
reagents used, table of specificities, **02**: 203-204
Drosophila melanogaster; biochemical mutants; enzyme and structural •, **04**: 848-849

Protein *(continued)*

Drosophila melanogaster; biochemical mutants; • synthesis, **04**: 849-851

egg white cross-reacting •
amino acid composition, complete data, **07**: 506

encephalitogenic A-1 •
average hydrophobicity value, **01**: 219

encephalitogenic •
amino acid composition, complete data, **07**: 506
circular dichroism in the UV region, **07**: 94
optical rotatory dispersion
UV region, **07**: 54
visible and near UV regions, **07**: 22

eukaryotic cytochromes *c*; amino acid sequences of •, tables, **07**: 268-285

familial • intolerance
characteristics of , **01**: 323

fiber •
circular dichroism in the UV region, **07**: 95

fibrous •
physical-chemical data for, index to ultracentrifuge studies, **02**: 229

flavo•
definition and nomenclature, **02**: 116
molar absorptivity and-or absorbance values, **02**: 428

fluorescent probes; naphthalene sulfonates, • structure, **07**: 604-606

fraction 1 •
amino acid composition, complete data, **07**: 507

fructosan-specific •
circular dichroism in the UV region, **07**: 96

globular •
physical-chemical data for, index to ultracentrifuge studies, **02**: 222-228

gonadotrophin-transporting •
plasma, nonhuman
carbohydrate content, **02**: 259

group specific •
amino acid composition, incomplete data, **07**: 513

guanidinyl • group, chemical modification of
reagents used, table of specificities, **02**: 203-204

high density
subunit, constitution of, **02**: 341

high potential iron •
molar absorptivity and-or absorbance values, **02**: 4

high potential iron sulfur •
average hydrophobicity value, **01**: 224

histidine-binding •
average hydrophobicity value, **01**: 224

hydroxyl • group, chemical modification of
reagents used, table of specificities, **02**: 203-204

imidazole • group, chemical modification of
reagents used, table of specificities, **02**: 203-204

incisor eruption accelerating •
amino acid composition, incomplete data, **07**: 513

indole • group, chemical modification of
reagents used, table of specificities, **02**: 203-204

isoelectric point; retinol-binding •, **02**: 304

β-ketoacyl acyl carrier • synthetase
amino acid composition, complete data, **07**: 508

kinase

subunit, constitution of, **02**: 344

kinase modulator
average hydrophobicity value, **01**: 230

lactose synthetase (A •)
circular dichroism in the UV region, **07**: 108
molar absorptivity and-or absorbance values, **02**: 463

leucine binding •
amino acid composition, complete data, **07**: 508

ligandin (Y •), **07**: 108
circular dichroism in the UV region, **07**: 108

M-
circular dichroism in the UV region, **07**: 111
optical rotatory dispersion in the UV region, **07**: 66

membrane •
circular dichroism in the UV region, **07**: 112

membrane •, mitochondria
circular dichroism in the UV region, **07**: 112
optical rotatory dispersion
UV region, **07**: 66
visible and near UV regions, **07**: 30

membrane •, mycoplasma
circular dichroism in the UV region, **07**: 112

membrane •, purple
circular dichroism in the UV region, **07**: 112

membrane •, thylakoid
circular dichroism in the UV region, **07**: 113

microtubule •
amino acid composition, complete data, **07**: 509

mitochondrial structural •
amino acid composition, complete data, **07**: 509

mitotic apparatus 22S •
amino acid composition, incomplete data, **07**: 513

Moffitt equation; for estimate or content in • molecule, **07**: 3-4

subunit, constitution of, **02**: 340

molybdenum-iron •
average hydrophobicity value, **01**: 227

myelin •
circular dichroism in the UV region, **07**: 113
optical rotatory dispersion in the visible and near UV regions, **07**: 31

myeloma •, *see* Immunoglobulin

naphthalene sulfonates; fluorescent probes of • structure, **07**: 604-606

nuclease-T; amino acid sequences of •, **07**: 310

P11
subunit, constitution of, **02**: 329

penton •
circular dichroism in the UV region, **07**: 117

phosphokinase
subunit, constitution of, **02**: 337

primary structure of a segment, definition, **01**: 73, **02**: 77

progesterone-binding •
average hydrophobicity value, **01**: 230

c-•
molecular parameters, **02**: 306

z-•, **07**: 129
circular dichroism in the UV region, **07**: 129

psoriatic scale •
amino acid composition, complete data, **07**: 509

Protein *(continued)*

quaternary structure of a molecule, definition, **02**: 77
quaternary structure of molecule, definition, **01**: 73
R17 coat-
  amino acid composition, complete data, **07**: 510
c-reactive •
  molar absorptivity and-or absorbance values, **02**: 409
  subunit, constitution of, **02**: 337
red-
  amino acid composition, complete data, **07**: 510
relaxing •
  molar absorptivity and-or absorbance values, **02**: 505
retinol-binding •
  average hydrophobicity value, **01**: 230
  circular dichroism
    UV and near UV region, **07**: 121, 160
  human, amino acid composition, **02**: 303
  molar absorptivity and-or absorbance values, **02**: 505
  optical rotatory dispersion in the UV region, **07**: 121
  properties of, **02**: 304
riboflavin-binding •
  average hydrophobicity value, **01**: 231
RNA, *see* Nucleic acids, Transfer RNA, TRNA
    (TRNA); • (wt %) in ribosomes from various
    sources, **04**: 472
RNA, *see* Nucleic acids, Transfer RNA, TRNA
    (TRNA); viral; code word table for the coat • gene,
    04: 340
30S ribosomal •
  amino acid composition, incomplete data, **07**: 514
spectrophotometric determination, • concentration,
    short-wavelength UV, **08**: 197
sulfate-binding •
  amino acid composition, complete data, **07**: 510
sulfhydryl • group, chemical modification of
  reagents used, table of specificities, **02**: 203-204
sweet-sensitive •
  amino acid composition, incomplete data, **07**: 514
Tamm-Horsfall glycoprotein, *see also* Glycoproteins
    Tamm-Horsfall; • composition, **02**: 303
tertiary structure of a molecule, definition, **02**: 77
tertiary structure of molecule, definition, **01**: 73
thio ether • group, chemical modification of
  reagents used, table of specificities, **02**: 203-204
tobacco mosaic virus, A •
  circular dichroism in the UV region, **07**: 125
tobacco mosaic virus •
  depolymerized, luminescence of, table, **01**: 206
  polymerized, luminescence of, table, **01**: 206
tobacco mosaic virus • subunit
  optical rotatory dispersion
    UV region, **07**: 76
    visible and near UV regions, **07**: 36
toxin B
  subunit, constitution of, **02**: 335
troponin Ca^{++}-binding • (Tn-C) rabbit skeletal
  amino acid sequence, **07**: 495
tryptophan synthetase A •
  amino acid composition, complete data, **07**: 510
  amino acid sequences of proteins, **07**: 313
tubulin (6S microtubule •)
  circular dichroism in the UV region, **07**: 128

UV spectra; • concentration determination in short-
    wavelength region, **08**: 197
virus, •
  molar absorptivity and-or absorbance values, **02**: 514
  physical-chemical data for, index to ultracentrifuge
    studies, **02**: 232
virus coat •
Y-Protein, *see* Ligandin, (y-protein)
Protein A
  aldehyde dehydrogenase, •
    average hydrophobicity value, **01**: 212
Protein biosynthesis
  althiomycin; origin, structure, and characteristic as • in-
    hibitor, **04**: 557
  fusidin, inhibitor of •, **04**: 575
Protein biosynthesis inhibitor
  abrin; origin, structure, and characteristics as •, **04**: 555
  acetoxy-cycloheximide, origin, structure, and character-
    istic as •, **04**: 555
  actinobolin; origin, structure, and characteristic as •,
    04: 556
  actinphenol; origin, structure, and characteristic as •,
    04: 556
  adrenochrome; origin, structure, and characteristic as •,
    04: 557
  allomycin; origin, structure, and characteristic as •, **04**:
    557
  amicetin; origin, structure, and characteristic as •, **04**:
    558
  aminoalkyl adenylate; origin, structure, and characteris-
    tic as •, **04**: 558
  DL-3-aminobutyramide; characteristics as •, **04**: 559
  aminochromes; origin, structure, and characteristics as
    •, **04**: 559
  angolamycin; origin, structure, and characteristic as •,
    04: 559
  anisomycin; origin, structure, and characteristics as •,
    04: 559
  Aureomycin®; origin, structure, and characteristic as •,
    04: 560
  aurintricarboxylic acid; origin, structure, and character-
    istic as •, **04**: 560
  avilamycin; origin, structure, and characteristic as •, **04**:
    561
  bacteriocin DF$_{13}$, origin, structure, and characteristic as
    •, **04**: 561
  bamicetin; origin, structure, and characteristic as •, **04**:
    561
  berninamycin; origin, structure, and characteristic as •,
    04: 562
  blasticidin S; origin, structure, and characteristic as •,
    04: 562
  bluensomycin; origin, structure, and characteristic as •,
    04: 563
  borrelidin; origin, structure, and characteristic as •, **04**:
    563
  bottromycin A$_2$; origin, structure, and characteristic as
    •, **04**: 563
  bryamycin; origin, structure, and characteristic as •, **04**:
    564
  carbomycin; origin, structure, and characteristic as •,
    04: 564

Protein biosynthesis inhibitor *(continued)*

celesticetin; origin, structure, and characteristic as •, **04:** 564

cephalosporin Pl; origin, structure, and characteristic as •, **04:** 565

chalcomycin; origin, structure, and characteristic as •, **04:** 565

chartreusin; origin, structure, and characteristic as •, **04:** 566

chloramphenicol; origin, structure, and characteristic as •, **04:** 566

chlortetracycline; origin, structure, and characteristic as •, **04:** 567

clindamycin; origin, structure, and characteristic as •, **04:** 567

colicin E3; origin, structure, and characteristic as •, **04:** 567

crotocin (Antibiotic T); origin, structure, and characteristic as •, **04:** 568

crotocol; origin, structure, and characteristic as •, **04:** 568

cryptopleurine; origin, structure, and characteristic as •, **04:** 569

cycloheximide; origin, structure, and characteristic as •, **04:** 569

deoxycycline, origin, structure, and characteristic as •, **04:** 570

dihydrostreptomycin; origin, structure, and characteristic as •, **04:** 570

diptheria toxin; origin, structure, and characteristic as •, **04:** 571

edeine; origin, structure, and characteristic as •, **04:** 571

emetine; origin, structure, and characteristic as •, **04:** 572

enomycin; origin, structure, and chracteristic as •, **04:** 572

erythromycin A; origin, structure, and characteristic as •, **04:** 573

fermicidin; origin and characteristic as •, **04:** 38

forocidin; origin, structure, and characteristic as •, **04:** 574

furanomycin; origin, structure, and characteristic as •, **04:** 574

fusarenone X; origin, structure, and characteristic as •, **04:** 574

fusidic acid; origin, structure, and characteristic as •, **04:** 575

gentamycin (C_1 and C_2); origin, structure, and characteristic as •, **04:** 575

gougerotin; origin, structure, and characteristic as •, **04:** 576

griseoviridine; origin, structure, and characteristic as •, **04:** 576

5′-guanylylmethylene diphosphate; origin, structure, and characteristic as •, **04:** 577

harringtonine; origin, structure, and characteristic as •, **04:** 577

homogentisic acid; origin, structure, and characteristic as •, **04:** 578

hydroxy-β-aminobutyramide; structure and mode of action as •, **04:** 578

hydroxylamine; structure and characteristic as •, **04:** 578

hydroxystreptomycin (Reticulin); origin, structure, and characteristic as •, **04:** 579

hygromycin B; origin, structure, and characteristic as •, **04:** 579

kanamycin A, B, and C; origin, structure, and characteristic as •, **04:** 580

kasugamycin, origin, structure, and characteristic as •, **04:** 581

kirromycin (Mocimycin), origin, structure, and characteristic as •, **04:** 581

lankamycin; origin, structure, and characteristic as •, **04:** 582

leucine; methyl and ethyl ester of, as •, **04:** 584

leucomycin A_3; origin, structure, and characteristic as •, **04:** 582

lincomycin; origin, structure, and characteristic as •, **04:** 583

lividomycin; origin, structure, and characteristic as •, **04:** 583

mannoside streptomycin; origin and characteristic as •, **04:** 584

MDMP; origin, structure, and characteristic as •, **04:** 584

6-methylenetetracycline; origin, structure, and characteristic as •, **04:** 584

methymycin; origin, structure, and characteristic as •, **04:** 585

micrococcin (Micrococcin P); origin, structure, and characteristic as •, **04:** 585

mikamycin A; origin, structure, and characteristic as •, **04:** 585

minosin (Minomycin); origin, structure, and characteristic as •, **04:** 586

multhiomycin; origin, structure, and characteristic as •, **04:** 586

Naramycin® B; origin, structure, and characteristic as •, **04:** 586

neomycin A, B, and C; origin, structure, and characteristic as •, **04:** 587

neospiramycin; origin, structure, and characteristic as •, **04:** 588

niddamycin; origin, structure, and characteristic as •, **04:** 588

niromycin A and B; origin of •, **04:** 588

nivalenol; origin, structure, and characteristic as •, **04:** 589

nucleocidin; origin, structure, and characteristic as •, **04:** 589

oleandomycin; origin, structure, and characteristic of •, **04:** 590

oxalysine, structure and mode of action as •, **04:** 593

PA 114-B; origin, structure, and characteristic as •, **04:** 594

pactamycin; origin, structure, and characteristic as •, **04:** 593

paromomycin; origin, structure, and characteristic as •, **04:** 594

pederin; origin, structure, and characteristic as •, **04:** 595

Protein biosynthesis inhibitor *(continued)*

phenomycin; origin, structure, and characteristic as ●, **04:** 595

phytolacca americana peptide (PAP); origin, structure, and characteristic as ●, **04:** 595

plicacetin; origin, structure, and characteristic as ●, **04:** 596

polydextran sulfate, characteristics as ●, **04:** 596

polyvinyl sulfate, mode of action as ●, **04:** 596

pristinamycin I, II; origin, structure, and characteristic as ●, **04:** 596-597

Protomycin®, origin and mode of action as ●, **04:** 597

puromycin; origin, structure, and characteristic as ●, **04:** 597

pyrocatechol violet; origin, structure, and characteristic as ●, **04:** 598

relomycin; origin, structure, and characteristic as ●, **04:** 598

ricin; origin, structure, and characteristic as ●, **04:** 598

rubradirin; origin, structure, and characteristic as ●, **04:** 599

sarkomycin origin, structure, and characteristic as●, **04:** 599

1-serine hydroxamate, characteristic as ●, 04: 599

showdomycin; origin, structure, and characteristic as ●, **04:** 599

siomycin; origin, structure, and characteristic as ●, **04:** 600

sodium fluoride; structure and characteristic as ●, **04:** 600

sparsomycin; origin, structure, and characteristic as ●, **04:** 600

spectinomycin; origin, structure, and characteristic as ●, **04:** 601

spiramycin I, II, and III; origin, structure, and characteristic as●, **04:** 601

sporangiomycin; origin, structure, and charateristic as ●, **04:** 602

Staphylomycin® S; origin, structure and characteristic as ●, **04:** 602

streptimidone; origin, structure, and characteristic as ●, **04:** 602

streptogramin A; origin, structure, and characteristic as ●, **04:** 603

streptogramin B₁; origin, structure, and characteristic as ●, **04:** 603

streptomycin; origin, structure, and characteristic as ●, **04:** 604

streptonigrin; origin, structure, and characteristic as ●, **04:** 604

streptovitacin A; origin, structure, and characteristic as ●, **04:** 605

Synergistin® A-1 (PA114-A-1); origin, structure, and characteristic as ●, **04:** 605

synergistin B-1, B-3; origin, structure, and charateristic as ●, **04:** 606

t2 toxin; origin, structure, and characteristic as ●, 04: 613

Telomycin® (Antibiotic A-128-OP); origin, structure, and characteristic as ●, **04:** 607

tenuazonic acid; origin, structure, and characteristic as ●, **04:** 607

Terramycin®; origin, structure, and characteristic as ●, **04:** 608

tetracycline; origin, structure, and characteristic as ●, **04:** 608

thermothiocin; origin, structure, and characteristic as ●, **04:** 608

thiactin; origin, structure, and characteristic as ●, **04:** 608

thiamphenicol (D-AMP-3); origin, structure, and characteristic as ●, **04:** 609

d-Thiocymetin®; origin, structure, and characteristic as ●, **04:** 609

thiopeptin B; origin, structure, and characteristic and ●, **04:** 609

thiostrepton; origin, structure, and characteristic as ●, **04:** 610

tobramycin; origin, structure, and characteristic as ●, **04:** 610

1-1-tosylamido-2-phenylethyl choloromethyl ketone (TPCK), origin, structure, and characteristic as ●, **04:** 611

translational control RNA; origin, structure, and characteristic as ●, **04:** 611

trichodermin; origin, structure, and characteristic as ●, **04:** 611

trichodermol; origin, structure, and characteristic as ●, **04:** 612

trichothecin; origin, structure, and characteristic as ●, **04:** 612

tubulosine; origin, structure, and characteristic as ●, **04:** 613

tylocrebrine; origin, structure, and characteristic as ●, **04:** 614

tylophorine; origin, structure, and characteristic as ●, **04:** 614

tylosin; origin, structure, and characteristic as ●, **04:** 615

tyramine; structure and characteristic as ●, **04:** 615

vernamycin A; origin, structure, and characteristic as ●, **04:** 615

vernamycin Ba, mode of action of ●, **04:** 615

verruacarins; origin, structure, and characteristic as ●, **04:** 616

verrucarol; origin, structure, and characteristic as ●, **04:** 616

viomycin; origin, structure, and characteristic as ●, **04:** 617

viridogrisein; origin, structure, and characteristic as ●, **04:** 618

d-Win-5094; origin, structure, and characteristic as ●, **04:** 571

Protein conjugates

dansyl; covalent ●, data, **01:** 208

pyrenebutyrate; covalent ●, data, **01:** 208

rhodamine B isothiocyanate; covalent ●, data, **01:** 208

Proteinase

Rhizopus acid ●

circular dichroism in the UV region, **07:** 121

optical rotatory dispersion in the UV region, **07:** 73

Aspergillus alkaline ●

optical rotatory dispersion

UV region, **07:** 48

UV region, **07:** 48

Proteinase *(continued)*
    visible and near UV regions, **07:** 18
  human serum, *see also* Serum, human; • inhibitors
    from, specificity and properties, **02:** 636-641
  Clostridium histolyticum • B
    optical rotatory dispersion
      UV region, **07:** 52
      visible and near UV regions, **07:** 21
  streptococcal •
    amino acid sequence, **07:** 356-357
Proteinase--alkaline, *Aspergillus, see Aspergillus* alkaline--
    proteinase
Proteinase, neutral, *see* Microbial metalloenzyme
Proteinase A and B--alkaline, thermophilic, *Streptomyces,*
    see Trypsin, thermophilic Streptomyces
Proteinase B
  alkaline
    circular dichroism intensities at maxima in near UV
      region, at room temperature, **07:** 159
  alkaline •
    average hydrophobicity value, **01:** 213
Proteinase inhibitor I
  subunit, constitution of, **02:** 327
Proteinase inhibitors
  animal sources
    amino acid composition, table, **02:** 649-653
    amino acid sequences, table, **02:** 656-659
    carbohydrate content, **02:** 618-628
    dissociation constant, **02:** 618-641
    isoelectric point, **02:** 618-641
    molecular weight, **02:** 618-641
    specificity, **02:** 618-641
  carbohydrate composition of selected, **02:** 666-667
  cereal grains, • from, specificities and properties, **02:**
    598-599
  egg whites, birds; • from, specificities and properties,
    02: 624-629
  human organs and secretions; • from, specificity and
    properties, **02:** 632-639
  legumes, • from, specificities and properties, **02:** 588-597
  mammalian organs and secretions; • from, specificity
    and properties, **02:** 630-635
  microbial sources
    amino acid composition, **02:** 664
    amino acid sequence, **02:** 665
    isoelectric point, **02:** 661-662
    molecular weight, **02:** 661-662
    specificity, **02:** 661-662
  plant sources
    amino acid composition, table, **02:** 605-610
    amino acid sequences, **02:** 611-617
    carbohydrate content, **02:** 598-599
    dissociation constant, **02:** 588-596, 600
    isoelectric point, **02:** 586-600
    molecular weight, **02:** 586-600
    specificity, **02:** 586-600
  potato tuber sources, • from, specificities and proper-
    ties, **02:** 586-587
Proteinase zymogen

amino acid composition, complete data, **07:** 509
Proteins, *see also* Bacteriophage Flavoproteins, Matrix
    protein, *also* Protein, individual proteins, Molybdo-
    proteins
  absorbance, UV and visible region, table of values, **02:**
    383-514
  amino acid; sequence data, ribosomal • from *Escheri-*
    chia coli, **04:** 479-481
  amino acid compositions; selected •, complete data, **07:**
    504
  amino acid sequence for selected •, **07:** 192-339
  aminopeptidase; enzymatic hydrolysis, conjugated •, **02:**
    211
  average hydrophobicity values for selected, table, **01:**
    210-235
  bacteriophage protein; amino acid sequence of coat •,
    07: 261-262
  blood coagulation, table of data and characteristics, **02:**
    254-255
  blood •, human, demonstrating quantitative abnormal-
    ity, **04:** 881
  blue copper •
    resonance raman spectra, **07:** 589
  carbohydrate content tables for glycoproteins from vari-
    ous sources, **02:** 257-274
  carbohydrate linkages, types of, **02:** 257
  carbohydrates
    physical-chemical data for, index to ultracentrifuge
      studies, **02:** 232
  catalase; amino acid sequences of •, **07:** 308
  chymotrypsin; enzymatic hydrolysis of •, **02:** 209
  chymotryptic hydrolysis, conditions for, **02:** 214
  circular dichroism; characteristics of a single aromatic
    side chain of • in near-ultraviolet region, Table 1,
    07: 142
  circular dichroism; intensities for native • at maxima in
    the near-ultraviolet region at room temperature,
    Table 2, **07:** 143-163
  circular dichroism; of various •, spectra, **07:** 8-13
  coat •
    amino acid sequences, **07:** 261
  concentration determination in short-wavelength UV re-
    gion, **08:** 197
  conformation; •, drawings illustrating, **02:** 760-766
  contractile, molecular parameters, **02:** 306
  covalent conjugates, *see also* Conjugated proteins;
    Covalent protein conjugates
  covalent conjugates, table of data, **01:** 208
  cyanogen bromide cleavage of, table, **02:** 199-202
  demonstrating genetically-determined structural varia-
    tion in man, **04:** 879
  electron-transfer, nomenclature, **02:** 114-121
  electrophoretic mobility; •
    human plasma, table of values, **02:** 242-250
  electrophoretic separation, *Escherichia coli* B 236 70 S
    ribosomal •, **04:** 474
  enamel •
    optical rotatory dispersion in the visible and near UV
      regions, **07:** 22
  entropies, absolute, for several, **06:** 110
  enzymatic cross-linking, **02:** 669-683

Proteins *(continued)*

enzymatic hydrolysis of, **02:** 209

enzymes, *see also* Coenzyme, Metalloenzyme, Multienzyme; amino acid sequences of •, **07:** 308-313

enzymes, *see also* Coenzyme, Metalloenzyme, Multienzyme; proteolytic, digestion cross-linked •, **02:** 669

Escherichia coli, see also E. coli; MRE 600 30 S ribosomal •, separation on cellulose phosphate Whatman® P 11, **04:** 475

fibrous, physical-chemical data for, index to ultracentrifuge studies, **02:** 229

globular, physical-chemical data for, index to ultracentrifuge studies, **02:** 222-228

heat capacities for several, **06:** 110

helical content; of some •, spectra, **07:** 8-13

heme •

resonance raman spectra, **07:** 589

histidine; pK values in various •, table, **02:** 689-692

histones, sequence and characterization tables, **02:** 294-299

human; genetically determined structural variations, • demonstrating, list of, **04:** 879

content in normal plasma, **02:** 242-250

molecular parameters, table, **02:** 242-250

hydrolysis, *see also* Peptic hydrolysis; acid, of •, data tables, **02:** 206-207

hydrolysis, *see also* Peptic hydrolysis; acid, recovery of tryptophan from various •, **02:** 207

hydrolysis of, tables of data for several, **02:** 206-221

infrared spectra, *see* IR spectra; of •, **07:** 596-597

inheritance, mode of; blood coagulation •, **02:** 255

iron, classification of, **02:** 90

iron-sulfur, *see also* Iron sulfur proteins

iron-sulfur, nomenclature recommendations, **02:** 89-90, 120

iron-sulfur primary structures
amino acid sequences, **07:** 425-427

iron-sulfur •
resonance raman spectra, **07:** 589

iron •
classification of, **02:** 90

iron transport •
resonance raman spectra, **07:** 589

isoelectric point; •, human plasma, **02:** 242-250

isoelectric point; *Escherichia coli* ribosomal • 30 S, **04:** 482-486

leucine aminopeptidase; enzymatic hydrolysis of •, **02:** 209

luminescence of some containing tryptophan, table, **01:** 205-207

luminescence of some lacking tryptophan, table, **01:** 204

lysozyme; amino acid sequences of •, **07:** 309

m-•
molecular parameters, **02:** 306

mean residue ellipticities; of three reference conformations based on five globular •, table, **07:** 138-139

mean residue rotation; of three reference conformations based on five globular •, table, **07:** 140

metalloproteins, table of molecular weights, sources, stoichiometry and function, **02:** 276-277

modification of, specificities of reagents used, **02:** 203-204

Moffitt equation; optical rotatory dispersion of • in visible and near UV regions, **07:** 15-38

molar absorptivity, UV and visible region, table of values, **02:** 383-514

molecular weight; •
carbohydrate, index to studies containing, **02:** 232

fibrous, index to studies containing, **02:** 229

globular, index to studies containing, **02:** 222-228

human plasma, table of values, **02:** 242-250

organelles, index to studies containing, **02:** 232

particles, index to studies containing, **02:** 222-228

subunits of, table, **02:** 326-351

table of values, **02:** 326-351

virus, index to studies containing, **02:** 232

molecular weight; *Escherichia coli* ribosomal • 30 S, **04:** 482-486

muscle contractile •
amino acid sequence, **07:** 490-496

near-UV region; circular dichroism for native • at maxima, at room temperature, table, **07:** 143-163

nonmuscle cells, identification of several in, **02:** 307-313

optical rotatory dispersion (ORD); spectra of various •, **07:** 8-11

organelles
physical-chemical data for, index to ultacentrifuge studies, **02:** 232

oxidation-reduction potentials of hemoproteins and metalloporphyrins, **06:** 132-144

particles, physical-chemical data for, index to ultracentrifuge studies, **02:** 232

penicillinase; amino acid sequences of •, **07:** 310

pK; histidine in; •, various, table of values, **02:** 692

pK values for several amino acids in, **02:** 689-696

plasma •
human, *see also* Human plasma proteins
refractive index increments, **02:** 380

raman lines, conformationally sensitive; •, **07:** 584-587

raman spectroscopy; •, **07:** 576-578

refractive index increments, table, **02:** 372-380

resonance raman spectra; •, discussion, **07:** 588

retinol-binding protein, properties, **02:** 304

ribonuclease, pancreatic; amino acid sequences of •, **07:** 311

ribosomal
amino acid composition of *Escherichia coli* 30 S, **04:** 476

amino acid composition of *Escherichia coli* 50 S, **04:** 477-478

electrophoretic separation, tracing, **04:** 474

Escherichia coli derivation, amino acid sequence data, **04:** 479-481

Escherichia coli MRE 600 30 S, separation on cellulose phosphate Whatman® P11, **04:** 475

Escherichia coli 30S, physical and functional characteristics, **04:** 482-486

sedimentation coefficient; intrinsic, contractile •, **02:** 306

serum vertebrate
sedimentation coefficients for, **02:** 230-231

stereo drawings of several •, **02:** 761, 763, 766

Proteins *(continued)*

structures, drawings of several, **02:** 760-766

substrates for enzymatic incorporation of amines, **02:** 680

subtilisin; amino acid sequences of •, **07:** 312

subunit constitution of, table, **02:** 326-351

symbols for, use of, **01:** 8-15, **02:** 8-15

techniques for determining pK values in, **02:** 689

tobacco mosaic virus; amino acid sequence of coat •, **07:** 261-262

tryptophan; recovery from various • after acid hydrolysis, **02:** 207

tryptophan synthetase A protein; amino acid sequences of •, **07:** 313

turnip yellow mosaic virus; amino acid sequences of virus coat •, **07:** 263-265

tyrosine; pK values in various •, tables, **02:** 694-695

UV absorption spectra; circular dichroism of • in, extrema between 185 and 250 NM, table, **07:** 82-129

UV absorption spectra; optical rotatory dispersion of • extrema between 185 and 250 NM^3, table, **07:** 44

visible, table, **07:** 15-38

viruses, physical-chemical data for, index to ultracentrifuge studies, **02:** 232

viscosity; intrinsic; contractile •, **02:** 306

viscosity; intrinsic; •, human plasma, **02:** 242-250

viscosity; intrinsic; • in native and denatured states, **02:** 721

viscosity, intrinsic, table for several in native and denatured states, **02:** 721

visible absorption spectra; optical rotatory dispersion of • in near UV and, table, **07:** 15-38

Proteins--nonheme

respiratory •

resonance raman spectra, **07:** 589

Proteoglycan

circular dichroism in the UV region, **07:** 120

Proteolipid

brain • protein

optical rotatory dispersion

UV region, **07:** 49

visible and near UV regions, **07:** 19

Prothrombin

amino acid sequence, **07:** 351-352

average hydrophobicity value, **01:** 230

beef

molar absorptivity and-or absorbance values, **02:** 503

circular dichroism intensities at maxima in near UV region, at room temperature, **07:** 160

general building plan, **07:** 350

human

molar absorptivity and-or absorbance values, **02:** 503

optical rotatory dispersion in the UV region, **07:** 73

physical data and characteristics, **02:** 254-255

plasma, human

carbohydrate content, molecular weights, sedimentation coefficients, **02:** 258

plasma, nonhuman

carbohydrate content, **02:** 260

Protists

DNA, *see also* Deoxyribonucleic acid; base composi-

tions of eucaryotic •, tables, **04:** 236-239

Protocatechuate

3,4-dioxygenase

amino acid composition, complete data, **07:** 509

Protomycin®

origin and mode of action as protein biosynthesis inhibitor, **04:** 597

Protoporphyrin IX

dimethyl ester

UV and visible absorption spectrum, **07:** 184

UV spectra, formula, molecular weight, **08:** 175

dimethyl ester dication

UV and visible absorption spectrum, **07:** 185

UV spectra, formula, molecular weight, **08:** 176

ε-Protoxin

optical rotatory dispersion in the UV region, **07:** 73

Protyrosinase

average hydrophobicity value, **01:** 230

Pseudoacetyl

cholinesterase

human

luminescence of, table, **01:** 206

Pseudomonas

cytochrome c_{551}

amino acid sequence, **07:** 292-294

Pseudouridine

composition in various tRNA's, **04:** 428-441

1-methyl-3-(3-amino-3-carboxypropyl) •

isolation and detection of, in RNA, general remarks, **03:** 240

RNA, various, natural occurrence in, **03:** 229

RNA, various, natural occurrence in, **03:** 228-229

β-ƒ-Pseudouridine 5'-diphosphate

physical constants and spectral properties, **03:** 194

Pseudouridine 5'-diphosphate

physical constants and spectral properties, **03:** 194

β-ƒ-Pseudouridine 3'(2')-phosphate

physical constants and spectral properties, **03:** 193

β-ƒ-Pseudouridine 5'-phosphate

physical constants and spectral properties, **03:** 194

Pseudouridine 3'(2')-phosphate

physical constants and spectral properties, **03:** 193

Pseudouridine 5'-phosphate

physical constants and spectral properties, **03:** 194

Pseudouridine and nucleoside derivatives

physical constants and spectral properties, index to, **03:** 70-71

Pseudouridine C 3'(2')-phosphate

physical constants and spectral properties, **03:** 193

Pseudouridine C 5'-phosphate

physical constants and spectral properties, **03:** 194

Pseudovitamin B$_{12}$ nucleoside

physical constants and spectral properties, **03:** 110

Psicofuranine

physicochemical constants, spectral chemotherapeutic and biological properties, **03:** 371

Psoriatic scale

protein

amino acid composition, complete data, **07:** 509

Purified lectins, *see also* Lectin, purified

isolectin content, •, **02:** 547-551

Purine, *see also* Purines

annelida; deoxyribonucleic acids from, • and pyrimidine distribution in, **04:** 265

arthropoda; deoxyribonucleic acids from, • and pyrimidine distribution in, **04:** 266

aschelminthes; deoxyribonucleic acids from, • and pyrimidine distribution in, **04:** 264

bacterial phages; deoxyribonucleic acids from, • and pyrimidine distribution in, **04:** 276-278

biosynthesis; pathways chart, **04:** insert

chordata; deoxyribonucleic acids from, • and pyrimidine distribution in, **04:** 268-273

coelenterata; deoxyribonucleic acids from, • and pyrimidine distribution in, **04:** 264

corn (Zea mays), *see also* Maize; deoxyribonucleic acids from, • and pyrimidine distribution in, **04:** 259

derivatives excreted in human urine, mg-day, **03:** 252-269

echinodermata; deoxyribonucleic acids from, • and pyrimidine distribution in, **04:** 267

Escherichia coli, see also E. coli; deoxyribonucleic acids from, • and pyrimidine distribution in, **04:** 247-248, 276

heat of proton ionization, pK, and related thermodynamic quantities, **06:** 240

mollusca; deoxyribonucleic acids from, • and pyrimidine distribution in, **04:** 265

mouse; deoxyribonucleic acids from, • and pyrimidine distribution in, **04:** 270

Neurospora crassa; deoxyribonucleic acids from, • and pyrimidine distribution in, **04:** 242

nucleoside phosphorylase
amino acid composition, complete data, **07:** 509

pK'_a values, **06:** 331, 337

phosphorylase, •-nucleoside
molar absorptivity and-or absorbance values, **02:** 497

porifera; deoxyribonucleic acids from, • and pyrimidine distribution in, **04:** 264

protozoa; deoxyribonucleic acids from, • and pyrimidine distribution in, **04:** 263

Salmonella typhimurium; deoxyribonucleic acids from, • and pyrimidine distribution in, **04:** 247

thallophyta; algae; deoxyribonucleic acids from, • and pyrimidine distributionin, **04:** 256-257

thallophyta; fungi; deoxyribonucleic acids from, • and pyrimidine distribution in, **04:** 242-253

tracheophyta; deoxyribonucleic acids from, • and pyrimidine distribution in, **04:** 258-261

viruses; chordate; deoxyribonucleic acids from, • and pyrimidine distribution in, **04:** 281

viruses; insect; deoxyribonucleic acids from, • and pyrimidine distribution in, **04:** 280

viruses; plant DNA; deoxyribonucleic acids from • and pyrimidine distribution in, **04:** 280

Purines, *see also* Purine

bond angles and distances, **08:** 224-227

distribution of, in deoxyribonucleic acids from diverse sources, **04:** 241-281

formula, molecular; •, index to table, **03:** 67-69

IR spectra, chart of characteristic frequencies between ~ 700-300 cm⁻¹, **08:** 243

melting point; •, index to table of values, **03:** 67-69

molal activity coefficients, **03:** 529

molal osmotic coefficients, **03:** 528

molecular weight; •, index to table of values, **03:** 67-69

nomenclature; • and pyrimidines, numbering schemes, **08:** 224

one-letter symbols; •, pyrimidines, nucleosides, and nucleotides index to table, **03:** 67-75

physical constants and spectral properties, index to, **03:** 67-69

pK; •, index to table of values, **03:** 67-69

specific rotation; •, index to table of values, **03:** 67-69

spectral data, *see also* IR spectra, PMR spectra, UV spectra, Circular dichroism; acidic; •, index to table of values, **03:** 67-69

spectral data, *see also* IR spectra, PMR spectra, UV spectra, Circular dichroism; alkaline; •, index to table of values, **03:** 67-69

spectral data, *see also* IR spectra, PMR spectra, UV spectra, Circular dichroism; neutral; •, index to table of values, **03:** 67-69

structure; •, index to table of values, **03:** 67-69

symbols; 1-letter; •, index to table, **03:** 67-69

symbols; 3-letter; •, index to table, **03:** 67-69

three-letter symbols; •, pyrimidines, nucleosides, and nucleotides, index to table, **03:** 67-65

Puromycin
origin, structure, and characteristic as protein biosynthesis inhibitor, **04:** 597

physicochemical constants, spectral, chemotherapeutic and biological properties, **03:** 373

Purothionin
circular dichroism in the UV region, **07:** 120

Purple membrane, *see* Membrane, protein, purple

Putidaredoxin
average hydrophobicity value, **01:** 230

bacterial
amino acid sequence, **07:** 428

β-Putreanine
physical and chemical properties, **01:** 121

Pyocyanine
UV spectra, formula, molecular weight, **08:** 186

Pyostacin A, B, *see* Pristinamycin II

Pyrazofuran, *see* Pyrazomycin

Pyrazofurin B, *see* Pyrazomycin B

β-Pyrazol-1-ylalanine
physical and chemical properties, **01:** 146

β-(1-Pyrazolyl)alanine
structure and symbols for those incorporated into synthetic polypeptides, **01:** 106

β-(3-Pyrazolyl)alanine
structure and symbols for those incorporated into synthetic polypeptides, **01:** 106

β-(4-Pyrazolyl)alanine
antagonism to phenylalanine, **01:** 179

structure and symbols for those incorporated into synthetic polypeptides, **01:** 106

Pyrazomycin
physicochemical constants, spectral, chemotherapeutic and biological properties, **03:** 375

Pyrazomycin B
physicochemical constants, spectral, chemotherapeutic and biological properties, **03:** 377

Pyrenebutyrate
covalent protein conjugates, data, **01**: 208

Pyridazine
pK'_a values, **06**: 331

Pyridine
hemochrome spectra, **08**: 280
hemochromogen
UV and visible absorption spectrum, **07**: 182
UV spectra, formula, molecular weight, **08**: 173
infrared correlation chart, **08**: 231, 234
IR spectra, chart of characteristic frequencies between ~ 700-300 cm^{-1}, **08**: 243
nucleotide
amino acid sequence, **07**: 314
pK'_a values, **06**: 331, 338-339
derivatives excreted in human urine, mg-day, **03**: 252-269

Pyridine derivatives
heat of proton ionization, pK, and related thermodynamic quantities, **06**: 240-243

Pyridine nucleotide transhydrogenase, *see* NAD(P)$^+$, trans-hydrogenase

Pyridosine
physical and chemical properties, **01**: 146

Pyridoxal
derivatives
structure, melting point, UV absorption data, **08**: 256-261
formula, empirical; pyridoxine, • and pyridoxamine derivatives, **08**: 252-266
melting point; pyridoxine, • and pyridoxamine derivatives, **08**: 252-266
molecular weight; pyridoxine, • and pyridoxamine derivatives, **08**: 252-266
properties of, **08**: 298

Pyridoxamine
derivatives
structure, melting point, UV absorption data, **08**: 261-263
formula, empirical; pyridoxine, pyridoxal and • derivatives, **08**: 252-266
melting point; pyridoxine, pyridoxal and • derivatives, **08**: 252-266
molecular weight; pyridoxine, pyridoxal and • derivatives, **08**: 252-266
properties of, **08**: 299

Pyridoxine
biological characteristics, **08**: 304
derivatives
structure, melting point, UV absorption data, **08**: 252-256
formula, empirical; •, pyridoxal and pyridoxamine derivatives, **08**: 252-266
melting point; •, pyridoxal and pyridoxamine derivatives, **08**: 252-266
molecular weight; •, pyridoxal and pyridoxamine derivatives, **08**: 252-266
nomenclature recommendations, **08**: 12

Pyridoxine hydrochloride
properties, **08**: 298

Pyridoxol
nomenclature recommendations, **08**: 12

β-2-Pyridylalanine
antagonism to phenylalanine, **01**: 179

β-4-Pyridylalanine
antagonism to phenylalanine, **01**: 179

Pyrimides
formula, molecular; •, index to table, **03**: 67-69
melting point; •, index to table of values, **03**: 67-69
molecular weight; •, index to table of values, **03**: 67-69
pK; •, index to table of values, **03**: 67-69
specific rotation; •, index to table of values, **03**: 67-69
spectral data, *see also* IR spectra, PMR spectra, UV spectra, Circular dichroism; acidic; •, index to table of values, **03**: 67-69
spectral data, *see also* IR spectra, PMR spectra, UV spectra, Circular dichroism; alkaline; •, index to table of values, **03**: 67-69
spectral data, *see also* IR spectra, PMR spectra, UV spectra, Circular dichroism; neutral; •, index to table of values, **03**: 67-69
structure; •, index to table of values, **03**: 67-69

Pyrimidine, *see also* Pyrimidines
abbreviations; • photoproducts, proposals for, **03**: 51-57
adducts, abbreviations for • photoproducts, **03**: 53-55
annelida; deoxyribonucleic acids from, purine and • distribution in, **04**: 265
arthropoda; deoxyribonucleic acids from, purine and • distribution in, **04**: 266
aschelminthes; deoxyribonucleic acids from, purine and • distribution in, **04**: 264
bacterial phages; deoxyribonucleic acids from, purine and • distribution in, **04**: 276-278
bond angles and distances, **08**: 224-227
chordata; deoxyribonucleic acids from, purine and • distribution in, **04**: 268-273
coelenterata; deoxyribonucleic acids from, purine and • distribution in, **04**: 264
corn (Zea mays), *see also* Maize; deoxyribonucleic acids from, purine and • distribution in, **04**: 259
deoxyribonucleosidase
Neurospora crassa mutant, **04**: 744
derivatives excreted in human urine, mg-day, **03**: 252-269
echinodermata; deoxyribonucleic acids from, purine and • distribution in, **04**: 267
Escherichia coli, *see also* E. coli; deoxyribonucleic acids from, purine and • distribution in, **04**: 247-248, 276
infrared correlation chart, **08**: 234
IR spectra, chart of characteristic frequencies between ~ 700 - 300 cm^{-1}, **08**: 243
mollusca; deoxyribonucleic acids from, purine and • distribution in, **04**: 265
mouse; deoxyribonucleic acids from, purine and • distribution in, **04**: 270
Neurospora crassa; deoxyribonucleic acids from, purine and • distribution in, **04**: 242
photobyproducts, proposed abbreviations for, **03**: 51-57
porifera; deoxyribonucleic acids from, purine and • distribution in, **04**: 264
protozoa; deoxyribonucleic acids from, purine and • distribution in, **04**: 263
Salmonella typhimurium; deoxyribonucleic acids from, purine and • distribution in, **04**: 247

Q

Quinoline, derivatives
    heat of proton ionization, pK, and related thermody-
        namic quantities, **06:** 245-247
Quinones
    nomenclature, journal references for, **02:** 87
    with isoprenoid side chains, nomenclature, **08:** 10-11
Quinonoid dihydropterin
    reductase
        average hydrophobicity value, **01:** 230

R

Rabbit aorta contracting substance, *see* RCS
Racemases
    definition and nomenclature, **02:** 98
    numbering and classification of, **02:** 108
Radio-opaque agents
    ligands binding to plasma albumin, **02:** 572
RCS
    biological activity of, **08:** 332
    nomenclature; •, suggested use of term in prostaglandin
        studies, **08:** 314
    prostaglandin nomenclature, suggested use of term, **08:**
        314
Reagents
    active site titrations; •, **02:** 681
    density; guanidine hydrochloride, aqueous solutions
        with added •, at 25°, **06:** 406
    density; urea, aqueous solutions with added •, at 25°,
        06: 406
    enzymes, *see also* Coenzyme, Metalloenzyme, Multien-
        zyme; immobilization of; fixation on solid supports,
        multifunctional • for, **02:** 735
    fixation of enzymes, multifunctional • for, **02:** 735
    guanidine hydrochloride; densities of aqueous solutions
        with added •, at 25°, **06:** 406
    guanidine hydrochloride; viscosities of aqueous solu-
        tions with added •, at 25°, **06:** 407
    hydrogen equivalents, oxidation and reduction •, **06:**
        352
    molecular weights; oxidation and reduction •, **06:** 352
    oxidation and reduction •, deci-normal solutions, table
        of data, **06:** 352
    protein modification, table of specificities for those in
        common use, **02:** 203-204
    reduction and oxidation •, deci-normal solutions, table
        of data, **06:** 352
    specificity; protein modification, table for • used in, **02:**
        203-204
    sulfhydryl protein group, chemical modification of; •
        used, table of specificities, **02:** 203-204
    thio ether protein group, chemical modification of; •
        used, table of specificities, **02:** 203-204
    urea; densities of aqueous solutions with added •, at
        25°, **06:** 406
    urea; viscosities of aqueous solutions with added •, at
        25°, **06:** 407
    viscosity; guanidine hydrochloride, aqueous solutions
        with added •, at 25°, **06:** 407

Receptor
    acetylcholine •
        average hydrophobicity value, **01:** 210
    acetylcholine • protein
        circular dichroism in the UV region, **07:** 82
    lipopolysaccharides •
        circular dichroism in the UV region, **07:** 109
Reductase
    adrenodoxin •
        average hydrophobicity value, **01:** 212
    danunorubicin •
        average hydrophobicity value, **01:** 218
    dehydroshikimic acid •
        Neurospora crassa mutant, **04:** 745
    dihydrofolate •
        average hydrophobicity value, **01:** 218
        molar absorptivity and-or absorbance values, **02:** 418
    glutathione •
        molar absorptivity and-or absorbance values, **02:** 433
        subunit, constitution of, **02:** 333
    glutathione • (NAD(P)H)
        amino acid composition, incomplete data, **07:** 512
        optical rotatory dispersion
            UV region, **07:** 57
            visible and near UV regions, **07:** 24
    glyoxylate •
        optical rotatory dispersion
            UV region, **07:** 58
            visible and near UV regions, **07:** 25
    hydroxypyruvate •
        amino acid composition, incomplete data, **07:** 513
        molar absorptivity and-or absorbance values, **02:** 451
        subunit, constitution of, **02:** 329
    malate-vitamin k •
        average hydrophobicity value, **01:** 226
    nitrate •
        cofactors, molecular weights, stoichiometry and
            sources, **02:** 285
        molar absorptivity and-or absorbance values, **02:** 484
        Neurospora crassa mutant, **04:** 740, 749, 750
        subunit, constitution of, **02:** 349
    pyrroline-5-carboxylate •
        Neurospora crassa mutant, **04:** 746
    quinonoid dihydropterin •
        average hydrophobicity value, **01:** 230
    ribonucleotide-diphosphate •
        molar absorptivity and-or absorbance values, **02:** 506
    ribonucleotide •
        amino acid composition, incomplete data, **07:** 514
        average hydrophobicity value, **01:** 231
        subunit, constitution of, **02:** 347
    rubredoxin •
        molar absorptivity and-or absorbance values, **02:** 507
    sulfite •
        Neurospora crassa mutant, **04:** 748, 750, 753, 755
    tartronic semialdehyde •
        amino acid composition, complete data, **07:** 510
        molar absorptivity and-or absorbance values, **02:** 509
    thioredoxin •
        amino acid composition, complete data, **07:** 510
        molar absorptivity and-or absorbance values, **02:** 509
        subunit, constitution of, **02:** 329

Ribosome
  binding sites, sequences,
    04: 354
  buoyant density; •, from various sources, **04**: 472
  physical characteristics of ribosomes from various
    sources, **04**: 472
  protein chemical data on *Escherichia coli* •, **04**: 471-486
  range of weights, **08**: 424
  RNA, *see* Nucleic acids, Transfer RNA, TRNA
    (TRNA); content in subunits of • from various
    sources, **04**: 472
O_2' (3′)-Ribosyladenosine
  isolation and detection of, in RNA, general remarks, **03**:
    236
  RNA, various, natural occurrence in, **03**: 221
6-Ribosylaminoisocytosine, 5-*N*-methylforamido-
  physical constants and spectral properties, **03**: 116
6-Ribosylaminoisocytosine 3′(2′)-phosphate
  derivatives
    physical constants and spectral properties, index to,
      03: 74
6-Ribosylaminopyrimidine, 2-Amino-4-hydroxy-5-*N*-
  methylformamido
  physical constants and spectral properties, **03**: 116
Ribosylpurine
  molal osmotic coefficients, **03**: 528
Ribosylthymine
  and nucleoside derivatives
    physical constants and spectral properties, index to,
      03: 71
Ribosylthymine 5′-diphosphate
  physical constants and spectral properties, **03**: 192
Ribosylthymine 3′(2′)-phosphate
  physical constants and spectral properties, **03**: 191
Ribosylthymine 5′-phosphate
  physical constants and spectral properties, **03**: 192
5-Ribosyluracil
  physical constants and spectral properties, **03**: 136
5-Ribosyluracil 5′-diphosphate
  physical constants and spectral properties, **03**: 194
5-Ribosyluracil 3′(2′)-phosphate
  physical constants and spectral properties, **03**: 193
5-Ribosyluracil 5′-phosphate
  physical constants and spectral properties, **03**: 194
Ribosylzeatin
  physical constants and spectral properties, **03**: 140
Ribothymidine
  physical constants and spectral properties, **03**: 131
Ribothymidine, O_2'-Methyl-
  physical constants and spectral properties, **03**: 134
L-Ribulokinase
  amino acid composition, incomplete data, **07**: 514
  molar absorptivity and-or absorbance values, **02**: 506
  subunit, constitution of, **02**: 333
Ribulose 1,5-diphosphate
  carboxylase
    amino acid composition, complete data, **07**: 510
L-Ribulose 5-phosphate
  4-epimerase
    amino acid composition, complete data, **07**: 510

Ribulose diphosphate
  carboxylase
    average hydrophobicity value, **01**: 231
Ricin
  origin, structure, and characteristic as protein biosynthe-
    sis inhibitor, **04**: 598
RNA, *see* Nucleic acids, Transfer RNA, TRNA (TRNA)
  N^4-Acetylcytidine; isolation and detection of, in •, gen-
    eral remarks, **03**: 237
  N^4-Acetylcytidine; •, various, natural occurrence in, **03**:
    222
  adenovirus 2--VA •, nucleotide sequence model, **04**: 349
  3-(3-Amino-3-carboxypropyl)uridine; isolation and de-
    tection of, in •, general remarks, **03**: 241
  3-(3-Amino-3-carboxypropyl)uridine; •, various, natural
    occurrence in, **03**: 229
  Bacillus subtilis; ribosomal • from, nucleotide composi-
    tion, **04**: 409
  bacteriophage types; viral •
    nucleotide sequences and models, **04**: 337-344
  bacteriophage types; virus-induced •
    nucleotide sequences and models, **04**: 346-348
  5-Carboxymethoxyuridine; isolation and detection of, in
    •, general remarks, **03**: 241
  5-Carboxymethoxyuridine; •, various, natural occur-
    rence in, **03**: 230
  5-Carboxymethyluridine; isolation and detection of, in
    •, general remarks, **03**: 241-242
  5-Carboxymethyluridine; •, various, natural occurrence
    in, **03**: 230
  chain termini in partially hydrolyzed, discussion of, **03**:
    403
  chloroplast ribosomal •, base composition, table, **04**:
    361-362
  circular dichroism parameters; oligonucleotides of •, **03**:
    461-465
  content in subunits of ribosomes from various sources,
    04: 472
  controlled partial hydrolysis of, discussion, **03**: 402-404
  5,6-Dihydrouridine; isolation and detection of, in •,
    general remarks, **03**: 243
  5,6-Dihydrouridine; •, various, natural occurrence in,
    03: 231-232
  N^6,N^6-Dimethyladenosine; isolation and detection of, in
    •, general remarks, **03**: 235
  N^6,N^6-Dimethyladenosine; •, various, natural occur-
    rence in, **03**: 220
  N^4,O^2-Dimethylcytidine; isolation and detection of, in
    •, general remarks, **03**: 237
  N^4,O^2-Dimethylcytidine; •, various, natural occurrence
    in, **03**: 223
  N^2,N^2-Dimethylguanosine; isolation and detection of, in
    •, general remarks, **03**: 238
  N^2,N^2-Dimethylguanosine; •, various, natural occur-
    rence in, **03**: 225-226
  $5,O^{2'}$-Dimethyluridine; isolation and detection of, in •,
    general remarks, **03**: 244
  $5,O^{2'}$-Dimethyluridine; •, various, natural occurence in,
    03: 233
  double-stranded, molar residue ellipticity, **03**: 601
  double-stranded, molar residue rotation, **03**: 599

RNA *(continued)*

double helices at atomic resolution, geometry of, **04:** 463-469

double helix; molecular structure, geometry of, for •, **04:** 363-369

E. coli, see also Escherichia coli; •s from; amino acid sequence, **04:** 333, 335

Escherichia coli, see also E. coli; • from, natural occurrence of the modified nucleosides in, **03:** 217-232

Escherichia coli, see also E. coli; • molecules from, physical properties, **04:** 406,409

Escherichia coli, see also E. coli; 4.5S • from, nucleotide sequence model, **04:** 331

Escherichia coli, see also E. coli; 6S • from, nucleotide sequence model, **04:** 332

extinction coefficients for single-strand types, **03:** 589

Flory-Fox equation for size of •, **04:** 405

fluorescent dyes bound to, data tables, **04:** 470

N^6-Glycinocarbonyladenosine; isolation and detection of, in •, general remarks, **03:** 234

N^6-Glycinocarbonyladenosine; •, various, natural occurrence in, **03:** 218

hydrolysis, limited, conditions for, **03:** 404

7-[(2-hydroperoxy)-3-(methoxycarbonyl)-3-(methoxyformamido)propyl] wyosine; isolation and detection of, in •, general remarks, **03:** 246

7-[(2-hydroperoxy)-3-(methoxycarbonyl)-3-(methoxyformamido)propyl] wyosine; •, various natural occurrence in, **03:** 233

N^6-(4-Hydroxyisopentenyl)-2-methylthioadenosine; isolation and detection of, in •, general remarks, **03:** 234

N^6-(4-Hydroxyisopentenyl)-2-methylthioadenosine; • various, natural occurrence in, **03:** 218

N^6-(*cis*-4-Hydroxyisopentenyl) adenosine; isolation and detection of, in •, general remarks, **03:** 234

N^6-(*cis*-4-Hydroxyisopentenyl) adenosine; •, various, natural occurrence in, **03:** 218

5-Hydroxymethyluridine; isolation and detection of, in •, general remarks, **03:** 242

5-Hydroxymethyluridine; •, various, natural occurrence in, **03:** 230

5-Hydroxyuridine; isolation and detection of, in •, general remarks, **03:** 242

5-Hydroxyuridine; •, various, natural occurrence in, **03:** 230

inosine; isolation and detection; in •, general remarks, **03:** 239-240

inosine; •, various, natural occurrence in, **03:** 227

N^6-(Δ^2-Isopentenyl)-2-methylthioadenosine; isolation and detection of, in •, general remarks, **03:** 234-235

N^6-(Δ^2-Isopentenyl)-2-methylthioadenosine; •, various,natural occurrence in, **03:** 219

N^6-(Δ^2-Isopentenyl) adenosine; isolation and detection of, in •, general remarks, **03:** 234

N^6-(Δ^2-Isopentenyl) adenosine; •, various, natural occurrence in, **03:** 219

7-[(3-methoxycarbonyl)-3-(methoxyformamido)propyl] wyosine; isolation and detection of, in •, general remarks, **03:** 245-246

7-[(3-methoxycarbonyl)-3-(methoxyformamido)propyl] wyosine; •, various, natural occurrence in, **03:** 233

5-(Methoxycarbonylmethyl)-2-thiouridine; isolation and detection of, in •, general remarks, **03:** 243

5-(Methoxycarbonylmethyl)-2-thiouridine; •, various, natural occurrence in, **03:** 231

1-Methyl-3-(3-amino-3-carboxypropyl) pseudouridine; isolation and detection of, in •, general remarks, **03:** 240

1-Methyl-3-(3-amino-3-carboxypropyl) pseudouridine; •, various, natural occurrence in, **03:** 229

5-Methyl-5,6-dihydrouridine; isolation and detection of, in •, general remarks, **03:** 244

5-Methyl-5,6-dihydrouridine; •, various, natural occurrence in, **03:** 232

5-Methyl-2-thiouridine; isolation and detection of, in •, general remarks, **03:** 243

5-Methyl-2-thiouridine; •, various, natural occurrence in, **03:** 231

N^6-Methyl-N^6-threoninocarbonyladenosine; isolation and detection of, in •, general remarks, **03:** 235

N^6-Methyl-N^6-threoninocarbonyladenosine; •, various, natural occurrence in, **03:** 221

N^6-Methyladenosine; isolation and detection of, in •, general remarks, **03:** 235

N^6-Methyladenosine; •, various, natural occurrence in, **03:** 219

O^2-Methyladenosine; isolation and detection of, in •, general remarks, **03:** 235-236

O^2-Methyladenosine; •, various, natural occurrence in, **03:** 221

1-Methyladenosine; isolation and detection of, in •, general remarks, **03:** 233-234

1-Methyladenosine; •, various, natural occurrence in, **03:** 216-217

2-Methyladenosine; isolation and detection of, in •, general remarks, **03:** 234

2-Methyladenosine; •, various, natural occurrence in, **03:** 218

5-(Methylaminomethyl)-2-thiouridine; isolation and detection of, in •, general remarks, **03:** 243

5-(Methylaminomethyl)-2-thiouridine; •, various, natural occurrence in, **03:** 231

$O^{2'}$-Methylcytidine; •, various, natural occurrence in, **03:** 223

3-Methylcytidine; isolation and detection of, in •, general remarks, **03:** 237

3-Methylcytidine; •, various, natural occurrence in, **03:** 222

5-Methylcytidine; isolation and detection of, in •, general remarks, **03:** 237

5-Methylcytidine; •, various, natural occurrence in, **03:** 222-223

N^2-Methylguanosine; isolation and detection of, in •, general remarks, **03:** 238

N^2-Methylguanosine; •, various, natural occurrence in, **03:** 224-225

$O^{2'}$-Methylguanosine; isolation and detection of, in •, general remarks, **03:** 239

$O^{2'}$-Methylguanosine; •, various,natural occurrence in, **03:** 227

RNA *(continued)*

1-Methylguanosine; isolation and detection of, in •, general remarks, **03**: 237-238

1-Methylguanosine; •, various, natural occurrence in, **03**: 224

7-Methylguanosine; isolation and detection of, in •, general remarks, **03**: 238-239

7-Methylguanosine; •, various, natural occurrence in, **03**: 226

1-Methylinosine; isolation and detection of, in •, general remarks, **03**: 240

1-Methylinosine; •, various, natural occurrence in, **03**: 2282′O-Methylpentose residue, UV absorbance of oligonucleotides containing, **03**: 448-449

$O^{2'}$-Methylpseudouridine; isolation and detection of, in •, general remarks, **03**: 240

$O^{2'}$-Methylpseudouridine; •, various, natural occurrence in, **03**: 229

$O^{2'}$-Methyluridine; isolation and detection of, in •, general remarks, **03**: 244

$O^{2'}$-Methyluridine; •, various, natural occurrence in, **03**: 232

3-Methyluridine; isolation and detection of, in •, general remarks, **03**: 240-241

3-Methyluridine; •, various, natural occurrence in, **03**: 229

5-Methyluridine; isolation and detection of, in •, general remarks, **03**: 242

5-Methyluridine; •, various, natural occurrence in, **03**: 230-231

molecular weights for several, **04**: 406-408

mouse; • from, natural occurrence of the modified nucleosides in, **03**: 217-232

Neurospora; • from, natural occurrence of the modified nucleosides in, **03**: 217-232

nucleosides, modified; isolation and detection of, in •, general remarks about several compounds, **03**: 233-246

nucleosides, modified, natural occurrence in various, **03**: 216-233

nucleotide; composition in high molecular weight ribosomal •, **04**: 409

nucleotide; composition in viral •, **04**: 410

nucleotide; sequences and models for several •s and DNAs, **04**: 324-353

nucleotide sequences and models for several, **04**: 324-349

nucleotidyltransferase
amino acid composition, complete data, **07**: 510
circular dichroism in the UV region, **07**: 123
optical rotatory dispersion
UV region, **07**: 75
visible and near UV regions, **07**: 35

oligonucleotides, circular dichroism parameters, **03**: 461-465

oligonucleotides, optical rotatory dispersion parameters, **03**: 450-458

optical rotatory dispersion parameters; oligonucleotides of •, **03**: 450-458

peroxywybutosine, *see* 7-[2-(Hydroperoxy)-3-

(methoxycarbonyl)-3-(methoxyformamido)propyl] wyosine; isolation and detection of, in •, general remarks, **03**: 240

physical properties, of, **04**: 405-410

polynucleotide double helices with Watson-Crick base pairs
atomic coordinates and molecular conformations for, **04**: 411-422

protein (wt %) in ribosomes from various sources, **04**: 472

pseudouridine; •, various, natural occurrence in, **03**: 228-229

raman spectral changes observed on melting, **03**: 545

ribosomal
chloroplast, base composition, **04**: 361-362
cytoplasmic, base composition, **04**: 361-362
molecular weights of some, **04**: 408
nucleotide composition of high molecular weight types, **04**: 409
nucleotide sequence data 5 S RNA from *Escherichia coli*, **04**: 473
5S type, nucleotide sequences for several, **04**: 324-327
5S type from *E. coli*, secondary structure model, **04**: 328
5.8S type from yeast, nucleotide sequence model, **04**: 330

ribosome binding sites, sequences, **04**: 354

O_2' (3′)-Ribosyladenosine; isolation and detection of, in •, general remarks, **03**: 236

O_2' (3′)-Ribosyladenosine; •, various, natural occurrence in, **03**: 221

sedimentation coefficient for several, **04**: 406-407

size of, Flory-Fox equation for, **04**: 405

structure, secondary, for *E. coli* 5S type, **04**: 328

synthesis; pathways chart, **04**: insert

2-Thiocytidine; isolation and detection of, in •, general remarks, **03**: 237

2-Thiocytidine; •, various, natural occurrence in, **03**: 221

4-Thiouridine; isolation and detection of, in •, general remarks, **03**: 241

4-Thiouridine; •, various, natural occurrence in, **03**: 229-230

N^6-Threoninocarbonyladenosine; isolation and detection of in •, general remarks, **03**: 235

N^6-Threoninocarbonyladenosine; •, various, natural occurrence in, **03**: 220

transfer type, *see also* Transfer RNA, TRNA (TRNA)
classes of sequences, **04**: 424-425
"cloverleaf" secondary configuration, generalized representation, **04**: 423
comparison of homology from prokaryotic and eukaryotic origins, **04**: 426
nucleoside composition of tables of values, **04**: 428-441
nucleoside in secondary structure; indentification, location, distribution, **04**: 427
nucleotide sequences, tables, **04**: 442-453
structure, three-dimensional, yeast phenylalanine transfer RNA, **04**: 457-461

RNA (continued)
translational control •; origin, structure, and characteristic as protein biosynthesis inhibitor, **04**: 611
$N^2,N^2,7$-Trimethylguanosine; isolation and detection of, in •, general remarks, **03**: 239
$N^2,N^2,7$-Trimethylguanosine; •, various, natural occurrence in, **03**: 226
viral
bacteriophage types, nucleotide sequences and models, **04**: 337-344
code word table for the coat protein gene, **04**: 340
nucleotide composition of some, **04**: 410
viral, buoyant density values, $Cs_2 SO_4$ gradient, **03**: 569
virus-induced
nucleotide sequences and models, **04**: 346-349
wyosine; isolation and detection of, in •, general remarks, **03**: 244-245
wyosine; •, various, natural occurrence in, **03**: 233
RNA molecules
bond angle; •, values for two fragments, **04**: 465-468
bond lengths; •, values for two fragments, **04**: 465-468
molecular weight; •, tables for several, **04**: 406-408
sedimentation coefficient of some •, **04**: 406-407
RNA polymerase, see RNA, nucleotidyltransferase
enzymatic activity, subcellular fractions, **02**: 700-701
molar absorptivity and-or absorbance values, **02**: 504
subunit, constitution of, **02**: 347-350
RNase A, see also Ribonuclease I
ribonuclease B′ (a glycosylated •)
circular dichroism at maxima in near UV region, at room temperature, **07**: 160
ribonuclease P (des-121-124 •)
circular dichroism in the UV region, **07**: 122
RNase B
optical rotatory dispersion in the visible and near UV regions, **07**: 35
RNase M, see Ribonuclease II
RNase S, see Ribonuclease S
RNase T, see Guanyloribonuclease
Roseanine
physical and chemical properties, **01**: 146
Rubradirin
origin, structure, and characteristic as protein biosynthesis inhibitor, **04**: 599
Rubredoxin
amino acid composition, complete data, **07**: 510
amino acid sequence, **07**: 429
average hydrophobicity value, **01**: 231
circular dichroism in the UV region, **07**: 123
molar absorptivity and-or absorbance values, **02**: 506
nomenclature recommendations, **02**: 89-90, 120
optical rotatory dispersion in the UV region, **07**: 75
reductase
molar absorptivity and-or absorbance values, **02**: 507
table of cofactors, molecular weights, stoichiometry and sources, **02**: 278

S

30S
proteins, ribosomal; *Escherichia coli* •, physical and

functional characteristics, **04**: 482-486
30S ribosomal
protein
amino acid composition, incomplete data, **07**: 514
5S RNA
E. coli, see also *Escherichia coli*; • from, secondary structure model, **04**: 328
RNA, see Nucleic acids, Transfer RNA, TRNA (TRNA); ribosomal; nucleotide sequence data • from *Escherichia coli*, **04**: 473
Saccharin
ligands binding to plasma albumin, **02**: 574
pK'_a values, **06**: 347
Saccharopine
physical and chemical properties, **01**: 151
saccharopinuria, effect of, **01**: 321
Sacromycin
physicochemical constants, spectral, chemotherapeutic and biological properties, **03**: 379
Salt
solutions
density calculation, coefficients for, from refractive indexes, **06**: 424
density gradient at equilibrium for some, **06**: 424
density values for some used for density gradients, **06**: 425
viscosities for some used for density gradients, **06**: 425
Salts
Spizizen's minimal •, preparation of, **04**: 649
Sangivamycin
physicochemical constants, spectral, chemotherapeutic and biological properties, **03**: 381
Sarcosine
pK'_a values, **06**: 319
physical and chemical properties, **01**: 151
sarcosinemia, effect of, **01**: 321
structure and symbols for those incorporated into synthetic polypeptides, **01**: 107
Sarkomycin
origin, structure, and characteristic as protein biosynthesis inhibitor, **04**: 599
Satellite DNA, see DNAs
Saturated fatty acids
solubility; water in •, table of values, **05**: 495
Scopolamine
pK'_a values, **06**: 327
Secretin
amino acid sequence, **07**: 376
Secretions
elastase inhibitor; mammalian organs and •, specificities and properties, **02**: 632-641
human organs and •
proteinase inhibitors from, specificity and properties, **02**: 632-639
kallikrein inhibitor; mammalian organs and •, specificity and properties, **02**: 630-631
Kunitz inhibitor; mammalian organs and •, specificity and properties, **02**: 630-631

Secretions *(continued)*
  mammalian organs and •
    proteinase inhibitors from, specificity and properties,
      02: 630-635
    trypsin inhibitor, *see also* Trypsin inhibitors; mam-
      malian organs and •, specificities and properties, 02:
      632-641
    urokinase inhibitor; mammalian organs and •, specifici-
      ties and properties, 02: 632-641
Segment
  protein, *see also* Bacteriophage protein, Conjugated
    proteins, Covalent protein conjugates, Covalent con-
    jugates, Flavoproteins, Glycoprotein listings, Human
    plasma proteins, Iron proteins, Iron-sulfur proteins,
    Lipoprotein, Matrix protein, Metalloproteins,
    Molybdoproteins, Mucoprotein, Plasma proteins,
    human, Proteins, conjugated, Proteins, iron-sulfur,
    Serum proteins, Tamm-Horsfall, Tamm-Horsfall
    glycoproteins, Tamm-Horsfall mucoprotein, *also*
    Proteins; primary structure of a •, definition, 01: 73,
    02: 77
Selenium
  amino acids, *see also* Aromatic amino acids, *also*
    specific acids; L-sulfur and •-containing, physical
    and chemical properties, 01: 151-158
Selenocystathionine
  physical and chemical properties, 01: 158
Selenocystine
  physical and chemical properties, 01: 158
Selenomethionine
  antagonism to methionine, 01: 178
  physical and chemical properties, 01: 158
Selenomethylselenocysteine
  physical and chemical properties, 01: 158
Semialdehyde
  tartronic • reductase
    amino acid composition, complete data, 07: 510
    molar absorptivity and-or absorbance values, 02: 509
Sephadex®
  filtration media, table of properties, 08: 133-134
Sepharose®
  filtration media, table of properties, 08: 135
Sequential polypeptides, *see* Polypeptides, sequential
Ser
  Ile oxytocin
    amino acid sequence, 07: 194-195
Serine
  active site peptides, 07: 186
  antagonism to α alanine, 01: 177
  antagonism to threonine, 01: 179
  antagonists of, 01: 179
  dehydratase
    molar absorptivity and-or absorbance values, 02: 507
    subunit, constitution of, 02: 328
  destruction of, during acid hydrolysis, 02: 206
  far ultraviolet absorption spectra
    aqueous solution at pH 5, 01: 184
    neutral water, table, 01: 185
    0.1 *M* sodium dodecyl sulfate, table, 01: 185
  free acid in amniotic fluid in early pregnancy and at
    term, 01: 327

free acid in blood plasma of newborn infants and
  adults, 01: 328
nucleoside composition, tables of values, 04: 438-439
nucleotide sequences of, 04: 450-451
pK'_a values, 06: 319
physical and chemical properties, 01: 128
proteases, trypsin-related
  amino acid sequence data, index to
    blood clotting factors, 07: 350-354
    explanation of tables, 07: 340-341
    sequence alignments, 07: 341-349
proteases, active, bearing the active site serine
  alignments of the chains of, 07: 344-349
requirements of, for growth of various microorganisms,
  table, 04: 630-643
d-• dehydratase
  average hydrophobicity value, 01: 231
  molar absorptivity and-or absorbance values, 02: 507
serine proteases, active, bearing the active site •
  alignments of the chains of, 07: 344-349
specific rotatory dispersion constants, 0.1 *M* solution,
  01: 244
spectra, far UV, 01: 184
symbols for atoms and bonds in side chains, 01: 69, 02:
  73
thumbprint, content in, 08: 121
transacetylase
  amino acid composition, incomplete data, 07: 514
D-Serine
  antagonism to β-alanine, 01: 177
L-Serine hydroxamate
  characteristic as protein biosynthesis inhibitor, 04: 599
Serotypic
  antigen 51A
    amino acid composition, incomplete data, 07: 514
Serratamolide
  proton NMR and suggested conformations, 07: 563
Serum
  albumin, *see also* Albumin, serum
    amino acid composition, complete data, 07: 510
    amino acid sequence, 07: 497
  albumin, bovine •
    heat of proton ionization, pK, and related thermody-
      namic quantities, 06: 161
  albumin; bovine •
    luminescence of, table, 01: 205
    heat capacity and entropy values, 06: 110
  albumin, horse •
    calorimetric Δ H values accompanying conformational
      changes, 06: 270
  albumin; human •
    luminescence of, table, 01: 205
    viscosity, intrinsic, 02: 721
  antibodies
    methods for detection, 07: 543-544
  ceruloplasmin; •, human
    subunit, constitution of, 02: 336
  content
    retinol-binding protein,
      02: 304

Serum (continued)
  human •
    proteinase inhibitors from, specificity and properties, 02: 636-641
    lipoprotein very low density, rat •
      molar absorptivity and-or absorbance values, 02: 467
    proteins, see also Bacteriophage Flavoproteins, Matrix protein, also Protein, individual proteins, Molybdoproteins; • vertebrate
      sedimentation coefficients for, 02: 230-231
    sedimentation coefficient; proteins; •, vertebrate, table of values, 02: 230-231
Shethna
  flavoprotein
    circular dichroism at maxima in near UV region, at room temperature, 07: 161
Short neurotoxins, see Neurotoxins, short
Showdomycin
  origin, structure, and characteristic as protein biosynthesis inhibitor, 04: 599
  physicochemical constants, spectral, chemotherapeutic and biological properties, 03: 383
Sialic acid
  content of, in glycoproteins, 02: 258-269, 271-274
  generic term usage, 05: 10
Side chain, see also Side chains
  arginine; bond distances and angles for •, 08: 222
  circular dichroism; characteristics of a single aromatic • of proteins in near-ultraviolet region, Table 1, 07: 142
  histidine; bond distances and angles for •, 08: 223
  pK; carboxyl •, values estimated in lysozyme, 02: 696
  tryptophan; bond distances and angles for •, 08: 223
Side chains, see also Chains, Side chain
  alanine; symbols for atoms and bonds in •, 01: 69, 02: 73
  amino acid •
    dimensions of, 02: 742-758
  amino acids, see also Aromatic amino acids, also specific acids; average hydrophobicity values for •, 01: 209
  bond angles and distances; amino acid • values for several, 08: 222-223
  quinones with isoprenoid •, nomenclature, 08: 10-11
  symbols; L-amino acids, • of, 02: 73-75
  vitamins; quinones with isoprenoid •, nomenclature, 08: 10-11
Siderophilin
  molar absorptivity and-or absorbance values, 02: 507
Silk
  fibroin
    circular dichroism in the UV region, 07: 123
    optical rotatory dispersion
      UV region, 07: 75
      visible and near UV regions, 07: 35
Siomycin
  origin, structure, and characteristic as protein biosynthesis inhibitor, 04: 600
Siromycin, see Toyocamycin
Snake venom toxins, see Toxins, snake venom
Sodium benzylpenicillin

UV spectra, formula, molecular weight, 08: 157
Sodium chloride
  refractive index; • versus concentration, 06: 387
Sodium dodecyl sulfate
  alanine; far ultraviolet absorption spectra; 0.1 M •, table, 01: 185
  amides; far ultraviolet absorption spectra; 0.1 M •, table, 01: 185
  arginine; far ultraviolet absorption spectra; 0.1 M •, table, 01: 185
  cysteine; far ultraviolet absorption spectra; 0.1 M •, table, 01: 185
  ½ cystine; far ultraviolet absorption spectra; 0.1 M •, table, 01: 185
  histidine; far ultraviolet absorption spectra; 0.1 M •, table, 01: 185
  leucine; far ultraviolet absorption spectra; 0.1 M •, table, 01: 185
  lysine; far ultraviolet absorption spectra; 0.1 M •, table, 01: 185
  methionine; far ultraviolet absorption spectra, 01: 185; 0.1 M •, table, 01: 185
  phenylalanine; far ultraviolet absorption spectra; 0.1 M •, table, 01: 185
  proline; far ultraviolet absorption spectra; 0.1 M •, table, 01: 185
  serine; far ultraviolet absorption spectra; 0.1 M •, table, 01: 185
  threonine; far ultraviolet absorption spectra; 0.1 M •, table, 01: 185
  tryptophan; far ultraviolet absorption spectra; 0.1 M •, table, 01: 185
  tyrosine; far ultraviolet absorption spectra; 0.1 M •, table, 01: 185
  UV spectra; amino acids, far absorption spectra, 01: 185; 0.1 M •, table, 01: 185
Sodium fluoride
  structure and characteristic as protein biosynthesis inhibitor, 04: 600
Solubilizers
  table of detergent properties, 08: 216
Solution, see also Solutions
  alanine; specific rotatory dispersion constants, 0.1 M •, 01: 244
  amides; far ultraviolet absorption spectra; aqueous • at pH 5, 01: 184
  asparagine; specific rotatory dispersion constants, 0.1 M •, 01: 244
  cesium chloride •, density values as a function of refractive index, 06: 419-423
  density; cesium chloride • as a function of refractive index, table of values, 06: 419-423
  fatty acids, see also Lipids, Wax fatty acids; methyl linoleate in carbon tetrachloride •, NMR spectrum, 05: 511
  free energy of •
    amino acids in aqueous solution at 25°C, 06: 118
  ornithine; specific rotatory dispersion constants, 0.1 M •, 01: 244
  phenylalanine; far ultraviolet absorption spectra; aqueous • at pH 5, 01: 184

Solution *(continued)*

 proline; far ultraviolet absorption spectra; aqueous • at pH 5, **01**: 184

 refractive index; density of cesium chloride • as function, table of values, **06**: 419-423

 serine; far ultraviolet absorption spectra; aqueous • at pH 5, **01**: 184

 threonine; far ultraviolet absorption spectra; aqueous • at pH 5, **01**: 184

 tryptophan; far ultraviolet absorption spectra; aqueous • at pH 5, **01**: 184

 tyrosine; far ultraviolet absorption spectra; aqueous • at pH 5, **01**: 184

 UV spectra; amino acids, far absorption spectra, **01**: 185; aqueous • at pH 5, **01**: 184

0.1 *M* Solution

 aspartic acid; specific rotatory dispersion constants, •, **01**: 244

Solutions, *see also* Solution

 absorption data; porphyrins in various •, **08**: 272

 buffer •

  amine types, table of structures and pK_a values, **06**: 368-369

  enzyme studies, preparation of buffers for, **06**: 370-377

  equilibrium data measurement, recommendations, **06**: 95

  histochemical studies, preparation of buffers for, **06**: 370-377

  pH values at varying temperatures for several, **06**: 360-361

  preparation data for several, **06**: 358-359

  preparation instructions for several, **06**: 362-363

  protonic activity for several, **06**: 529-539

  standard primary, pH values and preparation, **06**: 354-355

 density; coefficients for calculation of, from refractive indexes of • at 25°, **06**: 424

 density; guanidine hydrochloride, aqueous • with added reagents, at 25°, **06**: 406

 density; salt • used for density gradients, **06**: 425

 density, particle, of biological particles in sucrose •, **06**: 429

 density gradient; salt •, values for some at equilibrium, **06**: 424

 oxidation and reduction reagents, deci-normal •, table of data, **06**: 352

 porphyrins; absorption maxima; various •, data table, **08**: 272

 reduction and oxidation reagents, deci-normal •, table of data, **06**: 352

 salt •

  density calculation, coefficients for, from refractive indexes, **06**: 424

  density gradient at equilibrium for some, **06**: 424

  density values for some used for density gradients, **06**: 425

  viscosities for some used for density gradients, **06**: 425

 urea; refractive index of • at varying concentration, **06**: 387

Solvent systems

 refractive index; calculations, constants for several •, **06**: 389

Solvents

 absorption data; porphyrin spectra in organic •, **08**: 273-274

 density; organic •, calculations for change with temperature for some, **06**: 540

 density; •, mixed, for use in low temperature biochemistry, **06**: 520

 fluorescence; porphyrins, maxima in various •, **08**: 275

 lipids; solubility of selected, in chlorinated hydrocarbon •, **05**: 514

 lipids; solubility of selected, in organic •, **05**: 512

 metalloporphyrins; methyl esters; Soret band data using organic •, **08**: 278

 mixed, for use in low temperature biochemistry

  density table for several, **06**: 520

  dielectric constants and freezing points

   N,N-dimethylformamide-water mixtures, **06**: 528

   dimethylsulfoxide-water mixtures, **06**: 527

   ethylene glycol-methanol-water mixtures, **06**: 528

   ethylene glycol-water mixtures, **06**: 522

   glycerol-water mixtures, **06**: 526

   methanol-water mixtures, **06**: 523

   2-methyl-2-4-pentanediol-water mixtures, **06**: 524

   1-2-propanediol-water mixtures, **06**: 525

  ethylene glycol-methanol-water mixtures, viscosity, **06**: 521

 porphyrins; absorption maxima; organic •, data table, **08**: 273-274

 porphyrins; fluorescence maxima in various •, **08**: 275

 refractive index; dispersion of, for various •, tables, **06**: 388

 refractive index; •, various, calculations of, **06**: 386

 Soret band data; metalloporphyrins in organic •, **08**: 278

 Soret band data; porphyrins in organic •, **08**: 273-274

Somatomammotropin

 chorionic •

  circular dichroism

   UV and near-UV region, **07**: 89, 147

  hormone, *see also* Luteinizing hormone; chorionic •, human

  molar absorptivity and-or absorbance values, **02**: 450

Soybean

 trypsin inhibitor

  refractive index increments, **02**: 380

 trypsin inhibitor F$_3$

  amino acid composition, complete data, **07**: 510

Soybean leghemoglobin, *see* Leghemoglobin, soybean, aligned chains

Soybean 7S globulin, *see* γ-Conglycinin

Soybean 11S globulin, *see* Glycinin

Sparsomycin

 origin, structure, and characteristic as protein biosynthesis inhibitor, **04**: 600

Sparsomycin, A

 physicochemical constants, spectral, chemotherapeutic and biological properties, **03**: 385

Spectinomycin

 origin, structure, and characteristic as protein biosynthesis inhibitor, **04**: 601

Spectrin

 human erythrocytes

  molar absorptivity and-or absorbance values, **02**: 508

Sperm whale myoglobin
  conformation, three-dimensional, **02:** 760
Sphingoglycolipids
  nomenclature and classification, **05:** 416-421
Sphingolipid
  generic term usage, **05:** 9
  stereospecific nomenclature, **05:** 10
Sphingomyelin
  generic term usage, **05:** 10
Spiramycin I, II, and III
  origin, structure, and characteristic asprotein biosynthesis inhibitor, **04:** 601
Spirilloxanthin
  UV spectra, formula, molecular weight, **08:** 193
Spirostans
  names, new standard vs. old, **05:** 69-70
  steroid nomenclature, use of term, **05:** 66-68
  structures, **05:** 67, 70
Spleen acid DNase B, *see* Deoxyribonuclease II-B
Sporangiomycin
  origin, structure, and charateristic as protein biosynthesis inhibitor, **04:** 602
Stachydrine
  physical and chemical properties, **01:** 164
Staphylococcus aureus
  nuclease
    luminescence of, table, **01:** 206
Staphylomycin M$_1$ (PA114A), *see* Osteogrycin A, Virginiamycin M$_1$, **04:** 602
Staphylomycin® S
  origin, structure and characteristic as protein biosynthesis inhibitor, **04:** 602
Stellacyanin
  amino acid composition, incomplete data, **07:** 514
  carbohydrate content, **02:** 270
  molar absorptivity and-or absorbance values, **02:** 508
Stem bromelain, *see* Bromelain (stem)
Stendomycidine
  physical and chemical properties, **01:** 146
Stendomycin
  proton NMR and suggested conformations, **07:** 564
Stereochemistry
  fundamental, IUPAC rules for, nomenclature, **08:** 20-57
  fundamental; IUPAC rules for nomenclature, **04:** 13-50
Steroid, *see also* Steroids
  alkaloids, nomenclature rules, **05:** 83-85
  bufanolide; • nomenclature, use of term in, **05:** 65-66
  cardanolide; • nomenclature, use of term, **05:** 64-65
  derivatives, nomenclature rules, **05:** 71-73
  furostans; • nomenclature, use of term, **05:** 68-69
  Δ-isomerase
    circular dichroism in the UV region, **07:** 123
  spirostans; • nomenclature, use of term, **05:** 66-68
  systematic names vs. trivial names, • derivatives, **05:** 73
  trivial names vs. systematic names, • derivatives, **05:** 73
Steroids, *see also* Steroid
  formula, molecular, •, **05:** 531-588
  IR spectral data; •, table, **05:** 531-588
  ligands binding to plasma albumin, **02:** 563
  melting point; •, table, **05:** 531-588
  molecular weight; •, table, **05:** 531-588
NMR spectra; • table, **05:** 531-588
nomenclature; *abeo* system, usage for •, **05:** 81-83
nomenclature, IUPAC rules for, **05:** 56-88
nomenclature, journal references for, **02:** 87
pK'_a values, **06:** 348
potency, relative, for •, **05:** 531-588
specific rotation; •, table, **05:** 531-588
structures and properties, **05:** 531-558
abeo System, nomenclature usage for •, **05:** 81-83
systematic nomenclature; •, table, **05:** 531-588
UV spectral data; •, table, **05:** 531-588
Sterol
  fatty acids, *see also* Lipids, Wax fatty acids; wax esters and • esters from vernix caseosa and from human skin surface lipid, **05:** 509
  human skin surface; lipid, fatty acids from wax esters and • esters, **05:** 509-510
  lipids; human skin surface, fatty acids of wax esters and • esters, **05:** 509
  structures and properties, **05:** 544-558
  vernix caseosa; lipid, fatty acids from wax esters and • esters, **05:** 509-510
Stizolobic acid
  physical and chemical properties, **01:** 147
Stizolobinic acid
  physical and chemical properties, **01:** 147
Streptavidin
  circular dichroism at maxima in near-UV region, at room temperature, **07:** 161
  circular dichroism in the UV region, **07:** 124
  optical rotatory dispersion in the UV region, **07:** 75
Streptimidone
  origin, structure, and characteristic as protein biosynthesis inhibitor, **04:** 602
Streptococcal
  proteinase
    amino acid sequence, **07:** 356-357
Streptogramin A
  origin, structure, and characteristic as protein biosynthesis inhibitor, **04:** 603
Streptogramin B$_1$
  origin, structure, and characteristic as protein biosynthesis inhibitor, **04:** 603
Streptokinase
  amino acid composition, complete data, **07:** 510
  average hydrophobicity value, **01:** 231
  circular dichroism in the UV region, **07:** 124
  cyanogen bromide cleavage, **02:** 199
  molar absorptivity and-or absorbance values, **02:** 508
Streptolidine
  physical and chemical properties, **01:** 147
Streptomycin
  mannoside •; origin and characteristic as protein biosynthesis inhibitor, **04:** 584
  origin, structure, and characteristic as protein biosynthesis inhibitor, **04:** 604
Streptonigrin
  origin, structure, and characteristic as protein biosynthesis inhibitor, **04:** 604
Streptovitacin A
  origin, structure, and characteristic as protein biosynthesis inhibitor, **04:** 605

Strychnine
  pK'_a values, **06**: 327
Styrene-acronitrile
  chemical and physical properties, **08**: 427
Styrylacetic acid
  antagonism to trypotophan, **01**: 179
Substances
  ninhydrin reactive •, chromatographic positions, **08**: 126
Substrate
  concentration
    enzyme kinetics, definition, **02**: 112
  constant
    enzyme kinetics, definition, **02**: 112
  specificity
    myosins, nonmuscle, table of values,
      02: 319
  specificity; trypsin toward synthetic •, **02**: 211
  used in glycohydrolase reactions, **05**: 426-445
Subtilisin
  amino acid composition, complete data, **07**: 510
  amino acid sequences of proteins, **07**: 312
  circular dichroism
    UV and near-UV region, **07**: 124, 161
  conformation, stereo pair illustrating, **02**: 763
  enzymatic hydrolysis, conjugated proteins, **02**: 211
  enzymatic hydrolysis of proteins, **02**: 209
  molar absorptivity and-or absorbance values, **02**: 508
  optical rotatory dispersion in the UV region: extrema
    between 185 and 250 NM^3, **07**: 75
  specificity for hydrolysis of peptide bonds, **02**: 221
Subtilisin, Thiol-
  molar absorptivity and-or absorbance values, **02**: 508
Subtilisin BPN
  average hydrophobicity value, **01**: 231
  circular dichroism in the UV region, **07**: 124
  molar absorptivity and-or absorbance values, **02**: 508
  optical rotatory dispersion
    UV region, **07**: 75
    visible and near UV regions, **07**: 36
Subtilisin carlsberg
  luminescence of, table, **01**: 207
Subtilopeptidase A, *see* Subtilisin
Subunit
  tobacco mosaic virus protein •
    optical rotatory dispersion
      UV region, **07**: 76
      visible and near UV regions, **07**: 36
α Subunit
  chorionic gonadotropin; amino acid sequence; •, **07**:
    393-394, 402
  luteinizing hormone, *see also* Interstitial cell-stimulating
    hormone, **07**: 30, 66; amino acid sequence; •, **07**:
    393-394
β Subunit
  chorionic gonadotropin; amino acid sequence; •, **07**:
    402
  luteinizing hormone, *see also* Interstitial cell-stimulating
    hormone, **07**: 30, 66; amino acid sequence; •, **07**:
    395-397
Succinamic acid
  structure and symbols for those incorporated into syn-
    thetic polypeptides, **01**: 107

Succinate buffer
  preparation of, **06**: 373
Succinic acid
  heat of proton ionization, pK, and related thermody-
    namic quantities, **06**: 250-251
Succinyl
  coenzyme A synthetase
    average hydrophobicity value, **01**: 231
N-Succinyl-α-amino-ε-ketopimelic (15) acid
  properties of, **01**: 182
Succinyl-CoA
  synthetase
    molar absorptivity and-or absorbance values, **02**: 508
    subunit, constitution of, **02**: 337
  synthetase (ADP-forming)
    circular dichroism in the UV region, **07**: 124
O-Succinylhomoserine
  physical and chemical properties, **01**: 128
Succinyltransferase
  lipoate •
    circular dichroism in the UV region, **07**: 108
    optical rotatory dispersion in the UV region, **07**: 65
Sucrose
  Beckman rotors, construction data for isokinetic • and
    glycerol gradients, **06**: 432-464
  centrifugation, density gradient; isokinetic gradients, •
    and glycerol, data for construction
    Beckman rotors, **06**: 432-464
    Christ rotors, **06**: 465-479
    geometrical parameters used in calculations, **06**: 428
    International rotors, **06**: 480-488
    MSE rotors, **06**: 489-518
  Christ rotors, construction data for isokinetic • and
    glycerol gradients, **06**: 465-479
  density, particle, of biological particles in • solutions,
    06: 429
  International rotors, construction data for isokinetic •
    and glycerol gradients, **06**: 480-488
  MSE rotors, construction data for isokinetic • and
    glycerol gradients, **06**: 489-518
  pK'_a values, **06**: 317
  standard solution for calibrating spectropolarimeters,
    06: 390
  synthetase
    average hydrophobicity value, **01**: 231
  viral DNA molecules, relative content in, **03**: 551-556
  water solutions, viscosity and density tables, **06**: 415-418
Sugar, *see also* Amino sugar; specific sugar listings
  and sugar derivatives, use of symbols for, **05**: 8-9
  composition
    lipopolysaccharides of gram-negative bacteria, **05**:
      396-402
  Escherichia coli, *see also* E. coli; lipopolysaccharides of;
    • composition for O-type, **05**: 396-399
  Escherichia coli, *see also* E. coli; lipopolysaccharides of;
    • sequences, general structures, **05**: 406, 409-411
  fermentation, EMB medium for detection of, **04**: 650
  microorganisms; • fermentation, preparation of EMB
    medium for detecting, **04**: 650
  neutral, content of in glycoproteins, **02**: 259-274
  nucleases; nonspecific for the • moiety, functional
    characteristics, **04**: 518-523

Sugar *(continued)*
  nucleotide
    isolation and enzymatic synthesis of, **05**: 446-452
    x-ray crystal structure data; dimensions, average, of a •
      unit, **05**: 472
    salmonella; lipopolysaccharides of; • composition for
      O-group, **05**: 396-399
    salmonella; lipopolysaccharides of; • sequences, general
      structures, **05**: 403-406, 409, 412
  sequences
    lipopolysaccharides of gram-negative bacteria, **05**:
      403-412
  sugar and • derivatives, use of symbols for, **05**: 8-9
  unit
    bond lengths and angles, average, **05**: 472
    dimensions, average, **05**: 472
Sulfatase
  choline •
    Neurospora crassa mutant, **04**: 744
Sulfatase A
  amino acid composition, incomplete data, **07**: 514
Sulfate
  permease
    Neurospora crassa mutant, **04**: 744
Sulfate-binding
  protein
    amino acid composition, complete data, **07**: 510
Sulfhydrase A
  O-Acetylserine •
    molar absorptivity and-or absorbance values, **02**: 383
Sulfhydryl
  protein group, chemical modification of
    reagents used, table of specificities, **02**: 203-204
Sulfhydrylase A
  o-acetylserine •
    amino acid composition, complete data, **07**: 505
    average hydrophobicity value, **01**: 210
β-Sulfinyl-α-aminopropionic acid, *see* Cysteine sulfinic
      acid
Sulfite
  oxidase deficiency
    characteristics of, **01**: 322
  reductase
    Neurospora crassa mutant, **04**: 748, 750, 753, 755
β-Sulfo-α-amino-propionic acid, *see* Cysteic acid
S-Sulfo-L-cysteine
  sulfite oxidase deficiency, effect of, **01**: 322
Sulfonamides
  ligands binding to plasma albumin, **02**: 568
S-Sulfopepsin
  cyanogen bromide cleavage, **02**: 199
β-Sulfopyruvic acid
  properties of, **01**: 181
Sulfur
  adrenal iron-• protein
    amino acid composition, complete data, **07**: 505
  high-potential iron-•protein
    circular dichroism in near UV region, at room temper-
      ature, **07**: 154
  iron-• proteins
    resonance raman spectra, **07**: 589
  metabolism; pathways chart, **04**: wall chart

permease-I, conidial type
  Neurospora crassa mutant, **04**: 741
permease II
  Neurospora crassa mutant, **04**: 750
proteins, iron-• primary structures
  amino acid sequences, **07**: 425-427
L-sulfur
  amino acids, *see also* Aromatic amino acids, *also*
    specific acids; • and selenium-containing, physical
    and chemical properties, **01**: 151-158
Sulfuric acid
  heat of proton ionization, pK, and related thermody-
    namic quantities, **06**: 252
Sulfurous acid
  heat of proton ionization, pK, and related thermody-
    namic quantities, **06**: 252
Sulfurtransferase
  mercaptopyruvate •
    molar absorptivity and-or absorbance values, **02**: 471
    subunit, constitution of, **02**: 326
Sulfurylase
  adenosine triphosphate •
    molar absorptivity and-or absorbance values, **02**: 385
Sulphur, *see also* Sulfur
Sunflower hull
  wax fatty acids composition, **05**: 511
Superoxide
  dismutase
    amino acid composition, complete data, **07**: 506
    average hydrophobicity value, **01**: 231
    circular dichroism in the UV region: extrema between
      185 and 250 NM³, **07**: 124
    UV and near-UV region, **07**: 94, 124, 161
    optical rotatory dispersion in the UV region, **07**: 55
    subunit, constitution of, **02**: 326, 327
Surinamine, *see* N-Methyltyrosine
Sweet-sensitive
  protein
    amino acid composition, incomplete data, **07**: 514
Synergistin® A-1
  (PA114-A-1); origin, structure, and characteristic as
    protein biosynthesis inhibitor, **04**: 605
Synergistin B-1, B-3
  origin, structure, and charateristic as protein biosynthe-
    sis inhibitor, **04**: 606
Synthase
  anthranilate •
    molar absorptivity and-or absorbance values, **02**: 394
    subunit, constitution of, **02**: 331
  carbamoylphosphate •
    molar absorptivity and-or absorbance values, **02**: 400
    subunit, constitution of, **02**: 345
  citrate (si)-•
    circular dichroism in the UV region, **07**: 89
    optical rotatory dispersion in the UV region, **07**: 51
  cysteine •
    molar absorptivity and-or absorbance values, **02**: 412
  malate •
    circular dichroism in the UV region, **07**: 111
Synthetase, *see also* Synthetases
  anthranylate •, component I, II
    average hydrophobicity value, **01**: 213

Synthetase *(continued)*

arginine-specific carbamyl phosphate •
Neurospora crassa mutant, **04:** 740

argininosuccinase; •
Neurospora crassa mutant, **04:** 740

carbamyl phosphate •
average hydrophobicity value, **01:** 215

chorismic acid •
Neurospora crassa mutant, **04:** 745

cystathionine γ-•
amino acid composition, complete data, **07:** 506

cysteine •
subunit, constitution of, **02:** 345

dehydroquinic acid •
Neurospora crassa mutant, **04:** 745

3-deoxy-D-arabinoheptulosonate 7-phosphate
•-chroismate mutase
average hydrophobicity value, **01:** 218

3-enolpyruvylshikimic acid-5PO$_4$ •
Neurospora crassa mutant, **04:** 745

fatty acid •
amino acid composition, incomplete data, **07:** 512
molar absorptivity and-or absorbance values, **02:** 422
subunit, constitution of, **02:** 348, 350

formyltetrahydrofolate •
amino acid composition, incomplete data, **07:** 512

glutamine •
average hydrophobicity value, **01:** 222
circular dichroism in the UV region, **07:** 98
molar absorptivity and-or absorbance values, **02:** 433
Neurospora crassa mutant, **04:** 752
optical rotatory dispersion in the UV region, **07:** 57
subunit, constitution of, **02:** 345, 346, 347, 349

histidyl-tRNA •
average hydrophobicity value, **01:** 224

histidyl tRNA •
subunit, constitution of, **02:** 331

indole-3-glycerol phosphate •
amino acid composition, complete data, **07:** 508

α-IPM •
Neurospora crassa mutant, **04:** 740

α-isopropylmalate •
amino acid composition, complete data, **07:** 508

β-ketoacyl acyl carrier protein •
amino acid composition, complete data, **07:** 508

lactose •, A protein
molar absorptivity and-or absorbance values, **02:** 463

lactose • (A protein)
circular dichroism in the UV region, **07:** 108

leucyl tRNA •
Neurospora crassa mutant, **04:** 751

lysine tRNA •
subunit, constitution of, **02:** 336

lysyl tRNA •
molar absorptivity and-or absorbance values, **02:** 469

methionyl tRNA •
average hydrophobicity value, **01:** 227
molar absorptivity and-or absorbance values, **02:** 472

pyrimidine-specific carbamyl phosphate •; aspartate
transcarbamylase
Neurospora crassa mutant, **04:** 748

succinyl-CoA •
molar absorptivity and-or absorbance values, **02:** 508
subunit, constitution of, **02:** 337

succinyl-CoA • (ADP-forming)
circular dichroism in the UV region, **07:** 124

succinyl coenzyme A •
average hydrophobicity value, **01:** 231

sucrose •
average hydrophobicity value, **01:** 231

thymidylate •
average hydrophobicity value, **01:** 232
circular dichroism in the UV region, **07:** 124

tripeptide •
amino acid composition, complete data, **07:** 510

tryptophan •
average hydrophobicity values, **01:** 234
cyanogen bromide cleavage, **02:** 199
molar absorptivity and-or absorbance values, **02:** 512
Neurospora crassa mutant, **04:** 745
subunit, constitution of, **02:** 337, 338

tryptophanyl tRNA •
amino acid composition, complete data, **07:** 510
luminescence of, table, **01:** 206
molar absorptivity and-or absorbance values, **02:** 512
Neurospora crassa mutant, **04:** 753
subunit, constitution of, **02:** 330, 334

tyrosyl-tRNA •
average hydrophobicity value, **01:** 234

Synthetase A
tryptophan • protein
amino acid composition, complete data, **07:** 510
amino acid sequences of proteins, **07:** 313

Synthetases, *see also* Synthetase
definition and nomenclature, **02:** 98
numbering and classification of, **02:** 108

Synthetic
dehydroquinase
Neurospora crassa mutant, **04:** 745

Synthetic polypeptides, *see* Polypeptides, synthetic,
Polypeptides, synthetic

Synthetic substrates
trypsin; specificity toward •, **02:** 211

T

T2
toxin; origin, structure, and characteristic as protein biosynthesis inhibitor, **04:** 613

T-2 Tail sheath
refractive index increments, **02:** 380

Tabtoxinine
physical and chemical properties, **01:** 129

Taka-amylase A, *see* α-Amylase
carbohydrate content, **02:** 247

Tamm-Horsfall
glycoproteins; •, *see also* Tamm-Horsfall glycoprotein;
Tamm-Horsfall mucoprotein
molar absorptivity and-or absorbance values, **02:** 435

glycoproteins; •, human urine
glycoproteins; •, rabbit urine
molar absorptivity and-or absorbance values, **02:** 435

Thiazolidine-4-carboxylic acid
  structure and symbols for those incorporated into synthetic polypeptides, 01: 107
β-2-Thienylalanine
  antagonism to phenylalanine, 01: 179
  structure and symbols for those incorporated into synthetic polypeptides, 01: 107
β-3-Thienylalanine
  antagonism to phenylalanine, 01: 179
β-(2-Thienyl)serine
  structure and symbols for those incorporated into synthetic polypeptides, 01: 107
Thio
  ether protein group, chemical modification of
    reagents used, table of specificities, 02: 203-204
Thiocholine
  enhancement of the steady state formation of, 02: 683
D-Thiocymetin®
  origin, structure, and characteristic as protein biosynthesis inhibitor, 04: 609
2-Thiocytidine
  composition in various tRNA's, 04: 428-441
  isolation and detection of, in RNA, general remarks, 03: 237
  RNA, various, natural occurrence in, 03: 221
[ββ'-Thiodi-(α-aminopropionic acid)], *see* Lanthionine
Thioester
  β-hydroxydecanoyl • dehydrase
    amino acid composition, complete data, 07: 507
Thiogalactoside
  transacetylase
    amino acid composition, complete data, 07: 510
Thiol
  esters
    hydrolysis, kinetic constants, 02: 682
    free energy; hydrolysis; • esters, 06: 301
  pK'_a; •, 06: 346
Thiolhistidine
  physical and chemical properties, 01: 158
Thiopeptin B
  origin, structure, and characteristic and protein biosynthesis inhibitor, 04: 609
Thioredoxin
  amino acid composition, complete data, 07: 510
  amino acid sequence, 07: 500
  average hydrophobicity value, 01: 232
  cyanogen bromide cleavage, 02: 199
  molar absorptivity and-or absorbance values, 02: 509
  reductase
    amino acid composition, complete data, 07: 510
    molar absorptivity and-or absorbance values, 02: 509
    subunit, constitution of, 02: 329
Thioredoxin II
  average hydrophobicity value, 01: 232
Thiostreptine
  physical and chemical properties, 01: 158
Thiostrepton
  origin, structure, and characteristic as protein biosynthesis inhibitor, 04: 610

2-Thiouracil
  and derivatives
    physical constants and spectral properties, index to, 03: 68
Thiourea
  pK'_a values, 06: 345
2-Thiouridine
  and nucleoside derivatives
    physical constants and spectral properties, index to, 03: 71-72
4-Thiouridine
  composition in various tRNA's, 04: 428-441
  isolation and detection of, in RNA, general remarks, 03: 241
  physical constants and spectral properties, 03: 128
  RNA, various, natural occurrence in, 03: 229-230
4-Thiouridine 3'(2')-phosphate
  physical constants and spectral properties, 03: 188
4-Thiouridine 5'-phosphate
  physical constants and spectral properties, 03: 188
4-Thiouridine disulphide
  physical constants and spectral properties, 03: 128
2-Thiouridine nucleotide derivatives
  physical constants and spectral properties, index to, 03: 74-75
Thraustomycin
  physicochemical constants, spectral, chemotherapeutic and biological properties, 03: 387
Threo-α-amino-β,γγihydroxybutyric acid
  physical and chemical properties, 01: 122
Threo-β-hydroxyleucine
  physical and chemical properties, 01: 127
Threonine
  antagonism to methionine, 01: 178
  antagonism to serine, 01: 179
  antagonists of, 01: 179
  deaminase
    amino acid composition, complete data, 07: 510
    molar absorptivity and-or absorbance values, 02: 509
    subunit, constitution of, 02: 338, 340, 341
  destruction of, during acid hydrolysis, 02: 206
  far ultraviolet absorption spectra
    aqueous solution at pH 5, 01: 184
    neutral water, table, 01: 185
    0.1 M sodium dodecyl sulfate, table, 01: 185
  free acid in amniotic fluid in early pregnancy and at term, 01: 327
  free acid in blood plasma of newborn infants and adults, 01: 328
  nucleoside composition, tables of values, 04: 439
  nucleotide sequences of, 04: 450-451
  pK'_a values, 06: 319
  physical and chemical properties, 01: 129
  requirements of, for growth of various microorganisms, table, 04: 630-643
  spectra, far UV, 01: 184
  symbols for atoms and bonds in side chains, 01: 69, 02: 73
  thumbprint, content in, 08: 121
Threonine derivatives
  heat of proton ionization, pK, and related thermodynamic quantities, 06: 254-255

Thyroxine-binding
  globulin
    amino acid composition, incomplete data, **07:** 514
Thyroxine-binding prealbumin, *see* Prealbumin
    (thyroxine-binding prealbumin)
Tingitanine, *see* Lathytine
Tn-C
  troponin Ca^{++}-binding protein (•) rabbit skeletal
    amino acid sequence, **07:** 495
Tn-I
  troponin inhibitor (•), rabbit skeletal
    amino acid sequence, **07:** 494
Tobacco mosaic virus
  protein
    depolymerized, luminescence of, table, **01:** 206
    polymerized, luminescence of, table, **01:** 206
Tobramycin
  origin, structure, and characteristic as protein biosynthe-
    sis inhibitor, **04:** 610
Tocinamide
  proton NMR and suggested conformations, **07:** 572
Tocopherol
  lipids; vegetable oils, individual • contents, **05:** 512
  vegetable oils; • contents, individual, **05:** 521
DL-α-Tocopherol, *see also* Vitamin E
  properties, **08:** 289
  UV spectra, formula, molecular weight, **08:** 153-154
d-α-Tocopheryl acetate
  properties of, **08:** 289
DL-α-Tocopheryl acetate, *see also* Vitamin E
  UV spectra, formula, molecular weight, **08:** 155
d-α-Tocopheryl acid succinate
  properties of, **08:** 290
α Tocotrienol-TMS derivative
  mass spectra; •, **05:** 520
α-Toctrienol-TMS derivative
  lipids; mass spectrum of •, **05:** 520
Toluene derivatives
  heat of proton ionization, pK, and related thermody-
    namic quantities, **06:** 255-256
L-l-Tosylamido-2-phenylethyl choloromethyl ketone
  (TPCK), origin, structure, and characteristic as protein
    biosynthesis inhibitor, **04:** 611
Toxin, *see also* Neurotoxin, Toxins
  amino acid composition, complete data, **07:** 510
  animal sources, amino acid composition, **02:** 650
  average hydrophobicity values, **01:** 232
  c3a anaphyla•
    circular dichroism in the UV region, **07:** 84
  c5a anaphyla•
    circular dichroism in the UV region, **07:** 84
  cobro•
    circular dichroism
      UV and near-UV region, **07:** 89, 147
    optical rotatory dispersion in the UV region, **07:** 52
  diptheria •; origin, structure, and characteristic as
    protein biosynthesis inhibitor, **04:** 571
  lower animal sources, specificity and properties, **02:**
    622-623
  optical rotatory dispersion
    UV region, **07:** 76
    visible and near UV regions, **07:** 36

T2 •; origin, structure, and characteristic as protein bio-
    synthesis inhibitor, **04:** 613
tetanus •
  molar absorptivity and-or absorbance values, **02:** 509
ε-Toxin
  circular dichroism in the UV region, **07:** 125
  optical rotatory dispersion
    UV region, **07:** 76
    visible and near UV regions, **07:** 36
α-Toxin A
  average hydrophobicity value, **01:** 233
Toxin B
  protein •
    subunit, constitution of, **02:** 335
α-Toxin B
  average hydrophobicity value, **01:** 233
Toxin (type A)
  amino acid composition, complete data, **07:** 510
Toxins, *see also* Toxin
  angusticeps-type
    from venom of various snakes, amino acid sequence,
      07: 365
  snake venom, **07:** 360-373
Toyocamycin
  physiocochemical constants, spectral, chemotherapeutic
    and biological properties, **03:** 390
TPCK
  l-l-Tosylamido-2-phenylethyl choloromethyl ketone (•),
    origin, structure, and characteristic as protein bio-
    synthesis inhibitor, **04:** 611
Tranquilizers
  ligands binding to plasma albumin, **02:** 571
(*Trans*)-α-(Carboxycyclopropyl)
  glycine
    physical and chemical properties, **01:** 115
Transacetylase
  dihydrolipoyl •
    molar absorptivity and-or absorbance values, **02:** 419
    subunit, constitution of, **02:** 350, 351
  serine •
    amino acid composition, incomplete data, **07:** 514
  thiogalactoside •
    amino acid composition, complete data, **07:** 510
Transamidase
  activity
    detection of, **02:** 670
    inhibition of, **02:** 669-674
    sources of, **02:** 671
    tissues, list of references, **02:** 680
  α-dialkylamino •
    average hydrophobicity value, **01:** 218
  fibrinoligase, • activity, **02:** 671-681
  iodoacetamide; inhibition of • activity, **02:** 672
  molecular weight, subunit structure, **02:** 681
  subunit structures; •, purified, **02:** 681
Transamilase
  endo-γ-Glutamine: ε-lysine transferase; • activity, dis-
    cussion and data, **02:** 669-683
Transaminase
  imidazole acetol phosphate •
    Neurospora crassa mutant, **04:** 749

γ-Transaminase
  acetylornithine •
    average hydrophobicity value, **01**: 210
Transaminase B
  average hydrophobicity value, **01**: 233
Transamitase
  eDTA inhibition of • activity, **02**: 669-673
Transcarbamoylase
  aspartate •
    molar absorptivity and-or absorbance values, **02**: 397
Transcarbamylase
  aspartate •, average hydrophobicity values, **01**: 215
  ornithine •
    average hydrophobicity value, **01**: 228
    molar absorptivity and-or absorbance values, **02**: 485
    Neurospora crassa mutant, **04**: 745
    subunit, constitution of, **02**: 334
  pyrimidine-specific carbamyl phosphate synthetase; as-
    partate •
    Neurospora crassa mutant, **04**: 748
Transcortin
  amino acid composition, incomplete data, **07**: 514
  average hydrophobicity value, **01**: 233
  molecular parameters, **02**: 242
  plasma, human
    carbohydrate content, molecular weight, sedimentation
      coefficients, **02**: 258
    molecular absorptivity and-or absorbance values, **02**:
      510
Transcriptase
  enzymes, *see also* Coenzyme, Metalloenzyme, Multien-
    zyme; reverse •, sources of and reactions, **04**: 536
Transfer RNA, *see also* RNA, transfer type; TRNA
    (TRNA)
  hydrophobic stacking interactions, yeast phenylalanine
    •, **04**: 461
  RNA, *see* Nucleic acids, Transfer RNA, TRNA
    (TRNA); transfer type, *see also* Transfer RNA,
    TRNA (TRNA); structure, three-dimensional, yeast
    phenylalanine •, **04**: 457-461
Transferase
  alanine amino •
    amino acid composition, complete data, **07**: 505
    average hydrophobicity value, **01**: 212
  definition and nomenclature of, **02**: 96-97
  endo-γ-glutamine: ε-lysine •
    transamilase activity, discussion and data, **02**: 669-683
  enzymes, *see also* Coenzyme, Metalloenzyme, Multien-
    zyme; terminal •, sources of and reactions, **04**: 536
  γ-glutamyl •
    carbohydrate content, **02**: 274
  intramolecular, numbering and classification of, **02**: 108
  numbering and classification of, **02**: 106
  n-1-(5'-phosphoribosyl) adenosine triphosphate pyro-
    phosphate phosphoribosyl •
    amino acid composition, incomplete data, **07**: 513
  phosphoribosyl •
    viscosity, intrinsic, **02**: 721
  uridine diphosphate galactose: lipopolysaccharide
    α-3-galactosyl •
    amino acid composition, incomplete data, **07**: 514

Transferrin, *see also* Ovotransferrin
  amino acid composition, complete data, **07**: 510
  average hydrophobicity value, **01**: 233
  carbohydrate content, **02**: 268
  circular dichroism
    UV and near-UV region, **07**: 125, 162
  molecular parameters, **02**: 246
  molecular weight, stoichiometry, source, function, **02**:
    276
  optical rotatory dispersion
    UV region, **07**: 76
    visible and near UV regions, **07**: 36
  plasma, human
    carbohydrate content, molecular weights, sedimenta-
      tion coefficients, **02**: 258
    molar absorptivity and-or absorbance values, **02**: 510
  plasma, nonhuman
    carbohydrate content, **02**: 260
Transglutaminase
  amino acid composition, complete data, **07**: 510
Transhydrogenase
  malate-lactate •
    molar absorptivity and-or absorbance values, **02**: 470
  matate-lactate •
    average hydrophobicity value, **01**: 226
  NAD(P)+ •
    circular dichroism in the UV region, **07**: 115
    optical rotatory dispersion in the UV region, **07**: 68
Transketolase
  circular dichroism in the UV region, **07**: 125
  optical rotatory dispersion
    UV region, **07**: 76
    visible and near UV regions, **07**: 36
Transpeptidase
  DD-carboxypeptidase-•
    circular dichroism in near-UV region, at room temper-
      ature, **07**: 146
Trehalase
  Neurospora crassa mutant, **04**: 742
Triacanthine
  physical constants and spectral properties, **03**: 78
Triacylglycerol
  lipase
    circular dichroism in the UV region, **07**: 125
    optical rotatory dispersion
      UV region, **07**: 76
      visible and near UV regions, **07**: 36
1,2,4-Triazolealanine
  antagonism to Histidine, **01**: 178
Trichodermin
  origin, structure, and characteristic as protein biosynthe-
    sis inhibitor, **04**: 611
Trichodermol
  origin, structure, and characteristic as protein biosynthe-
    sis inhibitor, **04**: 612
Tricholomic acid
  physical and chemical properties, **01**: 147
Trichothecin
  origin, structure, and characteristic as protein biosynthe-
    sis inhibitor, **04**: 612
Tri(di)acylglycerol
  generic term usage, **05**: 9

5',5',5'-Trifluoroleucine
  antagonism to leucine, **01:** 178
Triglycerides
  lipids; surface areas for pure methyl esters and •, **05:** 515
  mixed triacid, solubility values, **05:** 497
  simple saturated, solubility values, **05:** 496
  surface areas, pure methyl esters and •, **05:** 515
Trigonelline
  physical and chemical properties, **01:** 164
3,5,3-Triiodothyronine
  physical and chemical properties, **01:** 160
Trimers
  proposal for use of abbreviations, **03:** 57
ϵ-N-Trimethyl-ϵ-hydroxylysine betaine
  physical and chemical properties, **01:** 164
2-Trimethylaminoethyl-betaine phosphonic acid
  physical and chemical properties, **01:** 161
(ϵ-Trimethylammonio)caproic acid, *see*
      ϵ-(Trimethylammonio)hexanoic acid
ϵ-(Trimethylammonio)hexanoic acid
  structure and symbols for those incorporated into syn-
      thetic polypeptides, **01:** 107
N^2,N^2,7-Trimethylguanosine
  isolation and detection of, in RNA, general remarks, **03:** 239
  RNA, various, natural occurrence in, **03:** 226
ϵ-N-Trimethyllysine betaine
  physical and chemical properties, **01:** 164
Trimethylpyruvic acid
  properties of, **01:** 182
Triosephosphate
  dehydrogenase
    average hydrophobicity value, **01:** 233
  isomerase
    amino acid composition, complete data, **07:** 510
    amino acid sequences, **07:** 324-326
    average hydrophobicity value, **01:** 233
    optical rotatory dispersion in the visible and near UV
        regions, **07:** 36
  isomerase-I, average hydrophobicity values, **01:** 233
  isomerase-III, average hydrophobicity values, **01:** 233
Tripeptide
  synthetase
    amino acid composition, complete data, **07:** 510
TRIS
  heat of proton ionization, pK, and related thermody-
      namic quantities, **06:** 236
Tris buffer
  protonic activity tables, **06:** 529-539
Trisaccharides
  chemical formula, **05:** 297-308, 334-340
  derivatives, **05:** 297-308, 334-340
  melting point, **05:** 297-308, 334-340
  nomenclature rules, **05:** 134-135
  specific rotation, **05:** 297-308, 334-340
  synonyms, **05:** 297-308, 334-340
Tris(hydroxymethyl)-amino methane-maleate (trismaleate)
      buffer
  preparation of, **06:** 374
Tris(hydroxymethyl)-aminomethane (tris) buffer
  preparation of, **06:** 375

TRNA, *see also* RNA, transfer type
  N^4-Acetylcytidine; composition in various •'s, **04:** 428-441
  adenosine; composition in various •'s, **04:** 428-441
  3-(3-Amino-3-carboxypropyl)uridine; composition in
      various •'s, **04:** 428-441
  5-Carboxymethoxyuridine; composition in various •'s,
      04: 428-441
  cytidine; composition in various •'s, **04:** 428-441
  N^2,N^2-Dimethylguanosine; composition in various •'s,
      04: 428-441
  guanosine; composition in various •'s, **04:** 428-441
  inosine; composition in various •'s, **04:** 428-441
  N^6-(^{2}-Isopentenyl)-2-methylthioadenosine; composition
      in various •'s, **04:** 428-441
  N^6-(^{2}-Isopentenyl)adenosine; composition in various •'s,
      04: 428-441
  leucyl • synthetase
    Neurospora crassa mutant, **04:** 751
  lysine • synthetase
    subunit, constitution of, **02:** 336
  lysyl: • ligase
    average hydrophobicity value, **01:** 226
  lysyl • synthetase
    molar absorptivity and-or absorbance values, **02:** 469
  methionyl • synthetase
    average hydrophobicity value, **01:** 227
    molar absorptivity and-or absorbance values, **02:** 472
  5-(Methoxycarbonylmethyl)-2-thiouridine; composition
      in various •'s, **04:** 428-441
  5-(Methoxycarbonylmethyl)uridine; composition in vari-
      ous •'s, **04:** 428-441
  N^6-Methyl-N^6-threoninocarbonyladenosine; composition
      in various •'s, **04:** 428-441
  methyladenosine; composition in various •'s, **04:** 428-441
  N^6-Methyladenosine; composition in various •'s, **04:** 428-441
  2-Methyladenosine; composition in various •'s, **04:** 428-441
  5-(Methylaminomethyl)-2-thiouridine; composition in
      various •'s, **04:** 428-441
  $O^{2'}$-Methylcytidine; composition in various •'s, **04:** 428-441
  3-Methylcytidine; composition in various •'s, **04:** 428-441
  5-Methylcytidine; composition in various •'s, **04:** 428-441
  N^2-Methylguanosine; composition in various •'s, **04:** 428-441
  $O^{2'}$-Methylguanosine; composition in various •'s, **04:** 428-441
  1-Methylguanosine; composition in various •'s, **04:** 428-441
  7-Methylguanosine; composition in various •'s, **04:** 428-441
  1-Methylinosine; composition in various •'s, **04:** 428-441
  $O^{2'}$-Methylpseudouridine; composition in various •'s,
      04: 428-441
  $O^{2'}$-Methyluridine; composition in various •'s, **04:** 428-441
  5-Methyluridine; composition in various •'s, **04:** 428-441

W

Water *(continued)*

amides; absorption data in • and in cyclohexane, **08:** 141-143

amides; far ultraviolet absorption spectra; neutral •, table, **01:** 185

amino acids, *see also* Aromatic amino acids, *also* specific acids; solubilities in • at various temperatures, table of values, **06:** 115

amino acids, *see also* Aromatic amino acids, *also* specific acids; solubility in •, equation coefficient values for several, **06:** 107-108

arginine; far ultraviolet absorption spectra; neutral •, table, **01:** 185

cysteine; far ultraviolet absorption spectra; neutral •, table, **01:** 185

½ Cystine; far ultraviolet absorption spectra; neutral •, table, **01:** 185

density; sucrose in •, tables at varying concentrations and temperatures, **06:** 415-418

dielectric constant; *N,N*-dimethylformamide-• mixtures, **06:** 528

dielectric constant; dimethylsulfoxide-• mixtures, **06:** 527

dielectric constant; ethylene glycol-methanol-• mixtures, **06:** 528

dielectric constant; ethylene glycol-• mixtures, **06:** 522

dielectric constant; glycerol-• mixtures, **06:** 526

dielectric constant; methanol-• mixtures, **06:** 523

dielectric constant; 2-methyl-2-4-pentanediol-• mixtures, **06:** 524

dielectric constant; 1-2-propanediol-• mixtures, **06:** 525

N-N-dimethylformamide-• mixtures, dielectric constants and freezing points, **06:** 528

dimethylsulfoxide-• mixtures, dielectric constants and freezing points, **06:** 527

ethylene glycol-methanol-• mixtures dielectric constants and freezing points, **06:** 528 viscosity table, **06:** 521

ethylene glycol-• mixtures, dielectric constants and freezing points, **06:** 522

fatty acids, *see also* Lipids, Wax fatty acids; freezing point, effect of addition of • upon, graph, **05:** 495

fatty acids, *see also* Lipids, Wax fatty acids; solubilities of some, in •, table of values, **05:** 495

fatty acids, *see also* Lipids, Wax fatty acids; solubilities of • in saturated fatty acids, table, **05:** 495

freezing point; fatty acids, effect of addition of •, graph, **05:** 495

heat of proton ionization, pK, and related thermodynamic quantities, **06:** 260-261

histidine; far ultraviolet absorption spectra; neutral •, table, **01:** 185

leucine; far ultraviolet absorption spectra; neutral •, table, **01:** 185

lysine; far ultraviolet absorption spectra; neutral •, table, **01:** 185

methionine; far ultraviolet absorption spectra, **01:** 185; neutral •, table, **01:** 185

optical rotatory dispersion; •, calculations of the refractive index, **06:** 385

phenylalanine; far ultraviolet absorption spectra; neutral •, table, **01:** 185

proline; far ultraviolet absorption spectra; neutral •, table, **01:** 185

refractive index, optical rotatory dispersion calculations, **06:** 385

refractive index, variation with temperature, **06:** 386

serine; far ultraviolet absorption spectra; neutral •, table, **01:** 185

solubility; amino acids in •, equations and coefficient values for several, **06:** 107-108

solubility; amino acids in • at various temperatures, **06:** 115

solubility; fatty acids in •, table of values, **05:** 495

solubility; • in saturated fatty acids, table of values, **05:** 495

threonine; far ultraviolet absorption spectra; neutral •, table, **01:** 185

tryptophan; far ultraviolet absorption spectra; neutral •, table, **01:** 185

tyrosine; far ultraviolet absorption spectra; neutral •, table, **01:** 185

UV spectra; amino acids, far absorption spectra, **01:** 185; neutral •, table, **01:** 185

viscosity; sucrose in •, tables at varying concentrations and temperatures, **06:** 415-418

Water, deuterated

heat of proton ionization, pK, and related thermodynamics quantities, **06:** 261

Water solutions

sucrose; •, viscosity and density tables, **06:** 415-418

Watson-Crick base pairs

DNA, *see also* Deoxyribonucleic acid; polynucleotide double helices with •

atomic coordinates and molecular conformations for, **04:** 411-412

RNA, *see* Nucleic acids, Transfer RNA, TRNA (TRNA); polynucleotide double helices with •

atomic coordinates and molecular conformations for, **04:** 411-422

Watson-Crick duplexes

viral DNA molecules, **03:** 549

Watson-Crick pairs

base stacking in standard models, diagrams, **04:** 414

standard polynucleotide double helices, values for constrained hydrogen bonds, **04:** 413

Wax

fatty acids, *see also* Lipids, Wax fatty acids; • esters and sterol esters from vernix caseosa and from human skin surface lipid, **05:** 509

human skin surface; lipid, fatty acids from • esters and sterol esters, **05:** 509-510

Wax esters

lipids; human skin surface, fatty acids of • and sterol esters, **05:** 509

vernix caseosa; lipid, fatty acids from • and sterol esters, **05:** 509-510

Wax fatty acids

sunflower hull, • composition, **05:** 511

Willardine

physical and chemical properties, **01:** 148

D-Win-5094

origin, structure, and characteristic as protein biosynthesis inhibitor, **04:** 571

Errata and Addenda

ERRATA AND ADDENDA

CRC HANDBOOK OF BIOCHEMISTRY AND MOLECULAR BIOLOGY, 3rd Edition
Dr. Gerald D. Fasman, Editor

Nucleic Acids, Volume I

Purines, Pyrimidines, Nucleosides, and Nucleotides: Physical Constants and Spectral Properties

Page 94   Compound 55. The alternative name based on Wye should be in normal type. The former designation should be "Y^+" not "$Y^\ddagger$". The systematic name should read: -α-(carboxyamino) . . . . imadazo[1,2-a] purine . . . . (added hyphen and change to square brackets).

Page 95   Compound 56. The alternative name based on Wye should be in normal type and end: -3-(methoxyformamido)propyl] wye^j; (change in "formamide" to end in o not e).

Page 141   The heading "Deoxyribonucleosides" should be all in capitals.

Page 196   The heading "Deoxyribonucleotides" should be all in capitals.

Natural Occurrence of the Modified Nucleosides

Page 216   Third paragraph, second sentence should read: "Particularly in earlier studies t and r represent more accurately the total low molecular weight and total high molecular weight RNA, respectively."

Page 233   General Remarks 1-Methyladenosine. The assumption made that 1-methyladenosine does not occur in tRNA of bacteria has been shown to be incorrect by recent work in several laboratories (Klagsbrun, *J. Biol. Chem.*, 248, 2612, 1973; Arnold and Kersten, *FEBS Lett.*, 36, 34, 1973; Romeo, Delk, and Rabinowitz, *Biochem. Biophys. Res. Commun.*, 61, 1256, 1974; Watanabe, Oshima, and Nishimura, *Nucleic Acids Res.*, 3, 1703, 1976).

Page 240   Addendum to Inosine. The $O^{2'}$-methyl-derivative of this nucleoside has been detected in rRNA from *Crithidia fasciculata* (Gray, *Biochim. Biophys. Acta*, 374, 253, 1974).

Page 241   Addendum to 3-(3-Amino-3-carboxypropyl)uridine. The $5'$-phosphate of this nucleoside is extremely resistant to hydrolysis by the $5'$-nucleotidase in snake venom (Gray, *Can. J. Biochem.*, 54, 413, 1976).

Page 242   Addendum to 5-Carboxymethyluridine. 5-Carbamoylmethyluridine has also been shown to occur in yeast tRNA as an $O^{2'}$-methyl-derivative (Gray, *Biochemistry*, 15, 3046, 1976).

Page 242   Addendum to 5-Hydroxyuridine. The methyl derivative: 5-methoxyuridine, has been shown to occur in tRNA from a number of *Bacilli* (Murao, Hasegawa, and Ishikura, *Nucleic Acids Res.*, 3, 2851, 1976).

Page 243   Addendum to 5-Methyl-2-thiouridine. This nucleoside completely replaces 5-methyluridine in tRNA of a thermophilic bacterium (Watanabe, Oshima, Saneyoshi, and Nishimura, *FEBS Lett.*, 43, 59, 1974).

Nucleoside Antibiotics

Page 391   The structural formula given for Toyocamycin is incorrect. The correct formula is given on page 390.

Spectrophotometric Constants of Ribonucleotides

Page 405   Values should be:
Cp pH12 λ min 249 λ max 271   (These errors were in *Analytical Biochemistry*. Corrected values are taken from Reference 212, p. 211).
Gp pH7 λ min 224 λ max 252
Gp pH12 λ min 230 λ max 258

Nucleic Acids, Volume II

Content of 6-Methylaminopurine and 5-Methylcytosine in DNA

Page 282   Values for 6-MeAde for the following should be replaced by ND^d:
Bacteriophage C20 (*Streptogriseus*)
Bacillus cereus
Baker's yeast
Staphylococcus aureus (Reference 2)
S. albus
Streptomyces griseus
Wheat germ
Calf
Horse

Proteins, Volume II

Through an editorial oversight the following contributor was inadvertently not identified:

Donald M. Kirschenbaum
Department of Biochemistry
State University of New York
Brooklyn, New York 11203

The material submitted by Dr. Kirschenbaum is "Molar Absorptivity and $A_{1cm}^{1\%}$ Values for Proteins at Selected Wavelengths of the Ultraviolet and Visible Region," pages 383 to 545.

Page 271   The intrinsic viscosity value for Tropomyosin in the native state should read as 45 (ml/g) instead of 4.5 (ml/g.)

Page 419   The $A_{1cm}^{1\%}$ values for diphtheria toxin should be 12.7, 12.9, and 14.1.

Proteins, Volume III

Optical Rotatory Dispersion and Circular Dichroism of Proteins

Page 46   Reference *32* (italic)

Page 53   Reference *84* (italic)

Page 82   Reference **2** (boldface)

Page 88   Reference **27** (boldface)
           Reference *62* (italic)

Page 97   Reference **57** (boldface)

Page 98   Reference **54** (boldface)

Page 110   Reference *171* (italic)

Page 121   **221** should appear in the reference column not in the $[\theta]_{max}$ column

Page 131   References 88a and 88b should be the following:
           88.   **D'Anna and Tollin,** *Biochemistry,* 11, 1073 (1972).
           89a.   **Tollin,** private communication.

CRC PUBLICATIONS OF RELATED INTEREST

CRC HANDBOOKS:

HANDBOOK OF ANALYTICAL TOXICOLOGY
Edited by **Irving Sunshine, Ph.D.**, Cuyahoga County Coroner's Office and Case Western Reserve University; ISBN- 0-87819-513-3.
Contains information on drugs, economic poisons, industrial chemicals, air pollution, water analysis, and more.

HANDBOOK OF CHEMISTRY AND PHYSICS, 58th Edition
Edited by **Robert C. Weast, Ph.D.**, Consolidated Natural Gas Co., Inc., ISBN-0-8493-0458.X.
The definative reference for chemistry and physics and maintains the tradition that has earned it the reputation as the best scientific reference in the world.

HANDBOOK OF CHROMATOGRAPHY
Edited by **Gunter Zweig**, U.S. Environmental Protection Agency and **Joseph Sherma, Ph.D.**, Lafayette College ; Vol. I, ISBN-0-8493-0561-6; Vol. II, ISBN-0-87819-562-9.
This two-volume set provides comprehensive information concerning chromatographic data, methods, and literature. It also contains a Compound Index that lists the more than 12,000 compounds referenced in this data collection.

HANDBOOK OF TABLES FOR ORGANIC COMPOUND IDENTIFICATION
Edited by **Zvi Rappoport, Ph.D.**, Hebrew University of Jerusalem; ISBN-0-8493-0303-6.
Compounds are divided in 26 groups with information on each compound including name, boiling or melting point, refractive index, density, and properties of up to eight derivatives.

CRC UNISCIENCE PUBLICATIONS:

ORGANOPHOSPHORUS PESTICIDES: ORGANIC AND BIOLOGICAL CHEMISTRY
By **Morifusa Eto**, Kyushu University, Japan; ISBN-0-8493-5201-2.
Organophosphorus pesticides are one of the most important and widely used pesticides in the world for agriculture and public health. This book reviews the chemical reactions, describes structure-activity relationships, and discusses important individual pesticides.

APPLICATION OF PROTEOLYTIC ENZYMES TO PROTEIN STRUCTURE STUDIES, 2nd Edition
By **Elemer Mihalyi, Ph.D.**, National Institute of Health; ISBN-0-8493-5189-8.
This Second Edition includes an overview of the new significance proteolytic enzymes have acquired over the past twenty years. Also included is a detailed author and subject index.

BIOCHEMISTRY OF WOMEN: CLINICAL CONCEPTS
By **A. S. Curry, Ph.D.**, Central Research Establishment and **J. V. Hewitt**, King Edward VII Hospital; ISBN-0-87819-041-4.
Includes chapters on The Ovarian Cycle, The Biochemistry of Infertility, The Biochemistry of Contraception, Biochemical Changes at the Menopause, as well as other chapters pertaining to the biochemistry of women.

BIOCHEMISTRY OF WOMEN: METHODS FOR CLINICAL INVESTIGATION
By **A. S. Curry, Ph.D.**, Central Research Establishment and **J. V. Hewitt**, King Edward VII Hospital; ISBN-0-87819-042-2.
A useful and definative manual for hospital laboratories where the authors wrote of the minutiae of their techniques and an interpretation of their results.

RECENT ADVANCES IN CANCER RESEARCH: CELL BIOLOGY, MOLECULAR BIOLOGY, AND TUMOR VIROLOGY
Edited by **Robert C. Gallo, M.D.**, National Cancer Institute and National Institutes of Health; ISBN-0-8493-51438-3.
A select group of papers by leading investigators from the diverse fields of cancer research is presented to illustrate and summarize the progress in this research.

CARBAMATE INSECTICIDES: CHEMISTRY, BIOCHEMISTRY AND TOXICOLOGY
By **H. Wyman Dorough, Ph.D.**, University of Kentucky, and **Ronald J. Kuhr, Ph.D.**, New York State Agricultural Experiment Station; ISBN-0-87819-052-X.
Contains a thorough discussion of carbamates, whose use has increased substantially in recent years.

CRC CRITICAL REVIEW JOURNALS:

CRITICAL REVIEWS IN BIOCHEMISTRY
Edited by **Gerald D. Fasman, Ph.D.,** Brandeis University.

Please forward inquiries to CRC Press, Inc., 18901 Cranwood Parkway, Cleveland, Ohio 44128, U.S.A.